BLUEPRINTS PEDIATRICS

Sixth Edition

BLUEPRINTS PEDIATRICS

Sixth Edition

Bradley S. Marino, MD, MPP, MSCE
Associate Professor of Pediatrics
Department of Pediatrics
University of Cincinnati College of Medicine
Divisions of Cardiology and Critical Care Medicine
The Heart Institute
Cincinnati Children's Hospital Medical Center
Cincinnati, Ohio

Katie S. Fine, MD
Pediatrician
Carolina Physicians Network
Carolinas Healthcare
Charlotte, North Carolina

Wolters Kluwer | Lippincott Williams & Wilkins
Health
Philadelphia • Baltimore • New York • London
Buenos Aires • Hong Kong • Sydney • Tokyo

Acquisitions Editor: Susan Rhyner
Product Manager: Jennifer Verbiar
Marketing Manager: Joy Fisher-Williams
Vendor Manager: Bridgett Dougherty
Manufacturing Coordinator: Margie Orzech
Design Coordinator: Terry Mallon
Production Services: S4Carlisle Publishing Services

Sixth Edition

351 West Camden Street,
Baltimore, MD 21201

Two Commerce Square
2001 Market Street
Philadelphia, PA 19103

Printed in China

Library of Congress Cataloging-in-Publication Data

Marino, Bradley S.
Blueprints pediatrics / Bradley S. Marino, Katie S. Fine.—6th ed.
p. ; cm.— (Blueprints)
Includes index.
ISBN 978-1-4511-1604-5
I. Fine, Katie S. (Katie Snead) II. Title. III. Series: Blueprints.
[DNLM: 1. Pediatrics—Examination Questions. WS 18.2]
618.9200076—dc23

2012049839

DISCLAIMER

Care has been taken to confirm the accuracy of the information present and to describe generally accepted practices. However, the authors, editors, and publisher are not responsible for errors or omissions or for any consequences from application of the information in this book and make no warranty, expressed or implied, with respect to the currency, completeness, or accuracy of the contents of the publication. Application of this information in a particular situation remains the professional responsibility of the practitioner; the clinical treatments described and recommended may not be considered absolute and universal recommendations.

The authors, editors, and publisher have exerted every effort to ensure that drug selection and dosage set forth in this text are in accordance with the current recommendations and practice at the time of publication. However, in view of ongoing research, changes in government regulations, and the constant flow of information relating to drug therapy and drug reactions, the reader is urged to check the package insert for each drug for any change in indications and dosage and for added warnings and precautions. This is particularly important when the recommended agent is a new or infrequently employed drug.

Some drugs and medical devices presented in this publication have Food and Drug Administration (FDA) clearance for limited use in restricted research settings. It is the responsibility of the health care provider to ascertain the FDA status of each drug or device planned for use in their clinical practice.

To purchase additional copies of this book, call our customer service department at **(800) 638-3030** or fax orders to **(301) 223-2320**. International customers should call **(301) 223-2300**.

Visit Lippincott Williams & Wilkins on the Internet: http://www.lww.com. Lippincott Williams & Wilkins customer service representatives are available from 8:30 am to 6:00 pm, EST.

9 8 7 6 5 4 3 2 1

RRS1212

Preface

Blueprints Pediatrics was first published almost 15 years ago as part of a series of books designed to help medical students prepare for USMLE Steps 2 and 3. Just as professional board evaluations have developed over time, and medical training continues to advance, so too has *Pediatric Blueprints* evolved to assist practitioners and students across multiple evaluation settings. Examination preparation remains a core component of the series; to that end, the authors review the subject parameters posted by the testing board before each edition. The authors and editors work together to organize the most important and factually current material into a complete yet concise review guide. Our ultimate goal remains integrating *depth* of factual knowledge with *breadth* of practice information in order to *optimize* both understanding and retention. We have been pleased to hear from our readers that the book is utilized by many medical students during their pediatric clinical rotations, as well as in preparation for shelf and board examinations. Residents in emergency medicine and family practice as well as nurse practitioners and physicians' assistants have found *Blueprints* helpful during the pediatric portion of their training. We believe the book's applications have broadened with each edition due to the quality of our guest authors and their dedication to highlighting and clarifying a targeted range of basic yet important topics that must be mastered in order to treat children.

Each chapter in the book consists of a single subject for review. Most can be read in less than an hour. The topics contained in each chapter are grouped in an orderly fashion, with an end-of-chapter "Key Points" section that permits instant review and highlights the concepts most frequently tested. This edition includes 100 questions and answers, as well as access to 50 more posted online. The questions are written in the "clinical vignette" style used on USMLE and Pediatric Board examinations. Thus, readers not only can evaluate their grasp of the material but also begin to acclimate themselves to the expected testing environment.

We are proud to offer this 6th edition of *Blueprints Pediatrics*. It incorporates suggestions we have received from medical students, faculty, providers, and even program directors with regard to content and organization. Virtually all of the chapters are coauthored by at least one pediatric expert in the respective content area. Utilizing authors with dual backgrounds in academic medicine and private practice for each chapter permits incorporation the most recent information and practice parameters available and accepted at publication.

We hope you find *Blueprints Pediatrics* to be a beneficial investment, regardless of how you use it.

Bradley S. Marino, MD, MPP, MSCE
Katie S. Fine, MD

Acknowledgments

This book is a tribute to our patients and their families. Each day we are reminded how truly precious children are and what an honor it is to care for them. We are grateful to our colleagues, including residents, fellows, attendings, providers, nurses, and support staff; we continue to learn from your knowledge of patient care and compassion for the human condition. Your enthusiasm and positive energy remind us both that we really do have "the best job in the world."

In addition, we would like to thank Emily Claybon and Katelyn Mellion for their help in formatting tables and figures, and their overall willingness to always lend a hand. This book has greatly benefited from the remarkable enthusiasm, support, and dedication of Jenn Verbiar, "managing editor extraordinaire."

We would like to dedicate this edition of *Blueprints Pediatrics* to our spouses and children, without whose support, forbearance, and encouragement none of this would be possible.

Bradley S. Marino
Katie S. Fine

Contents

Preface ... *v*
Acknowledgments ... *vi*
Contributors ... *viii*
Abbreviations ... *xi*
1 General Pediatrics ... 1
2 Neonatal Medicine ... 18
3 Adolescent Medicine ... 43
4 Nutrition ... 57
5 Fluid, Electrolyte, and pH Management ... 63
6 Dermatology ... 74
7 Cardiology ... 86
8 Pulmonology ... 114
9 Gastroenterology ... 134
10 Infectious Disease ... 154
11 Hematology ... 179
12 Oncology ... 205
13 Immunology, Allergy, and Rheumatology ... 224
14 Endocrinology ... 241
15 Neurology ... 256
16 Orthopedics ... 280
17 Nephrology and Urology ... 294
18 Genetic Disorders ... 315
19 Ophthalmology ... 327
20 Emergency Medicine: The Critically Ill and Injured Child ... 336
21 Poisoning, Burns, and Injury Prevention ... 354
Questions ... *367*
Answers ... *378*
Index ... *390*

Contributors

Shumyle Alam, MD
Assistant Professor of Surgery
Department of Surgery
University of Cincinnati College of Medicine
Division of Urology
Cincinnati Children's Hospital Medical Center
Cincinnati, Ohio

Melanie Bradley, MD
Fellow, Division of Pediatric Ophthalmology
Cincinnati Children's Hospital Medical Center
Cincinnati, Ohio

Rebecca C. Brady, MD
Associate Professor of Clinical Pediatrics
Department of Pediatrics
University of Cincinnati College of Medicine
Division of Infectious Diseases
Cincinnati Children's Hospital Medical Center
Cincinnati, Ohio

Karen Burns, MD
Assistant Professor
Department of Pediatrics
University of Cincinnati College of Medicine
Division of Oncology
Cincinnati Children's Hospital Medical Center
Cincinnati, Ohio

Kevin Carter, MD
Assistant Professor of Pediatrics
University of North Carolina School of Medicine
Pediatric Hospitalist
Levine Children's Hospital
Charlotte, North Carolina

Mitchell B. Cohen, MD
Professor and Vice Chair of Pediatrics
Department of Pediatrics
University of Cincinnati College of Medicine
Director, Division of Gastroenterology, Hepatology and Nutrition
Cincinnati Children's Hospital Medical Center
Cincinnati, Ohio

Kevin J. Downes, MD
Fellow, Division of Infectious Diseases
Cincinnati Children's Hospital Medical Center
Cincinnati, Ohio

Deborah A. Elder, MD
Assistant Professor of Pediatrics
Department of Pediatrics
University of Cincinnati College of Medicine
Division of Endocrinology
Cincinnati Children's Hospital Medical Center
Cincinnati, Ohio

Steven Frick, MD
Chair of Orthopedics Surgery
Nemours Children's Hospital
Orlando, Florida

Meera Patel Gallagher, MD
Private Pediatrician
Center for Pediatric and Adolescent Medicine
Mooresville, North Carolina

Paula Goldenberg, MD, MSW, MSCE
Assistant Professor
Department of Pediatrics
University of Cincinnati College of Medicine
Divisions of Cardiology and Human Genetics
The Heart Institute
Cincinnati Children's Hospital Medical Center
Cincinnati, Ohio

Jacqueline Grupp-Phelan, MD, MPH
Professor of Clinical Pediatrics
Associate Director, Division of Pediatric Emergency Medicine
Department of Pediatrics
University of Cincinnati College of Medicine
Cincinnati Children's Hospital Medical Center
Cincinnati, Ohio

Amy Harper, MD
Adjunct Assistant Professor of Pediatrics
UNC School of Medicine
Carolinas Pediatric Neurology Care/Levine Children's Hospital
Carolinas HealthCare System
Charlotte, North Carolina

Jennifer Huggins, MD
Associate Professor of Pediatrics
Department of Pediatrics
University of Cincinnati College of Medicine
Division of Pediatric Rheumatology
Cincinnati Children's Hospital Medical Center
Cincinnati, Ohio

Carolyn M. Kercsmar, MD
Professor of Pediatrics
Department of Pediatrics
University of Cincinnati College of Medicine
Director, Asthma Center
Division of Pulmonary Medicine
Cincinnati Children's Hospital Medical Center
Cincinnati, Ohio

Catherine Dent Krawczeski, MD
Associate Professor of Pediatrics
Department of Pediatrics
University of Cincinnati College of Medicine
Division of Cardiology
The Heart Institute
Cincinnati Children's Hospital Medical Director
Cincinnati, Ohio

Morissa J. Ladinsky, MD
Clinical Assistant Professor
Department of Pediatrics
University of Cincinnati College of Medicine
Cincinnati Children's Hospital Medical Center
Cincinnati, Ohio
Pediatrician, Group Health Associates/TriHealth
Mason, Ohio

Angela Lorts, MD
Assistant Professor of Pediatrics
Department of Pediatrics
University of Cincinnati College of Medicine
Division of Cardiology
The Heart Institute
Cincinnati Children's Hospital Medical Center
Cincinnati, Ohio

Anne W. Lucky, MD
Volunteer Professor
Departments of Dermatology and Pediatrics
University of Cincinnati College of Medicine
Divisions of Pediatric Dermatology and General and Community Pediatrics
Cincinnati Children's Hospital Medical Center
Cincinnati, Ohio

Preeti Matkins, MD
Clinical Professor of Pediatrics
University of North Carolina
Director, Adolescent Medicine
Teen Health Connection
Levine Children's Hospital
Charlotte, North Carolina

Rajaram Nagarajan, MD, MS
Associate Professor of Pediatrics
Department of Pediatrics
University of Cincinnati College of Medicine
Division of Oncology
Cincinnati Children's Hospital Medical Center
Cincinnati, Ohio

Daniel R. Neuspiel, MD, MPH
Clinical Professor of Pediatrics
University of North Carolina School of Medicine
Director, Ambulatory Pediatrics
Levine Children's Hospital
Charlotte, North Carolina

Marissa Perman, MD
Resident in Pediatrics
Department of Pediatrics
Cincinnati Children's Hospital Medical Center
Cincinnati, Ohio

Charles T. Quinn, MD, MS
Associate Professor
Department of Pediatrics
University of Cincinnati College of Medicine
Division of Hematology
Cincinnati Children's Hospital Medical Center
Cincinnati, Ohio

Marc Rothenberg, MD, PhD
Professor of Pediatrics
Department of Pediatrics
University of Cincinnati College of Medicine
Director, Division of Allergy and Immunology
Director, Cincinnati Center for Eosinophilic Disorders
Cincinnati Children's Hospital Medical Center
Cincinnati, Ohio

Franklin O. Smith, MD
Marjory J. Johnson Endowed Chair
Professor of Pediatrics
University of Cincinnati College of Medicine
Cincinnati Children's Hospital Medical Center
Cincinnati, Ohio

Brad Sobolewski, MD
Assistant Professor of Pediatrics
Department of Pediatrics
University of Cincinnati College of Medicine
Division of Emergency Medicine
Cincinnati Children's Hospital Medical Center
Cincinnati, Ohio

William Tsai, MD
Associate Professor
Critical Care and Emergency Medicine
Levine Children's Hospital at Carolinas Medical Center

Rene G. VanDeVoorde III, MD
Assistant Professor of Pediatrics
Department of Pediatrics
University of Cincinnati College of Medicine
Division of Nephrology and Hypertension
Cincinnati Children's Hospital Medical Center
Cincinnati, Ohio

Constance E. West, MD
Associate Professor of Pediatrics
Department of Pediatrics
University of Cincinnati College of Medicine
Director, Division of Pediatric Ophthalmology, and the Abrahamson Pediatric Eye Institute
Cincinnati Children's Hospital Medical Center
Cincinnati, Ohio

Robert E. Wood, PhD, MD
Professor of Pediatrics and Surgery
Departments of Pediatrics and Surgery
University of Cincinnati College of Medicine
Director, Pediatric Bronchology
Divisions of Pulmonary Medicine and Otolaryngology
Cincinnati Children's Hospital Medical Center
Cincinnati, Ohio

Abbreviations

ABG	arterial blood gas
ACTH	adrenocorticotropic hormone
AIDS	acquired immunodeficiency syndrome
ALL	acute lymphocytic leukemia
ALT	alanine transaminase
AMP	adenosine monophosphate
ANA	antinuclear antibody
AP	anteroposterior
ARDS	adult respiratory distress syndrome
ASD	atrial septal defect
ASO	antistreptolysin
AST	aspartate transaminase
AZT	zidovudine
BUN	blood urea nitrogen
CAVV	common atrioventricular valve
CBC	complete blood count
CDC	Centers for Disease Control and Prevention
CF	cystic fibrosis
CHF	congestive heart failure
CK	creatine kinase
CNS	central nervous system
CSF	cerebrospinal fluid
CT	computed tomography
DIC	disseminated intravascular coagulation
DMD	Duchenne-type muscular dystrophy
DTP	diphtheria/tetanus/pertussis
DTRs	deep tendon reflexes
DVT	deep venous thrombosis
EBV	Epstein-Barr virus
ECG	electrocardiography
ECMO	extracorporeal membrane oxygenation
EEG	electroencephalography
ELISA	enzyme-linked immunosorbent assay
EMG	electromyography
ESR	erythrocyte sedimentation rate
FEV	forced expiratory volume
FTA-ABS	fluorescent treponemal antibody absorption
FVC	forced vital capacity
G6PD	glucose-6-phosphate dehydrogenase
GI	gastrointestinal
Hgb	hemoglobin
Hib	Haemophilus influenzae type b
HIV	human immunodeficiency virus
HLA	human leukocyte antigen
IFA	immunofluorescent antibody
Ig	immunoglobulin
IM	intramuscular
INH	isoniazid
IV	intravenous
IVC	inferior vena cava
IVIG	intravenous immunoglobulin
JRA	juvenile rheumatoid arthritis
JVP	jugular venous pressure
KUB	kidneys/ureter/bladder
LDH	lactate dehydrogenase
LFTs	liver function tests
LP	lumbar puncture
L/S	lecithin-to-sphingomyelin (ratio)
LV	left ventricle
LVH	left ventricular hypertrophy
MMR	measles-mumps-rubella
MRI	magnetic resonance imaging
NG	nasogastric
NPO	nil per os (nothing by mouth)
NSAID	nonsteroidal anti-inflammatory drug
PCR	polymerase chain reaction
PDA	patent ductus arteriosus
PFTs	pulmonary function tests
PMI	point of maximal intensity
PPD	purified protein derivative
PT	prothrombin time
PTT	partial thromboplastin time
RBC	red blood cell
RF	rheumatoid factor
RPR	rapid plasma reagent (test)
RSV	respiratory syncytial virus
RV	right ventricle
RVH	right ventricular hypertrophy
SIDS	sudden infant death syndrome
s/p	status post
T3RU	tri-iodothyronine resin uptake
T4	thyroxine
TSH	thyroid-stimulating hormone
UA	urinalysis
URI	upper respiratory infection
US	ultrasound
VMA	vanillylmandelic acid
VSD	ventricular septal defect
vWF	von Willebrand factor
WBC	white blood cell

Chapter 1 General Pediatrics

Daniel R. Neuspiel • Katie S. Fine

In most pediatric practices in developed nations, infants and children are routinely examined several times in the first 2 months of life, every 2 to 3 months until 18 months, less often through age 3 years, and generally yearly thereafter, unless they have chronic conditions or are at high risk. Table 1-1 encompasses a list of items (categorized by age group) that should be considered in pediatric health supervision visits from ages 1 month through 10 years. Other age visits are considered elsewhere in this book (Chapters 2 and 3). This list is by no means exhaustive, but should provide a starting point and direction for further study. The steps do not have to be completed in any set order. For example, the sequence may change based on the age of the patient; older children may be embarrassed in a medical gown and are able to listen and respond more comfortably when they are fully dressed. A complete physical examination is needed at each health supervision visit, with key highlights noted in the table.

OBSERVING THE PARENT(S) AND CHILD

At every visit, it is important to closely observe the parent–child interaction to ascertain whether parental expectations for the child's behavior are in line with the developmental age. For instance, is the parent communicating in ways an infant or young child may understand? Does the child seek the attention of the parent prior to embarking on a new behavior? When the child misbehaves, how does the parent react? Does the parent of an older child give her or him appropriate freedom to respond to questions?

PARTNERING WITH FAMILIES IN A PATIENT-CENTERED MEDICAL HOME

In order to attain optimal health and illness prevention, clinicians must establish effective family-centered partnerships that encourage open and supportive communication with children and families. The general pediatric practice should affirm the strengths of individual family members. A health supervision partnership should be established between the child, family, community, and health care team. The pediatrician should provide the family and child with evidence-based information to assist them in making medical decisions.

In most cases, the primary care pediatrician should coordinate the care of children with significant medical problems and special needs. This responsibility extends beyond the time of a scheduled patient visit and may involve the assistance of other office staff. Ongoing communication with subspecialists, home care providers, and child care or school staff is essential in the management of care for children with complex health conditions.

EFFECTIVE COMMUNICATION SKILLS IN PEDIATRIC PRIMARY CARE

Some effective behaviors by the clinician include introducing oneself, greeting each family member, and sitting at the same level as the parent or older child. Patients and parents want to be listened to without interruption. Repeat the symptoms or questions of the patient or parent to make it clear you understand them correctly. It is useful to encourage questions and provide full answers in ordinary language free of medical jargon. Drawings may be helpful to illustrate your responses. If language barriers are evident at the beginning of the visit, make arrangements for appropriate translation before proceeding further.

GOAL SETTING DURING THE HEALTH SUPERVISION VISIT

To make most efficient use of time, it is helpful at the start of the visit to decide with the patient and parent on a mutual agenda. Ask the parent and/or patient what they would like to get out of the visit. Beyond the regular "checkup," do they have any concerns they would like addressed? Summarize their concerns and agree to address those that are realistic to cover at that visit, and make a plan to cover all concerns at either the current visit or in another setting.

ANTICIPATORY GUIDANCE

Primary care pediatrics focuses on health promotion and disease/injury prevention, and an important tool for this effort is **anticipatory guidance**, the advice that clinicians give to parents and children. Those offering this advice should be

TABLE 1-1 Health Supervision in Infancy and Childhood

Age	Nutrition	Developmental Surveillance	Key Items on Physical Examination	Anticipatory Guidance	Universal Screening[a]
1 mo	Encourage exclusive breast-feeding Correct formula preparation Vitamin D adequacy No water or solids	Calms when upset Follows parents with eyes Recognizes caregiver voice Starts to smile Lifts head when prone	Growth trajectory and percentiles Rashes, bruising Fontanelles Eye mobility, red reflexes Murmurs, pulses Hip stability Tone, strength	Back to sleep, tummy time when awake Rear-facing car seat in back Scald prevention: home water heater at 120°F, no hot beverage while holding infant Fall prevention Passive smoking Dealing with crying baby	Postpartum depression Review newborn screening results
2 mo	Encourage exclusive breast-feeding Correct formula preparation Vitamin D adequacy No water or solids	Social smile Self-comforts Holds head up Symmetric movements Begins push up when prone	Growth trajectory and percentiles Rashes, bruising Fontanelles Eye mobility, red reflexes Murmurs, pulses Hip stability Tone, strength	Back to sleep, tummy time when awake Encourage self-comforting to sleep Rear facing car seat in back Scald prevention Fall prevention Passive smoking Dealing with crying baby	Postpartum depression Review newborn screening results if not already done
4 mo	Encourage exclusive breast-feeding Correct formula preparation Vitamin D adequacy Cereal 4–6 mo, only with spoon No honey under 12 mo	Expressive babbling Pushes chest to elbows Begins to roll and reach	Growth trajectory and percentiles Rashes, bruising Fontanelles Skull shape Eye mobility, red reflexes, corneal light reflexes Murmurs, pulses Hip symmetry Tone, strength	Encourage self-comforting to sleep Stop night feedings Rear-facing car seat in back Scald prevention Fall prevention Passive smoking Keep small objects, plastic bags, poisons from baby	None routine

6 mo	Encourage exclusive breast-feeding Correct formula preparation Vitamin D adequacy Introduction of cereal, vegetables, fruits Solids only with spoon Start water, limit juice Introduce cup No honey under 12 mo Fluoride supplementation	Recognizes faces Babbles, vocal turn taking Responds to name Visual and oral exploration Hand to mouth Rolls over, sits with support, stands supported and bounces	Growth trajectory and percentiles Rashes, bruising Fontanelles Skull shape Eye mobility, red reflexes, corneal light reflexes Murmurs, pulses Hip symmetry Tone, strength	Assess fluoride source, clean teeth, avoid bottle propping and grazing Read picture books to baby Rear-facing car seat in back Scald prevention Fall prevention Passive smoking Keep small objects, plastic bags, poisons from baby Home safety check: gates, barriers, storage of dangerous items, no infant walkers Set water temperature <120°F, bath supervision Poison Control 1-800-222-1222	Oral health, development
9 mo	Encourage self-feeding Regular mealtime routines Vitamin D adequacy Table food introduction Cup drinking; plan to d/c bottle by 12 mo Continue nursing if desirable No honey under 12 mo	Stranger anxiety Points to objects Plays peek-a-boo Sits with no support Says "dada/mama" nonspecifically	Growth trajectory and percentiles Rashes, bruising Fontanelles Skull shape Eye mobility, red reflexes Murmurs, pulses Hip symmetry Tone, strength Parachute reflex	Keep consistent daily routines Read picture books; avoid TV, other screens Rear-facing car seat in back Scald prevention Fall prevention Passive smoking Keep small objects, plastic bags, poisons from baby Home safety check: gates, barriers, storage of dangerous items, no infant walkers Set water temperature <120°F, parent at arm's reach near water Poison Control 1-800-222-1222	Oral health, development

(continued)

TABLE 1-1 Health Supervision in Infancy and Childhood *(contined)*

Age	Nutrition	Developmental Surveillance	Key Items on Physical Examination	Anticipatory Guidance	Universal Screening[a]
1 y	Three meals, two snacks Whole milk 16–24 oz, cup only Limit juice Iron-rich foods Fruits/vegetables Avoid choking hazards	Waves bye-bye One to two words, "dada/mama" specific, imitates sounds Bangs two cubes Stands alone	Growth trajectory and percentiles Eye mobility, cover/uncover, red reflexes Dental caries, plaque Pulses Hip symmetry Testes descended Bruising	Apply fluoride varnish; dental referral Childproof home Rear-facing car seat Set water temperature <120°F, parent at arm's reach near water Read picture books; avoid TV, other screens Store guns unloaded and locked, with ammunition locked separately Poison Control 1-800-222-1222	Anemia, lead (high prevalence, Medicaid), development
15 mo	Three meals, two snacks Whole milk 16–24 oz, cup only Limit juice Iron-rich foods Fruits/vegetables Avoid choking hazards	Imitates activities Scribbles Walks well Two to three words	Growth trajectory and percentiles Eye mobility, cover/uncover, red reflexes Dental caries, plaque Pulses Bruising	Discipline, praise good behavior *How are you managing your child's behavior? Do you and your partner agree on how to do it?* Apply fluoride varnish; dental referral Read picture books; avoid TV, other screens Follow manufacturer's car seat instructions Store guns unloaded and locked, with ammunition locked separately Window guards above ground level Smoke detector; fire plan Poison Control 1-800-222-1222	

18 mo	Three meals, two snacks Whole milk 16–24 oz, cup only Limit juice Iron-rich foods Fruits/vegetables Avoid choking hazards	Six words Points to one body part Walks up steps, runs Stacks two to three blocks Uses spoon	Growth trajectory and percentiles Eye cover/uncover, red reflexes Dental caries, plaque Observe gait Birth marks, bruising	Discipline, praise good behavior Read picture books; avoid TV, other screens Apply fluoride varnish; dental referral Discuss toilet training readiness Follow manufacturer's car seat instructions Store guns unloaded and locked, with ammunition locked separately Window guards above ground level Smoke detector; fire plan Poison Control 1-800-222-1222	Development, autism
2 y	Three meals, two snacks Low-fat milk 16–24 oz, cup only, limit juice Iron-rich foods Fruits/vegetables Avoid choking hazards	At least 50 words, two-word phrases Stacks five to six blocks Throws ball overhand Jumps up	Growth trajectory and percentiles, including body mass index (BMI) Eye cover/uncover, red reflexes Dental caries, plaque Observe running, scribbling, socialization	Discipline, praise good behavior Read picture books; limit TV, other screens to 1–2 h and assess quality Encourage play with other children *How does your child act around other kids?* Discuss toilet training, personal hygiene Encourage physical activity Apply fluoride varnish; dental referral Car seat placed in back Bike helmet Supervise child outside Window guards above ground level Smoke detector; fire plan Store guns unloaded and locked, with ammunition locked separately	Development, autism Lead (high risk/Medicaid) Anemia (if high-risk or patient anemic at age 12 months)

(continued)

TABLE 1-1 Health Supervision in Infancy and Childhood *(contined)*

Age	Nutrition	Developmental Surveillance	Key Items on Physical Examination	Anticipatory Guidance	Universal Screening[a]
30 m	Three meals, two snacks Low-fat milk 16–24 oz, limit juice Iron-rich foods Fruits/vegetables Avoid choking hazards	Three- to four-word phrases, half of speech understandable *Is your child speaking in sentences?* Points to six body parts Dresses with help Copies vertical line	Growth trajectory and percentiles, including BMI Eye cover/uncover, red reflexes Observe coordination, language clarity, socialization	Read picture books; limit TV, other screens to 1–2 h and assess quality Encourage family physical activity *Tell me what you do together as a family.* Encourage independence by offering choices Discuss toilet training, personal hygiene Apply fluoride varnish; dental referral Car seat placed in back Bike helmet Dental referral Supervise child outside Window guards above ground level Smoke detector; fire plan Water safety, "touch" supervision Store guns unloaded and locked, with ammunition locked separately	Development
3 y	Three meals, two snacks Low-fat milk 16–24 oz, limit juice Iron-rich foods Fruits/vegetables	Feeds, dresses self Two to three sentences Speech 75% understandable Gender identity Tower of six to eight blocks Alternates feet up stairs Copies circle	BP, growth trajectory and percentiles, including BMI Fundoscopic exam Dental caries, plaque, gingivitis Speech clarity Adult–child interaction	Read books, limit TV, other screens Encourage interactive games, taking turns Family time and exercise Dental referral Car seat placed in back Bike helmet Supervise child outside Window guards above ground level Smoke detector; fire plan Store guns unloaded and locked, with ammunition locked separately	Development, visual acuity

4 y	Three meals, two snacks Low-fat milk 24 oz, limit juice Fruits/vegetables	Fantasy play Says full name Knows what to do if cold/tired/hungry (two out of three) Knows four colors Hops on one foot Copies cross Dresses self	BP, growth trajectories and percentiles, including BMI Fundoscopic exam Fine/gross motor skills Speech fluency/clarity Thought content/abstraction	Opportunities for play with other kids Read and talk together with child Regular bedtime rituals, meals without TV, limit TV to 1–2 hr daily, no TV in bedroom Family physical activities Use anatomic body terms Rules to be safe with adults: • No secrets from parents • No adult should be interested in child's private parts • No adult should ask child for help with his or her private parts Car seat in rear until maximum manufacturer limit, then belt-positioning booster seat Bike helmet Supervise child outside Window guards above ground level Smoke detector; fire plan Store guns unloaded and locked, with ammunition locked separately	Development, visual acuity, hearing
5–6 y	Low-fat milk 24 oz, limit juice Fruits/vegetables *What are your favorite foods?* *Does your child eat from all food groups?* *How much milk/juice/soda per day?*	Balances on one foot, hops, skips Able to tie knot Displays school-readiness skills Mature pencil grasp Draws person, six body parts Can copy square, triangle Good articulation/language skills Counts to 10	BP, growth trajectories and percentiles, including BMI Fundoscopic exam Dental caries, gingivitis, malocclusion Fine/gross motor skills Speech fluency/clarity Thought content/abstraction	School Readiness *Do you feel happy/safe at your school?* *What concerns do you have about your child's school work?* Mental Health *Does your family have chores/routines?* *How do you discipline your child? Is it effective?* *How does your child resolve conflict?*	Vision, hearing

(continued)

TABLE 1-1 Health Supervision in Infancy and Childhood *(contined)*

Age	Nutrition	Developmental Surveillance	Key Items on Physical Examination	Anticipatory Guidance	Universal Screening[a]
				How much exercise does your child average per day? *How much screen time (TV, video games, computer)?* Dental Care *Brushes how many times a day?* *Flosses daily?* *Visits dentist twice a year?* Safety *Booster/seat belt/rear seat of car?* *Stranger danger?* *Are there smokers in the home? Smoke alarms?* *Water safety/sunscreen?* Store guns unloaded and locked, with ammunition locked separately Rules to be safe with adults (see above)	
7–8 y	Low-fat milk 24 oz, limit juice Fruits/vegetables × 5 *What are your favorite foods?* *Does your child eat from all food groups?* *How much sweet drinks per day?* *What do you think of your child's growth over the past year?*	*How do you like school?* *Do others pick on you?* *How is your child doing in school?*	BP, growth parameters, including BMI Hip, knee, angle function Dental caries, gingivitis, malocclusion	Discuss rules and consequences *What types of discipline do you use?* Be aware of pubertal changes *What have you told your child about how to care for her or his changing body?* 1 hr of physical activity Eat meals as family Limit screen time to 2 hr daily Dental care Rules to be safe with adults (see above) *What would you do if you felt unsafe at a friend's house?*	

				Has anyone ever touched you in a way that made you feel uncomfortable? Booster seat until shoulder belt fits Safety equipment (helmet, pads, mouth guard) Smoke-free home Monitor Internet use Rules to be safe with adults (see above) Store guns unloaded and locked, with ammunition locked separately	
9–10 y	Low-fat milk 32 oz, limit juice Fruits/vegetables × 5	*What things are you good at in school?* *Any difficult things?*	BP, growth parameters, including BMI Dental caries, gingivitis, malocclusion Observe tattoos, piercings, signs of abuse, self-inflicted injuries, birthmarks Back exam	Promote independence, assign chores Be positive role model for respect, anger management Know child's friends Discuss puberty, sexuality, substance use *What questions do you have about the way your body is developing?* *How do you feel about how you look?* Rules to be safe with adults (see above) 1 hr physical activity Dentist twice a year Safety equipment (helmet, pads, mouth guard) Smoke-free home Monitor Internet use Store guns unloaded and locked, with ammunition locked separately Teach child to swim, use sunscreen	Vision and hearing (at 10)

[a]Selective screening for other conditions or at additional ages may be recommended if certain risk factors are present; see source below for details.
Adapted from Hagan JF, Shaw P, eds. *Bright Futures: Guidelines for Health Supervision of Infants, Children, and Adolescents*, 3rd ed. Elk Grove Village, IL: American Academy of Pediatrics, 2008.

aware that parents may have limited ability to retain long lists of recommendations, so it is useful to limit the number of items discussed at each visit. Some physicians integrate anticipatory guidance with the examination (e.g., while examining the mouth, "How many times a day does your child brush her or his teeth? Does he or she see a dentist every 6 months for routine evaluation?"). Many practices make use of written materials and ancillary staff to provide this preventive health information.

In deciding on the central issues to discuss at each health supervision encounter, it is useful to understand the main sources of morbidity and mortality at each age of a child.

In young infants, through 4 months of age, the leading cause of death is **sudden infant death syndrome**, which has declined significantly in incidence since the American Academy of Pediatrics began recommending "Back to Sleep" in 1994. Infants should be placed to sleep on their backs but should spend some time prone when awake and supervised in order to prevent positional brachycephaly and encourage strengthening of the upper extremities and posterior neck muscles.

After 4 months of age, and extending through the remainder of childhood, **traumatic injuries** cause most deaths. The mechanisms of these injuries change with age, and this knowledge has influenced the prioritization of issues to discuss at health supervision visits.

- **Motor vehicle injuries** are major causes of morbidity and mortality for all children and are the leading cause of injury death starting from age 3 years. Car safety seats have been found to prevent deaths in 71% of infants (birth to 1 year) and 54% of toddlers (1 to 4 years). Child car safety recommendations are undergoing modification; the most updated information may be found at http://www.aap.org. In addition, child pedestrian deaths may be prevented by careful supervision of children near traffic.
- In 2008, 13,000 children below 16 years were **injured while riding bicycles**; many of these injuries were preventable if helmets were used universally.
- **Falls** are the leading cause of nonfatal injuries in children. Many of these may be prevented by installing stairway gates, installing window guards on upper floors, avoiding infant walkers, employing safe playground design, and supervising children closely.
- Regrettably, **homicide and suicide** are leading causes of death throughout childhood and adolescence, and nonfatal firearms injuries are also very common. Half of US households have guns, and half of these are stored loaded. Homes with guns have three times the risk of homicide and five times the risk of suicide as those without firearms. In addition, children watch violent acts on TV an average of 45 times each day. Recommendations to store guns locked and unloaded, to store ammunition separately, and to monitor and reduce TV and other screen time may prevent many of these injuries.
- **Drowning** is the second leading cause of injury death in childhood. Many drowning deaths are due to lack of supervision in the bath tub, unprotected access to a pool, or lack of swimming skills. Toddlers and young children must be supervised at all times while in the bathtub or around pools or other bodies of water. Residential and commercial swimming pools should be fenced in (with unscalable fences) and have locked gates. Isolation fencing (fencing limited to the immediate pool area) is more effective at preventing accidental drowning than perimeter property fencing. CPR training is available to parents through the American Heart Association and many area hospitals. Learning to swim is an important preventive measure but does not take the place of close supervision.
- The third leading source of injury mortality is **fires and burns**. Forty percent of fire deaths occur in homes without smoke alarms. Most victims die from smoke or toxic gases rather than burns, and children are among the leading victims. Working smoke alarms, with batteries replaced annually, and home fire escape plans are helpful to reduce these hazards. Smoking cessation decreases the likelihood that matches or lighters will be left where children can experiment with them. Scald burns also cause significant morbidity and may be prevented by close supervision of young children near stoves and hot water faucets, as well as turning down home water heaters to 120°F.
- **Choking** is a leading cause of both illness and death in children. Choking risk starts when infants begin to grab small items and move them toward their mouths, around 6 months of age, and remains high through age 3 years. Many children do not have fully erupted second molars until age 30 months; inappropriate food choices include nuts, popcorn, hot dogs, hard vegetables, meat with bones, and seeds. Food, coins, and small toys constitute the most commonly aspirated objects. Inadequate supervision and pediatric anatomy result in increased risk.
- **Poisoning** is a major source of morbidity in childhood. Risk begins with the onset of hand-to-mouth behavior in infancy and increases as the child becomes mobile. Medications, cleaners, cosmetics, and plants are the leading poisons. Parents should keep these items out of reach of young children and have the National Poison Control hotline number accessible at all times (1-800-222-1222).
- **Dental caries** (tooth decay) is the most common chronic disease among US children. Untreated caries cause infection and pain, affecting speech, dietary intake, and learning. Proper dental care can prevent dental caries. A first dental checkup is recommended within 6 months of initial tooth eruption or at 12 months of age, whichever comes first. Many pediatric offices also apply fluoride topically to developing dentition in young children.

SCREENING

Many pediatric health supervision visits are associated with recommended screening tests. These tests are meant to identify treatable conditions that may benefit from early detection. In deciding which screening tests to recommend, there should be evidence that the screened condition is more treatable when detected early; that the treatment is available to the patient; and that the benefits of the treatment outweigh the risks of both the treatment and the screening program.

Due to the rarity of many conditions screened in pediatrics, the majority of positive tests are actually false positives, associated with no disease. A frequent problem in pediatrics is the negative psychological impact of labeling children with conditions they do not have, and false positive screening tests add to this burden. When conveying positive screening test results to parents, it is particularly important to be aware of this issue.

The American Academy of Pediatrics recommends universal screening for anemia at 1 year of age. Patients with hemoglobin levels <11.0 mg/dL require additional evaluation for iron deficiency (Chapter 11). Patients with low hemoglobin levels at 12 months of age and those at higher risk for iron deficiency anemia are tested again at age 2 years. This includes children with exposure to lead, children with iron-poor diets and/or who consume more than 24 oz/day of cow's milk, those with poor growth or inadequate nutrition associated with specific health problems, and children in families of low socioeconomic status.

Screening for lead poisoning used to be universal; however, the American Academy of Pediatrics developed new recommendations for lead screening in 2005 (Table 1-2). Management of elevated blood lead levels is described in Chapter 21.

Screening for tuberculosis (TB) via the purified protein derivative test (PPD) is recommended in certain populations at health maintenance visits. This includes children emigrating from countries where TB is endemic, children who visit such countries or have frequent visitors from those countries, and children with HIV.

VACCINATIONS

Vaccines contain all or part of a weakened or nonviable form of the infectious organism. Vaccination stimulates the recipient's immune system to develop a protective response that mimics that of natural infection but that usually presents little or no risk to the recipient. Figure 1.1 represents the current vaccination schedule recommended by the Centers for Disease Control and Prevention Advisory Committee on Immunization (ACIP) for children ages birth through 6 years in the United States. Most healthy children are then considered "up-to-date" on vaccinations until the age of 10 to 11 years, with the exception of annual influenza vaccination. Periodically, ACIP releases additional vaccine recommendations; these can be accessed at http://www.cdc.gov/vaccines/recs/acip/default.htm.

TABLE 1-2 Recommendations for Lead Screening

The following patients should have screening with a peripheral lead level at 12 and 24 mo of age:

- All Medicaid-eligible children
- All children whose families receive government assistance
- Children who live in communities with high rates of elevated pediatric blood lead levels (>12% above 10 mcg/dL)
- Many city/state health departments also have specific screening guidelines

Screening should be considered in the following pediatric patients at any age:

- Children with siblings with elevated blood lead levels (above 10 mcg/dL)
- Recent immigrants or adoptees

In the notes below the table, be aware that two vaccines are currently administered solely or on a different schedule to children with underlying health problems. The pneumococcal polysaccharide vaccine (PPSV) is recommended for the following patients ≥2 years of age: (1) immunocompetent children with chronic heart or lung disease, diabetes, or cochlear implants; (2) children with functional or anatomic asplenia (e.g., sickle cell disease); and (3) children who are immunocompromised (HIV infection, certain renal diseases, congenital immunodeficiencies, and immunocompromising treatments due to malignancies). The meningococcal conjugate vaccine (MCV) is recommended for children ≥2 years of age who have asplenia or inherited complement deficiencies.

Despite their long history of safe use and impressive cost-to-benefit ratio, there are some *contraindications* to use of certain vaccinations. A history of anaphylactic reaction to a component of a vaccine is an absolute contraindication; for instance, people who are allergic to egg or chicken protein should not receive the influenza vaccine. Contraindications are vaccine specific, and discussion of this topic is beyond the scope of this source. *Precautions* are generally temporary conditions under which administration of vaccines may be delayed (fever and/or moderate-to-severe illness).

DEVELOPMENTAL MILESTONES

Intellectual and physical development in infants and children occur in predictable, sequential patterns. Notable skills are subdivided into **gross motor**, **fine motor-adaptive** (or visual motor), **language** and **social** milestones. Key milestones for developmental surveillance are listed in Table 1-1. The American Academy of Pediatrics recommends that development be assessed with a formal screening tool at several health supervision visits in early childhood. This permits the early identification of potential delays in development and prompt referral for intervention. Some commonly used general developmental screening tests include the Denver Developmental Screening Test II (**Denver II**), the Parents Evaluation of Developmental Status (**PEDS**), and the Ages and Stages Questionnaire (**ASQ**). Each of these has its own strengths, and some rely more on parent report, but all of them provide useful information to assist in recommendations for further evaluation. However, even when the test identifies no areas of concern, if the pediatrician has concerns, the child should be more fully evaluated.

Developmental delay is diagnosed when performance lags significantly compared with average attainment in a given skill area for a child at the same age, adjusted for gestational age. In former preterm infants (under 36 weeks' gestation) up to 2 years of age, *developmental age* should be adjusted for *gestational age*. For example, a child born 3 months early should have 3 months subtracted from his or her chronological age before assessing developmental skills. Developmental delays may be **focal** (isolated to one domain among gross motor, fine motor-adaptive, language, or social) or **global**, crossing multiple domains.

Autism spectrum disorders (ASD) are a continuum of chronic, nonprogressive developmental disabilities that appear during the first 3 years of life. They represent a neurologic disorder that affects normal brain function, particularly in social interaction and communication skills (see Chapter 15). It is recommended that all children be screened for ASD at

<table>
<tr><th>Vaccine ▼ Age ►</th><th>Birth</th><th>1 month</th><th>2 months</th><th>4 months</th><th>6 months</th><th>9 months</th><th>12 months</th><th>15 months</th><th>18 months</th><th>19–23 months</th><th>2–3 years</th><th>4–6 years</th></tr>
<tr><td>Hepatitis B[1]</td><td>Hep B</td><td colspan="2">HepB</td><td></td><td colspan="4">HepB</td><td></td><td></td><td></td></tr>
<tr><td>Rotavirus[2]</td><td></td><td></td><td>RV</td><td>RV</td><td>RV[2]</td><td></td><td></td><td></td><td></td><td></td><td></td><td></td></tr>
<tr><td>Diphtheria, tetanus, pertussis[3]</td><td></td><td></td><td>DTaP</td><td>DTaP</td><td>DTaP</td><td></td><td>see footnote[3]</td><td colspan="2">DTaP</td><td></td><td></td><td>DTaP</td></tr>
<tr><td>Haemophilus influenzae type b[4]</td><td></td><td></td><td>Hib</td><td>Hib</td><td>Hib[4]</td><td></td><td colspan="2">Hib</td><td></td><td></td><td></td><td></td></tr>
<tr><td>Pneumococcal[5]</td><td></td><td></td><td>PCV</td><td>PCV</td><td>PCV</td><td></td><td colspan="2">PCV</td><td></td><td></td><td colspan="2">PPSV</td></tr>
<tr><td>Inactivated poliovirus[6]</td><td></td><td></td><td>IPV</td><td>IPV</td><td colspan="4">IPV</td><td></td><td></td><td>IPV</td></tr>
<tr><td>Influenza[7]</td><td></td><td></td><td></td><td></td><td colspan="7">Influenza (Yearly)</td></tr>
<tr><td>Measles, mumps, rubella[8]</td><td></td><td></td><td></td><td></td><td></td><td></td><td colspan="2">MMR</td><td></td><td>see footnote[8]</td><td></td><td>MMR</td></tr>
<tr><td>Varicella[9]</td><td></td><td></td><td></td><td></td><td></td><td></td><td colspan="2">Varicella</td><td></td><td>see footnote[9]</td><td></td><td>Varicella</td></tr>
<tr><td>Hepatitis A[10]</td><td></td><td></td><td></td><td></td><td></td><td></td><td colspan="4">Dose 1[10]</td><td colspan="2">HepA Series</td></tr>
<tr><td>Meningococcal[11]</td><td></td><td></td><td></td><td></td><td></td><td colspan="7">MCV4 — see footnote[11]</td></tr>
</table>

Range of recommended ages for all children

Range of recommended ages for certain high-risk groups

Range of recommended ages for all children and certain high-risk groups

This schedule includes recommendations in effect as of December 23, 2011. Any dose not administered at the recommended age should be administered at a subsequent visit, when indicated and feasible. The use of a combination vaccine generally is preferred over separate injections of its equivalent component vaccines. Vaccination providers should consult the relevant Advisory Committee on Immunization Practices (ACIP) statement for detailed recommendations, available online at http://www.cdc.gov/vaccines/pubs/acip-list.htm. Clinically significant adverse events that follow vaccination should be reported to the Vaccine Adverse Event Reporting System (VAERS) online (http://www.vaers.hhs.gov) or by telephone (800-822-7967).

1. **Hepatitis B (HepB) vaccine.** (Minimum age: birth)
   At birth:
   - Administer monovalent HepB vaccine to all newborns before hospital discharge.
   - For infants born to hepatitis B surface antigen (HBsAg)–positive mothers, administer HepB vaccine and 0.5 mL of hepatitis B immune globulin (HBIG) within 12 hours of birth. These infants should be tested for HBsAg and antibody to HBsAg (anti-HBs) 1 to 2 months after receiving the last dose of the series.
   - If mother's HBsAg status is unknown, within 12 hours of birth administer HepB vaccine for infants weighing ≥2,000 grams, and HepB vaccine plus HBIG for infants weighing <2,000 grams. Determine mother's HBsAg status as soon as possible and, if she is HBsAg-positive, administer HBIG for infants weighing ≥2,000 grams (no later than age 1 week).

   Doses after the birth dose:
   - The second dose should be administered at age 1 to 2 months. Monovalent HepB vaccine should be used for doses administered before age 6 weeks.
   - Administration of a total of 4 doses of HepB vaccine is permissible when a combination vaccine containing HepB is administered after the birth dose.
   - Infants who did not receive a birth dose should receive 3 doses of a HepB-containing vaccine starting as soon as feasible (Figure 3).
   - The minimum interval between dose 1 and dose 2 is 4 weeks, and between dose 2 and 3 is 8 weeks. The final (third or fourth) dose in the HepB vaccine series should be administered no earlier than age 24 weeks and at least 16 weeks after the first dose.
2. **Rotavirus (RV) vaccines.** (Minimum age: 6 weeks for both RV-1 [Rotarix] and RV-5 [Rota Teq])
   - The maximum age for the first dose in the series is 14 weeks, 6 days; and 8 months, 0 days for the final dose in the series. Vaccination should not be initiated for infants aged 15 weeks, 0 days or older.
   - If RV-1 (Rotarix) is administered at ages 2 and 4 months, a dose at 6 months is not indicated.
3. **Diphtheria and tetanus toxoids and acellular pertussis (DTaP) vaccine.** (Minimum age: 6 weeks)
   - The fourth dose may be administered as early as age 12 months, provided at least 6 months have elapsed since the third dose.
4. ***Haemophilus influenzae* type b (Hib) conjugate vaccine.** (Minimum age: 6 weeks)
   - If PRP-OMP (PedvaxHIB or Comvax [HepB-Hib]) is administered at ages 2 and 4 months, a dose at age 6 months is not indicated.
   - Hiberix should only be used for the booster (final) dose in children aged 12 months through 4 years.
5. **Pneumococcal vaccines.** (Minimum age: 6 weeks for pneumococcal conjugate vaccine [PCV]; 2 years for pneumococcal polysaccharide vaccine [PPSV])
   - Administer 1 dose of PCV to all healthy children aged 24 through 59 months who are not completely vaccinated for their age.
   - For children who have received an age-appropriate series of 7-valent PCV (PCV7), a single supplemental dose of 13-valent PCV (PCV13) is recommended for:
     — All children aged 14 through 59 months
     — Children aged 60 through 71 months with underlying medical conditions.
   - Administer PPSV at least 8 weeks after last dose of PCV to children aged 2 years or older with certain underlying medical conditions, including a cochlear implant. See *MMWR* 2010:59(No. RR-11), available at http://www.cdc.gov/mmwr/pdf/rr/rr5911.pdf.
6. **Inactivated poliovirus vaccine (IPV).** (Minimum age: 6 weeks)
   - If 4 or more doses are administered before age 4 years, an additional dose should be administered at age 4 through 6 years.
   - The final dose in the series should be administered on or after the fourth birthday and at least 6 months after the previous dose.
7. **Influenza vaccines.** (Minimum age: 6 months for trivalent inactivated influenza vaccine [TIV]; 2 years for live, attenuated influenza vaccine [LAIV])
   - For most healthy children aged 2 years and older, either LAIV or TIV may be used. However, LAIV should not be administered to some children, including 1) children with asthma, 2) children 2 through 4 years who had wheezing in the past 12 months, or 3) children who have any other underlying medical conditions that predispose them to influenza complications. For all other contraindications to use of LAIV, see *MMWR* 2010;59(No. RR-8), available at http://www.cdc.gov/mmwr/pdf/rr/rr5908.pdf.
   - For children aged 6 months through 8 years:
     — For the 2011–12 season, administer 2 doses (separated by at least 4 weeks) to those who did not receive at least 1 dose of the 2010–11 vaccine. Those who received at least 1 dose of the 2010–11 vaccine require 1 dose for the 2011–12 season.
     — For the 2012–13 season, follow dosing guidelines in the 2012 ACIP influenza vaccine recommendations.
8. **Measles, mumps, and rubella (MMR) vaccine.** (Minimum age: 12 months)
   - The second dose may be administered before age 4 years, provided at least 4 weeks have elapsed since the first dose.
   - Administer MMR vaccine to infants aged 6 through 11 months who are traveling internationally. These children should be revaccinated with 2 doses of MMR vaccine, the first at ages 12 through 15 months and at least 4 weeks after the previous dose, and the second at ages 4 through 6 years.
9. **Varicella (VAR) vaccine.** (Minimum age: 12 months)
   - The second dose may be administered before age 4 years, provided at least 3 months have elapsed since the first dose.
   - For children aged 12 months through 12 years, the recommended minimum interval between doses is 3 months. However, if the second dose was administered at least 4 weeks after the first dose, it can be accepted as valid.
10. **Hepatitis A (HepA) vaccine.** (Minimum age: 12 months)
    - Administer the second (final) dose 6 to18 months after the first.
    - Unvaccinated children 24 months and older at high risk should be vaccinated. See *MMWR* 2006;55(No. RR-7), available at http://www.cdc.gov/mmwr/pdf/rr/rr5507.pdf.
    - A 2-dose HepA vaccine series is recommended for anyone aged 24 months and older, previously unvaccinated, for whom immunity against hepatitis A virus infection is desired.
11. **Meningococcal conjugate vaccines, quadrivalent (MCV4).** (Minimum age: 9 months for Menactra [MCV4-D], 2 years for Menveo [MCV4-CRM])
    - For children aged 9 through 23 months 1) with persistent complement component deficiency; 2) who are residents of or travelers to countries with hyperendemic or epidemic disease; or 3) who are present during outbreaks caused by a vaccine serogroup, administer 2 primary doses of MCV4-D, ideally at ages 9 months and 12 months or at least 8 weeks apart.
    - For children aged 24 months and older with 1) persistent complement component deficiency who have not been previously vaccinated; or 2) anatomic/functional asplenia, administer 2 primary doses of either MCV4 at least 8 weeks apart.
    - For children with anatomic/functional asplenia, if MCV4-D (Menactra) is used, administer at a minimum age of 2 years and at least 4 weeks after completion of all PCV oses.
    - See *MMWR* 2011;60:72–6, available at http://www.cdc.gov/mmwr/pdf/wk/mm6003. pdf, and Vaccines for Children Program resolution No. 6/11-1, available at http://www. cdc.gov/vaccines/programs/vfc/downloads/resolutions/06-11mening-mcv.pdf, and *MMWR* 2011;60:1391–2, available at http://www.cdc.gov/mmwr/pdf/wk/mm6040. pdf, for further guidance, including revaccination guidelines.

This schedule is approved by the Advisory Committee on Immunization Practices (http://www.cdc.gov/vaccines/recs/acip), the American Academy of Pediatrics (http://www.aap.org), and the American Academy of Family Physicians (http://www.aafp.org).
Department of Health and Human Services • Centers for Disease Control and Prevention

Figure 1-1 • Recommended immunization schedule for persons aged 0 through 6 years—United States.

18 and 24 months of age. The most common screening tool is the Modified Checklist for Autism in Toddlers (**M-CHAT**). Toddlers identified as "at risk" on this screen should be referred for further evaluation, since intensive early intervention can improve socialization and communications skills in those affected by ASD.

LANGUAGE DELAY

Language is the best indicator of future intellectual potential, and **language delay** is the most commonly diagnosed form of developmental delay in preschool children. **Speech disorders** involve difficulty producing the sounds and rhythms of speech. **Phonetic disorders** are problems with articulation. Speech and phonetic difficulties are *expressive disorders*, while *language disorders* often affect both expressive and receptive language skills.

Dysfluency produces interruptions in the flow of speech. Developmental dysfluency is observed in many preschoolers, resolves by age 4 years, and is not pathologic. True dysfluency (**stuttering**) is characterized by signs of muscular tension and struggle when speaking, and/or complete speech blockage, accompanied by frustration in the child. Stuttering can significantly impede the ability of the affected child to communicate orally. Speech therapy is often quite effective for children who stutter.

Since young children may be uncomfortable speaking freely in front of strangers, a detailed history is often necessary to characterize the quantity and quality of the child's speech. Parental concern about a child's language development is a good predictor of the need for further evaluation, which should always begin with a full audiologic (hearing) assessment. Referral to a speech pathologist for evaluation and treatment (if indicated) should follow. The most frequent cause of mild-to-moderate hearing loss in young children is otitis media with effusion.

DENTAL DEVELOPMENT AND CARE

The first primary teeth to erupt are usually the lower central incisors (6 to 10 months), followed by upper central incisors (8 to 12 months), upper lateral incisors (9 to 13 months), and lower lateral incisors (10 to 16 months). These are followed by the canines (cuspids) and molars. The full set of 20 primary teeth will erupt by 25 to 33 months of age.

Primary teeth begin to exfoliate at 6 to 7 years of age, as permanent dentition begins to erupt, also beginning with the central and lateral incisors. Complete permanent dentition continues through adolescence.

At first tooth eruption, parents should be advised to clean teeth with a soft brush or cloth twice daily. In toddlers, a pea-sized amount of nonfluoridated toothpaste may be used. Pediatric providers should ascertain that children get adequate **fluoride supplementation** to protect their teeth. Fluoride combats tooth decay by incorporation into the structure of developing teeth and by contact with the dental surface. Approximately 60% of US communities are supplied with fluoridated tap water. Though most bottled water does not contain fluoride, some brands designed for infants do contain the recommended concentration of 0.7 to 1.2 ppm. Infants and children not receiving fluoride from water should be prescribed fluoride supplements as drops or tablets.

Too much fluoride may lead to **fluorosis**, with permanent dental enamel staining in children below 8 years of age, so clinicians should be careful in assuring that children get an appropriate amount of supplemental fluoride and that young children do not have access to ingesting significant amounts of fluoride toothpaste or mouthwashes. This may also be a problem in communities whose water supply has over 2 ppm of fluoride.

KEY POINTS

- The leading cause of death through 4 months of age is sudden infant death syndrome.
- After 4 months of age, the leading cause of childhood death is trauma.
- Motor vehicle injuries cause most traumatic deaths after age 3.
- Drowning is the second leading cause of injury death in childhood.
- Fires and burns are the third leading cause of injury death in children.
- Most fires occur in homes without working smoke alarms.
- Scald burns can be prevented by turning water heater temperature down to 120°F.
- Risk for choking and poisoning is highest between ages 9 months and 3 years.
- Falls are the leading cause of nonfatal injuries in children.
- Dental caries is the leading chronic illness in childhood.
- Until 2 years of age, a child's chronological age should be adjusted for gestational age at birth when assessing developmental milestones.
- The Denver II, PEDS, and ASQ are developmental screening tests used at several visits in early childhood to identify potential developmental delays.
- All children should be screened for autism spectrum disorders at 18 and 24 months.
- Language is the best indicator of intellectual potential.
- Any child with suspected speech or language disorder should be referred for a full audiology evaluation.
- The full set of 20 primary teeth should erupt by 25 to 33 months.
- Too much fluoride may cause fluorosis, which is irreversible staining of the enamel of the permanent dentition.

C Clinical Vignettes

Vignette 1

A 6-month-old infant is seen for a well visit, and his parents have lots of questions.

1. The parents ask you how to prevent scald burns. You recommend:
   a. Be in the next room when the infant is in the bath.
   b. Turn the water heater temperature to 120°F.
   c. Hold the baby in your opposite arm when you drink a hot beverage.
   d. Turn the water heater temperature to 130°F.
   e. Not an important issue for this age.

2. The parents ask about the infant's diet. Appropriate nutritional recommendations at this age include all *except*:
   a. Breastfed babies require vitamin D supplementation.
   b. Solid foods should be introduced and should only be given by spoon.
   c. Water should be added to the diet.
   d. Appropriate fluoride intake should be assured.
   e. Honey may be added to the diet.

3. They note that the baby is putting everything in his mouth. You use this as an opportunity to make which correct statement:
   a. Poisoning does not become an important risk until later, when children walk and climb.
   b. The best thing to do if they think their child has swallowed a poisonous substance is to call the pediatric office.
   c. Alcoholic beverages are the leading poison in children.
   d. All small objects, cosmetics, cleaners, medications, toxic plants and other poisonous substances should be kept out of reach.
   e. Parents should always try to induce vomiting immediately if their child is suspected of swallowing a poison.

Vignette 2

At a 9-month health supervision visit, you notice that the infant's first teeth have erupted.

1. You use this as an opportunity to discuss which of the following with the parent(s)?
   a. There is no need to clean baby teeth.
   b. Oral fluoride is dangerous for children below 1 year of age.
   c. An adequate fluoride source should be documented.
   d. Formal care by a dentist is not necessary until 4 years of age.
   e. Primary teeth continue to erupt until 5 years of age.

2. The parent asks you if fluoride drops should be given to the infant. Which of the following is the most appropriate response?
   a. Fluoride drops should be given to all infants after tooth eruption.
   b. Fluoride drops should only be given to infants who do not receive adequate amounts from fluoridated water.
   c. Most US communities do not supply fluoridated tap water.
   d. Most bottle water contains adequate fluoride.
   e. Too much fluoride does not cause significant problems.

3. The parent asks you when their child's full set of primary teeth should come in. Which of the following is correct?
   a. 12 to 17 months
   b. 18 to 24 months
   c. 25 to 33 months
   d. 3 years
   e. 4 years

Vignette 3

A neighbor of yours has three children.

1. The first child speaks in two-word phrases, can stack five blocks, jumps up and throws a ball overhand. This child's developmental age is closest of which of the following?
   a. 15 months
   b. 18 months
   c. 2 years
   d. 3 years
   e. 4 years

2. The second child speaks two sentences at a time and is mainly understandable, feeds and dresses independently, stacks seven blocks, alternates feet going upstairs and copies a circle. This child's developmental age is closest to which of the following?
   a. 15 months
   b. 18 months
   c. 2 years
   d. 3 years
   e. 4 years

3. The third child can say her full name, knows five different colors, hops on one foot and dresses herself. This child's developmental age is closest to which of the following?
   a. 2 years
   b. 3 years
   c. 4 years
   d. 5 years
   e. 6 years

Vignette 4

An 18-month-old child's parent is concerned because she says no words other than "mama" and "dada."

1. You should do all of the following *except*:
   a. Refer for audiology evaluation.
   b. Administer an M-CHAT screening test.
   c. Administer a developmental screening test, such as Denver-II, ASQ, or PEDS.
   d. Refer to a speech pathologist for evaluation.
   e. Do no further evaluation now, reassure the parent that the child is likely to catch up and arrange for a follow-up visit at age 2.

2. This child's audiology report shows a bilateral conductive hearing loss. Which of the following is the most likely cause of this?
   a. Otitis media with effusion
   b. Congenital infection
   c. A genetic condition
   d. Ear wax
   e. Excessive noise exposure

3. Which of the following is the most appropriate interpretation of a positive score on the M-CHAT test in this 18-month-old child?
   a. It is definitive proof of an autism spectrum disorder.
   b. It is not a significant indicator of abnormal behavior at this age.
   c. The parent should be reassured and the test repeated at 24 months.
   d. The child is at risk for a developmental disorder primarily affecting their motor development.
   e. The child is at risk for an autism spectrum disorder and should be referred for further evaluation.

Vignette 5

A parent of a 9-year-old asks about injury prevention. The parent reveals that there are firearms present in the home.

1. Which of the following represents appropriate advice to prevent firearm injuries and deaths?
   a. Store guns locked and unloaded, with ammunition stored in a separate location.
   b. Store loaded guns out of reach of children.
   c. Limit young children to violent TV programs and video games only on weekends.
   d. Do not be concerned when children have play dates in other homes, since very few other homes have loaded guns.
   e. Let your child take your gun to school for show-and-tell to promote gun safety.

2. The parent also asks you about preventing injuries from fires. Which of the following is *true*?
   a. Most child deaths in fires are due to burns.
   b. Smoke alarms are present in most house fires.
   c. All families should have working smoke alarms and home fire escape plans.
   d. Fires are the leading cause of injury deaths in children.
   e. Children are not the main victims of fire deaths because they typically are rescued early.

3. Other important safety advice for a 9-year-old includes all of the following *except*:
   a. Wear a helmet when riding a bicycle.
   b. Learn to swim.
   c. Replace smoke alarm batteries every 2 years.
   d. Wear appropriate protective padding when using skate boards, scooters, or roller skates.
   e. Apply sunscreen before going outside for more than 10 minutes.

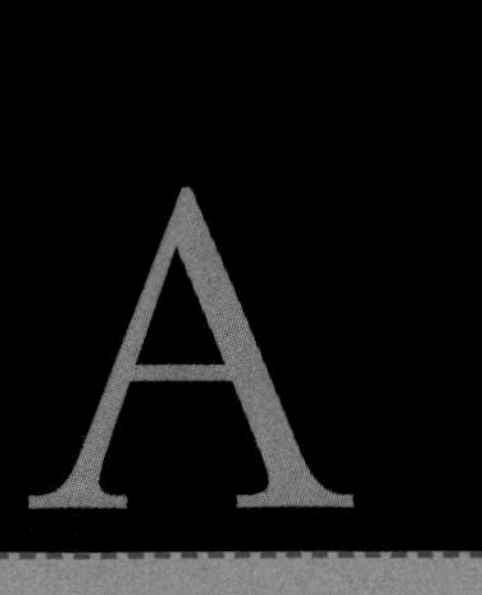

Answers

Vignette 1 **Question 1**

Answer B: Scald burns are an important source of injury at this age. Parents and caregivers should be at "touch distance" when bathing infants and toddlers. Hot beverages should not be held near infants. Water heaters should be turned down to 120°F to prevent significant scalding.

Vignette 1 **Question 2**

Answer E: Breast milk does not contain adequate vitamin D; infants require 400 IU of vitamin D daily from the first few days of life. Solids should be started by 6 months and only fed by spoon. Free water should also be introduced at this age. Fluoride may be supplied by fluoridated water or supplemental drops. Honey should not be given under 12 months because of risk of botulism.

Vignette 1 **Question 3**

Answer D: Poisoning and choking become important sources of injury starting when infants develop hand-to-mouth behavior at around 4 to 6 months, with a marked increase at age 9 months. If a poisonous ingestion is suspected, parents should call the Poison Control hotline immediately and should not induce vomiting. Cosmetics, cleaners, medications, and plants are the leading poisons in children. Prevention includes keeping dangerous substances and objects out of reach.

Vignette 2 **Question 1**

Answer C: Baby teeth should be cleaned twice daily from the time of eruption. Fluoride is effective in preventing dental caries. Dentist referral is recommended starting at 1 year. The 20 primary teeth should erupt by 25 to 33 months of age.

Vignette 2 **Question 2**

Answer B: Fluoride will help prevent caries and should be provided to all infants after tooth eruption. Approximately 60% of US communities are supplied with fluoridated water. Most bottled water does not have adequate fluoride, except for some brands designed for infants. Supplemental fluoride drops should only be provided if there is inadequate intake from water. Excess fluoride ingestion may cause fluorosis, a permanent staining of dental enamel.

Vignette 2 **Question 3**

Answer C: The first teeth usually erupt from 6 to 12 months of age. The full set of 20 primary teeth erupts by 25 to 33 months and begins to exfoliate at 6 to 7 years.

Vignette 3 **Question 1**

Answer C: A 2-year-old child who is developmentally normal should be able to speak at least 50 words, use two-word phrases, stack five to six blocks, throw a ball overhand, and jump up in the air.

Vignette 3 **Question 2**

Answer D: A developmentally normal 3-year-old should be able to feed and dress independently, speak two to three sentences with speech at least 75% understandable, know his or her gender, stack a tower of six to eight blocks, alternate feet going up stairs, and copy a circle.

Vignette 3 **Question 3**

Answer C: A developmentally normal 4-year-old child should be able to hop on one foot, know four colors, say her full name, dress herself, copy a cross, and respond correctly to the majority of questions such as, "what do you do when you are cold/tired/hungry?"

Vignette 4 **Question 1**

Answer E: Language delay is the most common type of developmental delay in early childhood. All 18-month-old children should be screened for developmental delay (with the Denver-II, ASQ, PEDS, etc.) and autism spectrum disorders (with the M-CHAT). All children with concerns about language delay should be referred for audiology and speech evaluations.

Vignette 4 **Question 2**

Answer A: Congenital infections and genetic conditions are important causes of *sensorineural* hearing loss, which may be detected by newborn hearing screening. The most common cause of *conductive* hearing loss in children after the neonatal period is otitis media with effusion.

Vignette 4 **Question 3**

Answer E: The M-CHAT is a screening test for ASD, which primarily affect social interaction and communication. It should be administered at 18 and 24 months, and a positive result should trigger referral for further evaluation, since it indicates increased risk for ASD.

Vignette 5 Question 1

Answer A: Guns should be stored locked, unloaded, and in a separate location from ammunition. All TV and other screen time should be limited to none before age 2 years, and maximum 2 hours daily thereafter. Content should be appropriate for age, and there should be no TV in the child's bedroom. Gun safety should be inquired about in all homes the child visits, since half of US homes have guns, and half of these are stored loaded.

Vignette 5 Question 2

Answer C: Fire is the third leading cause of injury death in children. Most deaths are due to smoke and toxic gas inhalation, not to burns. Only 40% of homes in fires have working smoke alarms. Children and the elderly are the main victims of fire deaths. Anticipatory guidance for having functional smoke alarms and a fire escape plan is recommended as part of health surveillance.

Vignette 5 Question 3

Answer C: Helmets should always be worn while riding bicycle to prevent serious head injuries. Learning to swim will help prevent drowning. Smoke alarm batteries should be replaced annually. Protective padding will help prevent injuries on various mobile devices. Sunscreen should always be applied prior to sun exposure to prevent damage due to ultraviolet rays, which increases the risk of skin cancer later in life.

Chapter

2 Neonatal Medicine

Katie S. Fine

With few exceptions, the information presented herein is limited largely to conditions encountered in term or near-term infants. This reflects the information that providers completing primary pediatric rotations and taking medical shelf and board examinations are expected to know. More specialized topics regarding neonatal intensive care can be found elsewhere.

PHYSICAL EXAMINATION OF THE INFANT

The physical examination of the term newborn as presented here is organized from head to toe. Many practitioners choose to examine the infant in a different order: starting with the heart, lungs, and abdomen, and ending with the back, hips, and oropharynx. This method permits auscultation of the aforementioned systems while the patient is (hopefully) quiet, delaying maneuvers which are more likely to elicit crying until the end. If the baby has already been given an initial antiseptic bath, it is likely that an antibiotic ointment has been instilled in the infant's eyes and that an intramuscular injection of vitamin K has been administered. Ophthalmic antibiotics are given universally in developed nations to prevent neonatal conjunctivitis, in particular infections due to *Neisseria gonorrhea* and *Chlamydia trachomatis*, still a leading cause of blindness in the developing world. Vitamin K prevents the development of hemorrhagic disease of the newborn.

GROWTH PARAMETERS

Weight, height, and head circumference are typically recorded in stable term newborns shortly after birth. Most nurseries also routinely assess newborns with both neuromuscular and physical maturity rating scales (i.e., Dubowitz or Ballard scoring). The scales are particularly significant when the mother did not receive prenatal care, does not know when she became pregnant, or when the scores diverge significantly from expected. The growth measurements and maturity scores are compared with those expected based on the newborn's recorded **gestational age** (via maternal dates and/or sonography). Weight, length, and head circumference assist in determining **appropriateness for gestational age.** The three data points are plotted and compared with expected ranges of values for that particular gestational age. In particular, the term "appropriate for gestational age" (AGA) typically refers primarily to an infant's weight. Fetal, maternal, and placental factors all influence fetal growth (see Table 2-1). Chromosomal anomalies, congenital malformations, and inborn errors of metabolism are discussed in their respective chapters.

Growth parameters may be less than expected because the baby is actually premature (i.e., the estimated gestational age is higher than the true gestational age). Newborns with weights less than the 10th percentile for gestational age are termed **small for gestational age** (SGA). Some of these infants followed a stable growth curve throughout fetal development and are simply in the lower percentiles. Others suffered abnormal growth restriction at some point in the pregnancy. Blood glucose levels should be monitored frequently in babies with SGA; decreased glycogen reserves increase the risk of hypoglycemia.

TABLE 2-1 Factors Contributing to Intrauterine Growth Retardation[a]
Fetal Factors
Chromosomal anomalies (Trisomy 13)
Congenital malformations (Potter syndrome)
Congenital infections (cytomegalovirus)
Inborn errors of metabolism (galactosemia)
Maternal Factors
Reduced or restricted uteroplacental flow (preeclampsia)
Maternal malnutrition
Multiple pregnancies
Maternal smoking
Maternal alcohol abuse
Maternal drug use (heroin)
Placental Factors
Placental insufficiency
Anomalies of the placenta or cord (two-vessel cord)
[a]Examples in parentheses.

Fetal demise, fetal distress, and neonatal death rates are higher in SGA babies as a group than the general birth population.

Intrauterine growth retardation (IUGR) is divided into two categories based on gestational age at onset. In *early onset (symmetric) IUGR*, the insult resulting in growth restriction begins prior to 28 weeks' gestation. At birth, length and head circumference are proportional to expected to weight. Chromosomal anomalies in particular often result in symmetric IUGR, for obvious reasons. Infants *with late onset (asymmetric) IUGR* have sparing of the (relatively normal) head circumference, but length and especially weight are reduced below what is expected. These babies had normal percentile growth early in the pregnancy but "fell off" the growth curve when placental function was insufficient to keep up with fetal requirements for growth. They often appear long and thin, even emaciated. This may occur in infants who become infected with a congenital pathogen after 28 weeks' gestation or experience late insufficiency of the cord or the placenta.

Newborns who are SGA due to incorrect dating of the pregnancy may actually be premature (gestational age <36 weeks). Findings consistent with prematurity include paucity of sole creases; absence or smaller-than-expected breast nodules; fine, fuzzy scalp hair; visible veins in the skin; absence of ear cartilage; and undescended testes.

Newborns with weights greater than the 90th percentile for gestational age are termed **large for gestational age** (LGA). Again, some of these infants are simply healthy babies with weights in the higher percentiles. Others are larger than expected because they are postterm (gestational age >42 weeks) or maternal dates are incorrect. Some have underlying conditions that contribute to their increased size. This is true for infants of diabetic mothers and neonates with Beckwith–Wiedemann syndrome. Birth trauma, polycythemia, and hypoglycemia are more common in LGA patients than the general neonatal population.

Infants thought to be "large for gestational age" who are actually postdates will have cracked, leathery, wrinkled skin which is usually peeling.

VITALS AND GENERAL APPEARANCE

The initial assessment is your first impression of the patient and includes appraisals of (1) overall appearance ("well" vs. "toxic"), (2) general body habitus, (3) comfort or level of distress, and (4) color. Is the infant active? Or, if sleeping, easily arousable and appropriately responsive? When provoked, is the cry strong or weak? Overall, is the infant the size, heft, and level of development that you are used to seeing from term neonates? Is the infant breathing easily, or is the respiratory rate increased and accompanied by signs of increased effort? The skin should be warm and may be ruddy but should not be pale or cyanotic. Parts of this initial evaluation become more intuitive over many years of practice, but the elements do not change.

SKIN

Following initial maternal–infant bonding, the well-term baby is unwrapped and placed under a warmer in the nursery to permit full examination and prophylactic interventions. The warmer reduces the amount of energy the infant needs to expend in order to maintain normal temperature when unwrapped, as evaporative and convective heat loss through the thin skin of the newborn is comparably quite high.

Common birthmarks include salmon patches and Mongolian spots. The **salmon patch** (nevus simplex), commonly termed a **stork bite**, is a superficial nonblanching hemangiotic lesion most commonly located on the eyelids and posterior neck at the hairline. The lesions become more prominent with bathing or crying but often fade greatly over time. **Mongolian spots** are flat, dark blue-black pigmented macules usually seen over the lower back and buttocks in 90% of African American, Indian, and Asian infants. The hyperpigmented areas fade as the child ages; they present no known long-term problems but may occasionally be mistaken for abusive trauma, as the appearance is somewhat similar to that of a bruise. Port wine stains, café-au-lait spots, and hypopigmented lesions are less common skin findings which may be associated with underlying neurologic conditions; these are discussed more fully in Chapter 15.

A few commonly acquired rashes often noted in the first month of life are milia, erythema toxicum neonatorum, seborrheic dermatitis, and neonatal acne. **Milia** is characterized by pearly white or pale yellow epidermal cysts found on the nose, chin, and forehead. The benign lesions exfoliate and disappear within the first few weeks of life. No treatment is necessary.

The extremely common rash of **erythema toxicum** consists of evanescent papules, vesicles, and pustules, each on an erythematous base, that usually occur initially on the trunk and spread outward to the extremities. The rash typically appears 24 to 72 hours after birth but may be seen earlier. Of note, the lesions "move around" over time; that is, they are visible in a particular spot for several hours only but may persist in a region for longer. The rash resolves over 3 to 5 days without therapy, and the condition is of no clinical significance.

Infantile seborrhea appears between 2 and 10 weeks and is commonly called "cradle cap" when it appears on the scalp. It may also involve the face and, less commonly, other areas rich in sebaceous glands (e.g., perineum, postauricular and intertriginous areas). It is characterized by erythematous, dry, scaling, crusty lesions. Affected areas are often sharply demarcated from uninvolved skin. For severe cradle cap, baby oil is applied to the scalp for 15 minutes, followed by washing with an anti-dandruff shampoo. Occasionally, 0.5% to 1% hydrocortisone cream may be indicated. If candidal superinfection occurs, nystatin ointment is recommended.

Neonatal acne typically develops on the cheeks and nose around age 3 to 4 weeks and persists for up to 3 months. The rash consists of small pustules and papules, with an appearance consistent with closed comedones in the adolescent. Like neonatal breast budding and vaginal bleeding, neonatal acne results from secondary maternal hormone stimulation and resolves gradually as these hormones are degraded in the infant. No treatment is required.

CARDIAC/PULSES

The heart examination in the infant is similar to that in any other patient. The heart sounds should be evaluated across the precordium as well as on the right (to diagnose situs inversus, if present) and in the back. Both heart sounds should be present and normal in character. It is often difficult to distinguish the S_2 split in infants due to rates which may range from 100 to 200 beats per minute or greater. Evaluate for extra heart sounds and murmurs. A murmur may be appreciated in the first few days of life as the ductus arteriosus closes, most often a continuous murmur over the second left intercostal space. It is important to palpate the brachial and femoral pulses for symmetry; both should be strong but not bounding. Coarctation of the aorta is associated with weak and/or delayed femoral pulses as compared with the right brachial pulse. See Chapter 7 for details regarding the presentations, differentiation, and management of congenital heart diseases.

LUNGS/CHEST

Rhonchi (transmitted upper airway sounds) are very common in the hours after delivery due to residual amniotic fluid. True crackles and wheezing are pathologic. Signs of respiratory distress, if present, are usually noted early in the examination of the infant. Increased respiratory rate, retractions, grunting, and nasal flaring are signs of neonatal distress, which may or may not be primarily respiratory in origin; neonatal sepsis and some congenital heart disorders present in an indistinguishable manner.

The character of the cry should be noted. Passage of a laryngoscope through the vocal cords in the delivery room to remove meconium with suctioning can result in hoarseness noted when the infant cries. Unexplained hoarseness warrants further investigation.

ABDOMEN

In an infant, the abdomen appears full due to as-yet-underdeveloped abdominal musculature. If present, abdominal distention suggests a congenital obstruction; scaphoid abdomen is more characteristic of diaphragmatic hernia (see Congenital Anomalies section). Typical bowel sounds are generally present within the first few hours of life. In neonates and older infants, the liver is often palpable up to a few centimeters below the anterior costal margin. The spleen tip should be only barely palpable, if at all. Hepatosplenomegaly is a common finding in babies with congenital infections and in some patients with congenital heart disease.

If the baby is newly born, the cord should be checked for the presence of a vein and two arteries. Two-vessel cords increase the likelihood of gastrointestinal and renal anomalies. The cord "dries" within days and typically falls off within 3 to 4 weeks. Persistence of the cord beyond 8 weeks is abnormal and may signify a neutrophil disorder. The inherent relative weakness of the abdominal wall around the cord insertion may result in intermittent protrusion of abdominal contents (covered by a membranous sac) through the space. These **umbilical hernias** are common, generally benign, and resolve in the majority of cases over time. They appear larger when the infant is crying or straining to stool. Those which are particularly large or persist beyond 3 to 4 years of age are repaired surgically.

GENITALIA

Female

While the labia majora typically cover the labia minora in newborn females, this is not always the case. Maternal estrogen stimulates growth of the labia minora, which may appear more prominent than expected in older children. For the same reason, mucoid vaginal secretions and occasionally blood may be noted in the introitus. These will resolve over time. The clitoris is also relatively larger at this age than in older children and adolescents. A clitoris which appears overly large and virilized may represent **ambiguous genitalia** (most commonly due to congenital adrenal hyperplasia in a genetic female). Both vagina and anus (in both females and males) should be patent and normally placed, and skin tags may be present in either region.

Male

In term neonates, the penis averages 3 to 4 cm long when stretched, and the testes are about 1 cm across. The uncircumcised penis has a foreskin which is minimally retractable; full retraction should never be attempted. The ventral surface of the penis should be inspected for any evidence of an (abnormal) urethral opening called **hypospadias**. **Chordae** is the fixed fibrotic ventral bowing of the penis; it is often associated with hypospadias. Urethral openings along the penile shaft should prompt a radiographic work-up of the genitourinary system to identify other associated anomalies, which are not uncommon. Chordae and hypospadias require urosurgical intervention, and the repair may need to be completed in stages. Children with either of these conditions should not be circumcised in the newborn nursery, as is routinely undertaken if the parents request, but instead managed by a surgical specialist.

Both testes are generally palpable in the scrotal sacs, but this may not be the case. If a testis is "missing," begin palpating for a testis-sized mass in the lower abdomen and proceed along the inguinal canal. **Retractile testes** are those which, when located, can be gently massaged into the associated scrotum. If no testis is found, or the mass is fixed, the testicle is termed *undescended*, a condition referred to as **cryptorchidism**. If the testis has not descended into the scrotal sac by age 1 year, it is surgically relocated there. Moving the testis does not decrease the associated risks of malignancy and sterility, but it does make the testis easier to examine and monitor. A mass that bulges from the groin area (possibly extending into the scrotal sac) which increases in size with crying and straining may represent an **inguinal hernia**.

The scrotal sacs should also be palpated for other masses, most notably **hydroceles**, which are fluid-filled remnants of the processus vaginalis. Hydroceles transilluminate, which helps differentiate them clinically from other masses. The great majority resolve by 1 year of age.

HEAD

Asymmetry of the newborn head is very common in the product of a vaginal birth. Molding is the slight cephalad-to-caudal elongation of the head due to pressure from the pelvic bones and narrow vaginal canal as the head "presents." **Caput succedaneum** is more marked, involving edema of the scalp tissues. The swelling often crosses the midline and/or suture lines and is firm but "pits" to gentle pressure. Bruising may or may not be present. Vacuum extractions are often followed by caput. A **cephalohematoma** involves bleeding into the subperiosteal space. Thus, the swelling is limited by sutures lines and therefore does not cross the midline.

The fetal skull bones are not fused at birth, which permits the brain and head to grow normally. Both an anterior and a posterior fontanelle are present. The suture lines may be slightly apart or mildly overlapping. Gaping sutures lines and/or a bulging (usually anterior) fontanelle are associated with hydrocephalus. Overlapping is common following vaginal deliveries but should normalize within a few weeks.

FACE

The face, too, is often asymmetric and may be bruised depending on the length and difficulty of the delivery. Looking at the face as a whole unit may permit you to identify when the appearance is syndromic, even if you are not yet certain what syndrome is represented.

EYES

Opening a newborn's eyes is difficult due to edema of the lids secondary to birth. Often the baby will open the eyes when the lights are dimmed and when the baby is held upright. In that few seconds, assess the symmetry of eye opening and pupils, if possible. Eyes which are too far apart, too close together, or abnormally slanted may signify a congenital syndrome. Epicanthal folds are found not only in children with Down syndrome but also in many unaffected babies. Dysconjugate gaze is a normal finding in infants prior to age 4 to 6 months.

If prophylactic antibiotic drops have recently been instilled in the newborn's eyes, it may be difficult to see bilateral clear red reflexes via fundoscopy. However, this finding is critical to assess and document. Congenital cataracts will cloud the red reflex; often these must be removed very early in life for the development of normal sight.

EARS

Ears should be examined for normal shape, placement, size, and rotation. Abnormalities in any of these are associated with numerous genetic and congenital conditions. The helix, antihelix, tragus, antitragus, and lobe should appear typical and symmetric between sides. Ear tags and ear pits are not uncommon. Preauricular pits may be associated with other branchial arch abnormalities, renal anomalies, and hearing loss.

NOSE

Examine the nose for obvious asymmetry. Mild asymmetry is common in the weeks after birth due to uterine compression. The length of the philtrum should also appear relatively normal.

Neonates are "obligate nose breathers." This means that they primarily breathe through the nose unless crying or distressed. **Choanal atresia**, a congenital condition, is the blockage of the posterior nasal airway by a membranous or bony obstruction. The obstruction may be partial/unilateral or complete. Infants with choanal atresia develop respiratory distress with cyanosis and may become apneic when the mouth is either occluded during feeding or simply closed while the infant is calm or resting. Infants who are cyanotic when calm or feeding but have improved color with crying should have a small catheter passed through each side of the nose. Failure of passage strongly suggests choanal atresia. In the short term, placement of an oral airway or even intubation may be indicated. Surgery restores patency of the nasal passages.

MOUTH/THROAT

Lip and mouth movement should be symmetric when the baby is crying. A bluish-gray tinge to the area around the lips may be observed; this is normal perioral cyanosis, resulting from the same *peripheral* vascular process as bluish palms and soles noted intermittently in newborns. However, this same discoloration of the lips and or tongue indicates *central* cyanosis due to arterial hypoxemia, a serious finding that warrants immediate intervention and rapid diagnostic procedures. The tongue should fit within the closed mouth, with the inferior frenulum long enough to permit easy movement of the tip of the tongue. The palate should be inspected and palpated. A cleft lip is obvious. A cleft palate is less so, although the condition will become clear once the infant attempts to feed. A bifid uvula may be accompanied by an abnormality of the soft palate which could affect feeding and, later, speech. Cleft lip and palate are discussed in more detail later in the chapter (see Congenital Anomalies section).

NECK

The newborn neck moves freely and is rather short. Restriction of head turning to either side may indicate **torticollis**, a unilateral congenital fibrotic shortening of the sternocleidomastoid muscle. Girls with Turner syndrome may have neck webbing with a low posterior hairline. Check the neck for masses or cysts.

UPPER EXTREMITIES

Palpate the entirety of the clavicles for crepitus indicating a **clavicle fracture**, present in up to 2% of deliveries. Clavicular fractures are more common in large infants and deliveries complicated by shoulder dystocia or other trauma. If crepitus is noted, radiographs are not generally indicated unless there are signs of gross deformity or asymmetric arm movements (more common in *complete* fractures). *Incomplete* fractures are usually missed at birth, with the diagnosis becoming evident when a reactive callus is noted in the area 2 to 4 weeks later. No specific treatment is necessary for simple clavicle fractures detected at birth. Complete fractures should be immobilized.

Movement at the arms and shoulders should be symmetric and generally free, excepting normal minor flexion contractures at the elbows, knees, and hips. Birth trauma can also result in Erb palsy (damage to C5–C6 nerve roots) and Klumpke paralysis (damage to C7, C8, and T1 nerve roots). The former is much more common. The infant with **Erb palsy** holds the affected arm close to the body, extended at the elbow, internally rotated, with the forearm fixed in pronation but hand movement preserved. In **Klumpke paralysis**, the upper arm is unaffected, but the hand muscles are weak, and the grasp reflex may not be present. Both conditions often resolve over the first 48 hours of life. In those that do not, improvement can be expected up to age 6 months. Thereafter, residual deficits may gradually improve for up to 18 months with intensive physical therapy. Surgery may be indicated for static cases.

Inspect the palmar creases. A single transverse crease is often noted in patients with Down syndrome, but most patients with this finding are typical, healthy infants. Examine and count fingers and fingernails.

LOWER EXTREMITIES

Anterior and posterior medial thigh creases and gluteal folds should be symmetric. If the "lines" do not match up, consider whether **hip dysplasia** may be a cause. Ortolani and Barlow maneuvers are discussed in detail in Chapter 16 and should be performed in all newborns and at all early infancy health maintenance visits. The feet should be examined for **metatarsus adductus** (medial curving of the forefoot), **talipes equinovarus** ("clubfoot"), and other anomalies. The diagnoses and treatments of these conditions are discussed in Chapter 16.

BACK

Palpate the entire length of the bony spine. Look for dimples, hair tufts, or hemangiomas overlying the spine. They may be associated with underlying neurologic anomalies (see Chapter 15). Small, shallow, solitary sacral dimples located within 2.5 cm of the anal verge are common and benign. If concerning signs are present, or there are associated neurologic functional deficits, radiographic imaging with MRI should be undertaken to assess for underlying anatomic abnormalities in the spine and/or neural tissue.

NEUROLOGIC (REFLEXES AND TONE)

The neonate should exhibit good tone, be rousable from sleep, and readily be calmed with feeding or sucking. A few beats of ankle clonus are found in many typical healthy newborns. Age-specific reflexes which should disappear over time include the rooting and sucking reflexes, the reflex grasp, and the Moro reflex, among others. When one cheek is lightly brushed from the corner of the mouth toward the ear, the neonate turns the head toward that side (rooting). The infant should have a strong suck from birth. When the examiner's finger is placed in the center of the open palm, the baby's fingers reflexively curl around it in a grip. To elicit the **Moro reflex**, lift the supine infant's chest and shoulders up slightly from a flat surface with your hands and forearms. Gently but suddenly allow your hands and arms to move back toward the bed. Both the infant's arms should abduct suddenly away from the midline with the fingers extended. If the response is asymmetric, there may be weakness on one side or abnormally increased tone on the other. Repeated asymmetric trials should prompt more thorough neurologic evaluation.

BEFORE THE DELIVERY: PRENATAL CONDITIONS

A wealth of important information can be gleaned from the prenatal and delivery records in a matter of minutes (Table 2-2). Knowledge of these factors can assist the pediatrician in uncovering subtle examination findings and suggest targeted laboratory and radiographic studies.

ABNORMALITIES IN AMNIOTIC FLUID VOLUME

Amniotic fluid balance is maintained through normal production of fluid and permeability across fetal (lung and skin) membranes and, later, release of adequate volumes of fetal urine. The most common cause of **polyhydramnios** (excess of fluid) is impaired fetal swallowing, which may occur in the setting of congenital gastrointestinal obstruction or malformation, conditions that interfere with neural function, and certain other congenital conditions (trisomies, Beckwith–Wiedemann, achondroplasia). Other etiologies to consider include excessive production of fetal (multiple fetuses, hydrops fetalis) or maternal origins (gestational diabetes).

TABLE 2-2 Review of the Prenatal and Delivery Records

Prenatal
Age of the mother (advanced maternal age, young mother)
Medical history of the mother (diabetes, mental illness, etc.)
Medications during the pregnancy (particularly those associated with birth defects)
Family history (bleeding disorders, heritable metabolic disorders and chromosomal anomalies, stillbirths, etc.)
Social history (cigarette smoking, alcohol use, drug use, domestic violence)
Initiation of prenatal care (adequate, sporadic, late, frequent missed appointments, none)
Number of pregnancies and live children
Prenatal screening results (spina bifida, Down syndrome, Trisomy 18)
Maternal prenatal laboratory results
Blood type (including Rh factor)
Rapid plasma reagin (RPR; screening test for syphilis)
Group B streptococcus culture
Hepatitis B surface antigen
Rubella immune status
Human immunodeficiency virus
Neisseria gonorrhoeae
Chlamydia trachomatis
Hepatitis C (if indicated)
Mantoux screening test (PPD) (if indicated)
Targeted genetic testing (cystic fibrosis, etc.)
Results of prenatal ultrasound (size, dates, estimated fetal weight, multiple fetuses, fetal movement, adequacy of amniotic fluid volume, and congenital anomalies of the palate, gastrointestinal, renal, skeletal, and urologic systems)
Delivery
Duration of rupture of membranes (< or ≥18 hr)
Characterization of amniotic fluid (clear, meconium-stained, purulent, foul-smelling)
Medications administered during delivery
Fetal heart rate monitoring and use of scalp electrodes
Route of delivery (vaginal or cesarean delivery)
If cesarean: elective, repeat, fetal distress, failure to progress, breech presentation
If vaginal: spontaneous, forceps, or vacuum extraction
Complications (twin gestation, nuchal cord, etc.)
APGAR scores
Resuscitation, if necessary (stimulation, oxygen, bagging, compressions, intubation)
Gestational age (via dates) at delivery

■ **TABLE 2-3** Transmission, Presentation, Identification, and Treatment of Perinatal Infections
Cytomegalovirus (CMV)
Transmission: Transmission anytime during the pregnancy or through exposure to maternal fluids during/after birth (including breast milk). Transmission rate significantly higher if the mother acquires the disease during pregnancy. Transmission possible even when the primary maternal infection occurred years before the pregnancy
Presentation *(Congenital):* Asymptomatic (90%) *or* combination of any of the following: preterm birth, intrauterine growth retardation (IUGR), microcephaly, poor feeding, lethargy, petechiae/purpura, "blueberry muffin" spots, jaundice, hepatosplenomegaly, elevated liver transaminases, anemia, thrombocytopenia, intracranial (particularly periventricular) calcifications, seizures, chorioretinitis. Acquired infections generally asymptomatic
Diagnosis: CMV detected in the urine (saliva, blood) within the first 2 wk of life is consistent with *congenital* infection
Treatment: Supportive care; ongoing trials with gancyclovir
Long-Term Sequelae: *Congenital CMV is the most common infectious cause of sensorineural hearing loss.* Seventy-five percent of infants with symptomatic congenital CMV will develop hearing loss. Hearing is often normal at birth, with progressive impairment over the first year. Other possible long-term complications include developmental delay, mental retardation, cerebral palsy (motor spasticity), and dental defects (abnormal enamel production). Acquired infections generally free of sequelae
Screening/Prevention: Antibody testing before or early in pregnancy to document prior infection
Herpes Simplex Virus (HSV)
Transmission: Perinatal infection acquired through exposure to organism in maternal genital tract during delivery. Transmission rate significantly higher if the mother contracts primary infection during pregnancy (up to 50% vs. <5% for infants born to mothers with recurrent infections). That being said, *most infants with neonatal HSV are born to women who have never experienced symptoms and do not know that they are infected.* Infants may also become infected through contact with herpetic breast lesions while feeding or from maternal oral secretions after birth.
Presentation: Neonatal HSV presents in the first 4 wk of life with any of the following three distinct clinical pictures:
Isolated mucocutaneous lesions (skin, eye, and/or mouth), including keratoconjunctivitis
Encephalitis
Disseminated disease involving multiple organs (lungs, liver, often CNS)
Infants with encephalitis and/or disseminated HSV disease may not manifest the characteristic vesicular skin lesions, leading to a delay in diagnosis.
Diagnosis: Viral culture or direct fluorescent antibody testing of vesicular scrapings. If no lesions present, virus also demonstrable in nasopharynx, conjunctivae, and urine; CSF infection: polymerase chain reaction (PCR) testing; EEG shows periodic epileptiform discharges.
Treatment: Intravenous acyclovir. Any neonate with vesicular lesions is presumed to have HSV, and acyclovir should be started pending laboratory confirmation.
Long-Term Sequelae:
Local disease: Recurrent mucocutaneous lesions
Encephalitis: Cataracts/blindness; microcephaly; developmental delay/learning disabilities
Disseminated disease: Severe neurologic impairment, death (50%)
Screening/Prevention: Deliver infants by C-section if genital lesions are present at the start of labor. If maternal lesions found after delivery, culture infant and treat with acyclovir if culture-positive or symptoms develop.
Parvovirus
Transmission: Congenital infection with vertical transmission
Presentation: Hydrops fetalis (risk increased if mother becomes infected during the first trimester)
Diagnosis: Maternal IgM, IgG levels
Treatment: Intrauterine blood transfusions; supportive care
Long-Term Sequelae: None, if fetus survives pregnancy and perinatal interventions
Screening/Prevention: None routine

■ **TABLE 2-3** Transmission, Presentation, Identification, and Treatment of Perinatal Infections *(continued)*
Human Immunodeficiency Virus
Transmission:
Congenital: Transmission may occur at any time during the pregnancy. Likelihood of vertical transmission increases with increasing maternal viral load.
Acquired: Transmission through exposure to the organism in maternal genital tract or breast milk
Presentation: Most infected infants are asymptomatic. Clinical manifestations which may develop over time include lymphadenopathy/hepatosplenomegaly, failure to thrive, developmental delay, encephalopathy, frequent bacterial infections, opportunistic infection (*Pneumocystis jiroveci*), and lymphoid interstitial pneumonitis.
Diagnosis: HIV culture; PCR
Treatment: Antiretroviral therapy
Long-Term Sequelae: All of the above listed under "Presentation"; death
Screening/Prevention: Antibody testing before or early in pregnancy to document infection. Zidovudine administered to the infected mother throughout pregnancy and delivery and zidovudine administered in the infant for the first 6 wk of life. This protocol decreases the rate of transmission from 25% to <2%. Breastfeeding is contraindicated.
Varicella Zoster Virus
Transmission
Congenital: Transmission may occur at any time during the pregnancy. Rash developing within the first 10 d of life is due to in utero infection.
Neonatal acquired: Infants with mothers who develop varicella lesions anytime from 5 d before delivery to 2 d after delivery are at high risk for severe (fatal) disease.
Acquired: Transmission through exposure to the organism in vesicular fluid, mucosa, or infected respiratory secretions
Presentation
Congenital: Congenital varicella syndrome includes any combination of the following: IUGR, cutaneous "zigzag" scarring, limb atrophy, ocular abnormalities (cataracts, chorioretinitis)
Neonatal acquired: Widespread cutaneous lesions, pneumonia, hepatitis; death in up to a third of affected infants
Acquired: mild clinical disease
Diagnosis: Generally clinical; immunofluorescent antibody testing of vesicular scrapings is confirmatory.
Treatment: Intravenous acyclovir for infants at risk for severe disease
Long-Term Sequelae: Early death (congenital varicella syndrome and about one-third of patients with neonatal-acquired varicella); otherwise minimal
Screening/Prevention: Vaccination prior to pregnancy; acyclovir for the mother if she develops primary disease during the pregnancy
Rubella
Transmission: Congenital infection may occur at any time during pregnancy; clinically worse if contracted during the first 20 wk
Presentation: Fetal demise, premature delivery, and/or *congenital rubella syndrome*, a constellation of any of the following: cataracts, sensorineural hearing loss (the most common impairment associated with congenital rubella syndrome), congenital cardiac defects, developmental delay (may be accompanied by IUGR, hepatosplenomegaly, thrombocytopenic purpura)
Diagnosis: Maternal antibody titers during pregnancy; after birth, the infant may be tested for the virus, rubella-specific IgM, or persistently elevated rubella-specific IgG.
Treatment: No specific treatment
Long-Term Sequelae: Hearing impairment, glaucoma, mental retardation
Screening/Prevention: All women of child-bearing age should have documented evidence of appropriate vaccination or immunity. Immunity should be confirmed with serology in all women who are considering becoming pregnant.

Syphilis
Transmission: Transplacental transmission of spirochetes and may occur at any time during the pregnancy, with highest transmission rates in first/second trimesters.
Presentation: Fetal demise; premature delivery; infants may be asymptomatic at birth but develop typical skin lesions, anemia, thrombocytopenia, jaundice, "snuffles," hepatosplenomegaly, elevated liver enzymes, and skeletal abnormalities, such as osteochondritis (inflammation of the cartilage and bone around a joint) and periostitis.
Diagnosis: Testing should be carried out in all symptomatic infants as well as asymptomatic infants of mothers with positive screens whose treatment occurred within 1 mo of delivery, was inadequate or undocumented, or did not result in a reduction in nontreponemal titers.
Treatment: Penicillin G. All infants should be presumed to have neurosyphilis and be treated with aqueous crystalline penicillin G (IV) or procaine penicillin (IM) for 10–14 d.
Long-Term Sequelae: Neurosyphilis (if untreated), deafness
Screening/Prevention: Routine maternal nontreponemal testing confirmed by a treponemal test; treatment of maternal disease during pregnancy.
Toxoplasmosis
Transmission: Transmission may occur at any time during the pregnancy. Fetal infection rates are lowest in the first trimester and highest in the third; conversely, disease severity is highest in the first trimester and lowest in the third.
Presentation: Intracranial calcifications and chorioretinitis; anemia, jaundice, hepatosplenomegaly, lymphadenopathy; infants may be asymptomatic at birth.
Diagnosis: Toxoplasma-specific antibody testing in the infant
Treatment: Multidrug therapy of the infant
Long-Term Sequelae: Blindness, developmental delay
Screening/Prevention: Keep cats indoors and change litter frequently; avoid eating undercooked meats; limit exposure to contaminated soil.
Adapted from Table 5-8, "Important Congenital and Perinatal Infections." Fine KS. *Pediatric Board Recertification*. Philadelphia, PA: Lippincott Williams & Wilkins, 2008:61–63.

Too little fluid, or **oligohydramnios**, restricts fetal movement, lung expansion, and (if severe) placental blood flow. The most common cause is renal disease, particularly bilateral renal agenesis, widespread multicystic disease, or severe obstruction of the urinary tract. Bilateral renal agenesis results in **Potter syndrome**, characterized by compression deformities of the face, limbs (clubbed feet), belly (scaphoid "prune belly" abdomen), and chest (pulmonary hypoplasia). The great majority of patients with Potter syndrome die of respiratory insufficiency in the neonatal period.

CONGENITAL/PERINATAL INFECTIONS

Congenital typically describes events that take place in utero, whereas *perinatal* encompasses the period just before, during, and after birth. However, the two terms are often used interchangeably when referring to maternally-derived infections. A congenital (perinatal) infection results when a neonate becomes infected with a pathogenic organism transmitted via the placenta (to the embryo or fetus) or via exposure in the birth canal during labor. Table 2-3 lists numerous key aspects regarding the identification and treatment of perinatal infections.

CONGENITAL EXPOSURE TO TERATOGENIC SUBSTANCES

Exposure to alcohol, prescription drugs, and illegal substances can lead to characteristic clinical presentations, syndromes, and/or birth defects. Table 2-4 overviews the most commonly used nonprescribed substances that are known to have effects on the fetus. Table 2-5 provides a list of several prescription agents that are associated with known birth defects.

IN THE DELIVERY ROOM

APGAR SCORES

In the delivery room, Apgar scores are assessed at 1 and 5 minutes based on defined physiologic responses to the birth process (see Table 2-6). The 1-minute score is generally considered to be reflective of the newborn's intrauterine environment and immediate response to delivery. The 5-minute score indicates the infant's adjustment to the extrauterine environment. If the 5-minute Apgar score is low, or there are ongoing resuscitation attempts, a 10-minute Apgar may be

TABLE 2-4 Maternal Substance Use: Associated Fetal Abnormalities/Neonatal Withdrawal Syndromes

	Fetal Abnormalities	Neonatal Withdrawal Syndromes	Increases Risk of:
Alcohol (onset 6–12 hr after birth) **Items in bold are characteristic findings of fetal alcohol syndrome**	– **Growth retardation** – Microcephaly – **Short palpebral fissures** – Midface hypoplasia – **Smooth philtrum** – **Thin, smooth upper vermillion border** – Joint anomalies – Altered palmar creases – Small distal phalanges – Hypoplastic nails – Fifth finger clinodactyly – Hirsutism – Congenital (septal) heart defects	Newborns with fetal alcohol syndrome are irritable and tremulous, regardless of whether they were exposed after the first trimester. If the mother is intoxicated at delivery, the infant may be lethargic and hypoglycemic. Withdrawal is uncommon but may include sweating, irritability, jitteriness, tachypnea, tremors, hypertonia, and seizures.	**Mental retardation** Impaired linear growth Sensorineural hearing loss Strabismus **Developmental delay** (motor, speech) **Learning disorders** Behavior problems (ADHD, conduct disorder)
Cocaine	– Intracranial hemorrhage – Seizures – Limb-reduction defects – Intestinal atresia – Gastroschesis – Urinary tract abnormalities	Irritability; otherwise none recognized	Increased incidence of sudden infant death syndrome; subtle abnormalities in attention/concentration
Marijuana	No known organ teratogenicity	Uncommon and mild; fine tremors, amplified Moro reflex	Under investigation; possibly measurable effects on IQ
Opiates: short-acting narcotics[a] (onset of withdrawal syndrome within 1–4 d)	No known organ teratogenicity – Impaired fetal growth	Hyperirritability, gastrointestinal dysfunction, respiratory distress, vague autonomic symptoms (yawning, sneezing, mottling, fever), tremulousness, jitteriness, high-pitched cry, increased muscle tone, irritability, loose stools	Developmental delay Behavioral problems
Opiates: methadone[a] (onset of withdrawal syndrome within 3 wk)	No known organ teratogenicity – Impaired fetal growth	Any combination of the above	Developmental delay Behavioral problems
Tobacco	No known organ teratogenicity – Intrauterine growth restriction – Low birth weight – Preterm labor – Late fetal demise	Fine tremors, hypertonia	Sudden infant death syndrome Developmental delay Asthma Otitis media

[a]Requires medical intervention with paregoric, phenobarbital, or methadone and assistance with feeding.
Adapted from Table 5-9, "Maternal Substance Use: Associated Fetal Abnormalities/Withdrawal Syndromes." Fine KS. *Pediatric Board Recertification*. Philadelphia, PA: Lippincott Williams & Wilkins, 2008:64–65.

TABLE 2-5 Prescription Medications Associated with Birth Defects

Teratogenic Medication	Effects
Carbazazepine	Anomalies of the neural tube, heart, urinary tract; cleft palate
Lithium	Ebstein anomaly of the tricuspid valve
Phenytoin	Fetal hydantoin syndrome (broad nasal bridge, cleft lip/palate, microcephaly, mental retardation)
Retinoic acid	Severe otic anomalies; thymic aplasia; anomalies of the heart and/or aorta; central nervous system defects
Valproic acid	Spina bifida; facial anomalies

TABLE 2-6 Apgar Scoring

Physical signs assessed at 1 and 5 min of life:

	0 Point	1 Point	2 Points
Heart rate	Absent	<100 bpm	≥100 bpm
Respiratory effort	Absent	Irregular, weak cry	Vigorous cry
Color	Pale, cyanotic	Cyanotic extremities	Pink throughout
Muscle tone	Absent	Weak, slightly flexed	Active extremities
Reflex irritability	Absent	Grimace	Active cry/ avoidance

recorded. Apgar scores are helpful in suggesting which infants are transitioning well and which will need ongoing support. However, it is imperative to remember that *the decision to institute resuscitation measures should be based on the patient's condition, rather than Apgar scores*. Infants with sustained low scores are virtually always acidotic, and the longer the Apgar score remains ≤3, the more likely the patient will have significant hypoxic injury and long-term neurologic damage.

MECONIUM-STAINED AMNIOTIC FLUID

Meconium is present in the fetal intestine by the second trimester. However, intrauterine passage of meconium is unusual before 37 weeks' gestation due to delayed smooth muscle and neural plexus maturation. Meconium-stained amniotic fluid at delivery is common (12% to 15% of all deliveries), with a higher incidence in African American and postterm infants. Often, intrauterine passage of meconium is associated with fetal stress; as a group, infants born through meconium-stained amniotic fluid have lower serum pH results and are more likely to have nonreassuring fetal heart tracings.

Evidence-based guidelines have resulted in subtle changes to the management of infants born through meconium-stained fluid. Recently, suctioning of the oropharynx at the perineum, before delivery of the shoulders, has fallen out of favor, as no benefit has been demonstrated in clinical trials. However, the practice has continued at many medical centers, on the basis that no harm has been associated with the procedure. Following delivery, if the infant is judged to be vigorous, with a good cry, good tone, and heart rate >100 beats per minute, only the mouth need be suctioned with a bulb syringe prior to stimulation. However, any newborn with a poor or no cry, poor tone, and heart rate <100 beats per minute should have both the oropharynx and trachea suctioned (via intubation and endotracheal suctioning as the tube is retracted). It is still unclear whether suctioning the nonvigorous infant results in any reduced morbidity, less respiratory distress, lower oxygen needs, or shorter hospital stays, nor has the complication rate been well studied. These recommendations may change as new data become available.

DISTRESS IN THE NEWBORN

Early in the first day of life, illness in the newborn often initially presents with respiratory distress. Distress may be due to a number of pathologic processes, several of which are life-threatening. While diagnosis is critical for guiding subsequent therapy, immediate medical intervention must take precedence. All infants in distress should be stabilized as quickly as possible; obtaining radiographic/laboratory/microbiology tests and results must not delay treatment. Many babies will only need oxygen via hood. When this is insufficient, nasal continuous positive airway pressure (CPAP) may suffice. A small minority of patients will need intubation, mechanical ventilation, and possibly even additional measures to maintain adequate oxygenation and acid–base balance. Table 2-7 summarizes the clinical, radiographic, and arterial gas findings associated with a few of the more common newborn diseases presenting with respiratory distress.

MECONIUM ASPIRATION SYNDROME

Although the immediate treatment and relative clinical significance of meconium-stained amniotic fluid are arguable and in flux, it is important to recognize **meconium aspiration syndrome (MAS)** in a susceptible neonate. MAS consists of delivery through meconium-stained amniotic fluid coupled with respiratory distress and characteristic chest radiograph findings (air trapping and patchy atelectasis). In affected infants, the large intrathoracic pressure that accompanies the first inspiration brings meconium from the oropharynx and trachea into the lungs. Only about 5% of infants born through meconium-stained amniotic fluid develop MAS. Severity ranges from mild (needing supplementary oxygen only) to severe disease, which requires intubation and positive pressure ventilation and is often complicated by **pulmonary hypertension**. Because meconium inactivates endogenous surfactant, surfactant administration may be beneficial in severely affected infants, who as a group suffer from high rates of morbidity (chronic lung disease) and mortality. That said, survival rates have improved markedly in recent years, due in part to the use of inhaled nitrous oxide to treat the associated pulmonary hypertension.

TABLE 2-7 Respiratory Distress in the Newborn

	Transient Tachypnea of the Newborn	Respiratory Distress Syndrome (RDS/HMD)	Pneumonia	Meconium Aspiration Syndrome
Definition	Transient pulmonary edema resulting from delayed clearance of fetal lung fluid	Newborn RDS resulting from insufficient surfactant	Lung infection acquired before, during, or after birth	Aspiration of meconium which results in obstructive lung disease, chemical pneumonitis, and inactivation of surfactant
Epidemiology	Occurs in both term and preterm infants; more common in infants delivered via C-section (especially if delivery takes place before the onset of labor)	More common in preterm infants	Varies depending on etiology (in utero infection, group B *Streptococcus*, bacterial pneumonia)	Uncommon before 37-wk gestation; more common in postterm pregnancies and infants with perinatal asphyxia
Presentation	Presents shortly after birth with tachypnea and occasionally grunting and nasal flaring	Presents shortly after birth with progressive tachypnea and respiratory distress	Signs of respiratory distress and/or sepsis; presentation may be virtually identical to that of RDS/HMD	Presents within 12 hr of birth with progressive tachypnea, flaring, grunting; rales/rhonchi on chest examination; "barrel" chest
Arterial blood gas changes	Respiratory acidosis (↓pH, ↑$PaCO_2$), mild-to-moderate hypoxemia (↓PaO_2)	Respiratory acidosis (↓pH, ↑$PaCO_2$), hypoxemia (↓PaO_2)	Respiratory acidosis, hypoxemia	Significant hypoxemia, hypercapnia
Chest radiograph	Prominent perihilar streaking, increased interstitial markings, fluid in the interlobar fissures	"Ground glass" appearance of lung fields due to air bronchograms superimposed on widespread atelectasis	Localized, patchy, or widespread consolidation; possibly pleural effusions; chest radiograph of pneumonia due to group B *Streptococcus* virtually identical to that for RDS/HMD	Areas of patchy atelectasis, coarse irregular densities interspersed with areas of hyperinflation
Treatment	O_2 therapy; continuous nasal positive airway pressure if needed	Respiratory support (e.g., mechanical ventilation) as needed	Empiric intravenous antibiotic therapy with ampicillin and cefotaxime until culture and sensitivity results are known; to complete a 10–21 d course	Mechanical ventilation with high concentration O_2 and high mean airway pressures
Prevention	None known; incidence lower in babies born vaginally, and those born via C-section following a period of labor	Antenatal steroids; exogenous surfactant administration at birth (prophylactic) or within 6 hr of birth (rescue therapy)	Prenatal screening and treatment of the mother before/during pregnancy; universal maternal group B *Streptococcus* screening	Antenatal amnioinfusion; removal of oropharyngeal/tracheal meconium in the delivery room if indicated (see text)
Complications/long-term prognosis	Spontaneous recovery within days with no long-term complications	Often minimal when recognized and treated; bronchopulmonary dysplasia when protracted mechanical ventilation with high oxygenation needs	Prognosis depends more on whether infection is present at other sites (CNS)	Acute: pulmonary air leaks. Long-term prognosis depends more on degree and duration of ventilatory support required; chronic lung disease is a known sequelae of severe meconium aspiration

RESPIRATORY DISTRESS SYNDROME

Respiratory distress syndrome (RDS), also referred to as **Hyaline membrane disease (HMD),** results from a deficiency of **surfactant**, a complex phospholipid and protein mixture produced by type II pneumocyte cells in the pulmonary epithelium. The surfactant lining the alveoli reduces surface tension, improving lung compliance and preventing full alveolar collapse during expiration. Thus, the infant can generate sufficient inhalation with lower intrathoracic pressures. Conversely, surfactant deficiency results in poor compliance, leading to progressive atelectasis, intrapulmonary shunting, hypoxemia, and cyanosis. Since fetal lung maturity is generally attained by 34 weeks' gestation, RDS is considered a disease of prematurity, and the incidence increases with decreasing gestational age. However, RDS does occur uncommonly in term and near-term infants, either through incorrect dating of the pregnancy or *delayed* cell maturation/surfactant production. For example, the combination of fetal hyperglycemia and hyperinsulinemia in maternal diabetes may result in delayed production of surfactant. Conversely, ongoing fetal stress (e.g., preeclampsia) is associated with *accelerated* lung maturation.

Affected infants characteristically present with tachypnea, grunting, nasal flaring, chest wall retractions, and cyanosis in the first few hours of life (see Table 2-7). Auscultation reveals poor air entry. The diagnosis is confirmed by chest radiograph that reveals a uniform **reticulonodular or ground-glass** pattern and air bronchograms that are consistent with diffuse atelectasis. Conventional therapy for the affected infant includes respiratory support with oxygen, CPAP, and/or mechanical ventilation, depending on the severity of respiratory compromise. The natural course is a progressive worsening over the first 24 to 48 hours of life. After the initial insult to the airway lining, the epithelium begins to repopulate with type II alveolar cells, which produce surfactant. Subsequently, there is increased production and release of surfactant, so there is a sufficient quantity in the air spaces by 72 hours of life. This results in improved lung compliance and resolution of respiratory distress.

The best form of treatment is prevention. When preterm delivery cannot be prevented, administration of corticosteroids to the mother 48 hours before delivery can induce or accelerate the production of fetal surfactant and minimize the incidence of RDS. In fact, antenatal steroids are administered to all women at risk for preterm delivery prior to 34 weeks' gestation. Surfactant can also be administered to infants soon after birth via endotracheal tube, with the goal of increasing lung compliance and preventing the onset or reducing the severity of RDS.

TRANSIENT TACHYPNEA OF THE NEWBORN

Transient tachypnea of the newborn (TTN) is relatively common, affecting up to 0.5% of term newborns. The condition, also termed *retained fetal lung liquid syndrome*, is thought to be due to delayed resorption of fetal pulmonary fluid. Normally, more than a third of fetal lung fluid is resorbed in the few days prior to the onset of labor. The remaining fluid must be cleared during labor and the first few hours of life. Disruption of this normal reabsorption results in excess fluid in the lungs. The respiratory distress is generally short lived, resolving in hours to a few days with minimal intervention. Large preterm infants are at increased risk, as are infants born by elective cesarean section without preceding labor. Multiple additional risk factors include macrosomia, significant maternal fluid overload, delayed cord clamping, precipitous delivery, multiple gestations, and infant of the diabetic mother.

The affected infant presents shortly after birth with obvious respiratory distress, including sustained tachypnea, nasal flaring, grunting, and chest wall retractions. Cyanosis is uncommon. Results of the arterial blood gas testing and chest radiograph are noted in Table 2-7. A complete blood count, when obtained, is not suggestive of infection. Although the studies listed are helpful, TTN is essentially a diagnosis of exclusion.

Management of the illness parallels the severity of the presentation. Mildly affected infants (the great majority) may need only supplemental oxygen delivered via hood. When hypoxemia persists despite 100% hood oxygenation, nasal CPAP is used. This is generally all that is needed. Rarely, intubation and mechanical ventilation may be necessary for a short time.

NEONATAL PNEUMONIA

Pneumonia is the most common neonatal infection. Pathogens may include many of those detailed in Table 2-3; however, the most common agents are bacterial (group B *Streptococcus*; *Escherichia coli*; *Klebsiella* species). Initial signs are generally those of respiratory distress; indeed, the clinical and radiographic presentation of pneumonia may be indistinguishable from MAS, RDS, and TTN. Chest radiograph findings are most likely to suggest widespread disease rather than a focal or lobar infiltrate. In other cases, early signs may instead be those of neonatal sepsis, including temperature instability, poor feeding, and lethargy. Because of the significant morbidity and mortality associated with neonatal bacterial infections, the most appropriate course of therapy is to obtain a complete blood count with differential and blood cultures. If the white blood count is concerning (e.g., high immature-to-mature cell ratio), or the infant appears ill, intravenous ampicillin and gentamycin should be started pending culture results.

NEONATAL SEPSIS

Neonatal sepsis is generally divided into early onset versus late onset sepsis. **Early onset** sepsis occurs anytime from birth to 5 or so days. **Late onset sepsis** affects babies after the first several days of life through 1 month of age. Both illnesses consist of bacterial infection of the blood associated with signs and symptoms of systemic compromise. Early subtle signs may hint at the diagnosis (temperature instability, poor feeding, decreased tone, apnea, irritability, lethargy, hypoglycemia). Often, however, neonatal sepsis presents suddenly and progresses rapidly, in severe cases culminating in respiratory failure, septic shock, meningitis (30%), disseminated intravascular coagulation (DIC), multisystem organ failure, and death.

EARLY NEONATAL SEPSIS

Pathogenesis/Epidemiology

In early onset sepsis, the infant becomes infected during the intrapartum period with bacteria residing in the mother's genitourinary tract. Group B *Streptococcus* is still the most common pathogen; however, universal antenatal screening at 35 to 37 weeks' gestation and intrapartum prophylactic administration to colonized women has decreased the incidence substantially. Two doses of the antibiotic (penicillin, ampicillin, or cefazolin) must be administered, at least 4 hours apart, prior to delivery for prophylaxis to be considered adequate. *Escherichia coli* and *Listeria monocytogenes* are also important pathogens in early onset neonatal sepsis.

Risk Factors

Predisposing factors for early onset sepsis include premature or prolonged rupture of the membranes (>18 hours), chorioamnionitis, maternal intrapartum fever or leukocytosis, and preterm birth.

Clinical Manifestations

Because the disease has a high mortality and is rapidly progressive, providers must maintain a high index of suspicion. Infants with subsequent decompensation may initially display the nonspecific signs mentioned above. Cyanosis, pallor, petechiae, vomiting, abdominal distension (ileus), respiratory distress/apnea, and hypotension are more worrisome signs. Respiratory manifestations in particular are extremely common; as previously noted, any infant presenting with respiratory distress in the newborn period warrants a septic work-up and treatment with broad-spectrum antibiotics until culture results are known.

Laboratory Evaluation

Seemingly unaffected infants who are at increased risk (suspected chorioamnionitis, maternal fever/leukocytosis, inadequate intrapartum prophylaxis, prolonged rupture of membranes) and afebrile infants with subtle/transient signs of possible early sepsis should have a complete blood count and blood culture drawn. Various algorithms exist regarding the use of the white blood cell count, differential, and serial C-reactive protein levels to guide "watchful waiting" versus 48 hours of antibiotic therapy until culture results are known. Infants with suspected sepsis should have blood and CSF sent for culture. CSF should also be tested for Gram stain, cell count and differential, and protein and glucose levels. A serum WBC <5,000 or >40,000, a total neutrophil count below 1,000, and a ratio of bands to neutrophils of >20% all correlate with an increased risk of bacterial infection. Neonates with organ-specific signs and symptoms will need additional testing (e.g., chest/abdominal radiographs).

Treatment

The treatment of early onset sepsis begins before the diagnosis is confirmed via laboratory data because the mortality rate is extremely high (up to 25%). If confirmed, the patient is treated with a combination of ampicillin and gentamicin for 10 to 14 days. This remains the most effective treatment against most organisms responsible for early sepsis and is the standard of care for initial management. If meningitis is present, the treatment is extended, and a third-generation cephalosporin is recommended for improved penetration across the blood–brain barrier. Once an organism is identified and antibiotic sensitivities are determined, antibiotic therapy may be tailored to treat the infecting organism. Infants with unstable vital signs and evidence of septic shock warrant transfer to a neonatal intensive care unit for more specialized management of their disease.

LATE ONSET NEONATAL SEPSIS

Late onset sepsis often occurs in a full-term infant who was discharged in good health from the normal newborn nursery. The infection may be isolated to the blood (bacteremia). However, it is not uncommon for hematogenous seeding to result in focal infections such as meningitis (25%, usually caused by group B streptococci or *E. coli*), osteomyelitis (group B streptococci and *Staphylococcus aureus*), arthritis (*Neisseria gonorrhoeae*, *S. aureus*, gram-negative bacteria), and urinary tract infection (*E. coli*, *Klebsiella* and other gram-negative rods). The presentation, work-up, and initial treatment of late onset sepsis is similar to that of early onset sepsis, with some variations depending on the most likely site of the infection.

JAUNDICE

Bilirubin is a bile pigment, formed from the degradation of heme derived from red blood cell (RBC) destruction and ineffective erythropoiesis. This initially unconjugated form must be conjugated in the liver to permit excretion in the bile, stool, and urine. **Hyperbilirubinemia** manifests as **jaundice**—a yellowing of the skin, mucous membranes, and sclerae. In neonates, jaundice becomes clinically apparent when serum bilirubin levels are >5 mg/dL. Hyperbilirubinemia may be classified as **unconjugated** (indirect), which in neonates can be physiologic or pathologic in origin, and **conjugated** (direct), which is always pathologic. Conjugated hyperbilirubinemia exists when the *direct* fraction of bilirubin in the blood exceeds 2 mg/dL or 15% of the total bilirubin; otherwise, the disorder is classified as "unconjugated." Expected levels of unconjugated bilirubin may top 12 mg/dL in healthy newborns, with "normal" values based on gestational and chronologic ages.

PATHOGENESIS

Physiologic jaundice and breast milk jaundice are by far the most common causes of hyperbilirubinemia in the neonate. **Physiologic jaundice** is due to indirect hyperbilirubinemia which occurs in the absence of any underlying abnormalities in bilirubin metabolism. The jaundice is never present before 24 hours of age and peaks between age of days 3 and 5, generally at or below 12 to 15 mg/dL. Values normalize by 14 to 21 days of life. Infants born before term have later and higher peak bilirubin levels.

Breast milk jaundice is similar to physiologic jaundice in terms of presentation, although bilirubin levels tend to peak slightly higher and remain elevated longer. The mechanism of breast milk jaundice is not completely understood. Some researchers have theorized that it is caused by an increase in enterohepatic circulation from an unknown maternal factor in breast milk. The American Academy of Pediatrics (AAP) recommends against routine interruption of breastfeeding in healthy, well-hydrated, term newborns with hyperbilirubinemia due to breast milk jaundice, even when serum bilirubin levels exceed numbers at which medical intervention (i.e., phototherapy) is recommended.

Jaundice due to a pathologic process does not appear any different on physical examination than physiologic or breast milk jaundice. However, identifying neonates with **nonphysiologic jaundice** is crucial to preventing long-term morbidity and complications from the underlying disease process (i.e., anemia, stroke, metabolic disease). Table 2-8 lists factors associated with an increased likelihood of pathologic jaundice. The most common cause of nonphysiologic *unconjugated* hyperbilirubenemia is ABO incompatibility. Frequent causes of *conjugated* hyperbilirubinemia are diseases involving liver

■ **TABLE 2-8** Factors Associated with Increased Risk that Jaundice/Hyperbilirubinemia Is Pathologic
• Evidence of jaundice prior to 24 hr of age (suspect hemolytic disease)
• Rise in serum bilirubin level faster than 0.5 mg/dL/hr
• Total serum bilirubin level ≥75th percentile for age in hours
• Jaundiced infant with history of traumatic delivery
• Need for phototherapy
• Persistent jaundice (longer than 8 d in a term infant or 14 d in a preterm infant)
• Jaundice in an ill-appearing infant
• Jaundice in an infant with microcephaly or petechiae
• Jaundice in an SGA infant
• Jaundice in an infant born to Mediterranean or Asian parents
• Family history of hemolytic anemia, liver disease, or sibling with nonphysiologic jaundice as a neonate

pathology (biliary atresia, neonatal hepatitis) and congenital infections; two additional causes to consider are α-antitypsin deficiency and galactosemia (Chapter 18).

ABO incompatibility is the most common cause of pathologic unconjugated hyperbilirubinemia. It is most common in infants with type A or B blood born to type O mothers. ABO incompatibility results in a *hemolytic anemia* in the newborn due to an isoimmune process. The direct Coombs test detects maternal antibody on the surface of the neonatal RBC and will be positive in infants with ABO incompatibility. The indirect Coombs test is used to identify the specific type of antibody (anti-A, anti-B, etc.). Additional laboratory indicators include an elevated reticulocyte count and a blood smear demonstrating hemolysis and microspherocytes. Hepatomegaly is uncommon but may be present. Approximately 1% of newborns develop clinically significant unconjugated hyperbilirubinemia from ABO incompatibility. Although the use of phototherapy is common in these infants, the incidence of severe hemolytic disease necessitating exchange transfusion is rare.

Rh incompatibility is a more serious type of isoimmune hemolytic anemia wherein an Rh-negative mother who has become sensitized to the antigen with a previous pregnancy produces antibodies that react with Rh-antigen on fetal RBCs. The fetus must be Rh-positive for the process to occur. Maternal Rh status is determined early in the prenatal period. RhoGAM, a solution of IgG antibodies to Rh-D antigen, binds fetal cells in maternal circulation and destroys them, preventing the development of isoimmunity. It is administered to Rh-negative mothers at 28 weeks' gestation. The hemolytic anemia resulting from Rh incompatibility is generally more severe than that from ABO incompatibility. Unlike Rh incompatibility, prior maternal antigen sensitization is not required for ABO incompatibility.

CLINICAL MANIFESTATIONS

History

It is important to determine the infant's diet (breastfed, formula-fed, or a relative mixture), the number of feeds in a 24-hour period (goal of 8 to 12), and the duration or volume of each feed. Inadequate intake is associated with delayed hepatic circulation and excretion of bilirubin, and more severe jaundice. The family history should include questions regarding heritable conditions in Table 2-8. Prenatal screens, the physical examination, and growth parameters should be reviewed for possible indications of congenital infection. The length of time the jaundice has been present, whether it is worsening or improving, and associated gastrointestinal or constitutional symptoms may assist in guiding the laboratory evaluation.

Physical Examination

In neonates, jaundice reliably progresses in a cephalopedal direction. Therefore, those infants with clinically apparent jaundice below the umbilicus are likely to have higher levels than those with only facial jaundice. It disappears in the opposite direction; scleral icterus is generally the last to resolve.

DIAGNOSTIC EVALUATION

Regardless of the presumptive etiology and classification (physiologic vs. pathologic), thoughtful stepwise evaluation of neonatal jaundice is imperative. Infants with significant clinical jaundice, jaundice in excess of expected based on age, and jaundice in the presence of risk factors noted above should have serum total and direct bilirubin measurements drawn. Published nomograms permit stratification of infants into risk categories based on gestational age, chronologic age in hours, and bilirubin levels. Infant who are in the category of high risk for development of excessive bilirubin levels should have serial measurements drawn every 4 to 12 hours. The utilization of transcutaneous measurement devices has decreased the need for frequent blood draws. The initial measurement should be a serum sample, as trancutaneous devices do not differentiate conjugated from unconjugated bilirubin. Similarly, a transcutaneous measurement that reaches the level at which medical intervention is recommended should be confirmed with a serum sample.

Figure 2-1 delineates the suggested work-up of an infant with suspected nonphysiologic jaundice which, as previously noted, may be either conjugated or unconjugated in origin. These additional studies should be selectively considered in infants with higher-than-expected peak bilirubin levels, rapidly rising levels, levels necessitating medical management, conjugated hyperbilirubinemia, or delayed resolution of jaundice.

TREATMENT

The goal in treating *unconjugated* hyperbilirubinemia is to avoid **kernicterus**, or sublethal bilirubin encephalopathy. Unconjugated bilirubin is normally bound tightly to albumin in the blood. However, when serum levels of unconjugated bilirubin exceed the binding capacity of albumin, excess free bilirubin can cross the blood–brain barrier. Kernicterus is characterized by yellow staining of the basal ganglia, hippocampus, cerebellum, and various additional brainstem

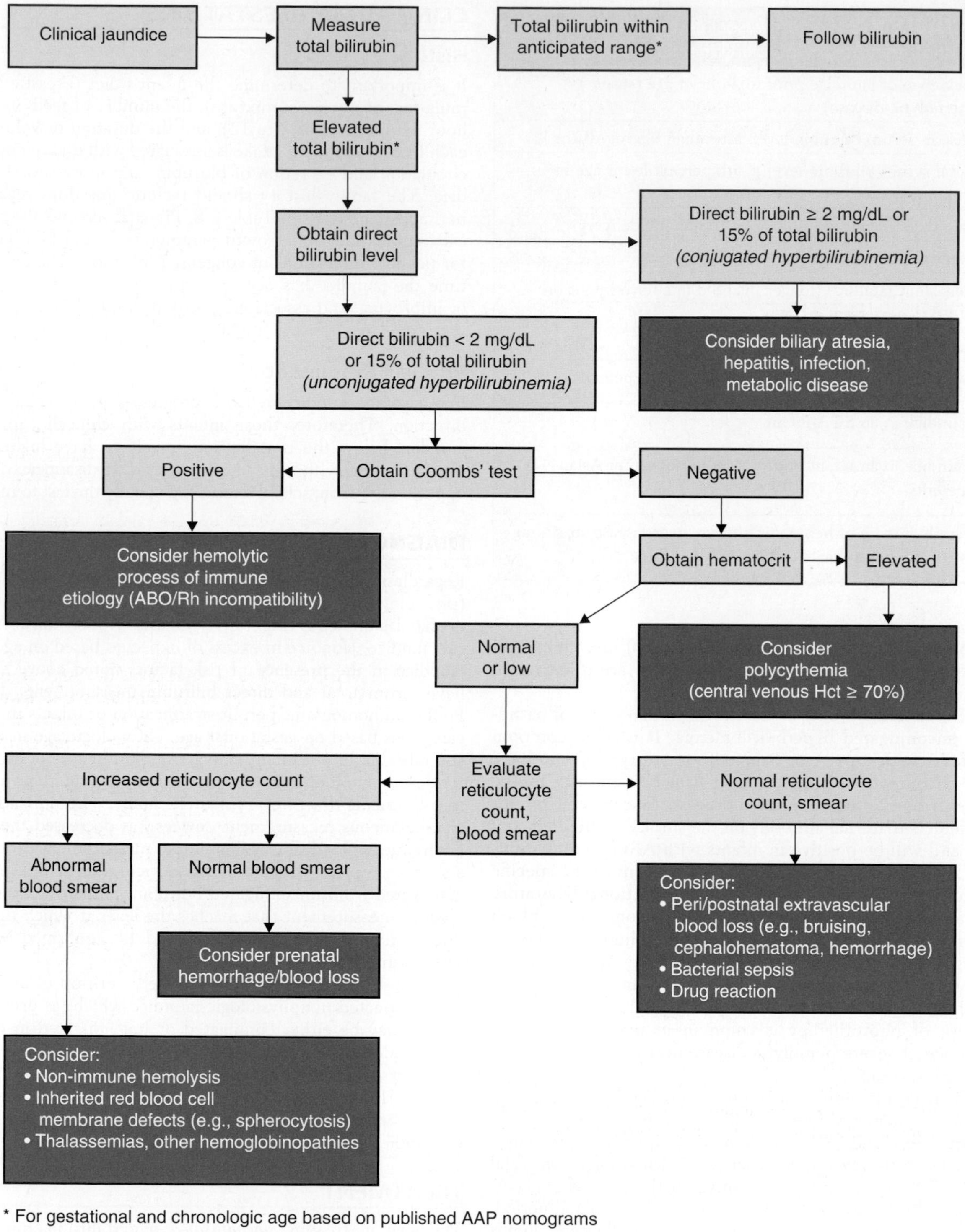

Clinical jaundice

Measure total bilirubin

Total bilirubin within anticipated range*

Follow bilirubin

Elevated total bilirubin*

Obtain direct bilirubin level

Direct bilirubin ≥ 2 mg/dL or 15% of total bilirubin *(conjugated hyperbilirubinemia)*

Consider biliary atresia, hepatitis, infection, metabolic disease

Direct bilirubin < 2 mg/dL or 15% of total bilirubin *(unconjugated hyperbilirubinemia)*

Obtain Coombs' test

Positive

Consider hemolytic process of immune etiology (ABO/Rh incompatibility)

Negative

Obtain hematocrit

Elevated

Consider polycythemia (central venous Hct ≥ 70%)

Normal or low

Evaluate reticulocyte count, blood smear

Increased reticulocyte count

Abnormal blood smear

Normal blood smear

Consider prenatal hemorrhage/blood loss

Consider:
- Non-immune hemolysis
- Inherited red blood cell membrane defects (e.g., spherocytosis)
- Thalassemias, other hemoglobinopathies

Normal reticulocyte count, smear

Consider:
- Peri/postnatal extravascular blood loss (e.g., bruising, cephalohematoma, hemorrhage)
- Bacterial sepsis
- Drug reaction

* For gestational and chronologic age based on published AAP nomograms

Figure 2-1 • Algorithm for the evaluation of suspected nonphysiologic jaundice in the neonate.

neurons, resulting in widespread cerebral dysfunction. Initial clinical features include lethargy and irritability, progressing to hypotonia, opisthotonos, and seizures. Infants who survive develop cerebral palsy and movement disorders and may also suffer from irreversible vision and hearing problems and/or mental retardation.

Orogastric feeding or intravenous fluids are beneficial when dehydration is present, although overhydration does not result in more rapid resolution of the jaundice. When additional intervention is needed or hydration status is normal, phototherapy and exchange transfusion are the treatment modalities used to lower serum unconjugated bilirubin levels.

In July 2004, the AAP Subcommittee on Hyperbilirubinemia published extensive and extremely helpful clinical practice guidelines regarding the management of hyperbilirubinemia and prevention strategies. In addition to the figures cited above, nomograms provide phototherapy and exchange transfusion treatment guidelines for infants in each risk group (http://aappolicy.aappublications.org/cgi/content/full/pediatrics;114/1/297).

Special blue fluorescent tubes are the most effective light source for providing *intensive phototherapy*. The light source is placed as close to the infant as practical, with lighting above and below if possible. The infant should be virtually naked and wearing eye protection. Since insensible losses are increased, adequate hydration is critical for assuring sufficient enterohepatic circulation and increasing urine and bile output. If possible, the infant should be allowed to breastfeed.

Exchange transfusion is recommended for infants with levels directed in the practice guideline nomograms mentioned above, as well as any infant with a total serum bilirubin >25 mg/dL or clinical manifestations of acute bilirubin encephalopathy. Infants with isoimmune hemolytic disease may respond to early intervention with intravenous gamma globulin therapy and avoid exchange transfusion.

As noted, elevated serum conjugated bilirubin levels are never physiologic. Every effort should be made to determine the cause, reverse the underlying process, and limit complications. Phototherapy in the setting of conjugated hyperbilirubinemia is not effective and causes "bronzing" of the skin that takes months to resolve.

CONGENITAL ANOMALIES

CLEFT LIP AND PALATE

Multiple genetic and environmental factors play a role in the etiology of cleft lip and cleft palate. Cleft lip (with or without cleft palate) occurs in 1 in 1,000 births and is more common in boys. Cleft palate occurs in 1 in 2,500 births.

Cleft *palates* are common in patients with chromosomal abnormalities. Malformations encountered more commonly in patients with cleft *lip* include hypertelorism, hand defects, and cardiac anomalies. In general, infants with isolated cleft lip do not need modifications to feed without respiratory difficulty. Patients with cleft palate are prone to choking when fed; most benefit from manually repositioning the tongue and feeding while side-lying. Many patients also do well with an elongated, soft nipple.

Most cleft lips are repaired shortly after birth or once the infant demonstrates steady weight gain. Cleft palate repair is usually undertaken at 9 to 12 months of age. Complications after cleft palate repair include speech difficulties, dental disturbances, and recurrent otitis media. Although two-thirds of palate-corrected children demonstrate acceptable speech, a hypernasal quality or muffled tone may persist in the voice.

TRACHEOESOPHAGEAL FISTULA

Incomplete anastomosis of the superior and inferior portions of the esophagus is known as *esophageal atresia*. Eighty-five percent of newborns with esophageal atresia also develop a **tracheoesophageal fistula (TEF),** which is an (abnormal) communication between the trachea and the esophagus. This connection is usually between the trachea and the lower portion of the esophagus (Fig. 2-2). Forty percent of patients with TEF have other congenital defects. For example, *VACTERL syndrome* describes the association of vertebral, anal, cardiac, tracheal, esophageal, renal, and limb anomalies.

Neonates with TEF have excessive oral secretions, inability to feed, gagging, and respiratory distress. Polyhydramnios often is noted on fetal ultrasound. Lateral and anteroposterior chest radiographs with a Replogle tube in the proximal esophagus reveal a superior blind pouch, with air in the GI tract. In isolated esophageal atresia *without* TEF, gas is absent from the GI tract. Infants with TEF but *without* associated esophageal atresia (H-type TEF) may have nonspecific symptoms for several months, including chronic cough with feeding and recurrent pneumonia.

Surgical correction involves division and closure of the TEF and end-to-end anastomosis of the proximal and distal esophagus. Esophageal strictures at the anastomosis site are a common complication requiring periodic dilation.

DUODENAL ATRESIA

Duodenal obstruction may be complete (atresia) or partial, resulting from a web, band, or annular pancreas. **Duodenal atresia** results from a failure of the lumen to recanalize during the 8th to 10th weeks' gestation. Polyhydramnios may be noted on prenatal ultrasound. Duodenal atresia is usually associated with other malformations, including cardiac anomalies and GI defects such as annular pancreas, malrotation of the intestines, and imperforate anus. Duodenal atresia occurs with increased incidence in patients with trisomy 21.

After birth, bilious emesis begins within a few hours of the first feeding. Abdominal radiographs typically demonstrate gastric and duodenal gaseous distention proximal to the atretic site. This finding is known as the **double bubble** sign. When

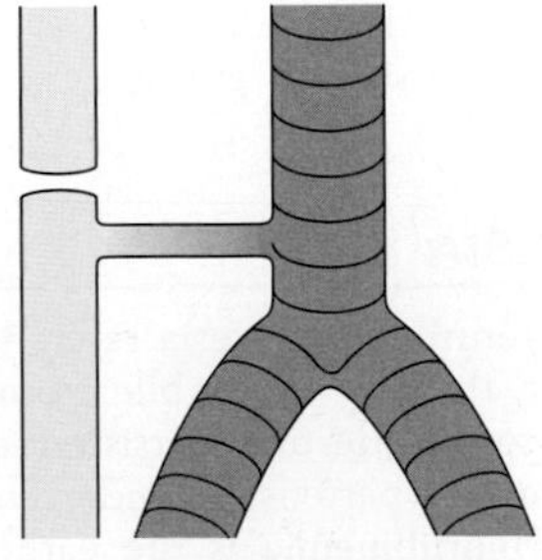

Figure 2-2 • Esophageal atresia with distal tracheoesophageal fistula.

present, gas in the distal bowel suggests *partial* obstruction. Surgical correction is necessary.

CONGENITAL DIAPHRAGMATIC HERNIA

Congenital diaphragmatic hernia results from a defect in the (usually left) posterolateral diaphragm that permits abdominal contents to enter the thorax and compromise early lung development. This defect is commonly referred to as a **Bochdalek hernia**. The combination of pulmonary hypoplasia and pulmonary arteriolar hypertension makes this congenital defect lethal in many cases. Early symptoms include respiratory distress with decreased breath sounds on the affected side, right-sided (shifted) heart sounds, and a scaphoid abdomen. Diagnosis is sometimes made via fetal ultrasound; after birth, the defect is obvious on chest radiograph.

Initial management consists of intubation and ventilation, and placement of a Replogle tube to minimize GI distention, which would further compromise effective lung volume. Sometimes conventional ventilation is not sufficient to provide adequate oxygen delivery and carbon dioxide excretion; in such cases, high-frequency ventilation or ECMO may be needed to manage the child's pulmonary hypertension. Ultimately, the defect requires surgical correction.

OMPHALOCELE AND GASTROSCHISIS

Omphalocele is an uncommon disorder in which the abdominal viscera herniate through the umbilical and supraumbilical portions of the abdominal wall into a sac covered by peritoneum and amniotic membrane. Large defects may contain the entire GI tract, the liver, and the spleen. The incidence of omphalocele is 1 in 6,000 births. Polyhydramnios is noted in utero, as is the omphalocele itself in many cases. Ten percent of infants with omphaloceles are born prematurely. The sac covering the defect is thin and may rupture in utero or during delivery. Associated congenital GI and cardiac defects are common. Ten percent of children with omphalocele have Beckwith–Wiedemann syndrome (exophthalmos, macroglossia, gigantism, hyperinsulinemia, and hypoglycemia).

In contrast, **gastroschisis** involves herniation of intestine through the abdominal wall (lateral to the umbilicus) with no covering peritoneal membrane. The eviscerated mass is adherent, edematous, dark in color, and covered by a gelatinous matrix of greenish material. The pathogenesis of this abdominal wall defect is not clear. Polyhydramnios is typically noted in utero. Gastroschisis is a surgical emergency, often with staged closure.

BILIARY ATRESIA

In newborns, the term biliary atresia refers to absence of the common bile duct, through which bile from the liver is normally transported to the intestine. Persistent cholestasis results in liver fibrosis, portal hypertension, and eventual liver failure. **Conjugated hyperbilirubinemia** is the earliest finding. Over the first few weeks of life, infants develop clay-colored (light) stools, dark urine, and hepatosplenomegaly. Liver enzymes are significantly elevated. Nuclear medicine scanning using technetium-99 can be used to confirm the absence of bile flow from the liver. Establishment of a conduit from the bile ducts into the intestine via surgery is beneficial in many children; however, the majority require liver transplantation.

BEFORE DISCHARGE HOME

Term, well-appearing newborn infants with no significant risk factors in the pre/perinatal period may be discharged at 48 hours of age. Discharge after 24 hours but before 48 hours of age may be permissible when sufficient time has elapsed to identify early problems and when the family is judged to be well prepared to care for the child at home (Table 2-9). Babies born via Caesarean section are not typically discharged prior to 72 hours of age due to maternal obstetrical considerations. The first vaccination against hepatitis B is typically administered prior to discharge.

At the hospital, a sample of infant blood is collected and sent to a state screening lab to test for a variety of illness, including some metabolic diseases (e.g., phenylketonuria), sickle cell disease, congenital adrenal hyperplasia, and congenital hypothyroidism (see Chapter 14). A hearing test is completed as well. These studies are undertaken in the nursery because early identification is relatively inexpensive compared with the cost of treating the disease at a later stage. The incidences of these conditions range from uncommon to rare, but all are associated with significant morbidity when left untreated.

TABLE 2-9 Newborn Early Discharge Criteria

Discharge prior to 48 hr of age may be considered appropriate if:
• the infant is full-term
• the infant has a normal physical examination
• the infant has maintained normal vital signs
• the infant is urinating and stooling
• the infant has had at least two consecutive successful feedings (breast or bottle)
• a risk assessment for hyperbilirubinemia has been completed and appropriate follow-up ensured (must be within 2 d of discharge)
• the circumcision site is healing without bleeding (if applicable)
• the risk for Group B streptococcal disease has been assessed and addressed
• maternal prenatal labs are negative/reassuring
• the parents have been educated regarding infant feeding expectations, the benefits of breastfeeding, skin/cord/circumcision care, car seat use, "Back to Sleep," prevention of shaken baby syndrome, etc.
• metabolic (state screening) and hearing screenings have been completed, and the first Hepatitis B vaccine has been administered
• the mother does not have a positive drug screen, is not an adolescent, and has a safe home to which to return

HEALTH-MAINTENANCE VISITS

Infants should be evaluated at a health-maintenance visit within a week of discharge. Many babies are seen earlier to make sure weight loss is not excessive and jaundice, if present, is resolving. Neonates typically lose 5% to 7% of their birth weight in the first few days. A 10% drop is within normal limits but warrants close monitoring and early follow-up. Babies should gain back to birth weight by 14 days of age.

The AAP recommends that breastfed infants be started on vitamin D drops (400 IU/day) beginning in the first few days of life. Although it is inarguable that breast milk provides the best nutrition for infants in the first year of life, to say nothing of its immunologic advantages, the adequacy of vitamin D in breast milk is not sufficient to prevent some infants from developing vitamin D deficiency and even rickets. The risk is highest in patients with dark skin who, due to their climate or otherwise, are exposed to very little sunlight.

Both breast milk and current commercial formulas provide sufficient iron to infants. Hemoglobin and hematocrit levels decrease slowly in the term infant to a "physiologic nadir" sometime between 8 and 12 weeks of life. During this period, hemoglobin values as low as 9 mg/dL are considered normal. Shortly thereafter, the hemoglobin begins to rise in response to infant marrow production of cells.

INFANT MORTALITY

The **infant mortality rate** is defined as the number of deaths prior to age 1 year per 1,000 live births. The infant mortality rate in the United States in 2005 was 6.86, statistically unchanged from 2000.

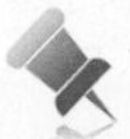

KEY POINTS

- Ophthalmic antibiotics are administered to newborns on day-of-life 1 to prevent conjunctivitis with *Neisseria gonorrhea* and particularly *Chlamydia trachomatis*, which is a leading cause of blindness in the developing world.
- Parenteral vitamin K prevents the development of hemorrhagic disease of the newborn.
- IUGR is divided into two categories based on gestational age at onset. In early onset (symmetric) IUGR, growth is restricted prior to 28 weeks' gestation, and birth length and head circumference are proportional to weight. Infants with late onset (asymmetric) IUGR have sparing of the (relatively normal) head circumference, but length and especially weight are reduced below what is expected.
- Common benign rashes in newborns and young infants include salmon patches, mongolion spots, milia, erythema toxicum, infantile seborrhea, and neonatal acne.
- Closure of the ductus arteriosus is often associated with a continuous murmur over the second left intercostal space.
- Persistence of the umbilical stump beyond 8 weeks of age is abnormal and may signify a neutrophil disorder.
- When the urethral opening is located along the penile shaft rather than at the tip, this is termed hypospadias. Chordae is fixed fibrotic ventral bowing of the penis; it is often associated with hypospadias. Hypospadias may be associated with other, less obvious genitourinary anomalies.
- Retractile testis will eventually relocate permanently to the scrotum; no intervention is necessary.
- Abnormal head shape in the newborn may be due to molding, caput seccedaneum, or cephalohematoma.
- Infants with choanal atresia develop respiratory distress with cyanosis and/or apnea when the mouth is occluded (during feeding) or closed (while the infant is calm or resting).
- Bilateral renal agenesis results in Potter syndrome, characterized by compression deformities of the face and limbs, "prune belly" abdomen, and severe pulmonary hypoplasia. Intrauterine bilateral renal agenesis results in oligohydramnios.
- The vast majority of infants with RDS/HMD are born prior to 34 to 35 weeks' gestation. The pathogenesis is lack of surfactant. The diagnosis is confirmed by a chest radiograph that reveals a uniform reticulonodular or "ground-glass pattern" and air bronchograms that are consistent with diffuse atelectasis.
- Pneumonia is the most common neonatal infection, and group B *Streptococcus* is the most common pathogen. Initial signs are generally those of respiratory distress; however, both the clinical and radiographic presentations of pneumonia may not differ significantly from neonatal sepsis, MAS, RDS/HMD, and TTN.
- Universal antenatal screening at 35 to 37 weeks' gestation for group B *Streptococcus* and intrapartum prophylactic administration to colonized women have decreased the incidence of early onset neonatal sepsis substantially. Two doses of an appropriate antibiotic must be administered at least 4 hours apart prior to delivery for prophylaxis to be considered adequate.
- Neonates with suspected bacterial infection, including neonatal sepsis and/or pneumonia, require emergent evaluation and coverage with ampicillin and gentamycin until culture results are known.
- Neonatal hyperbilirubinemia is classified as unconjugated (indirect), which can be physiologic or pathologic in origin, and conjugated (direct), which is always pathologic.
- Physiologic jaundice describes indirect hyperbilirubinemia which occurs in the absence of any underlying abnormalities in bilirubin metabolism. Physiologic jaundice and breast milk jaundice are by far the most common causes of hyperbilirubinemia in the neonate. The most common cause of nonphysiologic unconjugated hyperbilirubenemia is ABO incompatibility.
- Conjugated hyperbilirubinemia is often the result of diseases involving liver pathology, such as biliary atresia and neonatal hepatitis.
- Kernicterus results when high levels of unconjugated hyperbilirubinemia cross the blood–brain barrier, resulting in widespread cerebral dysfunction. Infants who survive the immediate effects

(continued)

develop cerebral palsy and movement disorders and may also suffer from vision/hearing problems and mental retardation.

- VACTERL syndrome describes the association of vertebral, anal, cardiac, tracheoesophageal fistula, renal, and limb anomalies.
- Infants with TEF in the absence of esophageal atresia may have nonspecific symptoms for several months, including chronic cough with feeding and recurrent pneumonia.
- Duodenal atresia is associated with a characteristic radiographic finding, the "double bubble" sign, consisting of gastric and duodenal gaseous distention proximal to the atretic site.
- Conjugated hyperbilirubinemia is the earliest sign of biliary atresia. This is followed by the development of clay-colored (light) stools, dark urine, and hepatosplenomegaly. Liver enzymes become significantly elevated early in life.
- Neonates may lose up to 10% of their birth weight within the first few days of life. Babies should gain back to birth weight by 14 days of age (21 days in breastfed infants).
- The AAP recommends that breastfed infants be started on vitamin D drops (400 IU/day) beginning in the first few days of life.
- Hematocrit levels in the term neonate decrease slowly to a "physiologic nadir" sometime between 8 and 12 weeks of life, when hemoglobin values as low as 9 mg/dL are considered normal. Iron supplementation before and/or during this nadir is neither indicated nor beneficial.

C Clinical Vignettes

CLINICAL VIGNETTES

Vignette 1

1. You are called to the nursery to evaluate a presumably term infant whose weight is at the 3rd percentile for gestational age. Which of the following history and/or physical findings is unlikely to suggest prematurity or a pathologic condition as the etiology of this child's "small for gestational age" weight?
   a. Prenatal care throughout pregnancy
   b. Fine, fuzzy scalp hair and visible veins in the skin
   c. Low Dubowitz/Ballard scores
   d. Hypoglycemia
   e. Head circumference at the 50th percentile
   f. Syndromic features
   g. Chronic preeclampsia
   h. a and d
   i. b and d
   j. b and c

2. The infant is calm when you arrive, so, following a general assessment and review of the vital signs, you conduct a cardiac examination. You note a normal cardiac rate. S1 and S2 are normal in placement, and the S2 is appropriately split. Femoral pulses are equal but not bounding. The palms and soles have a bluish tint to them, but the lips and tongue are pink. You appreciate a medium-pitched systolic ejection murmur, best heard at the left upper sternal border, with radiation to the back. The liver edge falls 1 cm below the costal margin. Given this clinical picture, the infant's murmur most likely results from which of the following?
   a. Peripheral pulmonic stenosis
   b. Critical pulmonary stenosis
   c. Tricuspid atresia
   d. Closure of the ductus arteriosus
   e. Tetralogy of Fallot

3. The infant has a sacral dimple within the anal verge. You are able to visualize the bottom of the dimple by abducting the gluteal folds. The Moro reflex is symmetric. Two to three beats of clonus are present in each ankle. Which of the following is the most appropriate next step in the evaluation of this infant's anomaly?
   a. Sonography of the spine, which should demonstrate any associated vertebral lesion given that the infant is <6 weeks of age
   b. Referral to a pediatric neurologist as an outpatient for a more thorough examination
   c. Referral to a pediatric neurosurgeon as an outpatient for a more thorough evaluation
   d. Magnetic resonance imaging of the lower spine to evaluate for spina bifida occulta prior to discharge
   e. This finding is not associated with underlying neurologic or bony abnormalities

4. The parents are concerned that their baby has an irregular head shape. The head is elongated, with a boggy area extending over the posterior parietal sutures. The protrusion is slightly more prominent on the left. Bruising is evident in the enlarged area. Gentle pressure to the area results in "pitting." Your parental counseling would include all but which of the following statements?
   a. The appearance of the head is due to pressure from the pelvic bones and the narrow vaginal canal on the head during the birth process.
   b. The infant has bleeding in the subperiosteal space.
   c. The infant is at no increased risk for hydrocephalus.
   d. The elongation will resolve without intervention.
   e. Bruising is not an uncommon finding in caput succedaneum.

Vignette 2

You are examining a 5-day-old AGA term newborn male in your office for his second health maintenance visit (the first being the initial hospital follow-up visit shortly after discharge). The mother had prenatal care throughout her pregnancy, the birth was via Caesarean section (due to a previous Caesarean delivery), and there were no significant pre- or perinatal complications. Weight, length, and head circumference progression are as expected. The baby is afebrile and acting normally. The infant is exclusively breastfed. There is a healthy older biological sister in the family.

Although they are not new to parenting, the parents have some questions about things they did not notice were present when their daughter was an infant.

The infant has five evanescent pustules, each on an erythematous base, scattered over the lower legs. A similar lesion is present on the left wrist and another on the right forearm. The parents note that the infant had similar "bumps" on his chest, abdomen, and back before leaving the hospital. Although he has fewer now, the parents are concerned that they are not gone yet, especially since the mother has a history of genital herpes. She did not have visible herpes lesions at the time of birth. This morning, the infant had the same bumps on the legs but in slightly different places.

1. This infant's rash is most consistent with which of the following?
   a. Transient neonatal pustular melanosis
   b. Erythema toxicum
   c. Infantile seborrhea
   d. Milia
   e. Superficial epidermal herpes

2. The infant's umbilical stump is dry. The mother states that, although she tries to be very gentle, she has bumped or pulled the cord accidently while dressing him a few times. She sees dried blood around the base. The bleeding was minor oozing only and stopped within minutes without pressure. She is afraid she is going to hurt the infant by traumatically dislodging the stump, and she wants to know when it will fall off on its own. All of the following represents appropriate advice except which of the following?
   a. Because the practice of saturating the cord stump with alcohol is no longer recommended, the cord is more susceptible to traumatic bleeding.
   b. Because the practice of saturating the cord stump with alcohol is no longer recommended, the skin at the base of the cord is more susceptible to bacterial infection.
   c. The cord should fall off within 3 to 4 weeks.
   d. If the cord persists beyond 6 to 8 weeks, the parents should bring it to the physician's attention.
   e. If an umbilical hernia becomes visible following separation of the cord, the hernia is likely to resolve within a few years without intervention.

3. The father rather sheepishly mentions that he has noticed that his son has firm "bumps" under both his nipples. Moreover, the examining physician in the hospital told him that only one testis was placed within the scrotum. During physical examination of the child, you note breast budding. Palpation of the scrotum reveals only the right testis. The left is located distal to the inguinal ligament, is equal in size to the right testis, and is easily manipulated into the left scrotum. Which of the following statements regarding this father's concerns is true?
   a. The breast budding, or gynecomastia, will resolve within 6 months but will reappear during puberty.
   b. There is a 50% chance that the retractile testis will need to be repositioned within the ipsilateral scrotum surgically.
   c. The child should not be circumcised until the retracted testis is permitted to "drop" in case the tissue of the prepuce is needed for repair.
   d. The breast budding results from the same underlying process as neonatal acne.
   e. Cryptorchidism carries an increased risk for breast budding and metastatic changes in the breast and testicular tissue later in life.

4. Which of the following is the most important supplement to provide for this infant at present?
   a. Prenatal vitamins through the mother
   b. Vitamin D
   c. Calcium
   d. Vitamin K
   e. Iron

Vignette 3

You are called to see a neonate in the newborn nursery who is about an hour old. The pregnancy was complicated by maternal gestational diabetes. Delivery was induced at 36 weeks' gestation due to difficulty managing the gestational diabetes. The infant was delivered by Caesarean section for failure to descend, although the obstetrician had to enlarge the initial incision to remove the infant due to size. Reassuring fetal heart tracings were documented throughout the labor and delivery. "Light meconium" was noted in the amniotic fluid. Apgar scores were 8 (–1 for color, –1 for respiratory effort) and 9 (–1 for color). He began to cry vigorously as he was dried, but calmed down in his mother's arms and was permitted to stay there and breastfeed as vital signs remained stable. Initial measurements placed the growth at "large for gestational age." Since admission to the nursery, the infant's respiratory rate has climbed steadily and is now at 70 breaths per minute. When you arrive, you note nasal flaring, grunting with each breath, and chest wall retractions. There is no cyanosis at present. You ask medical personnel present to administer oxygen via hood to keep saturations between 88% and 92% and order a STAT portable chest radiograph and arterial blood gas, complete blood count, differential, and cultures.

1. Which of the following conditions is least likely to be the source of this infant's respiratory distress?
   a. Neonatal pneumonia
   b. Choanal atresia
   c. Transient tachypnea of the newborn
   d. Respiratory distress syndrome
   e. Meconium aspiration syndrome

2. Which of the following chest radiograph findings would be most consistent with a diagnosis of meconium aspiration syndrome?
   a. Prominent perihilar streaking, increased interstitial markings, and fluid in the interlobar fissures
   b. Air bronchograms superimposed on widespread atelectasis, creating a "ground glass" appearance
   c. Areas of atelectasis, areas of coarse irregular densities, distinct areas of overinflation
   d. Symmetric, patchy consolidations with uni- or bilateral effusions
   e. Consolidation of one lobe or two contiguous lobes only

3. The infant is able to maintain oxygen saturation within the normal range when the hood environment is at 40% oxygen and the respiratory rate begins to decline. The ratio of immature-to-mature forms of white blood cells is low, and the total white blood count is normal for age. Ampicillin and gentamycin are administered while awaiting results of the blood culture. By 48 hours of age, the infant has been weaned to room air and is breastfeeding. Blood cultures are negative. This clinical picture is most consistent with which of the following?
   a. Nosocomial respiratory syncytial virus infection
   b. Transient tachypnea of the newborn
   c. Hyaline membrane disease
   d. Apnea of prematurity
   e. Meconium aspiration syndrome

4. The baby is discharged from the hospital and follows up at your clinic for regular health maintenance visits. Just before the 2-month visit, the mother calls about a large, hard bump she has noticed along the middle of the bone at the top of the chest on the right side. According to her, the child is moving both arms the same amount and with the same range of motion. Which of the following is the most likely cause of the abnormality prompting the mother's concern?
   a. Clavicular fracture at birth
   b. Erb palsy

c. Developmental shoulder dysplasia
d. Metatarsus adductus
e. Potter syndrome

Vignette 4

A Caucasian woman presents to the emergency department in labor. She is transferred to the delivery ward. There is no history of prenatal care other than a visit at an estimated 16 weeks' of pregnancy. The mother denies use of illicit drugs, prescription medications, and alcohol during the pregnancy. However, she is combative upon arrival to the delivery ward, and her breath smells of alcohol. Prenatal testing obtained at the obstetrics clinic is significant for: (–) HIV, (–) HBsAg, (–) hepatitis C, blood type A^+, (–) RPR, rubella immune, (+) CMV, (–) Swabs for *Chlamydia trachomatis* and *Neisseria gonorrhoeae*. Membranes are ruptured at the delivery, which is vaginal and uncomplicated. There is no clinical suspicion for chorioamnionitis.

1. Which of the following physical anomalies are most consistent with a diagnosis of fetal alcohol syndrome?
   a. Spina bifida, facial anomalies
   b. Broad nasal bridge, cleft palate, microcephaly
   c. Hepatosplenomegaly, lymphadenopathy, chorioretinitis
   d. Short palpebral fissures, midface hypoplasia, smooth philtrum, thin superior vermillion border
   e. Cataracts, hearing loss, thrombocytopenic purpura

2. Judging by the sonogram and results of the maturity and neuromuscular rating scales, the infant is full term and AGA. The infant's urine is positive for marijuana but no other drugs of abuse. The physical examination is entirely normal, and the infant formula-feeds well and maintains stable vital signs. Social work is consulted for support, discharge planning, follow-up, and appropriate referrals and notifications. At 30 hours of age, the infant is noted to be jaundiced. Which of the following represents the most appropriate screening laboratory work-up of this infant?
   a. Transcutaneous bilirubin measurement
   b. Serum total and indirect bilirubin levels
   c. Blood typing of the infant and direct Coombs testing
   d. Complete blood count and blood smear
   e. Maternal Rh antigen testing

3. The infant's direct bilirubin measurement is <1.5 mg/dL, but the total bilirubin level is plotted on the AAP graph and revels that the infant is within a group that has a high incidence of subsequent need for phototherapy. In addition to further work-up, you counsel the mother regarding the possibility of phototherapy for the infant. The risk of misunderstanding and misgivings is high with this mother, because based on social concerns, the phototherapy, if indicated, will have to take place in the hospital prior to discharge rather than at home. She is being discharged tomorrow, although the infant will remain hospitalized. There is some concern that she may attempt to remove the baby from the hospital without authorization or sign the baby out of the hospital "against medical advice." In counseling her regarding the risks of untreated hyperbilirubinemia, you are most likely to discuss which of the following conditions?
   a. Bronzing of the skin
   b. Polycythemia
   c. Slow growth
   d. Death
   e. Kernicterus

A Answers

Vignette 1 Question 1

Answer H: Newborns with weights less than the 10th percentile for length of gestation are termed *small for gestational age* (SGA). Infants can be SGA because of incorrect dating of the pregnancy; that is, the actual gestational age is lower than the recorded gestational age. This is true of infants who are premature or preterm; their weights may be appropriate for actual gestational age. Given that this mother had prenatal care starting early in her pregnancy, it is unlikely that the conception date is off by any significant degree. If other history, physical examination findings, and laboratory results are normal, the infant is (probably) just appropriately small, especially if the mother and father are both petite. Hypoglycemia is common in SGA infants, even those without pathology, due to finite glycogen stores.

The physical findings listed in B are consistent with prematurity, as are low scores on the neuromuscular and physical maturity rating scales. A head circumference at the 50th percentile suggests late onset intrauterine growth retardation (IUGR), which may be seen with preeclampsia. Specific chromosomal anomalies, congenital malformations, and inborn errors of metabolism can result in early onset, symmetric IUGR.

Vignette 1 Question 2

Answer A: As a functional heart murmur, peripheral pulmonic stenosis (PPS) may present in the newborn and persist until 2 months of age. The source is turbulent blood flow where the main pulmonary artery branches into left and right. The turbulence produces a medium-pitched systolic ejection murmur at the left upper sternal border, radiating to the back. PPS is a benign murmur which does not signify underlying anatomic disease. The liver edge in a term healthy infant may extend 1 to 2 cm below the anterior costal margin; as long as it is not firmer than expected, and there is no palpable spleen tip, this is a normal finding. In contrast, critical pulmonary stenosis is a life-threatening cardiac anomaly associated with central cyanosis in the newborn (evidenced by generalized cyanosis, including blueness of the lips and the tongue). This newborn has constriction of the distal peripheral vascular system, the end capillaries, which imparts a bluish tinge to the hands and feet. This is a normal finding in neonates. Tricuspid atresia and tetralogy of Fallot result in central cyanosis in the newborn.

The most commonly encountered murmur over the first 3 days in the life of the newborn is the continuous murmur associated with closure of the ductus arteriosus. It is best appreciated in the second left intercostal space, similar to PPS, but is continuous rather than limited to the systolic phase.

Vignette 1 Question 3

Answer E: Sacral dimples are not present in the majority of newborns; however, neither are they uncommon. Sacral dimples which are within 2.5 cm of the anal verge, which are shallow enough to see complete skin closure, which are not covered by hemangiomas or hair tufts, and which are not associated with abnormal neurologic function do not need to be evaluated further. A symmetric Moro reflex would not be considered particularly helpful, as the lesion associated with pathologic sacral dimples is usually limited to the pelvis and lower extremities early in life, and the Moro reflex examines primarily symmetry of the face and upper extremities. A few beats of ankle clonus is not uncommon in neonates and is without significance. Asymmetric tone in the lower extremities is a concerning finding which warrants further evaluation, regardless of the presence or absence of a sacral dimple. Similarly, a spine which does not extend caudally to a normally positioned coccyx bone must be studied further, preferably by magnetic resonance imaging.

Vignette 1 Question 4

Answer B: This infant has caput succedaneum, characterized by marked edema of the scalp tissues. The fact that it extends over suture lines rules out a cephalohematoma, or bleeding into the subperiosteal space, in which the swelling does not cross suture lines. Bruising is not uncommon in cases of caput succedaneum, especially when vacuum extraction is used or the birth process is prolonged. The elongation will resolve over time without intervention, and there is no associated increased risk of hydrocephalus.

Vignette 2 Question 1

Answer B: Erythema toxicum is an extremely common rash which is most visible and prominent in Caucasian newborns. It appears as described above, and the lesions disappear and reappear in different places on the skin. Overall, the rash begins centrally and spreads to the extremities before resolving. The cause has not been elucidated, and the condition has no known clinical significance and resolves without therapy.

Transient neonatal pustular melanosis, another benign neonatal dermatological condition, is more common in children with generously pigmented skin. Vesicles and pustules are similarly evident, but are more likely to present on the face as well as the rest of the body. Unlike those in erythema toxicum, the lesions rupture and then resolve over 48 to 72 hours. However, the condition is accompanied by small hyperpigmented macules which persist for the first several months of life.

Infantile seborrhea, also known as cradle cap when it is found on the scalp, is quite bothersome to many parents, who consider it cosmetically undesirable. However, it is harmless, generally easy to manage, and finite (lasting for at most several months). Milia are tiny waxy epidermal cysts located most often on the nose, but are found on the chin and forehead as well. They resolve as the skin naturally exfoliates.

Herpes is a life-threatening infection in neonates. However, symptoms of toxicity generally precede the rash, and the lesions themselves do not disappear and reappear, but remain fixed and scab over as they rupture. Moreover, this mother had no visible herpes lesions at the time of birth *and* had a caesarian section.

Vignette 2 Question 2

Answer B: The recommended "posthospital" care of the umbilical stump has changed in the past decade. Mothers are no longer encouraged to saturate the base of the stump several times a day to encourage detachment. No increase in bacterial infections has been reported, but there is some anecdotal evidence that the base of the cord is more susceptible to bleeding associated with the mild "trauma" of routine care (dressing, etc.). Continued oozing without resolution should prompt a visit for medical attention and possible evaluation. Most often, the stump detaches within 4 weeks, usually significantly earlier. Persistence beyond 8 weeks warrants evaluation of neutrophil activity.

Umbilical hernias may not become evident until separation of the cord, or even later (but usually within the first 2 to 3 months). The great majority resolve without intervention; those that persist beyond 3 to 4 years of age are repaired surgically.

Vignette 2 Question 3

Answer D: Neonatal breast budding, acne, and (in females) vaginal bleeding are all related to the presence of maternal estrogen. As the "exogenous" estrogen in the baby's system is broken down over the first few months, these findings resolve in both male and female infants. Gynecomastia is the presence of excessive breast tissue in the adolescent male and may be uni- or bilateral. As virtually all newborn males have breast budding, there is no association with breast enlargement during puberty. Retractile testes are a different matter than cryptorchidism. Retractile testes will locate themselves within the scrotum without intervention. Cryptorchidism signifies that the testicle is "fixed" outside the scrotum, whether palpable or not. These testicles are more likely to require surgical intervention, but even then the rate is much less than 50%. Prepucial tissue may be needed for repair in a male infant with significant hypospadias, but neither a fixed testicle nor a retractile one is a contraindication to circumcision. Cryptorchidism increases the risk of testicular cancer later in life, even if the testis is anatomically placed via surgery; however, there is no association with breast budding or the subsequent development of breast cancer.

Vignette 2 Question 4

Answer B: The American Academy of Pediatrics recommends universal administration of Vitamin D to infants who are breastfed in order to prevent the development of rickets. Many breastfeeding mothers are encouraged to continue taking prenatal vitamins while breastfeeding in order to ensure sufficient supplements for themselves and their children; however, these mothers should still provide vitamin D drops to their infants. Parenteral vitamin K is administered in the hospital to prevent hemorrhagic disease of the newborn. Breast milk provides the recommended levels of calcium and iron through at least 6 months of age.

Vignette 3 Question 1

Answer B: Factors in this infant's history which argue against a diagnosis include the ability to successfully breastfeed and stable vital signs noted when he was calm in his mother's arms. Infants with choanal atresia become apneic or drop their oxygen saturation levels when they attempt to feed, depending on whether the obstruction is total or partial. Moreover, since newborns are obligate nose-breathers, signs of distress improve when they are crying, which forces them to breathe through their mouths.

Any of the remaining conditions could cause this infant's distress. Respiratory distress syndrome (RDS) is most common in infants who are <34 weeks' gestation, but can occur in more advanced pregnancies. However, this child is large for gestational age, which is likely due to maternal diabetes but would also rule out incorrectly advanced dating of the pregnancy. Meconium aspiration syndrome (MAS) is also possible, although unlikely in this case given that only "light" meconium was present and the fetal heart tracings were reassuring. Neonatal pneumonia does not typically present this early, but if prolonged rupture of membranes or chorioamnionitis has gone unrecognized, early infection is plausible.

Vignette 3 Question 2

Answer C: Since meconium in the lungs causes airway plugging, usually a combination of distinct areas of atelectasis and overinflation are appreciated. The findings listed in answer B above create the "ground glass" appearance which is characteristic of RDS. Perihilar streaking with fluid in the interlobar fissures suggests that retained fetal lung fluid which is interfering with oxygenation. The findings in answer D are often associated with bacterial pneumonia; it is uncommon for neonates to have the appearance of true, isolated lobar consolidation unless there is an anatomic irregularity. It is important to note, however, that results of the radiograph should be interpreted with caution, as any of the first four answers above may be present with more than one condition and the quality of portable films is variable.

Vignette 3 Question 3

Answer B: Transient tachypnea of the newborn (TTN), also termed *retained fetal lung liquid syndrome*, is a relatively common condition in the term newborn. Most infants need only minimal support, such as oxygen via hood, to maintain saturations. Others may require nasal continuous positive airway pressure. In the rare case, further intervention is necessary, but the condition virtually always resolves within the first 48 to 72 hours of life, as the retained fluid is resorbed. This infant is at increased risk for TTN due to the maternal history of gestational diabetes. Elective caesarean section, without a trial at labor, and large for gestational age weight both increase the risk of TTN as well.

Nosocomial respiratory syncytial virus infection can be problematic in an infant ward but is unlikely in this newborn, which still has high maternal antibody load based on his age in days. Hyaline membrane disease is another, older name for RDS. RDS takes longer to resolve without intervention and usually requires more aggressive support measures, such as mechanical ventilation, unless treated with surfactant. Apnea implies periodic cessation of breathing; moreover, this child is not premature. While mild MAS could present and resolve in this manner, the preterm and perinatal history, along with the mildness of the illness and the rapid resolution, makes TTN more likely.

Vignette 3 Question 4

Answer A: Palpation of the clavicles in a newborn may produce crepitus, a creaking sensation under the fingertips consistent with a clavicular fracture. Clavicular fractures are more common in large infants born vaginally with associated trauma such as shoulder dystocia. This baby was not born vaginally, but the incision had to be widened to allow removal of the child, suggesting that the obstetrician was unable to maneuver the child out initially due to size. The "bump" the mother is describing is most likely a callus formed from healing bone.

Erb palsy is a neurologic deficiency of the upper extremity resulting from trauma to the nerve roots of C5–C6 during delivery. The affected patient holds the arm in an abnormal position, with extension at the elbow, internal rotation, and fixed pronation of the forearm. The arm is held close to the body on the involved side. Of note, the grasp reflex is preserved in these infants.

Developmental shoulder dysplasia is not a described condition in newborns; developmental hip dysplasia is, but this child's abnormality does not involve the hip. Metatarsus is medial curving isolated to the forefoot. Potter syndrome is a constellation of findings (compression deformities of the face and limbs, "prune" belly, and pulmonary hypoplasia) resulting from intrauterine bilateral renal agenesis.

Vignette 4 Question 1

Answer D: Fetal alcohol syndrome is the most common preventable congenital syndrome in the United States. Findings include those noted in answer D as well as growth retardation, microcephaly, and an increased incidence of joint and digit anomalies, hirsutism, and congenital heart defects. If the mother is intoxicated at delivery, the infant may be lethargic and hypoglycemic. Children with fetal alcohol syndrome may suffer a range of developmental problems as they age, from mental retardation to developmental delay, learning disabilities, and behavior disorders.

Spina bifida and facial anomalies can occur with maternal valproic acid use during pregnancy. Fetal hydantoin syndrome consists of broad nasal bridge, cleft lip/palate, microcephaly, and mental retardation. Hepatosplenomegaly, lymphadenopathy, and chorioretinitis can result from maternal toxoplasmosis or primary CMV infection during pregnancy. Cataracts, sensorineural hearing loss, IUGR, hepatosplenomegaly, and thrombocytopenic purpura are associated with maternal rubella infection.

Vignette 4 Question 2

Answer B: When an infant of Caucasian ancestry is noted to be jaundiced at >24 hours of age, is well appearing, AGA, and has no history of a traumatic delivery, then the likelihood of pathologic jaundice, be it direct or indirect, is low. Initial measurement of total bilirubin with a transcutaneous instrument is inappropriate because (a) a serum measurement is more accurate and (b) the direct fraction must be calculated from the total and indirect measurements to ensure that the patient does not have conjugated hyperbilirubinemia, which is always pathologic. The mother's blood type is A, so ABO incompatibility is not a concern (although there are other antigens on blood cells that can cause incompatibility and hemolytic jaundice, this is uncommon). Most physicians would order a blood type and Coombs test on the infant of a mother who is blood type O at the same time the serum bilirubin is drawn. Complete blood count and blood smear may be warranted if hemolysis is suspected because the bilirubin is much higher than expected, but this can be drawn later. Maternal Rh antigen testing takes place at the first prenatal visit and the status would not affect this pregnancy regardless because the parent is A^+ bloodtype.

Vignette 4 Question 3

Answer E: Although high levels of bilirubin can result in recalcitrant seizures and death, this is very rare and usually occurs late in the process, when it is obvious that there is something very wrong with the infant. Kernicterus is less common now than before the AAP recommendations were universally adopted in 2004, but the risk in this infant is higher given multiple less-than-ideal social factors. Kernicterus is sublethal bilirubin encephalopathy, which occurs when serum levels of unconjugated bilirubin cross the blood–brain barrier, affecting the basal ganglia, cerebellum, and hippocampus, among other cerebral area. Infants who survive the resulting lethargy, hypotonia, posturing, and possible seizures virtually always suffer from cerebral palsy and movement disorders and are at increased risk for mental retardation and vision/hearing deficiencies.

Chapter

3 Adolescent Medicine

Preeti Matkins • Katie S. Fine

Puberty is defined as the process of hormonal and physical changes whereby the body of a child matures into that of an adult, physiologically capable of sexual reproduction. **Adolescence**, on the other hand, encompasses the physical changes of puberty as well as the cognitive, social, and psychological advances that mark the transition from youth to adulthood. Some references further subdivide adolescence into an *early* period (middle school, age 10 to 13 years), a *middle* period (high school, age 14 to 17 years), and a *late* period (age 18 to 21 years). Developmental tasks of adolescence include the following:

- Development of a strong self-identity (defining the self, maintaining healthy self-esteem)
- Autonomy (self-governance, establishing autonomy)
- Achievement (recognizing talents, gifts, contributions)
- Establishing appropriate peer and sexual relationships (expression of relationships, intimacy, and expectations)
- Transition from relatively concrete thinking to more abstract concepts, such as cause/effect, long-term consequences, and complicated moral dilemmas.

Although adolescents are less likely than younger children to have regular health maintenance visits, regular contact with a primary care physician is particularly important in this age group. Many of the diseases and injuries that occur in adolescence result from lifestyle choices and risk taking that increase the risk of morbidity and mortality. Such behaviors include high-risk sexual activity, eating disorders, substance use and abuse, and actions resulting in accidental or intentional injury. Some intentional injury may be the result of depression, such as suicide. The leading causes of death in adolescents are motor vehicle crashes, suicide, and homicide.

THE ADOLESCENT OFFICE VISIT

Observing the parent–child interaction is informative, and the parent should be encouraged to raise any concerns with the clinician. However, it is imperative that *the majority of the interview and examination takes place without the parent present.* Teenagers may not be forthright or comfortable discussing certain health-related issues when they believe their parents may find out about their responses. While virtually all states mandate the reporting of suspected abuse, potential harm to self or others, and certain infectious diseases (including some sexually transmitted diseases [STDs]), most also provide for **confidentiality** of information related to sexual activity and substance use/abuse. Some states allow all adolescents access to medical care without their parents' knowledge; in other states, only emancipated minors are permitted this right. Emergency treatment should never be withheld pending parental notification or approval. Also, teens should be counseled about situations in which the clinician may break confidentiality. Some examples include teens disclosing plans to harm themselves or others or information related to mandated reporting of abuse.

Although studies show that adolescents are willing to discuss high-risk behaviors and preventative care issues with their physicians, most teens are uncomfortable initiating these conversations themselves. The acronym HEADSS (Table 3-1) is helpful in identifying pertinent areas in the adolescent social history. An indirect, nonjudgmental method of questioning may be more effective in eliciting an accurate history.

Height, weight, blood pressure, and body mass index (BMI) percentile should be recorded at every adolescent health maintenance visit. Other recommended procedures include vision screening every 3 years, hemoglobin/hematocrit (once in menstruating females), and lipid panel (at least once during adolescence). Every 3 years, teens should be assessed for increased risk of hearing loss, such as parental concern, family history of hereditary hearing loss, and excessive time listening to loud music via earbuds/headphones; such patients should have their hearing tested every 3 years. Tuberculosis testing is appropriate in individuals at high risk (see Chapter 1). The recommended examination and laboratory screening for sexually active patients is discussed in the following section.

Immunizations recommended during adolescence are listed in Figure 3-1. Of note, the Centers for Disease Control and Prevention Advisory Committee on Immunization Practices recommends that adolescents receive the tetanus and diphtheria toxoids and acellular pertussis (Tdap) vaccine and meningococcal conjugate vaccine (MCV) at the 11- to 12-year health maintenance visit. Human papillomavirus (HPV) vaccine is strongly recommended at the same visit for females and should be considered for males as well.

TABLE 3-1 The Adolescent Psychosocial History: HEADSS[a]

Home (family members, relationships, living arrangements)
Education (academic performance/educational goals)
Activities (peer relationships, work and recreational activities)
Drugs (substance use/abuse, including tobacco, alcohol, steroids, inhalants, and illicit drugs)
Sexuality (dating, sexual activity, contraception, sexual orientation)
Suicide (depression, anxiety, other mental health concerns)

[a]Some experts suggest that a second "E" should be added to remind physicians to screen for behaviors associated with **E**ating disorders and or **E**xercise and that a third "S" should be included to prompt questions concerning **S**afety (the potential for abuse or violent behavior [e.g., gang membership, owning a firearm]).

SEXUAL DEVELOPMENT/ REPRODUCTIVE HEALTH

As mentioned, **puberty** refers to those biologic changes that lead to reproductive capability. The events of puberty occur in a predictable sequence, but the timing of the initiation and the velocity of the changes are highly variable among individuals. The integration of the pubertal changes into the individual's self-identity is important to successful progression through adolescence.

In males, the initiation sequence of sexual development is testicular enlargement, followed by pubic hair growth, lengthening of the penis, and achievement of maximal height velocity. This progression is depicted in Figure 3-2.

In females, the order of pubertal events in sexual development is thelarche (breast budding), followed by pubarche, maximal height velocity, and menarche. Figure 3-3 shows these changes.

The **Sexual Maturity Rating** scale, or SMR (also called "Tanner Stages"), is used to determine where an individual is in the pubertal process. SMR stages for the male genitalia, female breasts, and male and female pubic hair are described in Table 3-2 and illustrated in Figures 3-4 through 3-6. Pubertal abnormalities are addressed in Chapter 14. All teens should have external genital exam yearly.

About half of high school students in the latest Centers for Disease Control and Prevention Youth Risk Behavior Survey reported that they had engaged in sexual intercourse. All teens should be asked if they are attracted to same gender, opposite gender, or both genders when taking a sexual history. Preventative health care for sexually active adolescents includes additional examination procedures and laboratory screening. Annual screening tests recommended for sexually active female adolescents include gonorrhea and chlamydia studies, serum testing for HIV and syphilis (rapid plasma regain [RPR]), careful visual examination of the external genitalia, and a wet mount of vaginal fluids for yeast, bacterial vaginosis (BV), and *Trichomonas vaginalis*. Rapid trichomonas testing should also be considered. Testing for chlamydia and gonorrhea may be vaginal or cervical nucleic acid amplification test (NAAT) or urine NAAT. Culture techniques are available but take longer for results and may not be as accurate. NAAT is not approved for testing oral or anal sites. HPV is the most common STD in adolescents. About 80% of sexually active persons will be exposed to HPV in their lifetime, and while most will resolve without symptoms, HPV may manifest as visible genital or oropharyngeal warts. The virus is responsible for almost all cases of cervical and anal cancers and is associated with vulvar, vaginal, penile, and non–tobacco-related oral cancers. Bimaual pelvic examinations are no longer recommended unless the pateint has symptoms of pelvic inflammatory disease, an abdominal mass, or uncontrolled bleeding. Papanicolaou smears are recommended starting at age 21 years. Adolescent males who are sexually active should have yearly sexually transmitted infection testing, including urine-based NAAT for gonorrhea and chlamydia and serum HIV and RPR. Rapid trichomonas testing or wet prep should be considered if penile discharge is present. Screening for young men who report same-gender sexual contact may include anal and pharyngeal cultures for STDs, and hepatitis B serology should be considered in nonimmunized patients. HIV and syphilis serology should be offered yearly to *all* sexually active adolescents. Per Centers for Disease Control guidelines, herpes testing should be limited to symptomatic patients. In addition, all patients who are sexually active should be offered use of condoms and contraception counseling at each health maintenance visit. Emergency contraception should be discussed with both male and female patients.

EATING DISORDERS

PATHOGENESIS

The need to be attractive to peers leads to a preoccupation with body image during adolescence. **Anorexia nervosa** is an eating disorder characterized by impaired body image and intense fear of weight gain, culminating in the refusal to maintain at least 85% of ideal body weight for age and height. It is postulated that external or internal psychological and/or social stressors superimposed on an inherited vulnerability lead to the development of anorexia.

Binge eating, followed by some compensatory behavior to rid the body of the ingested calories, is the hallmark of **bulimia nervosa**. To meet the criteria, patients must have at least two episodes of binge/purge a week for 2 months. Patients may purge (induce vomiting or take laxatives) or use other methods (fasting, intense exercise).

Many patients with eating disorders do not meet the *DSM-IV* criteria of anorexia nervosa or bulimia nervosa but have diordered thoughts about food, including dietary restrictions and/or binge/purge behavior. These patients are catagorized as "Eating Disorder Not Otherwise Specified (NOS)."

EPIDEMIOLOGY

Estimates of the incidence of anorexia in developed countries range from 1 in 200 to 1 in 2,000 adolescent females. Bulimia is more common, affecting 1% to 2% of Western young women. Depending on diagnostic criteria used, prevalence of Eating Disorder NOS is estimated to be between 0.8% and 14%. Up to 10% of patients with eating disorders are male, though the percentage may be higher; the data may reflect underrecognition or aversion to seeking care.

Vaccine ▼ Age ►	7–10 years	11–12 years	13–18 years
Tetanus, diphtheria, pertussis[1]	1 dose (if indicated)	1 dose	1 dose (if indicated)
Human papillomavirus[2]	*see footnote*[2]	3 doses	Complete 3-dose series
Meningococcal[3]	See footnote[3]	Dose 1	Booster at 16 years old
Influenza[4]	Influenza (yearly)		
Pneumococcal[5]	See footnote [5]		
Hepatitis A[6]	Complete 2-dose series		
Hepatitis B[7]	Complete 3-dose series		
Inactivated poliovirus[8]	Complete 3-dose series		
Measles, mumps, rubella[9]	Complete 2-dose series		
Varicella[10]	Complete 2-dose series		

Range of recommended ages for all children

Range of recommended ages for catch-up immunization

Range of recommended ages for certain high-risk groups

This schedule includes recommendations in effect as of December 23, 2011. Any dose not administered at the recommended age should be administered at a subsequent visit, when indicated and feasible. The use of a combination vaccine generally is preferred over separate injections of its equivalent component vaccines. Vaccination providers should consult the relevant Advisory Committee on Immunization Practices (ACIP) statement for detailed recommendations, available online at http://www.cdc.gov/vaccines/pubs/acip-list.htm. Clinically significant adverse events that follow vaccination should be reported to the Vaccine Adverse Event Reporting System (VAERS) online (http://www.vaers.hhs.gov) or by telephone (800-822-7967).

1. **Tetanus and diphtheria toxoids and acellular pertussis (Tdap) vaccine.** (Minimum age: 10 years for Boostrix and 11 years for Adacel)
   - Persons aged 11 through 18 years who have not received Tdap vaccine should receive a dose followed by tetanus and diphtheria toxoids (Td) booster doses every 10 years thereafter.
   - Tdap vaccine should be substituted for a single dose of Td in the catch-up series for children aged 7 through 10 years. Refer to the catch-up schedule if additional doses of tetanus and diphtheria toxoid–containing vaccine are needed.
   - Tdap vaccine can be administered regardless of the interval since the last tetanus and diphtheria toxoid–containing vaccine.
2. **Human papillomavirus (HPV) vaccines (HPV4 [Gardasil] and HPV2 [Cervarix]).** (Minimum age: 9 years)
   - Either HPV4 or HPV2 is recommended in a 3-dose series for females aged 11 or 12 years. HPV4 is recommended in a 3-dose series for males aged 11 or 12 years.
   - The vaccine series can be started beginning at age 9 years.
   - Administer the second dose 1 to 2 months after the first dose and the third dose 6 months after the first dose (at least 24 weeks after the first dose).
   - See *MMWR* 2010;59:626–32, available at http://www.cdc.gov/mmwr/pdf/wk/mm5920.pdf.
3. **Meningococcal conjugate vaccines, quadrivalent (MCV4).**
   - Administer MCV4 at age 11 through 12 years with a booster dose at age 16 years.
   - Administer MCV4 at age 13 through 18 years if patient is not previously vaccinated.
   - If the first dose is administered at age 13 through 15 years, a booster dose should be administered at age 16 through 18 years with a minimum interval of at least 8 weeks after the preceding dose.
   - If the first dose is administered at age 16 years or older, a booster dose is not needed.
   - Administer 2 primary doses at least 8 weeks apart to previously unvaccinated persons with persistent complement component deficiency or anatomic/functional asplenia, and 1 dose every 5 years thereafter.
   - Adolescents aged 11 through 18 years with human immunodeficiency virus (HIV) infection should receive a 2-dose primary series of MCV4, at least 8 weeks apart.
   - See *MMWR* 2011;60:72–76, available at http://www.cdc.gov/mmwr/pdf/wk/mm6003.pdf, and Vaccines for Children Program resolution No. 6/11-1, available at http://www.cdc.gov/vaccines/programs/vfc/downloads/resolutions/06-11mening-mcv.pdf, for further guidelines.
4. **Influenza vaccines (trivalent inactivated influenza vaccine [TIV] and live, attenuated influenza vaccine [LAIV]).**
   - For most healthy, nonpregnant persons, either LAIV or TIV may be used, except LAIV should not be used for some persons, including those with asthma or any other underlying medical conditions that predispose them to influenza complications. For all other contraindications to use of LAIV, see *MMWR* 2010;59(No.RR-8), available at http://www.cdc.gov/mmwr/pdf/rr/rr5908.pdf.
   - Administer 1 dose to persons aged 9 years and older.
   - For children aged 6 months through 8 years:
     — For the 2011–12 season, administer 2 doses (separated by at least 4 weeks) to those who did not receive at least 1 dose of the 2010–11 vaccine. Those who received at least 1 dose of the 2010–11 vaccine require 1 dose for the 2011–12 season.
     — For the 2012–13 season, follow dosing guidelines in the 2012 ACIP influenza vaccine recommendations.
5. **Pneumococcal vaccines (pneumococcal conjugate vaccine [PCV] and pneumococcal polysaccharide vaccine [PPSV]).**
   - A single dose of PCV may be administered to children aged 6 through 18 years who have anatomic/functional asplenia, HIV infection or other immunocompromising condition, cochlear implant, or cerebral spinal fluid leak. See *MMWR* 2010:59(No. RR-11), available at http://www.cdc.gov/mmwr/pdf/rr/rr5911.pdf.
   - Administer PPSV at least 8 weeks after the last dose of PCV to children aged 2 years or older with certain underlying medical conditions, including a cochlear implant. A single revaccination should be administered after 5 years to children with anatomic/functional asplenia or an immunocompromising condition.
6. **Hepatitis A (HepA) vaccine.**
   - HepA vaccine is recommended for children older than 23 months who live in areas where vaccination programs target older children, who are at increased risk for infection, or for whom immunity against hepatitis A virus infection is desired. See *MMWR* 2006;55(No. RR-7), available at http://www.cdc.gov/mmwr/pdf/rr/rr5507.pdf.
   - Administer 2 doses at least 6 months apart to unvaccinated persons.
7. **Hepatitis B (HepB) vaccine.**
   - Administer the 3-dose series to those not previously vaccinated.
   - For those with incomplete vaccination, follow the catch-up recommendations (Figure 3).
   - A 2-dose series (doses separated by at least 4 months) of adult formulation Recombivax HB is licensed for use in children aged 11 through 15 years.
8. **Inactivated poliovirus vaccine (IPV).**
   - The final dose in the series should be administered at least 6 months after the previous dose.
   - If both OPV and IPV were administered as part of a series, a total of 4 doses should be administered, regardless of the child's current age.
   - IPV is not routinely recommended for U.S. residents aged18 years or older.
9. **Measles, mumps, and rubella (MMR) vaccine.**
   - The minimum interval between the 2 doses of MMR vaccine is 4 weeks.
10. **Varicella (VAR) vaccine.**
    - For persons without evidence of immunity (see *MMWR* 2007;56[No. RR-4], available at http://www.cdc.gov/mmwr/pdf/rr/rr5604.pdf), administer 2 doses if not previously vaccinated or the second dose if only 1 dose has been administered.
    - For persons aged 7 through 12 years, the recommended minimum interval between doses is 3 months. However, if the second dose was administered at least 4 weeks after the first dose, it can be accepted as valid.
    - For persons aged 13 years and older, the minimum interval between doses is 4 weeks.

This schedule is approved by the Advisory Committee on Immunization Practices (http://www.cdc.gov/vaccines/recs/acip), the American Academy of Pediatrics (http://www.aap.org), and the American Academy of Family Physicians (http://www.aafp.org).
Department of Health and Human Services • Centers for Disease Control and Prevention

Figure 3-1 • ACIP-recommended vaccination schedule: ages 7 to 18 years.

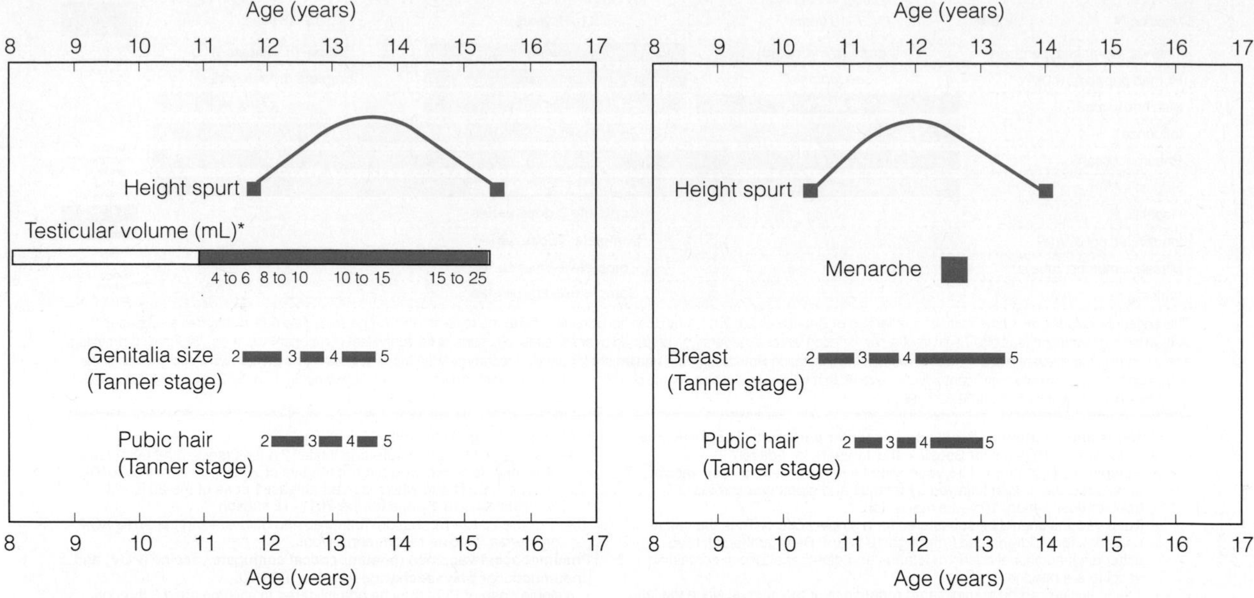

Figure 3-2 • Sequence of pubertal events in the average (American) male.

Figure 3-3 • Sequence of pubertal events in the average (American) female.

TABLE 3-2 Secondary Sex Characteristics: Tanner Sexual Maturity Rating (SMR) Scale

Breast Development (Female)	
Stage I	Preadolescent; elevation of papilla only
Stage II	Breast bud beneath the areola; enlargement of areolar diameter
Stage III	Further enlargement and elevation of breast and areola
Stage IV[a]	Projection of areola to form secondary projection above contour of breast
Stage V[a]	Mature stage; smooth breast contour
Genital Development (Male)	
Stage I	Preadolescent
Stage II	Enlargement of scrotum and testes; skin of scrotum reddens and changes in texture
Stage III	Enlargement of penis, particularly length; further growth of testes and scrotum
Stage IV	Increased size of penis with growth in thickness and development of glans; further enlargement of testes and scrotum and increased darkening of scrotal skin
Stage V	Adult genitalia
Pubic Hair (Male and Female)	
Stage I	Preadolescent (no pubic hair)
Stage II	Sparse growth of longer, slightly pigmented hair, chiefly at base of penis or along labia
Stage III	Increasingly darker, coarser, and more curled hair spreads over junction of pubis
Stage IV	Adult-type pubic hair with no spread to medial surface of thighs
Stage V	Adult in quantity and type with spread to thighs

[a]Stages IV and V may not be distinct in some patients.

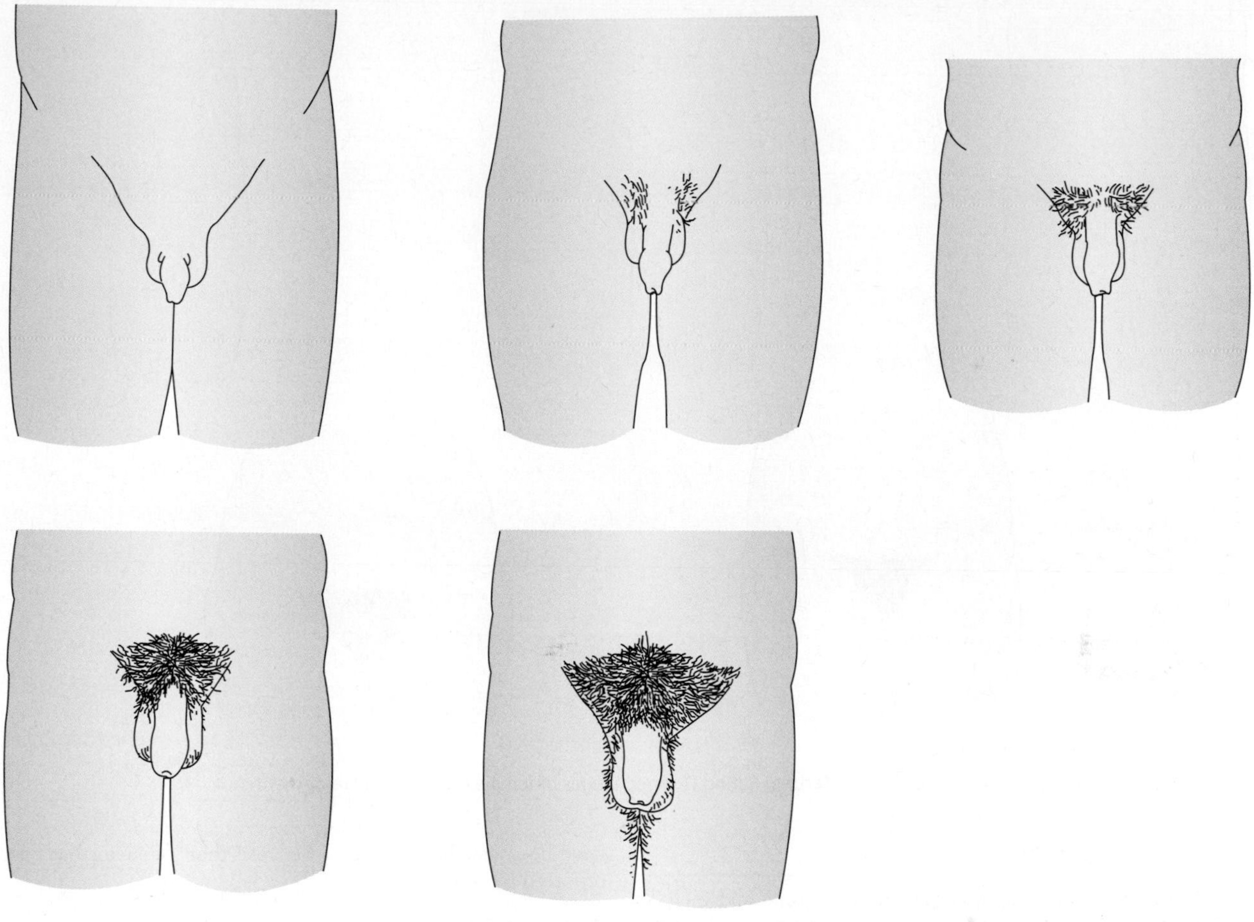

Figure 3-4 • Pictorial representation of Sexual Maturity Rating (Tanner) stages of male genital and pubic hair development.

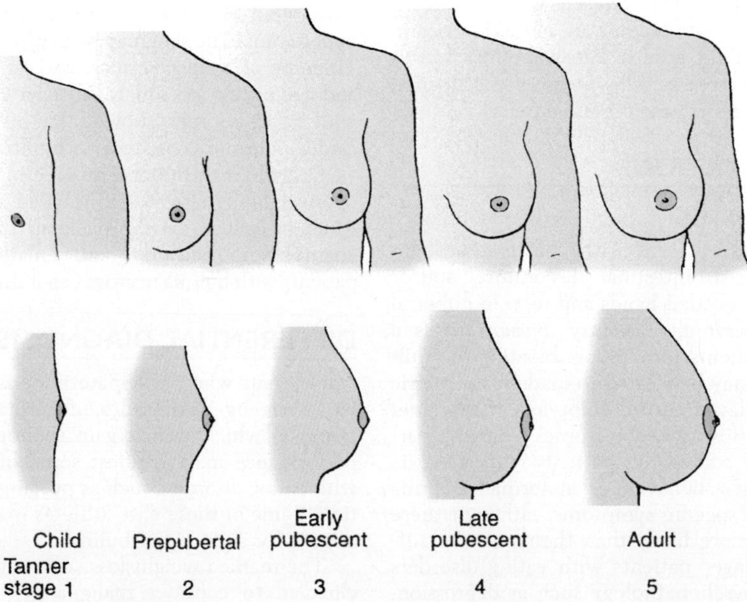

Figure 3-5 • Pictorial representation of Sexual Maturity Rating (Tanner) stages of female breast development.

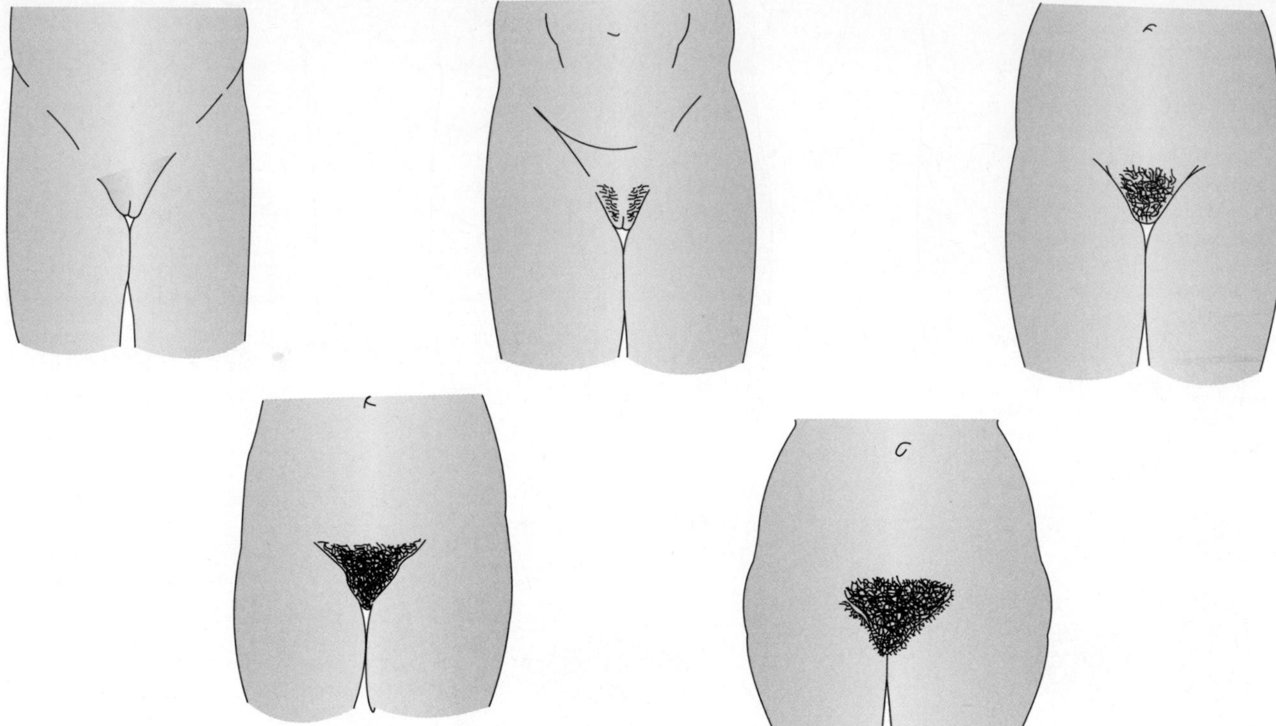

Figure 3-6 • Pictorial representation of Sexual Maturity Rating (Tanner) stages of female pubic hair development.

RISK FACTORS

Risk factors for eating disorders are multifactorial and include positive family history and female gender. There is a genetic component, but the mechanism of genetic influence is unknown. It is likely that the development of an eating disorder involves genetic factors, environment, and experience as well as neuroendocrine factors. Both anorexia and bulimia are more common in Caucasians than in other ethnic groups. Personality risk factors associated with anorexia nervosa include intense preoccupation with appearance, low self-esteem, and obsessive traits.

CLINICAL MANIFESTATIONS

History

Patients with anorexia may present with constipation, syncope, upper or lower gastrointestinal discomfort, and/or periodic episodes of cold, mottled hands and feet. In pubertal females with anorexia nervosa, *secondary amenorrhea* is a criterion for diagnosis. Patients may report bloating or "fullness" after eating, which may be related to inadequate caloric intake and subsequent delayed gastric emptying. If the chief complaint is weight loss, this invariably comes from the parents rather than from the adolescent; patients with anorexia generally do not view their behavior as abnormal. Bulimia does not usually produce specific symptoms, although these patients are significantly more likely than their peers to suffer from depression. Younger patients with eating disorders are more likely to have pyschopathology such as depression, obsessive compulsive disorder, and anxiety. All patients should be asked about self-harm (such as cutting) and suicidal ideation. Patients may be brought to the physician because they have been caught purging or because their behavior has been reported by someone else.

Physical Examination

Adolescents who suffer from anorexia may be severely underweight (usually with a BMI <17) and appear cachectic. Vital signs often reveal hypothermia, bradycardia, and orthostatic hypotension. The skin may be dry, yellowish, and hyperkeratotic. Thinning of scalp hair, increased lanugo hair, cool extremities, and nail pitting are additional signs. One study of adult patients with eating disorders showed that 30% to 40% of patients had a cardiac murmur consistent with mitral valve prolapse.

Patients with bulimia may be of normal weight or slightly overweight. Frequent self-induced vomiting (if present) may result in calluses on the backs of the knuckles, eroded tooth enamel, and parotid gland enlargement. However, many patients with bulmia nervosa can induce emesis without gagging.

DIFFERENTIAL DIAGNOSIS

Adolescents who participate in certain athletic activities (ballet, wrestling, gymnastics, cheerleading, cross country, and track) in which weight gain is thought to negatively impact performance may manifest some of the behaviors associated with eating disorders such as purging and severe calorie restriction. Some of these elite athletes may not meet the diagnostic criteria for anorexia or bulimia.

The marked weight loss seen with anorexia may cause the clinician to consider malignancy, inflammatory bowel disease or malabsorption syndromes, and other chronic diseases (infections, endocrine disorders). The differential diagnosis for vomiting (bulimia) is discussed in Chapter 9.

TABLE 3-3 Suggested Laboratory Tests for Adolescents with Eating Disorders

Study	Suspected Result
All Patients	
Complete blood count	Neutropenia; also anemia and thrombocytopenia
Serum electrolytes	Hypokalemia/hypochloremia/alkalosis (if purging or laxative or diuretic abuse); hyponatremia (due to manipulation of water intake or laxative use)
Blood urea nitrogen (BUN)	Increased BUN/creatinine (dehydration or renal dysfunction)
Glucose	Normal or low
Calcium/phosphate/magnesium	Normal or low (due to malnutrition)
Electrocardiogram	Bradycardia, T-wave inversions, ST depression (anorexia)
Prolonged QTc interval	Bulimia, if hypokalemic
Patients with Anorexia	
ESR[a]	Normal or low
Urinalysis	Proteinurea from muscle breakdown; decreased specific gravity from excessive water intake
Total protein, albumin, prealbumin	Low from poor nutrition
Liver function tests	Elevated
Cholesterol	Elevated
Serum protein/albumin, prealbumin	Low
TSH/fT_4[a]	Normal/normal to low
Patients with Bulimia	
Serum amylase, lipase	Elevated if vomiting

[a]Useful for ruling out other conditions in the differential.
ESR, erythrocyte sedimentation rate; TSH, thyroid stimulating hormone; fT_4, free thyroxine.

DIAGNOSTIC EVALUATION

Anorexia and bulimia are both clinical diagnoses. Laboratory studies are used to assess the need for specific medical intervention rather than to confirm the disease. Table 3-3 lists diagnostic tests that are used to rule out or quantify certain conditions associated with anorexia and bulimia.

TREATMENT

The treatment for eating disorders is multifactorial and includes nutritional support, behavioral and psychotherapy, and correction of any medical complications resulting from the severe weight loss or purging. Family-based treatment (Maudsley approach) is evidence-based treatment for anorexia or bulimia, and cognitive behavioral therapy may be used for patients with bulemia nervosa. Indications for hospitalization/inpatient therapy are noted in Table 3-4. Research is ongoing as to whether psychotropic medicines (particularly selective serotonin reuptake inhibitors) are useful in the treatment of these diseases. Psychotropic medication, if indicated, should start after some psychological therapy and nutritional management. Full recovery can take up to several years and should focus on strategies for ongoing disordered eating thoughts. The most recent published data indicate that the adolescent mortality rate for eating disorders is 1.8%.

TABLE 3-4 Anorexia and Bulimia: Indications for Possible Hospitalization

Both Conditions
Failure to improve with outpatient therapy
Hypokalemia (serum potassium <3.2 mmol/L)
Hypochloremia (serum chloride <88 mmol/L)
Cardiac arrhythmias/prolonged QTc interval/bradycardia
Medical complications requiring inpatient intervention such as esophageal tears
Syncope
Suicidal ideation
Anorexia
Unstable vital signs: pulse <50 in daytime; <45 when sleeping; orthostatic vital signs
Severe weight loss (BMI <75% for age and gender)
Need for enteral nutrition (food refusal)
Arrested pubertal development

SUBSTANCE USE AND ABUSE

Drug use is defined as the intentional use of any substance that results in alteration of the physical, psychological, cognitive, or mood state of the individual despite the potential for personal harm. Patients become addicted when they begin to use the drug in a compulsive, dependent manner despite significant functional impairment (**drug abuse**). This addiction can result from *physical dependence* (physiological symptoms of withdrawal when the drug is removed) or *psychological dependence*. Adolescents may have poor impulse control and prefer instant gratification, leading to high-risk behavior such as drug experimentation. The various substances that are used and abused by adolescents are listed in Table 3-5.

TABLE 3-5 Substance Use: Clinical Manifestations of Acute Intoxication and Chronic Use

Substance	Symptoms of Acute Use	Signs of Acute Use	Clinical Manifestations of Chronic Use
Alcohol	Decreased inhibition, impaired coordination, poor judgment; progressing to slurred speech, ataxia, confusion, coma, and respiratory depression	Nausea/vomiting, flushed skin, sluggish pupils, decreased reflexes, hypoglycemia	Poor coordination; nutritional deficiencies; cirrhosis of the liver; impaired cognition; physical dependency; impaired work, peer, family relationships
Marijuana	Euphoria, relaxation, loud talking, hunger, impaired cognition; progressing to mood instability and hallucinations	Drowsiness, slowed reaction times, tachycardia, orthostatic hypotension, injected conjunctiva, dry mouth	Decreased attention span; diminished short-term memory; impaired learning; psychological dependency
MDMA (ecstasy; 3,4 methylene-dioxy methylamphetamine)	Sense of happiness, enhanced well-being; progression to agitation, confusion, shock	Hyperthermia, hypertension, tachycardia, tachypnea, dilated pupils, agitation, hyponatremia	Impaired short-term and long-term memory; (rarely) hallucinogen persisting perception disorder
Cocaine/ amphetamines	Elation, increased alertness and activity, insomnia, anxiety; progressing to delirium, chest pain, psychosis, seizures, coma	Delirium, hyperthermia, dry mouth, tachycardia, hypertension, dilated pupils, hyperreflexia, tremors	Destruction of nasal septum (if nasal administration of cocaine); psychological addiction (amphetamines, prescription and otherwise, and cocaine)
Phencyclidine (PCP)	Euphoria or anxiety, passive to violent mood swings, impaired cognition, ataxia, hallucinations; progressing to psychosis, fear, respiratory depression, and death	Restlessness, labile affect, hyperthermia, tachycardia, hypertension, flushing, nystagmus, small pupils, impaired coordination, seizures	Depression; impaired memory and cognition; disordered articulation; physical dependency
Hallucinogens (including LSD; lysergic acid diethylamide)	Euphoria, increased alertness; progressing to nausea, anxiety, paranoia, hallucinations, seizures, coma	Restlessness, labile affect, hyperthermia, tachycardia, hypertension, flushing, warm skin, dilated pupils with injected conjunctiva, hyperreflexia	Emotional lability; exacerbation of depression, schizophrenia; flashbacks; ill-defined changes in the brain
Heroin	Euphoria followed by sedation; impaired cognition, nausea/vomiting, stupor, respiratory depression, coma	Altered (depressed) mental status, hypothermia, decreased respiratory rate, hypotension, pinpoint unresponsive pupils	Physical addiction with marked withdrawal syndrome of restlessness, insomnia, vomiting, muscle pain, leg shaking
Inhalants	Euphoria, impaired judgment; progressing to hallucinations, psychosis, seizures, coma	Agitation or stupor, slurred speech, nystagmus/eye watering, rhinorrhea, increased saliva	Short-term memory loss, cognitive impairment; loss of sense of smell; emotional lability; changes in articulation and gait
Anabolic steroids	Rapid increase in muscle mass, stamina (over months), mood instability	Gynecomastia, acne, hypertension, hair loss; aggressive behavior (over weeks/months)	Testicular shrinkage; jaundice; stunted height growth; psychological dependency

EPIDEMIOLOGY

Unfortunately, substance use among adolescents is not uncommon. In the 2009 Youth Behavior Surveillance System survey, 41.8% had drunk alcohol within the last 30 days, 20.8% had used marijuana, and 19.5% had used cigarettes. When asked if they had "ever" used the substance, 36.8% reported that they had tried marijuana; 6.4% had tried cocaine; 11.7% had tried inhalants; and 8.0% had used hallucinogenic drugs. Marijuana, a "gateway" drug, is the most commonly used "illicit" drug in the United States, but alcohol is the most commonly abused substance by teens in the country.

RISK FACTORS

Risk factors and protective factors related to substance use in adolescents are listed in Table 3-6.

CLINICAL MANIFESTATIONS

The clinical manifestations of acute intoxication with the substances of interest are listed in Table 3-5. Treatments are detailed in Chapter 21.

Adolescents should be asked and counseled at every maintenance visit regarding tobacco, alcohol, and substance use.

TABLE 3-6 Risk Factors for Substance Use

Illicit Drugs
Genetic predisposition (for addiction)
Use of drugs by family and friends
Easy access to drugs
Low levels of parental involvement and support
Poverty
Academic failure
Alcohol
Genetic predisposition (for alcoholism)
Use and abuse of alcohol by parents, peers
Low levels of parental involvement
Tobacco
Parental smoking and tobacco use
Easy access to cigarettes, other tobacco products
No restrictions on smoking in the home
Protective Factors
Stable home environment
Parental supervision
Membership in positive social organizations
Academic achievement
Association with abstinent peers

DIAGNOSTIC EVALUATION

Although drug testing is easily available through most labs and even over the counter, testing an adolescent at the request of the parents without the patient's knowledge is generally discouraged and potentially could be adverse to the patient–clinician relationship. Attempts should be made to involve the teen in the discussion and obtain consent for any recommended diagnostic studies.

MANAGEMENT

Patients suspected of drug/alcohol dependence should be referred to an addiction specialist and may require intensive inpatient or outpatient therapy. Adolescents who use tobacco must be encouraged to quit and supported in doing so. If the patient is interested in smoking cessation, nicotine replacement therapy ("the patch," gums, etc.) may be offered. Some adolescents may require more intensive behavioral therapy or prescription medication such as bupropion. Motivational interviews should be integrated into any discussion of behavioral changes.

VIOLENCE IN THE ADOLESCENT POPULATION

EPIDEMIOLOGY

Traumatic injury is the leading cause of death in the adolescent population. Homicide and suicide are second and third on this list, respectively. Adolescents may be victims of violence (including bullying), perpetrators of violence against others, and/or intentionally harmful to themselves.

RISK FACTORS

Individual risk factors for violent behavior include previous arrest for juvenile crime, early exposure to violence (interpersonal violence and in the media), being a victim of abuse, drug and alcohol use, and academic/school failure. While young women are more likely than young men to report experiencing sexual abuse, adolescent males are far more likely to be the victims and perpetrators of violent acts. Other factors associated with an increased likelihood of violent behavior include low socioeconomic status and easy access to guns.

The strongest risk factor associated with attempted suicide is a **prior attempt**. Other factors that increase the likelihood of attempted suicide include an existing psychiatric disorder (depression, etc.), substance abuse, a history of being abused, a family history of a major affective disorder and/or suicide, and a recent life stressor. *Adolescents who live in homes with firearms have a 10-fold greater risk of completed suicide than do their peers.*

CLINICAL MANIFESTATIONS

Physicians and other health care personnel who interact regularly with adolescents are in a position to question them about whether they feel safe and whether they have witnessed or been the victims of aggression. Asking how patients deal with anger, if they have ever been in a fight, if they have been suspended from school, and whether there is a gun in the home may also open avenues of discussion.

All adolescent patients should be screened for depression (sadness, despair, hopelessness) and, if these are positive, suicidal ideation. Several adolescent depressive screening tools have been validated in the clinical setting. Those patients who admit to having a plan for suicide are at particular risk.

MANAGEMENT

Encouraging parents to limit exposure to violence in the media should be part of preventive health counseling beginning in the toddler years. Securing mental health services for the affected adolescent (and social services for the family) may provide the support needed to make the transition to a productive adulthood and limit involvement with the juvenile justice system.

As previously mentioned, doctor–patient confidentiality does not extend to information which suggests the potential for immediate harm. Any patient who attempts suicide, even if the attempt is interpreted as merely a "gesture," should undergo immediate psychiatric evaluation and may need hospitalization.

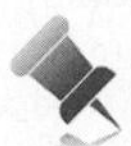

KEY POINTS

- It is recommended that adolescents receive a hearing screen, lipid panel, and hemoglobin/hematocrit (for menstruating females) at least once during adolescence. Vision should be assessed every 3 years. Height, weight, BMI, and blood pressure are assessed at each health maintenance visit.
- In males, the initiation sequence of sexual development is testicular enlargement, followed by pubic hair growth, penile lengthening, and attainment of maximal height velocity.
- In females, the order of pubertal events in sexual development is thelarche (breast budding), followed by pubic hair growth, attainment of peak height velocity, and menarche.
- Adolescents who are sexually active should be offered testing for gonorrhea and chlamydia, HIV, and syphilis (RPR) at least yearly. Screening for *Trichomonas vaginalis* is recommended for sexually active females. Contraception counseling should be conducted at each health maintenance visit.
- Secondary amenorrhea is a diagnostic feature of anorexia nervosa. Mitral valve prolapse is not uncommon.
- Marijuana is the most commonly used illicit drug in the United States; alcohol is the most commonly used substance by teens.
- Patients who are smokers should be encouraged to quit at each health visit. Those who express interest in doing so should be offered nicotine replacement therapy, behavioral therapy, social support, and (in some cases) bupropion.
- Traumatic injury is the leading cause of death in the adolescent population.
- Adolescents who live in homes with a firearm have a 10-fold greater risk of completed suicide than do their peers with depression and no firearm in their home.

C Clinical Vignettes

Vignette 1

A 15-year-old female comes into your clinic complaining of constipation. You note that she has lost 15 lb since her last clinic visit 8 months ago. She is 5′7″ and weighs 102 lb. Her current BMI is 16. When asked about it, she states, "I'm trying to be healthier." On her examination, her temperature is 97.4°F, respiratory rate is 14 breaths per minute, pulse is 40 bpm, and blood pressure is 110/82 mm Hg. Orthostatic blood pressures and pulses are as follows:

Lying: 105/70 mm Hg, pulse 40 bpm

Sitting: 100/65 mm Hg, pulse 55 bpm

Standing: 95/60 mm Hg, pulse 65 bpm

She is thin with cold extremities and light, downy hair on the back of her neck. On further investigation, you discover she has not had a period in 4 months.

1. What is the most likely diagnosis?
- **a.** Hyperthyroidism
- **b.** Irritable bowel syndrome
- **c.** Anorexia nervosa
- **d.** Bulimia nervosa
- **e.** Body dysmorphic disorder

2. What is the most appropriate next step in her care?
- **a.** Hospitalization
- **b.** Referral to a dietician
- **c.** Outpatient behavioral therapy
- **d.** Laboratory assessment including CBC and BMP
- **e.** Emergent psychiatric evaluation

3. The patient continues to return for follow-up after her initial treatment. Three months later, she remains amenorrheic. Which additional complication is she most at risk for?
- **a.** Infertility
- **b.** Polycystic ovarian syndrome
- **c.** Premature ovarian failure
- **d.** Osteopenia
- **e.** Anemia

Vignette 2

A 16-year-old female comes into your office complaining of vaginal discharge. She has regular periods, the last of which was 1 week ago. She has had three sexual partners in the last year. On physical examination, temperature is 98.7°F, respiratory rate is 15 breaths per minute, pulse is 72 bpm, and blood pressure is 102/78 mm Hg. Her abdominal examination is benign. On examination of the genitalia, a whitish, mucopurulent discharge is noted, but there are no lesions or ulcers on her vagina. On speculum examination, the cervix is edematous and friable.

1. Which of the following tests would most likely confirm the diagnosis?
- **a.** Wet mount
- **b.** Urine NAAT
- **c.** Rapid *Trichomonas* screen
- **d.** Urine pregnancy test
- **e.** RPR

2. Which of the following is the treatment of choice for this patient?
- **a.** Cefixime 200 mg by mouth once a day for 5 days *and* azithromycin 100 mg by mouth twice a day for 7 days
- **b.** Azithromycin 2 g by mouth, single dose
- **c.** Ceftriaxone 250 mg IM, single dose *and* azithromycin 1 g by mouth, single dose
- **d.** Ceftriaxone 250 mg IM, single dose and doxycycline 200 mg by mouth, single dose
- **e.** Doxycycline 100 mg by mouth twice a day for 7 days

3. Which of the following is the most likely complication of this illness if left untreated?
- **a.** Pelvic inflammatory disease
- **b.** Infertility
- **c.** Endometriosis
- **d.** Tubo-ovarian abscess
- **e.** Cervical cancer

4. Which of the following signs is pathognomonic for this complication?
- **a.** Dyspareunia
- **b.** Cervical motion tenderness
- **c.** Chronic pelvic pain
- **d.** Endocervical ulcers
- **e.** Dysmenorrhea

Vignette 3

A 14-year-old male comes to your office with his mother for a health maintenance visit. He has not been in the office since he was 9 years old. Before that time, he was seen regularly and was up-to-date on all immunizations. His mother states that he has been more distant than usual, but has no other concerns. On physical examination, his vital signs are normal and his examination is unremarkable.

1. Which of the following vaccinations should be offered at today's visit?
   a. Tdap, MCV, HPV, seasonal influenza
   b. Tdap only
   c. MCV only
   d. Tdap and HPV
   e. HPV, MCV, and seasonal influenza

2. Upon asking the mother to leave the room for confidentiality reasons, you conduct the remainder of the health maintenance interview. During the HEADSS assessment, you discover that your patient has had thoughts about suicide and has made a plan on how to do so in the past. What is the largest risk factor for attempting suicide?
   a. History of abuse
   b. Having a gun in the home
   c. Depression
   d. A prior suicide attempt
   e. History of parent committing suicide

3. Your patient asks you not to tell his mother about his suicidal thoughts. He states that this "would really upset her." Prior to the visit, you had reviewed your confidentiality policy with both the patient and the parent. What is your role as the physician in this situation?
   a. Report the patient to the police
   b. Reveal the information to the parent and refer for emergent psychiatric evaluation
   c. Uphold the patient request
   d. Encourage the patient to tell his mother
   e. Consult the ethics committee emergently

Vignette 4

You are in the emergency department on a Friday night when a 17-year-old male with altered mental status is brought in by his mother. His mother states that she heard him come home after his curfew and found him in the kitchen. He seemed somewhat disoriented and was snacking on dinner leftovers. On physical examination, his temperature was 99°F, respiratory rate 20 breaths per minute, pulse 112 bpm, and blood pressure 130/90 mm Hg. He responds very slowly to your questions, and you note that his eyes are injected and his oral mucosa is dry.

1. Which of the following is the most likely diagnosis?
   a. Acute psychosis
   b. Alcohol ingestion
   c. Cannabis ingestion
   d. Amphetamine ingestion
   e. Inhalant use

2. Which of the following samples provides the most likely confirmatory test?
   a. Blood
   b. Urine
   c. Hair
   d. Oral secretions
   e. Skin

3. If this patient continues to engage in use of the drug in question, he is at increased risk for which of the following?
   a. Dropping out of school
   b. Use of other illicit drugs
   c. Criminal behavior
   d. a and b only
   e. a, b, and c

4. You see the patient 6 months later in clinic. He reports that his grades are dropping, yet he does not seem bothered by this change. On further questioning the patient states that he has continued to use the drug recreationally but does not spend excessive time acquiring the drug. In between uses of the drug, he does not experience any sleep or mood disturbances. What condition best characterizes our patient?
   a. Repeated intoxication
   b. Drug abuse
   c. Drug dependence
   d. Conduct disorder
   e. Dysthymia

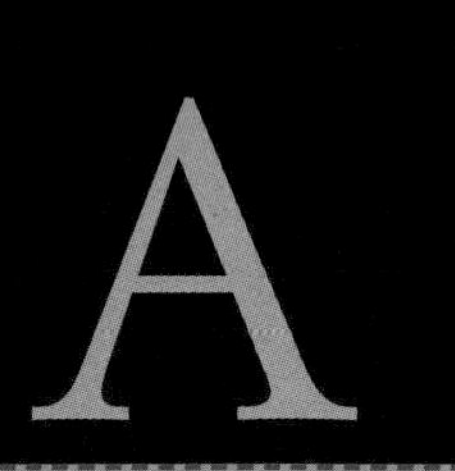

Answers

Vignette 1 Question 1
Answer C: The *DSM-IV* criteria for anorexia nervosa includes the following: the refusal to maintain body weight at or above minimally normal body weight for age and height; intense fear of gaining weight or becoming fat despite being underweight; distorted perception of body weight and shape; and amenorrhea. Many patients will have a BMI below normal; this patient's BMI is less than the 3rd percentile for age. Associated symptoms include fatigue, dry skin, lanugo, hypoactive bowel sounds, constipation, early satiety, bradycardia, orthostatic hypotension, sensitivity to cold, and difficulty concentrating.

Patients with bulimia nervosa are often of normal weight, but see themselves as overweight. On physical examination, they may have dental caries/enamel erosion, swollen parotid glands, and calluses across the knuckles from forceful vomiting (Russell's sign). Irritable bowel syndrome is considered in the differential diagnosis, but these patients will often also have issues with diarrhea and abdominal pain. They do not have amenorrhea. In hyperthyroidism, patients may have irregular periods and weight loss, but they generally have an increased appetite, heat intolerance, an increase in bowel movements, and possibly a goiter on exam. Lastly, body dysmorphic disorder is defined as a preoccupation with an imagined defect in one's body or a disproportionate concern with a very slight physical anomaly. These patients generally have completely normal vitals and physical examinations.

Vignette 1 Question 2
Answer A: The following criteria qualify a patient with anorexia nervosa to be admitted to the hospital: severe malnutrition, dehydration, electrolyte instability, cardiac dysrhythmia, arrested growth and development, failure of outpatient treatment, acute food refusal, psychogenic emergencies, and/or physiologic instability. Physiologic instability is defined as the following:

- Severe bradycardia (heart rate $<$50 bpm during day or $<$45 bpm at night)
- Hypotension (blood pressure $<$80/50 mm Hg)
- Hypothermia (temperature $<$96°F)
- Orthostatic changes in pulse ($>$10 bpm) or blood pressure ($>$20 mm Hg).

Complete blood count (CBC) and basic metabolic panel (BMP) are helpful baseline labs to look for anemia and electrolyte abnormalities, but the patient's bradycardia and positive orthostasis are of greater concern. All eating disorder patients should have a dietician, therapist, and sometimes even a psychiatrist involved in their care, but the most important thing to do first for this patient is to hospitalize her for unstable vital signs.

Vignette 1 Question 3
Answer D: Osteopenia is a medical complication of anorexia nervosa. Peak bone mass develops during adolescence and inadequate intake of nutrients, minerals, and vitamins in patients with eating disorders affect bone development. Furthermore, the loss of bone mineral density is correlated with the duration of amenorrhea. Patients who remain amenorrheic for 6 months or greater are at an increased risk of osteopenia and osteoporosis.

It is still possible for a patient to become pregnant despite an amenorrheic state. Furthermore, fertility is generally restored in recovered anorexics. Polycystic ovarian syndrome and premature ovarian failure may be causes of secondary amenorrhea, but should not result from anorexia nervosa. Anemia is present in roughly one third of anorexic patients but is not associated with the status of amenorrhea.

Vignette 2 Question 1
Answer B: The patient most likely has cervicitis caused by either *Neisseria gonorrhoeae* or *Chlamydia trachomatis*. These organisms are often co-pathogens. This diagnosis is more likely due to the history of multiple partners, the type of discharge, and the friable cervix. Urine nucleic acid amplification test (NAAT) is the best method for diagnosing *N. gonorrhoeae* and *C. trachomatis*. It is more rapid and sensitive than cultures.

While any of the tests would be beneficial as screening exams in a sexually active teenager, not all of them would lead to the most likely diagnosis in this patient. A wet mount would be helpful to look for bacterial vaginosis (BV), which usually presents with a fishy-smelling, thin, white discharge. Clue cells on the wet mount would be diagnostic of BV. A rapid trichomonas test would diagnose *Trichomonas vaginalis*, which tends to cause a green, frothy, foul-smelling discharge. Patients with *Trichomonas* are less likely to have a friable cervix. Due to the recent history of menses, she is less likely to be pregnant. On examination, our patient did not have the classic painless chancre on her vagina (sign of primary syphilis); thus the rapid plasma regain (RPR) will not confirm the most likely diagnosis.

Vignette 2 Question 2
Answer C: First-line treatment for chlamydial infections is azithromycin, 1 g orally in a single dose *or* Doxycycline 100 mg orally BID for 7 days. First-line treatment for gonococcal infections is ceftriaxone 250 mg IM in a single dose or cefixime 400 mg orally in a single dose. Due to the high likelihood of coinfection with both *C. trachomatis* and *N. gonorrhoeae*, it is recommended that both infections be empirically treated.

Vignette 2 Question 3

Answer A: Pelvic inflammatory disease (PID) is an acute infection of the upper genital tract in women and results from sexually transmitted infection. The most likely causative agents are *N. gonorrhoeae* and *C. trachomatis*. Early treatment of both infections can help prevent this complication.

Infertility may be a complication of untreated *N. gonorrhoeae* and *C. trachomatis* in that both can cause PID, singly or in combination. Endometriosis is the presence of endometrial glands and stroma in extrauterine sites. This disorder is caused by genetic and immune factors as well as possibly retrograde menstruation. It is not associated with cervical infections. A tubo-ovarian abscess may not only result from PID but also arise as a complication of other abdominal infections. Cervical cancer is a complication of infection with HPV.

Vignette 2 Question 4

Answer B: Cervical motion tenderness is defined as unpleasant or severe discomfort during bimanual examination of the cervix and is indicative of an inflammatory process of the pelvic organs. It is also called the "chandelier sign" because patients may "jump off the table" due to the pain. Dyspareunia (pain with coitus) may certainly be associated with PID but also occurs with urinary tract disease, poor lubrication, endometriosis, and a wide variety of other disorders. Chronic pelvic pain may result not just from gynecological causes, but also from urinary, gastrointestinal, somatic, and oncogenic causes. Endocervical ulcers may occur in PID as well as in simple cervicitis. Dysmenorrhea (pain with periods) is caused by prostaglandin production during menstruation and is not a sign of PID.

Vignette 3 Question 1

Answer A: Between the ages of 11 and 12 years, the recommended vaccinations are the Tdap (tetanus and diphtheria toxoids and acellular pertussis), MCV4 (meningococcal conjugate vaccine, quadrivalent), human papillomavirus (HPV), and the seasonal influenza vaccine. The Tdap should be followed by a tetanus and diphtheria toxoids (Td) booster every 10 years thereafter; administration of the Td for an interval <10 years, even in response to a tetanus-prone injury, is unnecessary. The HPV vaccine is generally started at or after 11 years of age and is a three-shot series. A yearly influenza vaccine is also recommended.

Recommendations regarding the administration schedule for MCV4 have recently been updated. Adolescents should initially be vaccinated at 11 to 12 years of age, followed by a booster at age 16 years. If the adolescent receives the first does at 13 to 15 years, a one-time booster should be administered at age 16 to 18 years (or up to 5 years after the first dose).

Vignette 3 Question 2

Answer D: The last S in the HEADSS assessment stands for suicide. Risk factors for suicide include mental illness, family history of mood disorder or suicide, and history of physical or sexual abuse. However, the largest risk factor for suicide is a prior suicide attempt. Previous attempts at suicide can increase an individual's risk of suicide by 30 to 40 times. Precipitating factors for suicide include access to means (such as having a gun), exposure to suicide, alcohol and drug use, social stress and isolation, and behavioral factors.

Vignette 3 Question 3

Answer B: Confidentiality is an important component of the adolescent health visit. It builds trust and fosters an environment in which the teen can begin to manage his or her own health care. However, if certain information is reported that puts the patient at risk, confidentiality may be broken. Cases for which confidentiality may be broken include child abuse/neglect, reportable sexually transmitted infections, homicidal ideation, violent injuries, rape, and suicidal ideation or plans to commit suicide. Laws regarding confidentiality vary by state, so it is important to review the laws in your state. All states permit break in confidentiality if the patient is judged to be an imminent danger to him- or herself or others.

The patient in question has confessed to suicidal ideation as well as a plan. It is important to refer him for emergent psychiatric evaluation, which would also require revealing the information. This information cannot be kept secret. The police do not need to be involved, as they would be in a case of child abuse. Trusting the child to tell his or her mother is not appropriate because the child needs immediate help. Waiting on a decision from the ethics committee would delay treatment.

Vignette 4 Question 1

Answer C: Cannabis, when either inhaled or ingested, can cause symptoms of euphoria, impaired cognition, slowed reaction times, and increased appetite. Physiologic signs include tachycardia, orthostatic hypotension, injected conjunctiva, and dry mouth.

Acute psychosis is the disruption of perception of reality characterized by thought disorganization, hallucinations, and/or delusions. This patient's history does not support this. Alcohol will cause impaired judgment and coordination, slurred speech, nausea/vomiting, sluggish pupils, and flushed skin. Amphetamine ingestion may cause acute anxiety, insomnia, tachycardia, hypertension, and dilated pupils. Last, with inhalant use teens may experience euphoria, impaired judgment, agitation, nystagmus, and increased secretions (eye, nose, mouth).

Vignette 4 Question 2

Answer B: Urine, blood, hair, and oral fluid can all be used to test for cannabis intake. Urine tests are inexpensive and widely available and therefore are the most commonly used. The screen is first performed with a sensitive immunoassay. Positive results are followed up with more specific tests such as gas chromatography or mass spectrometry. Skin sampling is not used to test for cannabis. However, sweat patch testing may be used. Marijuana can be detected for 7 to 10 days after use in a nonchronic user.

Vignette 4 Question 3

Answer E: Marijuana is considered the "gateway drug" because users are more likely to try additional illicit drugs. Chronic use of marijuana also results in decreased attention span, diminished short-term memory, and impaired learning. These symptoms place the patient at increased risk for school dropout. Last, some studies have shown significant correlation between increased marijuana use and number of crimes.

Vignette 4 Question 4

Answer B: Abuse implies that the patient's use of the drug is interfering with work, school, and home. It also can include recurrent legal problems, use in hazardous situations, and persistent use despite problems with interpersonal relationships.

Dependence, on the other hand, is marked by tolerance to the drug, increased time spent acquiring the drug, unsuccessful attempts to stop, and persistent use despite knowledge that adverse physical/psychological symptoms are caused by the drug. Because our patient is showing significant impairment in school, he is beyond the classification of repeated intoxication. Children with conduct disorder also will generally engage in repeated delinquent activities such as fighting, acts of cruelty, arson, and stealing. Dysthymic disorder is characterized by depressed mood for at least 2 years that is present most of the day and more days than not. Patients with dysthymia can also develop poor school performance.

Chapter

4 Nutrition

Meera P. Gallagher • Katie S. Fine

Good nutrition is essential for optimal physical growth and intellectual development. A healthy diet protects against disease, provides reserve in times of stress, and contains adequate amounts of protein, carbohydrates, fats, vitamins, and minerals. Children with vegan diets (ingesting no animal products) are at risk for vitamin B_{12} deficiency and, if exposed to inadequate sunlight, vitamin D deficiency as well. Iron supplementation/fortification should be considered for both vegan and lacto-ovo vegetarians. Infant feeding intolerance, failure to thrive (FTT), iron-deficiency anemia (Chapter 11), and obesity are the most common pediatric conditions associated with malnutrition in the developed world.

In order to assess a child's nutritional status and growth, pediatricians follow the patient's **growth chart**. Growth charts represent cross-sectional data from the National Center for Health Statistics. The patient's weight, height, weight-for-length (prior to 2 years of age) and **body mass index** (BMI; weight in kilograms divided by height in meters squared, after 2 years of age) are recorded as points on the chart at each health maintenance visit. Separate growth charts are generated for preterm infants and children with certain genetic disorders, including Down syndrome and Turner syndrome.

INFANT FEEDING ISSUES

Infant feeding addresses the physical and emotional needs of both mother and child. Babies double in weight by age 4 to 5 months and typically triple their birth weight by their first birthday. Height reaches twice birth length by age 3 to 4 years. Although breastfeeding is almost always preferable, many commercially prepared iron-fortified formulas provide appropriate calories and nutrients. Preterm infants require specifically balanced formula or breast milk with added fortifier. Newborns feed on demand, usually every 1 to 2 hours. Neonates typically lose up to 10% of their birth weight over the first several days; formula-fed babies regain that weight by the second week of life, whereas breastfed babies may take about a week longer. Healthy infants automatically regulate intake to meet caloric demand for basic metabolism and growth.

All infant formulas contain the recommended amounts of vitamins and minerals. Iron-fortified cereals should be added to the infant diet between 4 and 6 months of age. Cereal and baby foods should only be fed by spoon, rather than mixed in a bottle of formula. When the infant is taking cereal well, other baby foods may be started, including meats, fruits, and vegetables. When introducing new foods, only one novel product should be introduced at a time to evaluate for potential adverse reactions. Whole-fat cow milk may be introduced at age 12 months and should continue until age 24 months, when skim milk should be substituted. Infants and children sent to bed with a bottle containing anything but water are at risk for **milk-bottle teeth caries**.

BREASTFEEDING

The American Academy of Pediatrics recommends **exclusive breastfeeding** during the first 6 months of life and continuation of breastfeeding during the second 6 months for optimal infant nutrition. Studies have shown that breastfed infants have a lower incidence of infections, including otitis media, pneumonia, sepsis, and meningitis. Human milk contains bacterial and viral antibodies (secretory IgA) and macrophages. **Lactoferrin** is a protein found in breast milk that increases the availability of iron and has an inhibitory effect on the growth of *Escherichia coli*. Breastfed infants are less likely to experience feeding difficulties associated with allergy (eczema) or intolerance (colic).

Breastfed infants should receive oral **vitamin D supplementation** beginning within a week after birth to prevent **rickets**, a condition in which developing bone fails to mineralize due to inadequate 1,25-dihydroxycholecalciferol. Dark-skinned infants and those at extreme latitudes are at increased risk. Rickets in breastfed infants becomes clinically and chemically evident in late infancy (Table 4-1). Rickets due solely to vitamin D deficiency begins to respond to supplementation within weeks. It is recommended that all children receive a minimum of 400 IU of vitamin D daily. According to the American Academy of Pediatrics, breastfed infants may require fluoride supplementation if the concentration of the mineral in their main water source is extremely low.

In developed countries, mothers with human immunodeficiency virus (HIV) infection or untreated active tuberculosis and those who are using illegal drugs should not breastfeed. Other contraindications include infants with galactosemia and certain maternal medications (antithyroid agents, lithium, isoniazid, and most chemotherapy drugs).

TABLE 4-1 Clinical and Laboratory Manifestations of Rickets

Clinical and Laboratory Manifestations of Rickets
Craniotabes (thinning of the outer skull layer)
Rachitic rosary (enlargement of the costochondral junctions)
Epiphyseal enlargement at the wrists and ankles
Delayed closing of abnormally large fontanelle
Bowlegs
Delayed walking
Normal-to-low serum calcium
Low serum phosphorus
Elevated serum alkaline phosphatase
Low serum 25-hydroxycholecalciferol

INFANT FEEDING INTOLERANCE

Feeding intolerance may lead to food aversion and FTT; the most significant cause is cow milk–protein intolerance or allergy.

Clinical Manifestations

History and Physical Examination

Feeding intolerance may present with any number of clinical manifestations. **Malabsorption** is characterized by poor growth and chronic, nonbloody diarrhea. **Allergy** may be accompanied by eczema or wheezing. A severe local allergic reaction within the bowel results in **colitis**, indicated by anemia and/or obvious blood in the stools. Other possible nonspecific symptoms include vomiting, irritability, and abdominal distention.

Differential Diagnosis

Infectious gastroenteritis, necrotizing enterocolitis, intussusception, intermittent volvulus, celiac disease, cystic fibrosis, chronic protein malnutrition, aspiration, and eosinophilic enteritis should be considered. The most common condition mistaken for milk–protein intolerance is colic, which is generally limited to infants 3 weeks to 3 months of age. **Colic** is a syndrome of recurrent irritability that persists for several hours, usually in the late afternoon or evening. During the attacks, the child draws the knees to the abdomen and cries inconsolably. The crying resolves as suddenly and spontaneously as it begins.

Treatment

Exclusive breastfeeding during the first year of life eliminates the problem posed by cow milk–protein intolerance, except in severely allergic infants. If there is no evidence of any underlying disease in formula-fed infants with characteristic symptoms, substitution of a protein hydrolysate (extensively hydrolyzed) formula is recommended because as many as 10% to 17% of children with cow milk protein allergy are also intolerant of soy protein.

FAILURE TO THRIVE

Failure to thrive is defined here as persistent weight below the third percentile or falling off a previously established growth curve. It is not uncommon for a child to cross a growth percentile curve between 9 and 18 months of age, as growth begins to relate more closely to genetic potential rather than maternal nutrition during pregnancy. In particular, breastfed infants have steeper weight curves than formula-fed infants initially, but often have a normal and anticipated percentile drop in weight once cow's milk and solid foods are started. However, a growth curve which flattens or decreases across one or more growth percentile curves is cause for concern. Risk factors for FTT include low birth weight, low socioeconomic status, physical or mental disability, and caretaker neglect. FTT is often associated with developmental delay, particularly if it occurs during the first year of life when brain growth is maximal.

Differential Diagnosis

FTT may result from inadequate caloric intake, excessive caloric losses, or increased caloric requirements. **Most cases of FTT in developed countries are nonorganic (or psychosocial) in origin**; that is, there is no coexistent medical disorder. Neglect is a common form of psychosocial FTT. The list of organic diagnoses predisposing to FTT is extensive, and virtually all organ systems are represented (Table 4-2). **Organic** FTT virtually never presents with isolated growth failure; other signs and symptoms are generally evident with a detailed history and physical examination.

Clinical Manifestations

History

The caretaker must be questioned in detail about the child's diet, including how often the child eats, how much is consumed at each feeding, what the child is fed, how the formula is prepared, and who feeds the child. Information regarding diarrhea, fatty stools, irritability, vomiting, food refusal, ability to vigorously complete a feeding, and polyuria should be documented. Recurrent infections suggest congenital or acquired immunodeficiency. Constitutional growth delay can usually be diagnosed by family history alone. Foreign and domestic travel, source of water, and developmental delay are occasionally overlooked topics. The psychosocial history includes questions concerning the caretaker's expectations of the child, parental and sibling health, financial security, recent major life events, and chronic stressors.

Physical Examination

Weight, height, and head circumference should be recorded on an appropriate growth chart. Relatively recent growth failure is usually limited to weight alone, whereas height and (later) head circumference are also affected in chronic deficiency. Severely deprived children may present with lethargy, edema, scant subcutaneous fat, atrophic muscle tissue, decreased skin turgor, coarsened hair, dermatitis, and distended abdomen.

Observation of caretaker–child interactions and feeding behavior is critical. Children who are listless, minimally responsive to the examiner and/or caretaker, withdrawn, or excessively fearful often have contributing psychosocial issues. Findings suggestive of physical abuse or neglect (see Chapter 21) should be sought and documented.

A complete physical examination, with careful attention for dysmorphism, pallor, bruising, cleft palate, rales or crackles, heart murmurs, and muscle tone may suggest the etiology.

TABLE 4-2 Differential Diagnosis of FTT

Nonorganic	
Neglect	Inadequate amount fed
Abuse	Incorrect preparation of formula
Cardiac	
Congenital heart malformations	
Gastrointestinal	
Malabsorption	Inflammatory bowel disease
Cow milk–protein intolerance/allergy	Celiac disease
Gastroesophageal reflux	Hirschsprung disease
Pyloric stenosis	
Pulmonary	
Cystic fibrosis	Chronic aspiration
Bronchopulmonary dysplasia	Respiratory insufficiency
Infectious	
HIV	Intestinal parasites
Tuberculosis	Urinary tract infection
Chronic gastroenteritis	
Neonatal	
Prematurity	Congenital or perinatal infection
Low birth weight	Congenital syndromes
Endocrine	
Diabetes mellitus	Adrenal insufficiency or excess
Hypothyroidism	Growth hormone deficiency
Neurologic	
Cerebral palsy	Degenerative disorders
Mental retardation	Oral-motor dysfunction
Renal	
Renal tubular acidosis	Chronic renal insufficiency
Other	
Inborn errors of metabolism	Immunodeficiency syndromes
Malignancy	Collagen vascular disease
Cleft palate	

Diagnostic Evaluation

Information obtained from the history and physical examination determines the direction of further diagnostic workup. Any child with FTT should receive a complete blood count, serum electrolytes, blood urea nitrogen and creatinine, protein and albumin measurements, urinalysis, and urine culture. Bone age films may also be helpful in children beyond infancy. Severely malnourished children and patients with suspected nonorganic FTT should be admitted to the hospital. Adequate catch-up growth during hospitalization on a regular diet is virtually diagnostic of psychosocial FTT.

OBESITY

When a pediatric patient's BMI is greater than the 95th percentile for age, that individual is considered **obese**. A child whose BMI falls between the 85th and 95th percentiles is considered **overweight**. According to the most recent US National Health and Nutrition Examination Survey, about 17% of 2- to 19-year-old children are obese and 32% of all children are overweight. A period of adipose cell proliferation occurs from age 2 to 4 years and again during puberty, placing pediatricians in an ideal position to affect their patients' health well into adulthood.

Clinical Manifestations

While the root cause is simply caloric intake in excess of expenditure, several factors contribute to the risk of becoming obese, including genetic, parental, family, and lifestyle issues (Table 4-3). Therefore, it is critical to obtain a detailed history and perform a complete physical examination. The history should consist of a thorough review of systems and relevant family history. In addition, the social history should include not only dietary history but also activities and self-esteem. The social and psychological consequences of being a "fat" child may be particularly damaging to self-esteem at a critical age. Weight-for-length or BMI should be calculated, and blood pressure should be obtained. A physical examination should be completed to screen for comorbidities, although obese patients of normal or above-average height are unlikely to have a predisposing health condition.

TABLE 4-3 Risk Factors for Obesity in Children
Overweight parent(s)
Large birth weight
Diabetic mother
Low parental education level
Poverty
Overweight child at age 3 y
Increased length of TV viewing
Poor dietary choices
Lower activity levels

Diagnostic Evaluation

Although there are no universally accepted current guidelines, if there is a clinical suspicion or strong family history of comorbidities, a laboratory workup should be considered. This would include a fasting lipid protein analysis and metabolic profile with fasting glucose, liver, and renal function tests. The workup of the short obese child should include consideration of endocrine disorders (hypothyroidism, Cushing syndrome), genetic syndromes, and hypothalamic tumors.

Complications

Metabolic syndrome is the combination of **obesity, hypertension, insulin resistance, and dyslipidemia** (increased triglycerides, decreased HDL levels, and relatively high levels of abnormally dense LDL particles). Rates of type 2 diabetes, cardiovascular disease, and fatty liver disease are increased in patients with metabolic syndrome. Other potential complications of obesity include depression, hypertension, obstructive sleep apnea, gallbladder disease, slipped capital femoral epiphysis, and early onset puberty in females.

Treatment

Obesity is treated by setting reasonable goals for the patient, by altering caloric intake/dietary habits, developing a regular exercise program, decreasing screen time (television, video games, computers), and behavioral modification (setting limits and monitoring self-control). Careful attention must be paid to maintaining patients' growth and development while at the same time decreasing their BMI over time. Surgical options and appetite suppressants are currently considered inappropriate for use in the pediatric population.

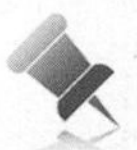

KEY POINTS

- The American Academy of Pediatrics recommends exclusive breastfeeding during the first 6 months of life, with continued breastfeeding through age 12 months.
- Exclusively breastfed infants should be supplemented with 400 IU vitamin D beginning in the first week of life.
- Newborns initially lose weight, but should ultimately gain in weight back to birthweight by the third week of life.
- Cow milk–protein intolerance can result in colitis and FTT.
- The sporadic nature and sudden onset of colic usually distinguish this condition from feeding intolerance.
- The healthy formula-fed infant with presumed cow milk–protein intolerance should be switched to a protein hydrolysate formula rather than one formulated with soy protein.
- Most cases of FTT in developed countries are due wholly or in large part to neglect.
- Children with BMIs greater than the 85th percentile for age are considered overweight.
- Metabolic syndrome (obesity, insulin resistance, dyslipidemia, and hypertension) increases the risk for development of type 2 diabetes and cardiovascular disease.

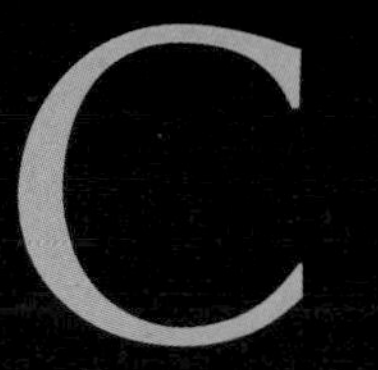

Clinical Vignettes

Vignette 1

A 6-day-old term newborn comes to your office for a well-child check. The infant had no problems at birth and was released from the hospital with his mother. His birth weight was 2.5 kg. The mother is exclusively breastfeeding every 1 to 2 hours and each feeding takes approximately 30 minutes. She feels that her milk has come in and believes the breast empties after each feed. Today, the infant appears well with normal stools and urine output. His weight today is 2.37 kg. This is the mother's first child and she has several questions.

1. The mother is concerned that her baby has lost weight since birth. How can this best be explained?
- **a.** The infant is not receiving enough milk and the mother needs to breastfeed more often
- **b.** The infant is not receiving enough milk and the mother needs to supplement with formula
- **c.** The infant is not receiving enough milk and the mother needs to feed for a longer period of time
- **d.** The infant is feeding appropriately, and there is no reason to be concerned at this time

2. The mother has always heard that breastfeeding is best. She wonders if she needs to supplement her breast milk with anything at this time. What would most likely be your response?
- **a.** The infant does not need any supplements
- **b.** The infant needs 400 IU of vitamin D daily
- **c.** The infant needs meats, fruits, and vegetables three times a day
- **d.** The infant should be supplemented with formula

3. The mother returns at the infant's 2-month visit. She returned to work and stopped breastfeeding 2 weeks ago. She is feeding the infant formula, but is concerned because she noticed streaks of blood in his stool. Otherwise, the infant has been well, and the mother has no other concerns. You suspect milk-protein intolerance. What would most likely be your recommendation at this time?
- **a.** Start breastfeeding again
- **b.** Replace the infant's formula with a soy-based formula
- **c.** Replace the infant's formula with a protein hydrolysate formula
- **d.** Replace the infant's formula with cow's milk

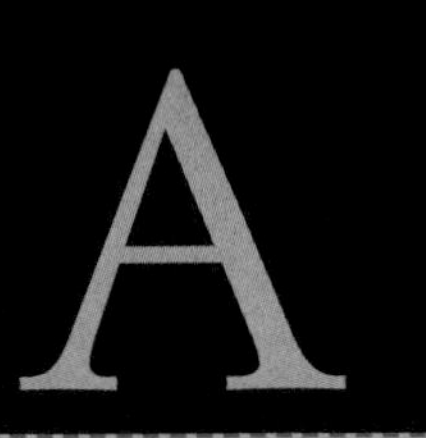

Answers

Vignette 1 Question 1

Answer D: In this case, the mother appears to be feeding the infant normally. Neonates typically lose up to 10% of their birth weight over the first several days; formula-fed babies regain that weight by the second week of life, whereas breastfed babies may take about a week longer.

Healthy infants automatically regulate intake to meet caloric demand for basic metabolism and growth. Typically, infants feed on demand every 1 to 2 hours. This mother is feeding her infant in this manner. Thirty minutes is sufficient time to empty milk from breasts. In general, there are very few indications to supplement breast milk with formula. As previously noted, this infant's weight is within a normal range for his age, and the mother is breastfeeding appropriately.

Vignette 1 Question 2

Answer B: All infants require supplementation of vitamin D to prevent rickets. The recommended value is 400 IU of vitamin daily. This is almost always added to infant formulas; however, exclusively breastfed infants require supplementation from birth.

Additional foods should not be added until 4 to 6 months of age, when the infant may begin to take baby food (cereal, vegetables, fruits, and meats) by spoon. The infant is not developmentally ready to coordinate swallowing solid foods until this time. Finger food is added around 9 months of age. As previously noted, this infant is sufficiently fed, and does not require supplemental formula.

Vignette 1 Question 3

Answer C: The infant's history suggests milk-protein intolerance, given that his symptoms started after beginning infant formula. The first-line treatment is replacing the infant's formula with protein hydrolysate formula.

Infants who are being breastfed exclusively can sometimes show signs of milk-protein intolerance if the mother ingests milk products. Even if the mother was not ingesting milk products, she quit breastfeeding several weeks ago. Breastfeeding requires a demand to make a supply, and it is likely that the mother is no longer able to produce milk. Soy-based formulas are not the recommended treatment for milk-protein intolerance. Many patients with milk-protein intolerance also have an intolerance to soy protein. Cow's milk is also not an option, as this is what is causing the intolerance. In babies without cow milk protein allergy, regular cow's milk (rather than formula) is started at age 1 year.

Chapter 5 Fluid, Electrolyte, and pH Management

Kevin S. Carter • Katie S. Fine

Electrolyte homeostasis, **fluid distribution**, and **pH balance** are critical to the maintenance of normal physiology. Organs that provide compensation for disturbances in these systems are less effective in pediatric patients due to their relative immaturity, especially infants. The younger the patient, the more intolerant he or she is to challenges to these systems.

At birth, free water accounts for 90% of body weight, due largely to proportionally higher extracellular fluid (ECF) volume. Body composition changes dramatically over the first year of life as muscle mass increases. By 1 year of age, a child's total body water (TBW) approaches the adult level of 60% body weight.

MAINTENANCE FLUIDS

Fluid losses may be categorized as either sensible or insensible. Sensible losses include water and solute lost from urine, stool, and other measurable losses. Unmeasurable losses from skin and lungs are classified as insensible; these are relatively consistent from day to day. Insensible losses can be estimated at 400 mL/m^2 body surface area per day.

The amount of fluid needed to maintain normal body function is directly related to caloric expenditure, which in turn is related to a child's weight. The **Holliday-Segar method** is useful for approximating daily maintenance fluids: 100 mL/kg/day for the first 10 kg, plus 50 mL/kg/day for the next 10 kg, plus 20 mL/kg/day for each additional kilogram thereafter. The "4-2-1 rule" is often more practical to calculate an hourly rate: 4 mL/kg/hr (first 10 kg body weight), 2 mL/kg/hr (second 10 kg body weight), 1 mL/kg/hr (each additional kilogram).

An example of calculating maintenance fluid requirements for a 22-kg child follows:

Daily rate: (100 mL/kg/day × 10 kg) + (50 mL/kg/day × 10 kg) + (20 mL/kg/day × 2 kg) = 1,540 mL/day

Hourly rate: 1,540 mL/day ÷ 24 hr/day = 64 mL/hr

"4-2-1" Short-cut method: (4 mL/hr × 10 kg) + (2 mL/hr × 10 kg) + (1 mL/hr × 2 kg) = 62 mL/hr

For each 100 mL of maintenance fluids, a child needs 3 mEq of sodium and 2 mEq of potassium, as well as a carbohydrate source (dextrose). For the example above, the child would require 46 mEq of sodium (3 mEq × 1,540 mL/100) and 31 mEq of potassium (2 mEq × 1,540 mL/100). In general, one-fourth normal saline with 5% dextrose (10% in infants) and 20 mEq/L KCl meets maintenance electrolyte needs and provides enough calories to prevent catabolism for several days. One-half normal saline with 5% dextrose and 20 mEq/L KCl is often used in adolescents and adults, although this provides more sodium than is required for maintenance needs.

DEHYDRATION

Dehydration in the pediatric patient is usually secondary to acute losses, typically from **vomiting** and/or **diarrhea**. Infants and toddlers are particularly susceptible because of the limited ability of the immature kidney to conserve water and electrolytes and because of the child's dependence on caretakers to meet his or her needs. When addressing dehydration, it is important to consider **maintenance fluid** needs as well as **replacement** of the initial deficit and **ongoing losses**.

Clinical Manifestations

History

A careful history limits the differential diagnosis list and provides information concerning the acuity, source, and quantity of fluid lost, all of which influence treatment. Recent **weight loss** and **decreased urine output** are important benchmarks of the degree of deficiency. The color, consistency, frequency, and volume of stool and/or emesis may influence initial diagnostic and therapeutic measures.

Many chronic medical illnesses may present acutely with dehydration, including diabetes, metabolic disorders, cystic fibrosis, and congenital adrenal hyperplasia. Polyuria in the presence of physical signs of dehydration may indicate diabetes mellitus, diabetes insipidus, or renal tubular acidosis. Children who are neglected or refuse to drink because of severe oropharyngeal pain may also become significantly dehydrated.

Physical Examination

There is no single physical or laboratory finding that will accurately assess a patient's degree of dehydration (Table 5-1). It is important to remember that a child's primary initial mechanism of compensation for decreased plasma volume is **tachycardia**. **Hypotension**, a sensitive early indicator in adults, is a very late and ominous finding in children.

TABLE 5-1 Clinical Estimation of Degree of Dehydration[a]

	Mild	Moderate	Severe
Weight loss (%)	<5	5–10	>10
1. Vital signs			
Heart rate	Increased	Increased	Greatly increased
Respiratory rate	Normal	Normal	Increased
Blood pressure	Normal	Normal (orthostasis)	Decreased
2. Skin			
Capillary refill (s)	<2	2–3	>3
Mucous membranes	Normal/dry	Dry	Dry
Anterior fontanelle	Normal	Depressed	Depressed
3. Eyes			
Tearing	Normal/absent	Absent	Absent
Appearance	Normal	Sunken	Sunken
Mental status	Normal	Altered	Depressed
4. Lab values			
Urine osmolarity	600 mOsm/L	800 mOsm/L	Maximal
Urine specific gravity	1.020	1.025	Maximal
Blood urea nitrogen	<20	Elevated	High
Blood pH	Normal	Mildly acidotic	Moderate/profound acidosis
Stage of shock	Not in shock	Compensated shock	Uncompensated shock

[a]Infants will exhibit greater weight loss per degree of dehydration (5% mild, 10% moderate, 15% severe), whereas adolescents will exhibit less weight loss per degree of dehydration (3% mild, 5% to 6% moderate, 7% to 9% severe).

Diagnostic Evaluation

Serum electrolyte levels help guide the *choice* of fluid composition and *rate* of replacement. Dehydration may be isotonic, hypotonic (hyponatremic), or hypertonic (hypernatremic), depending on the nature of the fluid lost and the replacement fluids provided by the caretaker.

Isotonic dehydration is the most common form and suggests that either compensation has occurred or that water losses roughly parallel sodium losses. **Hypotonic (hyponatremic) dehydration** is defined by a serum sodium <130 mEq/L. Children who lose electrolytes in their stool and are supplemented with free water or very dilute juices may present in this manner. **Hypertonic (hypernatremic) dehydration** (Na ≥150 mEq/L) is uncommon in children, but implies an excessive loss of free water compared with electrolyte loss (e.g., diabetes insipidus). Of note, patients with hyponatremic dehydration tend to appear more dehydrated than they truly are, while those with hypernatremic dehydration may not appear as clinically compromised because intravascular volume is preserved.

Other electrolyte and osmotic abnormalities are frequently present in dehydration states. Usually, the serum bicarbonate concentration is decreased secondary to metabolic acidosis from relative underperfusion and generation of lactate. Conditions with bicarbonate losses will result in acidosis with a normal anion gap (see **Metabolic Acidosis** below). Conversely, protracted vomiting may result in metabolic alkalosis and a high bicarbonate level due to acid lost from gastric secretions (see **Metabolic Alkalosis** below). With significant dehydration, perfusion of the kidneys may be impaired. This will be reflected in elevations of the serum blood urea nitrogen (BUN) and creatinine (Cr) levels as glomerular filtration rate falls. A BUN/Cr ratio >20 is consistent with intravascular depletion and prerenal failure.

Treatment

Oral rehydration therapy (ORT) is the preferred treatment for mild-to-moderate dehydration. The World Health Organization recommends that ORT solutions contain 90 mEq/L sodium, 20 mEq/L potassium, and 20 g/L glucose. Commercial preparations that approximate these concentrations are available. Free water may precipitate hyponatremia and is contraindicated. ORT is particularly labor intensive, requiring small volumes of fluid given very frequently, particularly in the child with nausea and vomiting. Administered correctly, it is extremely effective.

Severe dehydration leads to life-threatening **hypovolemic shock**. Children in hypovolemic shock should receive 20 mL/kg intravenous (IV) boluses of isotonic fluid (normal saline or Ringer's lactate) until their blood pressure normalizes (see Chapter 20). Both fluids are isotonic, resulting in improved intravascular volume without fluid shifts. Clinical estimation of degree of dehydration and serum electrolyte studies tailor subsequent management.

Most **deficits** are replaced over 24 hours, with half given in the first 8 hours and the rest over the next 16 hours. One notable exception is the child with hypernatremic dehydration, in whom the deficit should be replaced over 48 to 72 hours to prevent excessive fluid shifts and cerebral edema. **Ongoing losses** (usually in stool) are replaced milliliter for milliliter with IV fluid comparable in electrolyte content to that being lost.

For example, an 18-kg infant with a normal serum sodium who is judged to be 10% dehydrated has lost an estimated 2,000 mL of fluid (1,000 mL = 1 kg). Half the deficit is replaced over the first 8 hours, with the balance given over the next 16 hours. Maintenance therapy must also be included. The child received a 20-mL/kg bolus initially.

1. 2,000 mL ÷ 2 = 1,000 mL (one-half the total deficit); 360 mL (20 mL/kg) has already been replaced. Therefore, 640 mL is given over the first 8 hours at 80 mL/hr. This should be added to the 56 mL/hr the child requires to meet maintenance needs. Rate = 80 mL/hr + 56 mL/hr = 136 mL/hr.
2. The second half (1,000 mL) is replaced over the next 16 hours (63 mL/hr) along with the maintenance rate (56 mL/hr). Rate = 63 mL/hr + 56 mL/hr = 119 mL/hr.

The composition of the **replacement fluid** varies depending on the initial laboratory values. Intravenous fluid should not contain potassium until the patient urinates. Replacement of bicarbonate may be indicated if there is a known loss of bicarbonate or if the pH and serum bicarbonate levels remain dangerously low after initial isotonic boluses. In general, ongoing gastrointestinal losses are replaced with one-half normal saline. Urine electrolyte and osmolality studies should be obtained if ongoing losses result from an abnormal renal process.

Patients with profound hyperglycemia or electrolyte disturbances due to an ongoing underlying pathologic process (e.g., diabetic ketoacidosis [DKA]) may require more specialized management discussed elsewhere in this text.

HYPONATREMIA

Hyponatremia (serum sodium level <130 mEq/L) may occur in the face of decreased, normal, or increased total body sodium content, reflected in the volume status of the patient. In children, the most common setting is **dehydration**, a hypovolemic state. Euvolemic causes include syndrome of inappropriate secretion of antidiuretic hormone (SIADH), adrenal insufficiency, and excessive free water intake (as can be seen with dilution of infant formula). Chronic renal insufficiency, congestive heart failure, and cirrhosis are volume-expanded states associated with hyponatremia.

Clinical Manifestations

History and Physical Examination

The severity of clinical manifestations depends on both the **level of sodium** in the extracellular space and the **rate of change** from normal. Falling levels that occur over several days are better tolerated than rapid losses. Anorexia and nausea are early, nonspecific complaints. Neurologic findings include confusion, lethargy, and decreased deep tendon reflexes. **Seizures** and **respiratory arrest** are late, life-threatening complications which are more likely to be present as serum sodium falls below 125 mEq/L.

Diagnostic Evaluation

The laboratory workup of hyponatremia should include serum electrolytes, glucose, BUN and Cr, serum osmolality, liver function tests, protein, and lipid levels. Urine studies can also be helpful, particularly specific gravity and urine sodium and Cr concentrations. These laboratory values quantitate the severity of the deficit and may suggest an underlying cause. The measured serum sodium needs to be "corrected" in the setting of hyperglycemia. For every 100 mg/dL rise in glucose above a normal blood glucose of 100 mg/dL, 1.6 mEq Na must be added to the *measured* value to get the *true* serum sodium.

Treatment

Dehydration is treated with fluid resuscitation as discussed previously, with additional attention to the replacement of the sodium deficit. Hyponatremia due to normal or increased TBW states such as SIADH or renal failure requires fluid restriction and treatment of the underlying disorder. Adrenal insufficiency is treated with fluid resuscitation and stress-dose hydrocortisone. The cautious use of 3% hypertonic saline is limited to life-threatening situations (i.e., intractable seizures). Serum sodium correction should not exceed 1 to 2 mEq/L/hr because of the risk of central-pontine myelinolysis.

HYPERNATREMIA

Hypernatremia is uncommon in children in the absence of dehydration. The infant with congenital diabetes insipidus frequently presents in this manner. Either the lack of antidiuretic hormone (ADH) or the kidney's inability to respond to the hormone results in inappropriately dilute urine and excessive free water loss. Signs and symptoms include muscle irritability, weakness, and lethargy. Seizures and coma are the major complications. Hypernatremic dehydration is treated with infusion of isotonic saline. Serum sodium correction should not exceed 1 to 2 mEq/L/hr due to the risk of cerebral edema.

HYPERKALEMIA

Normal serum potassium values range from 3.5 to 5.7 mEq/L; a measurement of 5.8 mEq/L or greater is considered **hyperkalemia**. In children, the most common cause of an abnormally high potassium level is artifactual hyperkalemia, due to hemolysis of red cells during sample collection. Transcellular shifts in hydrogen ions increase serum potassium without changing total body content; for every unit reduction in arterial pH, plasma potassium increases 0.2 to 0.4 mEq/L. Disorders and medications that interfere with renal excretion of the electrolyte precipitate true hyperkalemia.

Differential Diagnosis

Common causes of hyperkalemia include the following:

- Acidosis
- Severe dehydration
- Potassium-sparing diuretics (spironolactone)
- Excessive parenteral infusion
- Renal failure

Other less common but important conditions to consider include the following:

- Adrenal corticoid deficiency (i.e., Addison disease)
- Renal tubular acidosis

- Massive crush injury with rhabdomyolysis
- β-blocker or digitalis ingestions
- Excessive supplementation

Clinical Manifestations

Paresthesias and weakness are the earliest symptoms; flaccid paralysis and tetany occur late. Cardiac involvement produces specific progressive **ECG changes**; T-wave elevation ("peaking") is followed by loss of P waves, widening QRS complexes, and ST segment depression (see Fig. 5-1). Ventricular fibrillation and cardiac arrest occur at serum levels >9 mEq/L.

Treatment

True hyperkalemia represents a medical emergency. **Calcium gluconate** infusion protects the heart by stabilizing the myocyte cell membrane. Infusion of sodium bicarbonate or insulin (and glucose) drives potassium into the cells. Hyperventilation prompts the transfer of hydrogen ions out of the cell in exchange for potassium ions, effectively lowering the serum potassium. Cation exchange resins (e.g., Kayexylate) and hemodialysis are the only measures that actually remove potassium from the body.

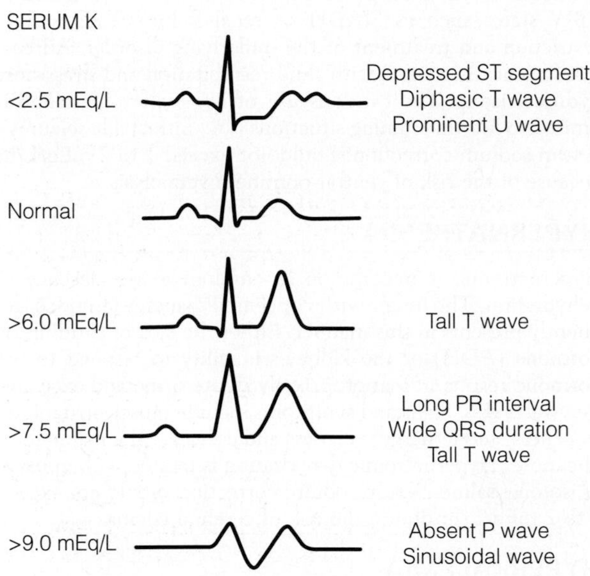

Figure 5-1 • ECG findings consistent with hyperkalemia (Lead II).

HYPOKALEMIA

Hypokalemia in the pediatric population is usually encountered in the setting of alkalosis secondary to vomiting, administration of loop diuretics (furosemide), or DKA. Signs and symptoms include weakness, tetany, constipation, polyuria, and polydipsia. Muscle breakdown leading to myoglobinuria may compromise renal function. ECG changes (prolonged Q-T interval, T-wave flattening) are noted at levels ≤2.5 mEq/L; cardiac arrhythmias (ventricular tachycardia/fibrillation) can occur and are more likely if the patient is being treated with digoxin. Blood pressure changes and urine electrolyte content assist in diagnosis (Fig. 5-2). Treatment consists of correcting pH (when increased) and replenishing potassium stores orally or intravenously.

CALCIUM AND MAGNESIUM HOMEOSTASIS

Calcium has several different functions in the body, ranging from key roles in intracellular signaling and muscle contraction to providing the mineral matrix of the skeleton. Calcium regulation and associated disorders are discussed in detail in Chapter 14.

Like calcium, **magnesium (Mg)** is a divalent cation found both intracellularly and in the serum, as well as complexed within the skeletal system. Mg is frequently used as a cofactor in several enzymatic processes, notably those involved with use and generation of adenosine triphosphate (ATP). It also plays a role in membrane potential, making it important in neuromuscular and cardiovascular function. Normal serum Mg is typically 1.6 to 2.4 mg/dL, though about two-thirds of total

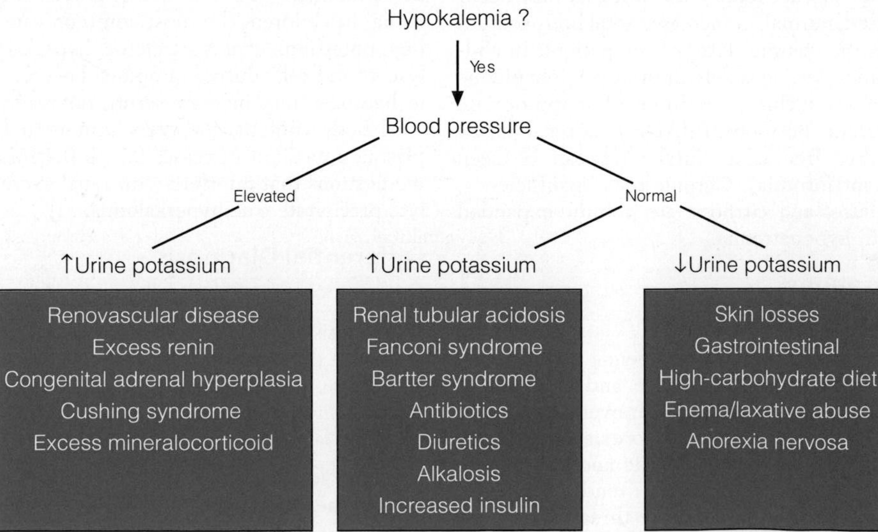

Figure 5-2 • Evaluation of hypokalemia.

body Mg is stored within bone, where it is available for release when needed.

Hypomagnesemia can be a result of inadequate intake or absorption or increased renal losses. Depletion of magnesium frequently leads to both hypocalcemia and hypokalemia. Thus, signs of hypomagnesemia can include neuromuscular irritability and tetany normally associated with hypocalcemia. ECG changes such as flattened T waves and a widened QRS complex can be seen. Careful review of the patient's history and measurement of serum and urine electrolytes can aid in the diagnosis of the underlying cause, and replacement therapy is then tailored according to whether the problem is acute or chronic in nature.

The kidney is able to excrete excess Mg easily, making hypermagnesemia a relatively uncommon problem provided renal function is normal. Infants born to mothers receiving Mg therapy for preeclampsia or tocolysis frequently show signs of hypermagnesemia at delivery, including muscle weakness, respiratory depression, and lethargy. Intravenous calcium infusion may help mitigate symptoms of hypermagnesemia, but in cases of toxic overload or renal failure hemodialysis may be necessary.

ACID/BASE PHYSIOLOGY

The ECF **pH** (the negative logarithm of the hydrogen ion concentration) is maintained in a very narrow range (normal 7.4), largely as a result of the **bicarbonate buffer system**. Hydrogen ions (H^+) combine with bicarbonate (HCO_3^-) to form H_2CO_3, which is transformed into water and CO_2 (carbon dioxide). Maintenance of the molecular components of this buffer system is performed by the *kidneys*, which control excretion of HCO_3^-, and the *lungs*, which expire CO_2. The physiologic responses to challenges of acid/base equilibrium is termed **compensation**.The addition or production of excessive H^+, the loss of HCO_3^-, or abnormal renal or pulmonary function can all affect this buffering system and lead to acid–base disturbances.

METABOLIC ACIDOSIS

Metabolic acidosis (pH ≤7.35) results from the loss of HCO_3^- *or* the addition of H^+ in the ECF. It is the most common acid–base disorder encountered in the pediatric population. Causes include increased acid intake or production, decreased renal excretion of acid, and increased renal or gastrointestinal bicarbonate loss. Respiratory compensation begins almost immediately as $PaCO_2$ falls due to increased ventilation; maximal compensation is complete within 24 hours. In the presence of a metabolic acidosis, the expected $PaCO_2 = 1.5 \times HCO_3^- + 8\ (\pm 2)$. If the measured $PaCO_2$ is higher than expected, then there is a concurrent primary respiratory acidosis. If it is lower than expected, there is a concurrent primary respiratory alkalosis (see Respiratory Acidosis and Alkalosis section).

Clinical Manifestations

Hyperpnea is the most consistent clinical finding in metabolic acidosis, as demonstrated by Kussmaul breathing in DKA. Severe acidemia affects multiple organ systems: cardiac contractility is impaired, cardiac output is reduced, and the heart becomes vulnerable to arrhythmias. Protein breakdown is accelerated, and mental status changes occur. Other signs and symptoms are specific to the underlying disorder. Important laboratory studies include serum electrolytes, BUN, Cr, glucose, venous or arterial blood gas, and urine dipstick for pH and glucose. These studies help quantify the acidosis and may suggest the causative condition. The difference between the sums of the measured cations ($Na^+ + K^+$) and anions ($Cl^- + HCO_3^-$), termed the **anion gap**, is normally 12 ± 4; Table 5-2 lists conditions associated with changes in the anion gap. A normal anion gap in the setting of acidosis suggests gastrointestinal losses of HCO_3^- or renal wasting, as in the case of renal tubular acidosis.

Treatment

Management of the child with metabolic acidosis is tailored to correction of the underlying cause, especially in cases with an elevated anion gap. Sodium bicarbonate therapy should be reserved for extreme cases in which the serum pH is <7.0 and the cause is unknown or slow to reverse (i.e., many forms of normal anion gap acidosis). Boluses of sodium bicarbonate are reserved for extreme situations; in general, the infusion should be slow and relatively isotonic. Patients receiving alkali therapy require frequent monitoring of blood pH, sodium, potassium, and calcium. Complications include alkalosis

TABLE 5-2 Changes in the Anion Gap

Increased Anion Gap[a]	Normal Anion Gap	Decreased Anion Gap
Hypokalemia	Diarrhea	Hyperkalemia
Hypocalcemia	Renal tubular acidosis	Hypercalcemia
Hypomagnesemia	Hyperalimentation	Hypermagnesemia
Hyperphosphatemia	Hypoaldosteronism	Hypoalbuminemia
Lactic acidosis	Lithium ingestion	
Diabetic ketoacidosis		
Renal failure/uremia		
Salicylate ingestion		
Ethylene glycol, ethanol, methanol ingestion		

[a]The mnemonic **MUDPILES** is helpful for recalling several clinical conditions that result in metabolic acidosis with a high anion gap: **m**ethanol ingestion; **u**remia; **d**iabetic ketoacidosis; **p**araldehyde ingestion; **i**soniazid ingestion, **i**ron ingestion, and **i**nborn errors of metabolism; **l**actic acidosis; **e**thanol or **e**thylene glycol ingestion; and **s**alicylate ingestion.

(overcorrection), hypokalemia, hypernatremia/hyperosmolarity, and hypocalcemia.

METABOLIC ALKALOSIS

Metabolic alkalosis (pH ≥7.45) is much less common than acidosis in children. "Contraction" alkalosis results from the loss of fluid high in H^+ or Cl^-, as may occur with protracted gastric vomiting (pyloric stenosis, bulimia) or chronic thiazide or loop diuretic administration. Patients with cystic fibrosis may develop metabolic alkalosis due to excessive chloride losses in the sweat. Other causes include laxative abuse and other chloride-wasting diarrheas.

Diagnosis and resolution of the underlying disorder guide management decisions. Volume expansion and chloride replacement correct the alkalosis unless it results from disorders of mineralocorticoid excess (e.g., renal artery stenosis, adrenal disorders, steroid use); potassium supplements are also necessary in these cases. Complications of severe alkalosis include reduction in coronary blood flow and arrhythmias, hypoventilation, seizures, and decreased potassium, magnesium, and phosphate levels.

RESPIRATORY ACIDOSIS AND ALKALOSIS

Normal $PaCO_2$ levels range from 35 to 45 mm Hg. Any process that causes respiratory insufficiency (central nervous system [CNS] depression, chest wall muscle weakness, pulmonary or cardiopulmonary diseases) results in CO_2 retention and a primary elevation in the $PaCO_2$, termed respiratory acidosis. The kidney responds by generating new bicarbonate in the collecting duct and distal tubule, producing a rise in the serum bicarbonate measurement (compensatory metabolic alkalosis). This process is slower than the respiratory compensation that occurs in metabolic acidosis, taking several days to complete. Thus, severe acidosis due to acute respiratory failure may require ventilatory support.

Respiratory alkalosis results from a primary reduction in the $PaCO_2$, typically as a result of increased ventilation. Common etiologies include hypoxia, restrictive lung disease, medications (particularly aspirin toxicity), and CNS abnormalities that result in an elevated respiratory rate. The kidney responds by increasing the urine bicarbonate concentration (compensatory metabolic acidosis). Management consists mainly of identifying and treating the underlying cause.

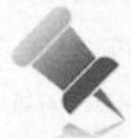

KEY POINTS

- Tachycardia is an early sign of dehydration in children. Hypotension occurs very late in children, and its absence does not rule out significant dehydration requiring intervention.
- If IV fluids are required, initial 20 mL/kg boluses of normal saline or Ringer's lactate should be given until the patient's condition stabilizes.
- In the dehydrated child unable to take fluids by mouth, the fluid and electrolyte deficit must be replaced, in addition to providing daily maintenance fluid and the replacement of ongoing losses.
- Potassium should not be added to replacement or maintenance fluids until urine output is assured.
- Hyponatremia in the pediatric patient is most frequently due to dehydration; other causes include SIADH, water intoxication, renal or heart failure, and adrenal insufficiency.
- Serum sodium levels need to be "corrected" in the setting of hyperglycemia.
- Neither hyponatremia nor hypernatremia should be corrected too quickly due to the risk of severe central nervous system complications.
- Progressive ECG changes associated with hyperkalemia include peaked T waves, loss of P waves, and widening of the QRS complex.
- Emergent treatment for life-threatening hyperkalemia includes hyperventilation and calcium gluconate, sodium bicarbonate, and/or insulin/glucose infusion.
- The equation $PaCO_2 = 1.5 \times HCO_3^- + 8\ (\pm 2)$ can help distinguish between primary and secondary metabolic acidosis.
- An increased respiratory rate is the most consistent physical finding in metabolic acidosis.
- Intravenous $NaHCO_3$ (sodium bicarbonate) should be used only when acidosis is severe or difficult to correct.

C Clinical Vignettes

Vignette 1

A 2-month-old female infant is brought to the emergency department for lethargy. The baby was born at term and has been in good health until today. There has been no fever or other sign of infection. Upon reviewing the family's social situation you discover that they have recently become homeless and are "stretching out" the infant's powdered formula to make it last longer. She weighs 5.5 kg (75th percentile). On physical examination, she is thin and difficult to arouse. She is tachycardic but has brisk capillary refill and does not appear dehydrated. Her muscle tone is noticeably diminished with decreased deep tendon reflexes.

1. Which of the following is a good estimate of this infant's daily fluid and electrolyte requirements?
   a. 220 mL water, 16.5 mEq sodium, 11 mEq potassium
   b. 220 mL water, 6.6 mEq sodium, 4.4 mEq potassium
   c. 550 mL water, 16.5 mEq sodium, 11 mEq potassium
   d. 550 mL water, 6.6 mEq sodium, 4.4 mEq potassium
   e. 1,100 mL water, 33 mEq sodium, 22 mEq potassium

2. You ask the mother to clarify how she is preparing the formula and learn that she is diluting the formula to less than half its recommended concentration. Based on this information and the presentation of the baby, which of the following electrolyte abnormalities is most likely to be present?
   a. Hypocalcemia
   b. Hyperglycemia
   c. Hyponatremia
   d. Hypomagnesemia
   e. Hyperchloremia

3. The infant suddenly begins to have a generalized tonic-clonic seizure. You and the staff begin stabilization as laboratory results return: sodium 120 mEq/L, potassium 4.9 mEq/L, chloride 92 mEq/L, bicarbonate 18 mEq/L, calcium 9.4 mg/dL, magnesium 2.1 mEq/L, glucose 84 mg/dL. Which of the following is the most appropriate method for correcting the electrolyte deficit in this patient?
   a. Water restriction
   b. 2 mL/kg bolus of 10% dextrose in water
   c. Intravenous normal saline at maintenance rate over a 3- to 4-day period
   d. Administration of desmopressin
   e. Infusion of hypertonic saline

Vignette 2

A father brings his 18-month-old son to the emergency department with a chief complaint of vomiting. The child has had four bouts of emesis beginning this morning and has been able to take only a few sips of juice by mouth without vomiting. He has had no fever, but had one loose bowel movement just prior to arrival. His weight is 12 kg. On physical examination, you see an alert but tearful child. His heart rate is 110 beats per minute and blood pressure is 98/62 mm Hg. His oral mucosa is tacky, his diaper is wet, and his abdominal examination is unremarkable. After a thorough review of systems and physical examination, you feel he most likely has viral gastroenteritis.

1. Which of the following is the most appropriate initial approach to fluid and hydration management in this child?
   a. Water in small sips with a goal of 1.5 oz/hr
   b. Electrolyte solution in small sips with a goal of 1.5 oz/hr
   c. Electrolyte solution in small sips with a goal of 5 oz/hr
   d. Immediate intravenous (IV) access for fluid resuscitation
   e. Placement of a nasogastric tube for enteral feeding

2. Two days later, he returns to the emergency department with continued vomiting and now frequent watery diarrhea. He now weighs 10.8 kg, his heart rate is 145, and his blood pressure is 92/58. He has dry mucous membranes and his extremities are slightly mottled with capillary refill at about 3 to 4 seconds. Which of the following fluids and routes is most appropriate for initial management of this patient?
   a. Oral rehydration solution in small, frequent volumes
   b. One-half normal saline with 5% dextrose at 44 mL/hr
   c. One-half normal saline with 5% dextrose, 240 mL bolus
   d. 10% Dextrose in water, 240 mL bolus
   e. Normal saline, 240 mL bolus

3. You opt to continue this patient's fluid and electrolyte management with IV rehydration. You plan to replace half of his deficit over the first 8 hours and the second half over the next 16 hours. What fluid and rate will best replace his losses and account for maintenance needs for the first 8 hours?
   a. One-half normal saline with 20 mEq/L KCl and 5% dextrose, 45 mL/hr
   b. One-half normal saline with 40 mEq/L KCl and 5% dextrose, 90 mL/hr

c. One-half normal saline with 5% dextrose, 150 mL/hr
d. Normal saline with 10% dextrose, 90 mL/hr
e. Normal saline with 80 mEq KCl and 10% dextrose in water, 150 mL/hr

Vignette 3

You are called to examine a 6-year-old girl in the emergency department for a chief complaint of abdominal pain and fatigue. On taking the history from the parents, you learn that the child has had urinary frequency for several days, and today developed vague abdominal pain with nausea and vomiting. You note on entering the room that the child is sleeping deeply, but breathing rapidly at about 30 breaths per minute. On examination, you note tachycardia, delayed capillary refill, and dry mucous membranes and tell her parents she looks dehydrated. This surprises them, as they feel like "she is always drinking." A nurse brings you the girl's urinalysis results, which are strongly positive for glucose and ketones. You decide to confirm your diagnostic suspicion with further laboratory testing.

1. The electrolyte panel returns with the following results: sodium 132 mmol/L, potassium 5.0 mmol/L, chloride 104 mmol/L, bicarbonate 10 mmol/L. What is this child's anion gap?
   a. 4
   b. 8
   c. 15
   d. 23
   e. 42

2. An arterial blood gas is obtained, with the following results: pH 7.24, pCO_2 19 mmHg, bicarbonate 8 mEq/L, pO_2 95 mmHg. Which of the following best describes this child's acid–base status?
   a. Respiratory acidosis, compensated
   b. Metabolic acidosis, compensated
   c. Respiratory alkalosis, overcompensated
   d. Metabolic acidosis with concurrent respiratory acidosis
   e. Respiratory acidosis, uncompensated

3. A fingerstick blood glucose returns with a result of 400 mg/dL. What impact, if any, does this information have on the previously reported electrolyte results?
   a. The sodium is artificially low and should be corrected to a value of 137 mEq/L
   b. The sodium is artificially high and should be corrected to a value of 127 mEq/L
   c. The potassium is artificially high and should be corrected to a value of 2.5 mEq/L
   d. The bicarbonate is artificially low and should be corrected to a value of 16 mEq/L
   e. There is no effect on the previously reported results

Vignette 4

A 16-year-old male is admitted to the hospital with rhabdomyolysis after starting football practices. He had been having severe muscle pain for 3 days prior to presentation but did not tell his parent or coach for fear of losing his spot on the team. He had a particularly strenuous practice last night. He was brought to the emergency department this morning after finally telling his mother that he had voided only a small amount of urine, which was deep brown in color. He also complains of muscle tenderness, as well as weakness which seems much worse than the previous day. The patient's initial laboratory studies return with the following results: Sodium 136 mEq/L, potassium 7.3 mEq/L, chloride 104 mEq/L, bicarbonate 19 mEq/L, blood urea nitrogen (BUN) 38, Cr 2.8, glucose 138 mg/dL, calcium 8.4, magnesium 1.9 mEq/L, phosphate 5.1 mEq/L, CK (creatine kinase) 30,000.

1. Which of the following metabolic disturbances notable in this patient presents the greatest risk for immediate, life-threatening complications?
   a. Hyperglycemia
   b. Elevated Cr
   c. Hyperkalemia
   d. Hypocalcemia
   e. Hyperphosphatemia

2. You obtain an ECG which reveals tall, peaked T waves. The patient remains alert and without significant distress other than his pain and weakness. Which of the following is the most appropriate next step in his management?
   a. Infusion of calcium gluconate
   b. Administration of furosemide
   c. Infusion of sodium bicarbonate
   d. Immediate hemodialysis
   e. Consultation with a pediatric nephrologist

3. The patient's ECG normalizes after initial therapy. Of the following therapeutic options for managing hyperkalemia, which is the only intervention that will actually remove excess potassium from the body?
   a. Infusion of insulin and glucose
   b. Nebulized albuterol
   c. Infusion of sodium bicarbonate
   d. Infusion of calcium chloride
   e. Administration of a cation exchange resin

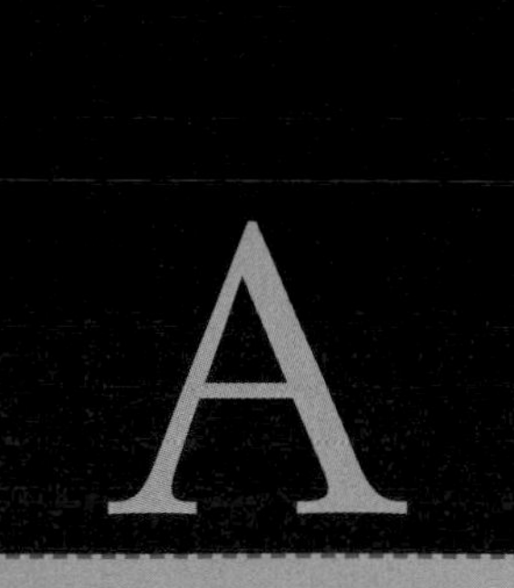

Answers

Vignette 1 Question 1
Answer C: Maintenance fluid requirements can be estimated based on body weight using the Holliday-Segar method. An individual requires 100 mL/kg/day for the first 10 kg of body weight, 50 mL/kg/day for the next 10 kg, and 20 mL/kg/day thereafter. This patient, weighing 5.5 kg, requires $100 \times 5.5 = 550$ mL daily. Sodium and potassium are estimated based on this fluid requirement. For every 100 mL fluid per day, 3 mEq sodium is required ($5.5 \times 3 = 16.5$) and 2 mEq potassium is required ($5.5 \times 2 = 11$).

Vignette 1 Question 2
Answer C: Dilution of formula is an unfortunate cause of hyponatremia in infants. The electrolyte imbalance results from a combination of immature kidney function and excessive free water intake. The symptoms of hyponatremia may be subtle but become more apparent as the deficit grows. Hypotonia and hyporeflexia are common. Lethargy (confusion in older children) may also be seen. Seizures and coma are late findings and imply a large sodium deficit.

Both hypocalcemia and hypomagnesemia are characterized by hyperreflexia and paresthesias. Hyperglycemia may go undetected in children and adults, with fatigue and polyuria being the most common signs. Hyperchloremia is typically asymptomatic and is either the result of concomitant hypernatremia or loss of bicarbonate (in the case of a metabolic acidosis with a normal anion gap).

Vignette 1 Question 3
Answer E: In cases of hyponatremia that have progressed to serious central nervous system symptoms, such as seizures or coma, the use of hypertonic saline to rapidly increase the serum sodium is indicated. Raising the serum sodium by 4 to 6 mEq will typically stop seizure activity. Correction should progress slowly from that point at a rate of about 10 mEq/day to avoid central pontine myelinolysis.

Water restriction is useful in treatment of hyponatremia resulting from syndrome of inappropriate secretion of antidiuretic hormone (SIADH) but not for a solute-depleted state as is presented here. Provision of dextrose intravenously is appropriate in symptomatic hypoglycemia, which can present with seizures, but this child's glucose level is normal. Slow correction over 2 to 3 days is a good strategy for managing hyponatremia without severe neurologic symptoms but will not acutely help this patient. Desmopressin (a synthetic form of antidiuretic hormone [ADH]) will decrease the sodium further as it increases water reabsorption in the renal collecting ducts.

Vignette 2 Question 1
Answer B: The child described in the vignette is certainly at risk for developing dehydration, but at this point he can only be described as mildly dehydrated. His vital signs are all within normal limits and he continues to produce tears and urine. The preferred method for fluid management in this scenario is the use of an oral solution to provide maintenance fluid and electrolytes. Many commercially prepared solutions are available for use. The child's hourly maintenance fluid rate as estimated by the Holliday-Segar method is (100 mL/kg $\times$ 10 kg + 50 mL/kg $\times$ 2 kg) / 24 hours = 46 mL/hr, which is approximately 1.5 oz (30 mL = 1 oz). It is reasonable to monitor the parent's ability to provide the solution in the acute care setting. If the child tolerates the solution without vomiting, he or she can be discharged home with close follow-up.

Pure water should not be used for maintenance hydration, as it lacks the solutes needed for homeostasis and can precipitate hyponatremia. A goal of 5 oz every hour is excessive and might precipitate more vomiting in this case. Nasogastric administration of fluid or formula is not recommended, and it would be unreasonable to expect the parent to maintain the tube as an outpatient. IV fluid hydration would be appropriate if oral rehydration fails, but is not first-line treatment in cases of mild dehydration.

Vignette 2 Question 2
Answer E: The child in the vignette is appropriately assessed as being moderately dehydrated. His somnolence and tachycardia with normal blood pressure suggest that he is already in compensated hypovolemic shock. Correction of diminished intravascular volume is best accomplished with bolus infusions of isotonic fluid, such as normal saline or lactated Ringer's. Colloidal solutions such as albumin can also be used. Twenty milliliter of fluid per kilogram of weight should be used as an initial volume expanded; repeat boluses may be necessary to stabilize the patient.

Oral rehydration is effective in a mildly to moderately dehydrated patient who is stable, but is not appropriate for a hypovolemic patient who requires rapid intravascular expansion. Likewise, placing the child on maintenance IV fluids does not provide the necessary volume to stabilize the patient. The fluid chosen for volume replacement should not contain dextrose. Dextrose is rapidly taken up by the cells, resulting in an effectively hypotonic solution that could lead to complications including cerebral edema.

Vignette 2 Question 3

Answer B: A plan for IV rehydration begins with calculation of maintenance needs. Based on his 12-kg "rehydrated" weight, he requires 1,100 mL/day, or about 45 mL/hr, for maintenance (100 mL/kg for the first 10 kg, 50 mL/kg for the next 2 kg). Sodium and potassium requirements for the day are 33 and 22 mEq, respectively (3 mEq per 100 mL fluid for sodium, and 2 mEq per 100 mL fluid for potassium); 33 mEq sodium per 1,100 mL is equal to 30 mEq/L, or approximately one-fifth normal saline and 22 mEq potassium per 1,100 mL is equal to 20 mEq/L.

Next the deficit must be accounted for. Using his weight loss as a guide, his deficit is approximately 1,200 mL, which is divided into two 600 mL deficits for your plan. A total of 240 mL was given as bolus fluid, so 360 mL remains to be given over the first 8 hours, resulting in an additional 45 mL/hr. Adding this to the maintenance rate gives a total rate of 90 mL/hr.

Electrolyte content in a replacement fluid for a dehydrated patient is estimated based on the nature of fluid losses. In general, isotonic dehydration from gastrointestinal losses results in electrolyte deficits comparable to a fluid between half normal and normal saline. The use of half normal saline is a good approximation of the final fluid accounting for both the deficit replacement and maintenance needs. Additional potassium above maintenance needs can be added to the fluid to account for potassium losses, but should not exceed 40 mEq/L in acute dehydration. Five percent dextrose is added as a caloric substrate to prevent catabolism.

Vignette 3 Question 1

Answer D: The anion gap conceptually represents the unmeasured anions in the serum. The anion gap is calculated as the difference between the measured cations (sodium and potassium) and anions (chloride and bicarbonate). In the example above, the gap is $(132 + 5) - (104 + 10) = 23$. The anion gap is typically 12 ± 4. This patient has a high anion gap; the differential diagnosis for an elevated anion gap in the setting of acidosis can be found in Table 5-2.

Vignette 3 Question 2

Answer B: The determination of an acid–base abnormality is greatly aided by the clinical scenario. Polyuria, polydipsia, and hyperglycemia are symptoms suggestive of type 1 diabetes mellitus, and in this case ketonuria and decreased pH indicate the child is in diabetic ketoacidosis (DKA). The blood gas should be evaluated with this information in mind. The reduced pH indicates an acidemia, and decreased bicarbonate and PCO_2 suggest that the process is metabolic in origin. Appropriate respiratory compensation can be determined with the formula $PCO_2 \pm 2 = 1.5 \times \text{bicarbonate} + 8$, which is satisfied in this example. While mixed acid–base derangements are common, a concurrent respiratory acidosis with this patient's metabolic acidosis would result in a higher PCO_2 than would be expected based on the above formula.

A respiratory acidosis would result in an elevated PCO_2 on blood gas analysis. Acute renal compensation for a respiratory acidosis results in an increase in bicarbonate concentration by 1 mEq/L for every 10 mm Hg rise in PCO_2. Maximal compensation over 3 to 4 days allows an increase in the bicarbonate concentration of 4 mEq/L for every 10 mm Hg rise in PCO_2. While a respiratory alkalosis would result in a decreased PCO_2 and bicarbonate, the kidneys will not "overcompensate" for the alkalosis.

Vignette 3 Question 3

Answer A: Extreme alteration in serum solutes can disrupt routine laboratory testing, particularly in the case of sodium. In the case of hyperglycemia, the sodium is artificially low. The value can be corrected by adding 1.6 to the measured sodium value for every 100 mg/dL glucose above the normal value of 100. In the example above, this results in a value of 4.8 added to the measured sodium, or a corrected sodium of 137 mEq/L. Additional states in which the measured sodium is artificially low include other hyperosmolar states, such as in the administration of mannitol, or in hyperproteinemia or hypertriglyceridemia.

The child with DKA, as in the vignette, suffers from several electrolyte derangements. However, laboratory measurement of the serum electrolytes is only confounded by hyperglycemia in the case of sodium. In truth, whole body potassium is depleted as a result of the child's diuresis, but potassium is shifted to the extracellular space as a result of the ongoing acidosis. The acidosis likewise depletes serum bicarbonate, but measurement of this and potassium are both accurate in the setting of hyperglycemia.

Vignette 4 Question 1

Answer C: Rhabdomyolysis and resultant acute renal failure can be responsible for alterations in many electrolytes. While all of the answer choices are present in this scenario, it is hyperkalemia that should be considered a medical emergency. Initial symptoms of elevated serum potassium include weakness and paresthesias of the extremities. Untreated, it can lead rapidly to ventricular tachyarrhythmias and cardiac arrest.

Hyperglycemia is common in patients with severe illness, but is not life threatening. Serum Cr is a useful marker to estimate renal function and, when elevated, suggests renal insufficiency. This patient's renal failure must be addressed as it likely is contributing to hyperkalemia, but management of the potassium must be handled first. Hypocalcemia and hyperphosphatemia are frequently encountered in rhabdomyolysis, as free serum calcium binds to damaged muscle fibers and phosphate is released from the muscle cells. Hypocalcemia may also lead to widening of the QRS complex and development of arrhythmias, but not as acutely as in cases of hyperkalemia. Hyperphosphatemia can worsen acidosis, but not to a life-threatening extent.

Vignette 4 Question 2

Answer A: ECG changes in a patient with hyperkalemia are ominous findings requiring immediate intervention. The earliest sign of cardiac involvement is typically the development of peaked T waves, followed by disappearance of P waves and widening of the QRS complex. Ultimately, a sinusoidal pattern or ventricular fibrillation evolves if the hyperkalemia continues. Stabilization of cardiac muscle cell membranes is accomplished with infusion of calcium salts and should be the first priority in treating the hyperkalemia.

Diuresis with furosemide in the healthy patient can decrease potassium, but does not have any immediate benefit in stabilizing the patient. Sodium bicarbonate temporarily drives potassium from the serum into the intracellular space by treating the acidosis, but does not reduce myocardial excitability. Hemodialysis is one method by which excess potassium can be removed from the body, but is reserved for cases in which medical management and temporizing measures fail. The patient in the vignette may require the attention of a specialist for his acute renal injury, but needs immediate therapy for his current condition.

Vignette 4 Question 3

Answer E: Once cardiac membrane potentials have been restored with IV calcium, potassium must be shifted out of the ECF space, either into the cells or out of the body. A cation exchange resin, such as Kayexelate, can be given orally or rectally to eliminate potassium from the colon. Hemodialysis or hemofiltration can also be used to remove potassium but carry higher risk, require greater resources, and thus are reserved for extreme situations.

Both insulin and albuterol stimulate the action of the sodium–potassium ATPase that exchanges intracellular sodium for extracellular potassium. These effects are temporary, and excess potassium will eventually return to the serum. Sodium bicarbonate indirectly acts to increase the sodium/potassium gradient by relieving acidosis and thus improves the exchange. Calcium chloride can be used to reduce myocardial excitability but has no effect on the serum potassium directly.

Chapter

6 Dermatology

Marissa J. Perman • Anne W. Lucky • Bradley S. Marino

SKIN MANIFESTATIONS OF VIRAL INFECTIONS

Hand-foot-and-mouth disease is a common acute disease of young children during the spring and summer caused by Coxsackie A viruses. There is usually a prodrome of fever, anorexia, and oral pain, followed by crops of ulcers on the tongue and oral mucosa and a vesicular rash on the hands, feet, and occasionally the buttocks and thighs. The individual vesicles often have a "football" shape with surrounding erythema. Diagnosis is made by the history and the constellation of symptoms. Treatment is supportive.

Giannoti-Crosti Syndrome or papular acrodermatitis of childhood is a typically asymptomatic erythematous papular eruption occurring commonly from 1 to 6 years of age following an upper respiratory illness. It is symmetrically distributed on the face, extensor surfaces of the arms, legs, and buttocks, and strikingly spares the trunk (Color Plate 1). Papules may coalesce into larger edematous plaques or become purpuric. Several viruses have been associated with this syndrome including hepatitis B (rare in the United States), Epstein–Barr virus (EBV), and varicella. Treatment is supportive, and the rash typically resolves without treatment, but resolution may take up to 8 weeks. A thorough history and physical examination to assess for signs and symptoms associated with hepatitis B should be obtained, and if suggestive, hepatitis B serologies should be ordered.

Varicella (chickenpox) is a highly contagious disease caused by primary infection with varicella-zoster virus (VZV). It is usually a mild, self-limited disease in immunocompetent children. Its severity can range from a few lesions and a low-grade fever to hundreds of lesions and a temperature up to 105°F (40.6°C). Fatal disseminated disease may occur in immunocompromised children or in neonates whose mothers develop the infection within 1 week of delivery. Adolescents and adults often have a more severe clinical course. After an incubation period of 10 to 21 days, there is a prodrome consisting of mild fever, malaise, anorexia, and occasionally a scarlatiniform or morbilliform rash. The characteristic pruritic rash occurs the following day, appearing first on the trunk and then spreading peripherally. The rash begins as red papules which develop rapidly into clear vesicles that are approximately 1 to 2 mm in diameter (the so-called "dewdrop on a rose petal"). The vesicles then become cloudy, rupture, and form crusts (Fig. 6-1). The lesions occur in widely scattered "crops," so several stages are usually present at the same time. Vesicles often are present on mucous membranes as well. Patients are infectious from 24 hours before the appearance of the rash until all the lesions are crusted, which usually occurs 1 week after the onset of the rash.

Primary varicella is a clinical diagnosis. In unclear cases, a Tzanck smear, looking for multinucleated giant cells, can be performed on a vesicle or a pharyngeal swab, or a swab of vesicular fluid can be sent for viral identification. Most centers now perform direct fluorescent antibody (DFA) testing, which can rapidly identify the presence of infected cells. Other confirmatory techniques include viral culture for varicella (which may take as long as a week) and polymerase chain reaction (PCR) testing. Progressive varicella with meningoencephalitis, hepatitis, and pneumonitis may occur in immunocompromised children and is associated with a 20% mortality rate. Immunization with varicella vaccine has significantly reduced the frequency of this infection in the United States.

Treatment of varicella is supportive and includes antipyretics and daily bathing to reduce the risk of secondary bacterial infection. In some patients, ibuprofen has been associated with an increased risk of streptococcal cellulitis when given in the setting of primary varicella. In addition, Reye syndome is a rare complication seen in patients with primary varicella taking aspirin. Oral antihistamines for pruritus are safe to use. Immunocompromised children who are exposed to VZV are given varicella-zoster immune globulin within 96 hours of the exposure and observed closely. Administration of the varicella vaccine within 72 hours of exposure may prevent or lessen disease severity. Systemic antiviral medications such as acyclovir, valacyclovir, or famciclovir are not indicated for children with uncomplicated primary varicella but may be administered in children with varicella pneumonia or encephalitis and immunocompromised patients.

Herpes zoster (shingles) represents a reactivation of VZV infection and occurs predominantly in adults who previously have had varicella and have circulating antibodies. However, if varicella occurs early in life, the risk for shingles in childhood is higher. After primary infection, VZV retreats to the dorsal

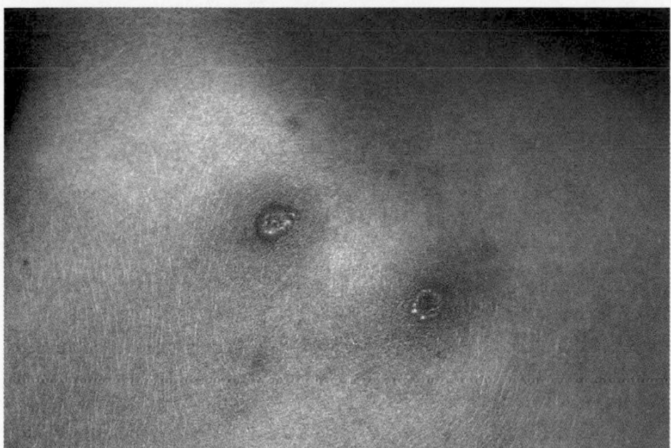

Figure 6-1 • Ruptured, crusted vesicles from varicella.
(Image courtesy of Dr. Anne W. Lucky.)

root ganglia; as a result, it follows a dermatomal distribution when reactivated. Although herpes zoster occurs in children, it is uncommon in healthy children <10 years of age. An attack of zoster begins with pain and/or pruritus along the affected sensory nerve and is accompanied by fever and malaise. A vesicular eruption then appears in crops confined to the dermatomal distribution and clears in 7 to 14 days. Typical of all herpes virus infections, the lesions are grouped vesicles on an erythematous base (Color Plate 2). The rash may last as long as 4 weeks, with pain persisting for weeks or months (postherpetic neuralgia). Other complications from herpes virus include encephalopathy, aseptic meningitis, Guillain-Barré syndrome, pneumonitis, thrombocytopenic purpura, cellulitis, and arthritis.

Herpes zoster can be quite painful, and narcotics are sometimes needed. Systemic administration of antivirals, such as acyclovir, may be considered for use in immunocompromised patients, patients older than 12 years, children with chronic disease, and those who have received systemic steroids for any reason.

Molluscum contagiosum is a cutaneous viral infection caused by a poxvirus and is very common in childhood. It is manifested by small, flesh-colored, pearly, umbilicated, dome-shaped papules in moist areas such as the axillae, buttocks, and groin region, but they can appear anywhere (Fig. 6-2). The papules spread via touching, auto-inoculation, and scratching. They are often seen in wrestlers and sauna bathers. Lesions may resolve spontaneously over 1 to 2 years, but families typically request treatment sooner. Treatment depends on the experience of the practitioner and includes curettage, crythotherapy, cantharidin (an extract from the blister beetle that causes blistering of the epidermis), oral cimetidine, and imiquimod cream.

Verrucae, commonly known as warts, are caused by the human papillomavirus (HPV). Warts are typically benign in otherwise healthy individuals and are spread by skin-to-skin contact or fomites. They may also develop at sites of trauma. There are four common types including verruca vulgaris (common wart) (Fig. 6-3), verruca plantaris (plantar wart), verruca plana (flat wart), and condyloma accuminata (genital warts).

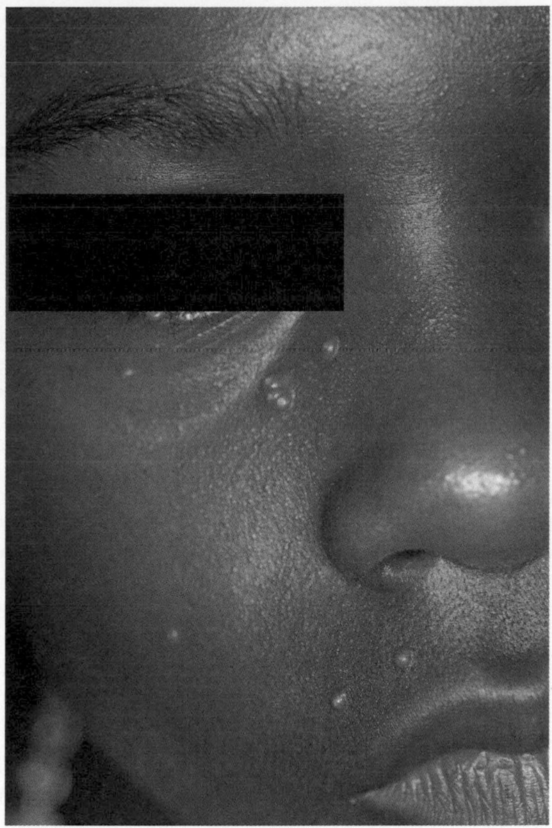

Figure 6-2 • Molluscum on the face. Note how the lesions have central umbilication.
(Image courtesy of Dr. Anne W. Lucky.)

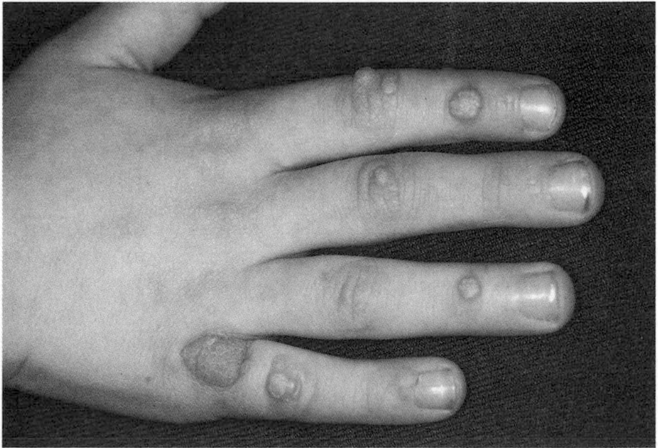

Figure 6-3 • Verruca vulgaris on the dorsal surface of the digits.
(Image courtesy of Dr. Anne W. Lucky.)

Treatment of warts in the pediatric population is based on the type and location of the wart and includes topical salicylic acid, liquid nitrogen, imiquimod cream, oral cimetidine, oral zinc sulfate, injected immunotherapies such as intralesional *Candida* antigen, and squaric acid dibutylester. Patients may require multiple treatments, especially in the case of recalcitrant warts.

PRESUMED VIRAL EXANTHEMS

Pityriasis Rosea is an exanthem of unknown etiology, but a viral prodrome, often upper respiratory in nature, is sometimes found in the history. The rash has a distinct morphology that typically begins with a herald patch, a 2 to 10 cm oval salmon-pink plaque on the trunk, neck, upper extremities, or thigh (Color Plate 3). This is followed by several smaller lesions often distributed in a "Christmas tree pattern" over the trunk and upper extremities that develop over days to weeks. The lesions often have a "collarette" of scale which may cause the lesions to be confused with tinea corporis. Some patients develop lesions with a more papular appearance, especially younger children and African Americans. The rash fades over 4 to 12 weeks and is typically asymptomatic in most patients but can be pruritic in some. Usually, pityriasis rosea is self-limited, and no treatment is needed. Topical and oral antihistamines as well as mild topical steroids can be used for pruritus. Sunlight has been shown to hasten resolution of the lesions.

Unilateral thoracic exanthem (asymmetric periflexural exanthem of childhood) is a rash with varying morphologies that occurs in children ages 1 to 5 years and begins as an exanthem on one side of the trunk that spreads centripetally. The rash is seen more commonly in the winter and spring months and may follow symptoms of low-grade fever, lymphadenopathy, respiratory, or gastrointestinal complaints. A viral etiology has been presumed, although no specific virus has been implicated. Often confused with contact dermatitis, the lesions vary from erythematous macules or papules with a surrounding halo to morbilliform, eczematous, scarlatiniform, or reticulate configurations that may spread to the opposite side from initial involvement (Fig. 6-4). Pruritus is common and can be treated in the same manner as pityriasis rosea-associated pruritus. Lesions resolve over 6 to 8 weeks without treatment and may desquamate or leave postinflammatory pigmentary changes.

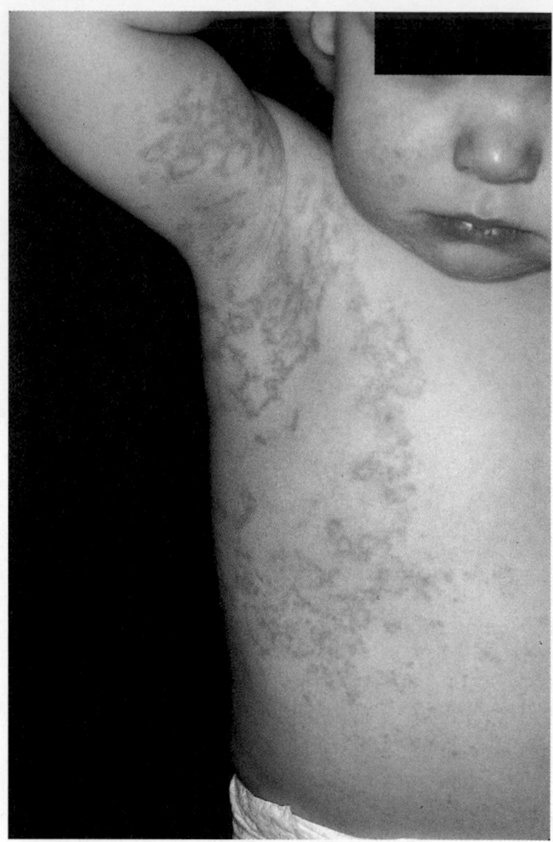

Figure 6-4 • Erythematous reticulated plaques with central clearing and scattered erythematous papules involving the right trunk and periflexural region following a viral URI. The unilateral thoracic exanthem lesions subsequently desquamated before resolving completely over several weeks. (Image courtesy of Dr. Anne W. Lucky.)

SKIN MANIFESTATIONS OF BACTERIAL INFECTIONS

Bacterial infections of the skin are common, and in most cases they are the result of group A β-hemolytic streptococcal or *Staphylococcus aureus* infection.

Bullous impetigo, which is caused by a toxin-producing strain of *S. aureus*, begins as red macules that progress to bullous (fluid-filled) eruptions on an erythematous base (as seen on Color Plate 4). These lesions range from a few millimeters to a few centimeters in diameter. After the bullae rupture, a clear, thin, varnish-like coating forms over the denuded area. *S. aureus* can be cultured from the vesicular fluid. Bullous impetigo lesions can be mistaken for cigarette burns, raising the suspicion for abuse.

Nonbullous impetigo, which is caused by both group A β-hemolytic streptococci and *S. aureus*, begins as papules that progress to vesicles and then to pustules measuring approximately 5 mm in diameter with a thin erythematous rim. The pustules rupture, leaving a honey-colored thin exudate that then forms a crust over a shallow ulcerated base (Color Plate 5). Local lymphadenopathy is common with streptococcal impetigo. Fever is uncommon. The causative organism can usually be isolated from the lesions.

Limited nonbullous impetigo can be treated with topical antibiotics such as mupirocin ointment. If the lesions of bullous and/or nonbullous impetigo are numerous, they can be treated with a first-generation cephalosporin such as cephalexin, an oral drug that is effective against both *Staphylococci* and group A *Streptococcus*. In settings where methicillin-resistant *S. aureus* (MRSA) is suspected, agents such as clindamycin or trimethoprim-sulfamethoxazole may be more appropriate. The caretaker can remove any honey-colored crusts with twice-daily warm compresses.

Staphylococcal scalded skin syndrome (SSSS), which is caused by exfoliative toxin-producing isolates of *S. aureus*, is most common in infancy and rarely occurs beyond 5 years of age. Onset is abrupt, with diffuse erythema, marked skin tenderness, irritability, and fever. Within 12 to 24 hours of onset, superficial flaccid bullae develop and then rupture almost immediately, leaving a beefy red, weeping surface (Color Plate 6). Although widespread areas may be affected, accentuation is seen on periorificial areas of the face, as well as flexural areas around the neck, axillae, and inguinal creases. Exfoliation is caused by a Staphylococcal toxin and may affect most of the body. There is usually a positive Nikolsky sign (separation of the epidermis after light rubbing). The initial focus of staphylococcal infection may be minor such as conjunctivitis or rhinitis or inapparent. Unruptured bullae contain sterile fluid.

Mild to moderate cases of SSSS are treated with an oral antistaphylococcal medication. Children with severe cases should be treated as though they have a second-degree burn, with meticulous fluid management and intravenous oxacillin or clindamycin.

Folliculitis is an infection of the shaft of the hair follicle, usually with *S. aureus*. Superficial folliculitis is common and easily treated. The buttocks and the lower legs in girls who shave are frequent sites of infection. Deep forms of this infection include furuncles (boils) and carbuncles. Furuncles begin as superficial folliculitis and are most frequently found in areas of hair-bearing skin that are subject to friction and maceration, especially the scalp, buttocks, and axillae. Carbuncles are collections of furuncles.

Superficial folliculitis responds to aggressive hygiene with antiseptic cleansers and topical mupirocin. Folliculitis of the male beard is unusually recalcitrant and requires an oral antistaphylococcal drug. Simple furunculosis is treated with moist heat. Larger and deeper furuncles, which are becoming increasingly more common in the community (particularly with the spread of MRSA), may need to be incised and drained. There is debate regarding oral antibiotic therapy following incision and drainage. Rarely, folliculitis can be caused by *Pseudomonas aeuroginosa* in the specific setting of bathing in contaminated hot tubs. These lesions are self-limited when the exposure is discontinued.

SUPERFICIAL FUNGAL INFECTIONS

Essentially, two fungal species cause the most common superficial infections: *Trichophyton* and *Microsporum*, although *Trichophyton tonsurans* is the most common cause of **tinea capitis** in the United States. *Microsporum canis* is also common and is spread from animals, especially kittens and puppies. On the scalp, tinea capitis manifests as patches of scaling and hair loss, broken off hairs known as "black dots," (Fig. 6-5) and boggy, pustular masses known as kerions. The latter can be associated with pain, itching, a diffuse morbiliform eruption, and lymphadenopathy. On the skin, **tinea corporis** frequently manifests as annular plaques with peripheral scaling, giving the appearance of rings (hence the name "ring-worm"). **Tinea pedis**, usually an infection with *Trichophyton rubrum* classically presents as scaling in a "moccasin" distribution, and frequently also involves the interdigital spaces of the toes. **Tinea cruris**, also caused by *T. rubrum*, presents with erythema, scaling, and maceration in inguinal creases. Most superficial skin infections can be treated with topical antifungal agents. However, systemic antifungal drugs are necessary to eradicate dermatophyte infections of the nails or hair. Table 6-1 presents tinea infections and their treatments.

Tinea (pityriasis) versicolor is caused by infection with a yeast, *Malassezia furfur*, and is characterized by superficial tan or hypopigmented oval scaly patches on the neck, upper part of the back, chest, and upper arms. Dark-skinned individuals tend to have hypopigmented lesions during the summer when uninfected skin tans from sunlight exposure. However, individual patients may demonstrate both dark- and light-colored lesions at the same time (hence the name versicolor). Treatment includes selenium sulfide shampoo or other topical or systemic antifungal agents. Recurrence in the summertime is common.

Diaper rash may result from atopic dermatitis, primary irritant dermatitis, or primary or secondary *Candida albicans* infection. Eighty percent of diaper rashes lasting more than 4 days are colonized with *Candida*. Fiery red papular lesions with peripheral papules, pustules, and scales in the skin folds and satellite lesions are typical for candidal diaper rash. Barrier creams along with topical antifungal or ny-statin creams are the first-line treatments of choice. Recalcitrant diaper rash may indicate more severe problems such as Langerhans Cell Histiocytosis or metabolic disorders like zinc deficiency.

ACNE VULGARIS

Acne vulgaris is a very common, self-limited, multifactorial disorder of the pilosebaceous unit that begins in adolescence. Lesions may begin as early as 8 to 10 years of age. Prevalence increases steadily throughout adolescence and then decreases in adulthood. Although girls often develop acne at a younger

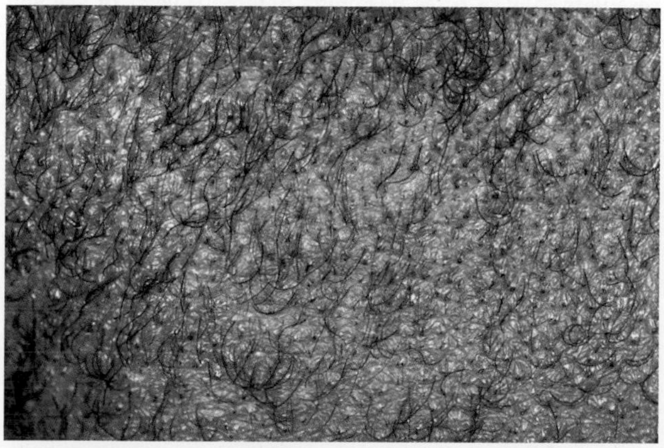

Figure 6-5 • Tinea capitis causing characteristic "black dot" alopecia. (Image courtesy of Dr. Anne W. Lucky.)

TABLE 6-1 Common Tinea Infections and Their Treatments

Infection	Treatment
Tinea capitis (scalp)	Oral griseofulvin, 6–8 wk
	Selenium sulfide shampoo to kill spores; does not eradicate infection
Tinea corporis (body)	Topical antifungals (e.g., clotrimazole) for at least 4 wk; oral griseofulvin if refractory
Tinea cruris (genitocrural) "jock itch"	Same as tinea corporis
Tinea pedis ("athlete's foot")	Same as tinea corporis, plus proper foot hygiene

age than boys, severe disease affects boys 10 times more frequently because of higher androgen levels. In fact, 15% of all teenage boys have severe acne (Fig. 6-6).

The **pathogenesis** of acne includes multiple factors such as androgen stimulation of the sebaceous glands, follicular plugging, proliferation of *Propionibacterium acnes*, and inflammatory changes. There is a predilection for the sebaceous follicle-rich areas of the face, chest, and back. Closed comedones (whiteheads) and open comedones (blackheads) are noninflammatory and nonscarring. Pustules, papules, and nodules (formerly called cysts) are inflammatory and carry the potential for scarring. Atrophic and hypertrophic scars or keloids may occur. At puberty, there is androgen-dependent sebaceous follicle stimulation leading to increased sebum production. Female patients with severe acne often have high levels of circulating androgens.

Risk factors include family history and puberty. In girls, **polycystic ovary syndrome** (PCOS) is a common underlying factor. Rarely, Cushing disease or any other condition that results in androgen excess can predispose to acne. Poor hygiene and food intake are *not* risk factors for acne.

It is important to obtain a good **medical history** including when the acne started and whether there is a family history of acne. A full menstrual history should be taken to determine whether there is a hormonal pattern to flares associated with the menstrual cycle. It is also important to discuss the patient's skin care, including how the patient's acne has been treated in the past, and any medications the patient is currently taking as some drugs can cause or exacerbate acne.

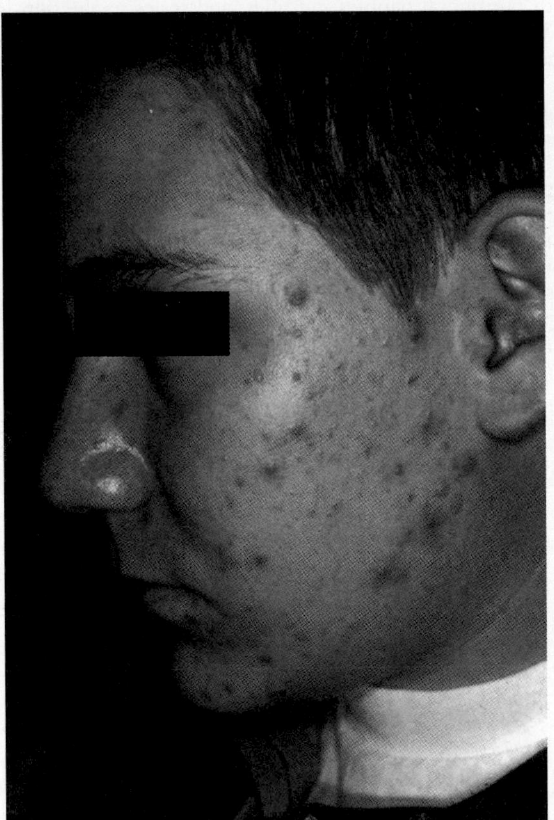

Figure 6-6 • Typical inflammatory acne lesions. (Image courtesy of Dr. Anne W. Lucky.)

A thorough **physical examination** including distribution, morphology, and severity of lesions should be recorded. The back and chest should be examined and treated as well as the face. Severe inflammatory and especially nodular acne may result in hypertrophic or pitted scarring.

Treatment should be individualized depending on the patient's gender and the severity, type, and distribution of lesions. Mild acne generally responds to topical therapy without scarring. Benzoyl peroxide works by decreasing the colonization of *P. acnes*. Topical retinoids (e.g., tretinoin, adapalene, and tazarotene) have strong anticomedogenic activity; however, side effects may limit use and include dryness, burning, and photosensitivity by reducing the thickness of the stratum corneum layer. The use of sunscreen with a sun protection factor (SPF) of at least 15 is necessary. Topical antibiotics (clindamycin and erythromycin) are used to prevent and decrease colonization of *P. acnes*, but their sole use for acne treatment promotes bacterial resistance. Topical antibiotics are also available in combination with benzoyl peroxide, which prevents bacterial resistance. Dapsone gel is a newer topical agent with anti-inflammatory and possibly antibacterial properties as well. Other newer topical therapies include retinoids combined with benzoyl peroxide or topical antibiotics.

There is growing bacterial resistance to antibiotic therapy for acne, and oral antibiotics should be used only in severely affected patients or those who do not respond to conventional topical therapy. Systemic antibiotics for acne include tetracycline, doxycycline, minocycline, and erythromycin. In females, oral contraceptives may also be helpful by suppressing androgen production and are now approved for acne therapy. In addition, spironolactone, an aldosterone antagonist with antiandrogen properties, although not FDA-approved for acne, is useful in hormone-related acne. Oral isotretinoin is very effective for acne, but because of its teratogenicity and high adverse effect profile, strict monitoring is needed through the I-pledge system. Isotretinoin is usually prescribed by a dermatologist. See Figure 6-7 for a guide to acne therapy.

PSORIASIS

Psoriasis is a common but often undiagnosed childhood disease with 10% of cases beginning before 10 years of age and 35% before 20 years of age. There is often a positive family history, and human leukocyte antigen inheritance is part of the mode of transmission.

This nonpruritic, papulosquamous eruption consists of erythematous papules that coalesce to form dry plaques with sharply demarcated borders and silvery scales. The scales tend to build up into layers, and their removal may result in pinpoint bleeding (**Auspitz sign**). Psoriasis often appears at sites of physical, thermal, or mechanical trauma. This is known as the **Koebner phenomenon**, a diagnostic feature of the disease. It is usually symmetric, with plaques appearing over the knees, elbows, and in childhood, the scalp, periocular, and genital areas. The nails often demonstrate punctate stippling or pitting, distal detachment of the nail plate (onycholysis), and accumulation of subungual debris. Examination of the palms and soles reveals scaling and fissuring.

Psoriatic arthritis may also be present in a subset of patients. Occasionally, atopic dermatitis may be confused with

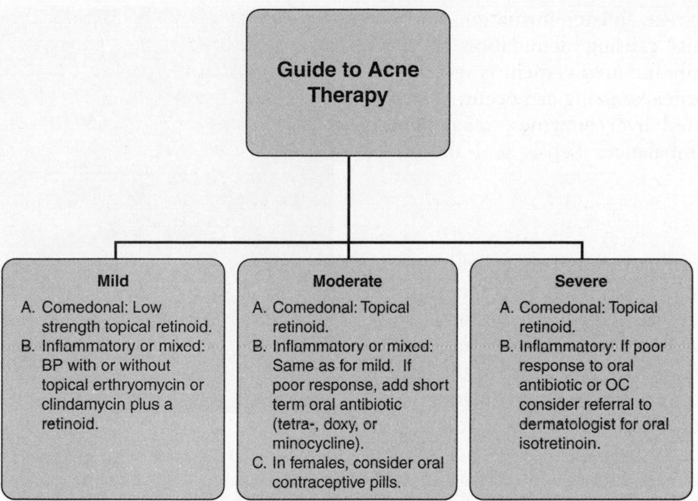

Figure 6-7 • Therapy for mild, moderate, and severe acne.
BP, benzoyl peroxide; OC, oral contraceptive.

psoriasis; however, eczema is often pruritic and concentrated in flexural creases, whereas psoriasis is not usually pruritic and favors extensor surfaces. Scalp lesions may be confused with seborrheic dermatitis or tinea capitis.

Psoriasis is characterized by remissions and exacerbations. Group A β-hemolytic streptococcal infections are a common exacerbating cause of psoriasis in a genetically susceptible individual. The most important aspect of treating psoriasis is to educate the patient and family that the disease is chronic and recurrent. It cannot be cured but can be controlled with conscientious therapy. No matter the location or severity of the rash, the goal of psoriasis therapy is to keep the skin well hydrated. Topical steroids are the mainstay of therapy; the least potent but effective dose should be used because adrenal suppression can occur. Topical vitamin D cream or ointment and tar can also be helpful. For more severe cases, natural sunlight or ultraviolet B (UVB) light is useful. In severe cases, methotrexate and biological immunosuppressants such as etanercept can be tried under the supervision of a dermatologist.

ERUPTIONS SECONDARY TO ALLERGIC REACTIONS

Atopic dermatitis, urticaria, and angioedema are discussed in Chapter 13.

ERYTHEMA MULTIFORME

Erythema multiforme (EM) is an acute, self-limited, hypersensitivity reaction that is uncommon in children. The most frequent etiologic agents include viral infections such as herpesvirus, adenovirus, and EBV.

Clinical Manifestations

In EM, a symmetric distribution of lesions evolves through multiple morphologic stages: erythematous macules, papules, plaques, vesicles, and target lesions. The lesions evolve over days, not hours and often have a target-like appearance. EM is often confused with polycyclic urticaria which also can appear targetoid, but urticarial lesions are not fixed and do not have necrotic centers. Urticarial lesions tend to have edematous, erythematous borders with central clearing, and individual lesions resolve within 12 to 24 hours. In contrast, lesions in EM are typically fixed and develop dusky, necrotic centers. EM lesions also tend to occur over the dorsum of the hands and feet, palms and soles, and extensor surfaces of extremities, but may spread to the trunk. Burning and itching are common. Systemic manifestations include fever, malaise, and myalgias. The most common cause of recurrent EM in children is herpes simplex virus type I.

Stevens–Johnson syndrome (SJS) is a distinct hypersensitivity reaction and a variant of toxic epidermal necrolysis (TEN). There is a prodrome for 1 to 14 days of fever, malaise, myalgias, arthralgias, arthritis, headache, emesis, and diarrhea. This is followed by the sudden onset of high fever, erythematous and purpuric macules with dusky centers, and inflammatory bullae of two or more mucous membranes (oral mucosa, lips, bulbar conjunctiva, and anogenital area; Color Plate 7). In the most severe cases, involvement of most of the gastrointestinal, respiratory, or genitourinary tracts may be seen. Untreated, this syndrome has a mortality rate of approximately 10%. The most common causes of SJS include drugs such as nonsteroidal anti-inflammatory drugs, penicillins, sulfonamides, and many antiepileptic medications, mycoplasma infections, and rarely immunizations.

TEN is the most severe form of cutaneous hypersensitivity and likely a more severe variant of SJS involving more than 30% body surface area. Although its occurrence in children is rare, it is associated with a 30% mortality rate. The pathogenesis appears to be related to upregulated expression of Fas ligand in the epidermis, a mediator of apoptosis. The etiology is similar to SJS. Onset is acute, with high fever, a burning sensation of the skin and mucous membranes, and/or oral and conjunctival erythema and erosions. The presentation of the skin resembles that of staphylococcal scalded skin, with widespread erythema, tenderness, blister formation, and full detachment of the epidermis causing denudation (positive Nikolsky sign). Mucous membrane involvement is severe, and the nails may be shed and corneal scarring can occur. Systemic complications include elevated liver enzymes, renal failure, and fluid and electrolyte imbalance. Sepsis and shock are frequent causes of death.

Treatment

For uncomplicated EM, symptomatic treatment and reassurance are all that are necessary. Oral antihistamines, moist compresses, and oatmeal baths are helpful. The lesions resolve over a 1- to 3-week period, with some hyperpigmentation. The use of corticosteroids is controversial. Treatment of the patient with SJS includes hospitalization with barrier isolation, fluid and electrolyte support, treatment of common secondary infections of the skin, moist compresses on bullae, and colloidal oatmeal baths. For oral mucosal lesions, mouthwashes with viscous lidocaine, diphenhydramine, and Maalox (aluminum hydroxide, magnesium hydroxide) are comforting. Because corneal ulceration, keratitis, uveitis, and panophthalmitis are possible, an ophthalmology consultation is recommended. Children with TEN are treated as though they had a full-body second-degree burn. Fluid therapy and reverse barrier isolation are critical to survival; many patients are treated in an intensive care or burn center unit. Intravenous immunoglobulin has been used with some success in several series of patients with TEN, presumably because of its effects of binding or modulating the effect of Fas ligand.

ALLERGIC DRUG REACTIONS

Allergic reactions to drugs typically present as urticarial or morbilliform exanthems which can develop within 1 to 2 weeks of starting a new medication. The risk of an allergic drug reaction may be increased if the patient has a concurrent viral illness similar to patients with mononucleosis treated with ampicillin. The eruption may clear after the inciting agent is removed, but it may take several days to weeks. Following the acute eruption, many patients tend to desquamate. Treatment is based on symptoms. The decision to discontinue the medication is based on the risks and benefits of the need for treatment in the primary illness and possible alternative medications.

HYPERPIGMENTED LESIONS

With the incidence of melanoma increasing, it is very important to identify suspicious lesions and understand risk factors. Children with fair skin, excessive sun exposure, and multiple nevi are at increased risk for both melanoma and nonmelanoma skin cancer such as basal cell and squamous cell carcinomas.

Congenital nevi are usually larger than acquired nevi and can vary considerably in color and shape. They tend to get darker, thicker, and more hairy with time, although giant nevi often will become lighter. Congenital nevi are classified based on their size. Large or giant nevi are >20 cm^2 (Fig. 6-8), small nevi are <2 cm^2, and intermediate nevi are in between in size. Congenital nevi must be followed annually for changes and may require complete excision. Although there is controversy about the magnitude, large- and medium-sized congenital nevi appear to have a small increased risk of developing melanoma. The increased lifetime risk of melanoma in giant nevi is estimated to be between 5% and 15%. There is also an association with neurocutaneous melanosis; thus patients with large lesions over the head and spine, or with multiple associated satellite nevi, require a magnetic resonance imaging (MRI) of the brain and spinal cord to evaluate for central nervous system (CNS) involvement. Any nevi over the sacral spine may indicate underlying spinal abnormalities, especially tethered cord.

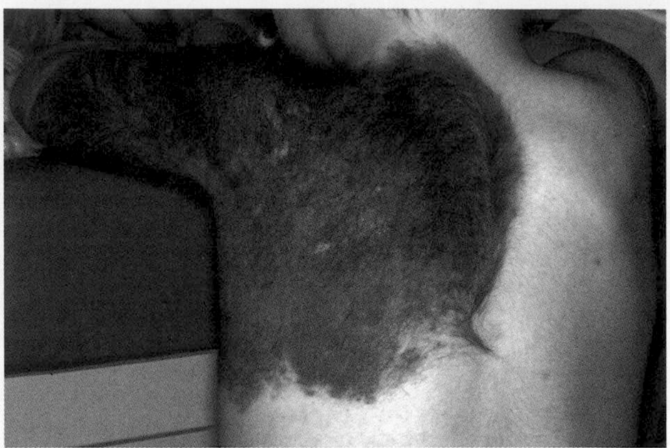

Figure 6-8 • Giant congenital (hairy) nevus on the back. (Image courtesy of Dr. Anne W. Lucky.)

Many children develop **acquired nevi** during infancy and childhood, reaching a maximum number in early adulthood. Patients with more than 15 common acquired moles may have an increased risk for melanoma in the future. Nevi need to be assessed by using the ABCDE rules: watching for **A**symmetry, irregular **B**orders, variations in **C**olor, **D**iameter >6 mm, and **E**volution of the nevus. Nevi that change rapidly or exhibit atypical features may need to be excised.

A **Spitz** (spindle and epithelial cell) nevus is a smooth pink to brown to jet black dome-shaped papule which usually enlarges rapidly after its appearance. These nevi are usually benign but may need to be removed if they grow rapidly as malignant forms have been reported rarely.

Halo nevi are moles which develop up to 1 cm depigmented surrounding rings. These represent an immune reaction against the pigment cells. Halo nevi may completely regress, leaving a white macule that eventually fills in. They are generally benign in children but may be associated with the presence of vitiligo or melanoma at another site.

PREVENTION

A large amount of childhood sun exposure and frequent sunburns are associated with increased risk for the development of moles and skin cancer. Sun protection with a sunblock having an SPF of 30 or more against UVB as well as protection against ultraviolet A (UVA) light is recommended. Many sunscreens now contain physical sunblockers such as titanium dioxide or zinc oxide which provide UV scatter rather than absorption. Reapplying sunscreen during exposure, avoiding long periods of sun exposure in midday, and sun-protective clothing are equally important for adequate protection.

INFANTILE HEMANGIOMAS

Infantile hemangiomas are vascular tumors which are common in infancy, noted in 1% to 2% of neonates. They are more common in females, Caucasians, and premature infants. They are classified as superficial, deep, or mixed, and are generally not present at birth. Superficial hemangiomas are bright red and noncompressible, whereas deep hemangiomas are subcutaneous, compressible, and often have a bluish hue and superficial telangiectasias. Mixed lesions have characteristics of both superficial and deep hemangiomas (Color Plate 8). Infantile hemangiomas can be found in any location but are commonly seen on the head and neck. Hemangiomas must be distinguished from more aggressive vascular tumors, such as hemangioendotheliomas, and from vascular malformations which may involve capillaries, veins, arteries, lymphatics, or combinations of these. Vascular malformations tend not to resolve and become more troublesome with time.

The evolution of infantile hemangiomas is generally predictable. They present during the first month of life, maintain a period of growth over the next several months to a year, and then begin to slowly involute. Involution is marked by decreasing size and change in color from a bright to duller red or purple to grey. Involution may take many years; however, most lesions typically resolve by 10 years of age. There may be residual textural change in the skin or superficial telangiectasias.

Treatment is based on individual findings including: size, location, overlying changes, and rate of growth. The most common management is to provide anticipatory guidance and support to the family while following the lesion on a regular basis. Lesions requiring active intervention are those that pose life-threatening or functional risks. Large hemangiomas may cause heart failure; lesions involving the airway may cause obstruction; periocular lesions are mandatory to treat to prevent astigmatism or blindness; facial lesions may produce severe disfigurement or interfere with eating; genital and perianal lesions may ulcerate and cause significant pain; lumbosacral lesions may indicate underlying spinal abnormalities (SACRAL syndrome); facial segmental hemangiomas may be associated with CNS, cardiovascular, eye, and sternal anomalies (PHACE syndrome) and multiple (>5) lesions may be associated with liver and other internal hemangiomas.

Treatment varies with each situation, but may include oral propranolol, local or systemic corticosteroids, antibiotics and dressings, or excision where indicated. Laser treatment has a limited role, often improving ulceration. In severe cases, vincristine or alpha interferon may be necessary.

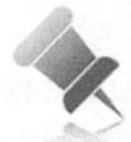

KEY POINTS

- Children with chickenpox are contagious from 24 hours before the onset of rash until all lesions have crusted over.
- *Staphylococcus aureus* and Group A β-hemolytic *Streptococcus* cause most bacterial skin infections.
- *Trichophyton tonsurans* is the most common cause of tinea capitis in the United States.
- Severe inflammatory and nodular acne are associated with scarring.
- Acne is best treated with combination therapy, and choice of therapy depends on the type of acne.
- Psoriasis can be treated but not cured and is characterized by remissions and exacerbations that may be precipitated by streptococcal infections. Psoriasis occurs at sites of trauma (Koebernization) and, unlike atopic dermatitis, is nonpruritic.
- EM is most commonly caused by herpes simplex virus type I.
- Nevi need to be assessed for change as well as asymmetry, irregular borders, color, and size.
- Sun protection against ultraviolet B and A (UVB and UVA) light is recommended to decrease the risk of melanoma as well as nonmelanoma skin cancer.
- Infantile hemangiomas are vascular tumors that appear in the first month of life and often regress without treatment over the first several years of life.

C Clinical Vignettes

Vignette 1

A healthy 4-year-old presents with fever, malaise, and a new-onset pruritic erythematous papulovesicular eruption involving the trunk, face, and extremities (Figure 1).

1. Which of the following is the most likely diagnosis in this patient?
   a. Herpes zoster
   b. Pityriasis rosea
   c. Rubella
   d. Primary varicella
   e. Molluscum contagiosum

2. What is the incubation period for the eruption described in Question 1?
   a. 10 to 21 days
   b. 3 to 10 days
   c. 21 to 28 days
   d. 3 to 4 months
   e. 24 to 96 hours

3. Which of the following is the best treatment for this eruption?
   a. Oral acyclovir
   b. Ibuprofen
   c. Aspirin
   d. Varicella zoster–immune globulin
   e. Supportive therapy

Vignette 2

A 5-month-old white female presents to your clinic with a 1-cm enlarging red nodule on her neck. The family is highly concerned as the "bump" was not present at birth and continues to grow slowly. There is no bleeding, and the child appears to be asymptomatic.

1. Which of the following is the most appropriate next step in the evaluation of this patient?
   a. Referral to surgery for excision
   b. Referral to oncology for evaluation of a malignancy
   c. Reassurance that this is a nevus. It will stop growing by 12 to 18 months of age, then slowly regress over several years.
   d. Reassurance that this is a hemangioma. It will stop growing by 12 to 18 months of age, then slowly regress over several years.
   e. Biopsy for definitive diagnosis

2. What would be the most appropriate next step in the management of this patient if the nodule was located in the lumbosacral region?
   a. Anticipatory guidance and support
   b. Magnetic resonance imaging (MRI) of the spine
   c. Oral prednisone
   d. Surgical excision
   e. Oral propranolol

Vignette 3

A 3-year-old African American boy presents with a few focal areas of asymptomatic scalp alopecia associated with mild scale and black dots. The lesions have been present for several weeks. He also has shotty posterior cervical lymphadenopathy.

1. Which of the following is the most likely cause of this scalp eruption?
   a. *Trichophyton tonsurans*
   b. *Microsporum canis*
   c. *Trichophyton rubrum*
   d. *Candida albicans*
   e. *Epidermophyton floccosum*

2. Which of the following is the most likely complication of this eruption?
   a. Osteomyelitis
   b. Meningitis
   c. Kerion
   d. Cellulitis
   e. Progressive secondary alopecia

3. Which of the following is the best treatment for this eruption?
   a. Topical ketoconazole cream
   b. Selenium sulfide lotion
   c. Oral griseofulvin
   d. Observation
   e. Oral doxycycline

Vignette 4

A 15-year-old male presents with a 9-month history of several nonpruritic well-defined, round, silver scaling, erythematous papules, and plaques on his elbows, knees, and scalp. He has an uncle with similar skin findings. You make the diagnosis of psoriasis.

1. Infection with which of the following bacterial agents is most likely to trigger psoriasis?
   - **a.** *Staphylococcus aureus*
   - **b.** *Klebsiella pneumoniae*
   - **c.** *Hemophillus influenza*
   - **d.** Group A streptococcus (*Streptococcus pyogenes*)
   - **e.** *Bartonella henslae*

2. Psoriasis often appears at sites of physical, mechanical, or thermal trauma. This tendency is known as which of the following?
   - **a.** Auspitz sign
   - **b.** Koebner phenomenon
   - **c.** Nikolsky sign
   - **d.** Herald sign
   - **e.** Onycholysis sign

3. Which of the following is NOT an appropriate treatment for uncomplicated chronic plaque psoriasis?
   - **a.** Topical steroids
   - **b.** Etanercept
   - **c.** Oral antibiotics
   - **d.** Ultraviolet B phototherapy
   - **e.** Methotrexate

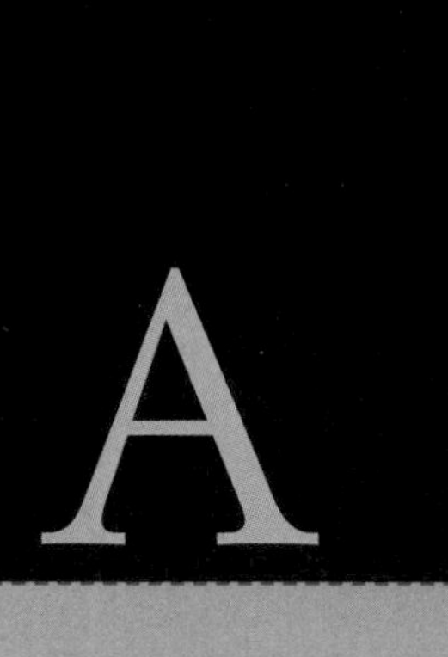

Answers

Vignette 1 Question 1

Answer D: The image depicts the classic eruption seen in primary varicella, or chickenpox. Varicella occurs in a centrifugal manner, with lesions starting on the head and trunk and spreading to the extremities. The papulovesicles seen in varicella are often described as "dewdrops on a rose petal." The individual lesions should be present in all stages including erythematous papules, papulovesicles, and crusted papules. Fever and malaise are common prodromal symptoms.

Herpes zoster usually occurs in a dermatomal distribution (unless disseminated) and may or may not be associated with systemic symptoms such as fever. Pityriasis rosea often involves the trunk and flexural regions and begins with a single, larger lesion known as the herald patch. The individual lesions of pityriasis rosea are ovoid, pink to violaceous patches, or thin plaques with a collarette of scale. Rubella may present in newborns as violaceous papules and nodules ("blueberry muffin" rash) or as enumerable erythematous macules and papules coalescing on the face and trunk. Molluscum are pearly, translucent, umbilicated papules most commonly found in moist areas such as the axillae, groin, and buttocks but can be found anywhere on the skin.

The patient played with her 3-year-old cousin the day prior to developing her rash.

Vignette 1 Question 2

Answer A: The incubation period for varicella is 10 to 21 days. The virus is spread via airborne droplets and colonizes the respiratory tract. The virus then replicates in the regional lymph nodes over the next 2 to 4 days, followed by spread to the reticuloendothelial system over 4 to 6 days, resulting in a primary viremia. A secondary viremia develops over the next week, with the virus spreading to viscera and skin, at which time the classic skin lesions develop. Patients are contagious from 24 hours before the rash until all lesions crust over, which usually takes place within 5 to 7 days. The other choices do not fit the time period for incubation of varicella.

Vignette 1 Question 3

Answer E: Treatment of varicella is based on several factors. Most uncomplicated cases of varicella are treated with supportive therapy that may include antipyretics, daily "oatmeal" baths, and oral antihistamines for pruritus. Ibuprofen may be associated with an increased risk of streptococcal cellulitis in the setting of primary varicella. Aspirin should be avoided to prevent the rare complication of Reye syndrome. Oral acyclovir should be considered for patients at risk for or with more severe disease including adolescents, those with chronic medical conditions, or those who are immunocompromised. Varicella zoster–immune globulin should be given within 96 hours to susceptible individuals (those who have not had primary varicella or immunization and are at high risk for serious disease or are pregnant) exposed to varicella.

Vignette 2 Question 1

Answer D: Infantile hemangiomas are common benign cutaneous vascular tumors (rather than nevi) seen in infancy with a predictable growth pattern of proliferation for 6 to 12 months, followed by a slow regression over several years. Therefore, the best answer is reassurance that this is a hemangioma that will stop growing by 12 to 18 months and regress over several years. The history and clinical photo support the diagnosis; therefore, a biopsy is not required. An uncomplicated hemangioma involving a low-risk site does not require any further treatment at this time. High-risk sites include the face (especially lesions that obscure vision by enlarging the skin or lids around the eye), genital, and lumbosacral regions; options for these patients include surgery, laser, or systemic therapy. Oncology referral would be inappropriate as this is a benign lesion that can be followed clinically by the primary physician or a dermatologist.

Vignette 2 Question 2

Answer B: Infantile hemangiomas located in the lumbosacral region may be associated with spinal dysraphism including tethered cord, myelomeningocele, lipoma, and other spinal abnormalities. MRI to evaluate the spinal canal is essential for early diagnosis and management to avoid serious complications at a later age. Therefore, anticipatory guidance and support would be inappropriate. The other treatment options listed should be deferred until the imaging study confirms or rules out associated anomalies of the spine.

Vignette 3 Question 1

Answer A: Tinea capitis can be identified by one or several patches of scalp alopecia that are often associated with scale, crust, and black dots. The black dots represent broken hair shafts which occur when dermatophytes weaken the shaft and allow breakage. *Trichophyton tonsurans* accounts for more than 90% of tinea capitis infections in the United States. *Microsporum canis* is the most common cause of tinea capitis worldwide. *Trichophyton rubrum* does not cause tinea capitis;

however, it is the most common cause of tinea corporis and tinea pedis. *Epidermophyton floccosum* causes tinea pedis. *Candida albicans* does not cause tinea capitis.

Vignette 3 Question 2

Answer C: A kerion is a severe inflammatory reaction presenting as a boggy, pustular, alopecic eruption at the site of tinea capitis due to an aggressive host immune response toward the dermatophyte. Kerions require systemic therapy with oral antifungal agents; oral prednisone is also administered to decrease inflammation. None of the other choices occur with tinea capitis, although a secondary bacterial folliculitis can develop and requires antibiotic therapy.

Vignette 3 Question 3

Answer C: Dermatophytes invade the hair follicle in tinea capitis; therefore, systemic antifungal therapy is required for penetration of the hair follicle. Oral griseofulvin is the only systemic antifungal agent listed and is the most commonly used antifungal to treat tinea capitis in children. Griseofulvin is FDA approved for tinea capitis in children, has an excellent safety record, and is well tolerated. Most cases of tinea capitus require 4 to 8 weeks of oral therapy. The medicine must be taken with or directly following a meal and is best absorbed with fatty foods. Topical ketoconazole cream will not penetrate the hair follicle. Selenium sulfide lotion can be used as an adjunctive to systemic antifungal therapy to decrease shedding of viable spores but is not a primary treatment. Antibiotics are not indicated for tinea capitis, and observation would not be appropriate.

Vignette 4 Question 1

Answer D: Group A streptococcus (GAS; *Streptococcus pyogenes*) is the most likely bacteria to trigger psoriasis. GAS can induce guttate psoriasis or cause a flare of existing psoriasis. Psoriasis may be triggered by any stress on the immune system including illness and psychological stress, GAS is the most likely bacteria to trigger/worsen psoriasis.

Vignette 4 Question 2

Answer B: Psoriasis developing at sites of trauma is an isomorphic response known as the Koebner phenomenon. It is often related to minor trauma or sunburn. The mechanism for this reaction is not known. The Auspitz sign refers to pinpoint bleeding when scale is removed from a psoriasis plaque. The Nikolsky sign refers to separation of the superficial layers of the epidermis with light pressure, a finding seen in staphylococcal scalded skin syndrome. A herald *patch* is the first, and often largest, characteristic lesion seen in pityriasis rosea. There is no "Herald sign." Onycholysis refers to separation of the distal nail plate from the nail bed, a common finding in psoriatic nail disease. There is no "Onycholysis sign."

Vignette 4 Question 3

Answer C: While oral antibiotics may be used to treat a streptococcal infection associated with guttate psoriasis or a flare of plaque psoriasis, they are not beneficial as primary therapy for psoriasis. There are many treatment options for psoriasis, including topical steroids, phototherapy, topical vitamin D creams and ointments, tar, systemic immunosupressants (such as methotrexate or cyclosporine), and biologic therapy such as etanercept, infliximab, and adalimumab.

Chapter

7 Cardiology

Angela Lorts • Catherine D. Krawczeski • Bradley S. Marino

The field of pediatric cardiology has experienced a remarkable evolution over the past half century due to advances in diagnostic techniques, interventional cardiac catheterization and cardiac surgical procedures, pediatric anesthesia, neonatal medicine, and intensive care. **Functional heart murmurs** are very common in childhood and do not signify disease. The incidence of structural heart disease is approximately 8 in 1,000 live births. Critical **congenital heart disease** (CHD), requiring cardiac surgery or an interventional cardiac catheterization procedure in the neonatal period, occurs in approximately 1 in 400 live births. Children may acquire **structural heart disease, functional heart disease** (i.e., myocarditis or cardiomyopathy), or **arrhythmia**.

HEART MURMURS

Heart murmurs are common in children; they are heard on routine physical examinations in approximately one third of patients. **Functional ("innocent") heart murmurs** are the result of normal physiologic flow turbulence. Each of these murmurs has specific characteristics that usually allow it to be confidently diagnosed by physical examination alone (Table 7-1). It is equally important to recognize the signs and symptoms of potentially pathologic murmurs to facilitate rapid diagnosis and intervention, if necessary (Table 7-2).

CLINICAL MANIFESTATIONS

History

Infants with heart disease may have a history of difficulty feeding, tachypnea, irritability, diaphoresis, cyanosis, and/or failure to thrive. Significant symptoms in older patients include shortness of breath, dyspnea on exertion, exercise intolerance, palpitations, paroxysmal nocturnal dyspnea, orthopnea, and syncope. Chest pain is a frequent complaint in older children and adolescents; however, it is rarely cardiac in origin. Children who have syndromes associated with heart disease (e.g., Turner, Down, William, Noonan, DiGeorge/velocardiofacial) are at a higher risk for a pathologic murmur. The family history should include questions regarding syncope, sudden death, heart attacks, or stroke before 50 years of age; connective tissue disorders (Marfan syndrome); hyperlipidemia; hypercholesterolemia; arrhythmia; valvular disease; cardiomyopathy; and CHD.

PHYSICAL EXAMINATION

The physical examination includes a comparison of the child's weight and height to normal values for age and gender and to previous measurements on a growth curve. Careful attention should be paid to vital signs, including heart rate (Table 7-3), respiratory rate, and blood pressure. The examiner should assess for cyanosis and digital clubbing (indicating a right-to-left shunt), as well as signs of congestive heart failure (edema and hepatomegaly). Pulses should be palpated in both upper and lower extremities and compared. The examiner should inspect and palpate the chest for placement of the apical impulse and any heaves or thrills. Auscultation allows detection and characterization of heart sounds (normal and extra) and murmurs. Murmurs may be systolic, diastolic, or continuous and should be graded according to their intensity.

DIAGNOSTIC EVALUATION

Pulse oximetry assesses oxygen saturation in the blood. The chest radiograph evaluates heart size and pulmonary vascularity. The heart size should be less than 50% of the chest diameter in children above age 1 year. Pulmonary vascularity is usually increased in lesions with large left to right shunts, for example, ventricular septal defects, and may be diminished in lesions such as tetralogy of Fallot. All patients with suspected pathologic murmurs should receive an electrocardiogram (ECG) and echocardiogram (ECHO).

TREATMENT

The treatment of heart disease may be medical, surgical, interventional (cardiac catheterization), or a combination of these, depending on the specific abnormality.

EVALUATION OF THE CYANOTIC NEONATE

Cyanosis is a physical sign characterized by a bluish tinge of the mucous membranes, skin, and nail beds. Cyanosis results from hypoxemia (decreased arterial oxygen saturation). Cyanosis does not become clinically evident until the absolute concentration of deoxygenated hemoglobin is at least 3.5 g per dL. Factors that influence the degree of cyanosis include the total hemoglobin concentration (related to the hematocrit)

TABLE 7-1 Functional Heart Murmurs

Murmur	Typical Age at Presentation	Characteristics	Source
Peripheral pulmonary artery (PPS)	Neonate (birth to 2 mo)	Medium-pitched systolic ejection murmur best heard at the left upper sternal border, through to the back	Turbulence of flow where the main pulmonary artery branches into left and right arteries
Vibratory (still murmur)	2 to 8 yr	Grade II to III midsystolic musical or vibratory murmur heard best near the left lower sternal border and apex	Vibrations in ventricular or mitral structures caused by flow in the left ventricle
Venous hum	3 to 7 yr	Continuous, soft humming murmur heard at the neck or right upper chest that disappears in the supine position	Turbulent flow in the jugular venous/superior vena cava systems
Carotid bruit	3 to 8 yr	Systolic ejection murmur heard best at the neck	Turbulence of flow where the brachiocephalic vessels attach to the aorta
Pulmonary flow murmur	6 yr to adolescence	Systolic ejection murmur best heard at the left upper sternal border	Turbulence of flow where the main pulmonary artery connects to the right ventricle (across the pulmonary valve)

TABLE 7-2 Concerning Signs on Cardiac Examination

Heaves, thrills, or other abnormal or increased precordial activity
Brachiofemoral delay and/or decreased femoral pulses
Abnormal first or second heart sound (abnormal splitting)
Extra heart sounds
Gallop rhythms (S_3, S_4, or summation gallop)
Ejection click
Opening snap
Pericardial rub
Murmurs
Very loud, harsh, or blowing
Does not change in intensity relative to patient positioning

TABLE 7-3 Resting Heart Rates

Age	Low	High
<1 mo	80	160
1 to 3 mo	80	200
2 to 24 mo	70	120
2 to 10 yr	60	90
11 to 18 yr	40	90

and factors that affect the O_2 dissociation curve (pH, PCO_2, temperature, and ratio of adult to fetal hemoglobin). Cyanosis will be evident sooner (and more pronounced) under the following conditions: (a) high hemoglobin concentration (polycythemia), (b) decreased pH (acidosis), (c) increased PCO_2, (d) increased temperature, and (e) increased ratio of adult to fetal hemoglobin. Cyanosis should not be confused with acrocyanosis (blueness of the distal extremities only). Acrocyanosis is caused by peripheral vasoconstriction and is a normal finding during the first 24 to 48 hours of life.

DIFFERENTIAL DIAGNOSIS

Cyanosis in the newborn may be cardiac, pulmonary, neurologic, or hematologic in origin (Table 7-4). Cyanosis is one of the most common presentations of CHD in the newborn (Table 7-5). Pulmonary disorders may lead to cyanosis as a result of primary lung disease, airway obstruction, or extrinsic compression of the lung. Neurologic causes of cyanosis include central nervous system dysfunction and respiratory neuromuscular dysfunction.

CLINICAL MANIFESTATIONS

History and Physical Examination

A complete birth history that includes maternal history; prenatal, perinatal, and postnatal complications; history of labor and delivery; and neonatal course should be obtained. Exactly when the child developed cyanosis is critical because certain congenital heart defects present at birth, whereas others may take as long as 1 month to become evident.

The initial physical examination should focus on the vital signs and the cardiac and respiratory examinations, assessing for evidence of right, left, or biventricular congestive heart failure and respiratory distress. Blue or dusky mucous membranes are consistent with cyanosis. Rales, stridor, grunting, flaring, and retractions should be evaluated on pulmonary examination. On cardiovascular examination, the precordial

TABLE 7-4 Differential Diagnosis of Cyanosis in the Neonate

Cardiac	Pneumonia
Ductal-independent mixing lesions	Persistent pulmonary hypertension of the newborn
Truncus arteriosus	***Airway obstruction***
Total anomalous pulmonary venous return	Choanal atresia
D-transposition of the great arteries[a]	Vocal cord paralysis
Lesions with ductal-dependent PBF	Laryngotracheomalacia
Tetralogy of Fallot with pulmonary atresia[b]	***Extrinsic compression of the lungs***
Critical pulmonic stenosis	Pneumothorax
Tricuspid valve atresia[b] with normally related great arteries[b]	Chylothorax
	Hemothorax
Pulmonic valve atresia with intact ventricular septum	**Neurologic**
Lesions with ductal-dependent SBF	***CNS dysfunction***
Hypoplastic left heart syndrome	Drug-induced depression of respiratory drive
Interrupted aortic arch	Postasphyxial cerebral dysfunction
Critical coarctation of the aorta	Central apnea
Critical aortic stenosis	***Respiratory neuromuscular dysfunction***
Tricuspid valve atresia with transposition of the great arteries[b]	Spinal muscular atrophy
	Infant botulism
Pulmonary	Neonatal myasthenia gravis
Primary lung disease	**Hematologic**
Respiratory distress syndrome	Methemoglobinemia
Meconium aspiration	Polycythemia

[a]A patent ductus arteriosus may improve mixing, especially with an intact ventricular septum.
[b]Most forms.
PBF, pulmonary blood flow; SBF, systemic blood flow.

TABLE 7-5 Most Common Congenital Heart Disease Leading to Cyanosis in the Newborn

Tetralogy of Fallot
Transposition of the great vessels
Tricuspid atresia
Pulmonary atresia with intact ventricular septum
Truncus arteriosus
Total anomalous pulmonary venous connection
Critical pulmonary stenosis

impulse is palpated, and the clinician should evaluate for systolic or diastolic murmurs, the intensity of S1, S2 splitting abnormalities, and the presence of a S3 or S4 gallop, ejection click, opening snap, or rub. Examination of the extremities should focus on the strength and symmetry of the pulses in the upper and lower extremities, evidence of edema, and cynaosis of the nail beds. Hepatosplenomegaly may be consistent with right ventricular or biventricular heart failure.

DIAGNOSTIC EVALUATION

The goal of the initial evaluation of the cyanotic neonate is to determine whether the cyanosis is cardiac or noncardiac in origin. Preductal and postductal oxygen saturation and four extremity blood pressures should be documented. An ECG, chest radiograph, and hyperoxia test should be performed.

Preductal (right upper extremity) and postductal (lower extremity) oxygen saturation measurements permit evaluation for *differential* cyanosis and reverse *differential* cyanosis. When the preductal saturation is higher than the postductal measurement, differential cyanosis exists. Possible diagnoses associated with differential cyanosis include persistent pulmonary hypertension of the newborn (PPHN; see Chapter 2) and left ventricular outflow tract obstructive lesions such as interrupted aortic arch, critical coarctation of the aorta, and critical aortic stenosis. Deoxygenated blood from the pulmonary circulation enters the descending aorta through a patent ductus arteriosus (PDA), decreasing the postductal oxygen saturation. When the preductal saturation is lower than the postductal saturation, reverse differential cyanosis exists. In the absence of a measurement error, this can only occur in the presence of transposition of the great arteries *with* either PPHN or coarctation of the aorta. In this situation, oxygenated blood from the pulmonary circulation enters the descending aorta through a PDA, increasing the postductal oxygen saturation.

Four extremity blood pressure measurements that show a systolic blood pressure in the upper extremities greater than 10 mm Hg, higher than that in the lower extremities are consistent with coarctation of the aorta, or other lesions with ductal-dependent systemic blood flow with a restrictive ductus arteriosus. The **ECG** evaluates the heart rate, rhythm, axis, intervals, forces (atrial dilatation, ventricular hypertrophy), and repolarization (abnormal Q-wave pattern, ST/T wave abnormalities, and corrected QT interval).

A **hyperoxia test** should be carried out in all neonates with a resting pulse oximetry reading less than 85%.The hyperoxia test consists of obtaining a baseline right radial (preductal) arterial blood gas measurement with the child breathing room air (FIO_2 = 0.21), and then repeating the measurement with the child inspiring 100% oxygen (FIO_2 = 1.00). PaO_2 should be measured directly via arterial puncture. **Pulse oximetry measurements are not appropriate for interpretation of the hyperoxia test.** A PaO_2 greater than 250 mm Hg on 100% oxygen essentially rules out cardiac disease. These patients are more likely to have a pulmonary cause for their cyanosis. A PaO_2 less than 50 mm Hg on 100% oxygen is very suggestive of a cardiac lesion.

The combined results of the tests described will typically point the clinician in the right direction as to the source of the cyanosis and may also suggest a specific diagnosis. If a cardiac cause is deemed likely, an echocardiogram **(ECHO)** and cardiology consultation should be obtained.

TREATMENT

Cyanotic infants require immediate assessment of the ABCs (Chapter 20) and stabilization. **Prostaglandin E1** (PGE1) administration, via continuous intravenous infusion, should be started in any unstable infant with a strong suspicion of CHD. In newborns with mixing lesions or defects that have ductal-dependent pulmonary or systemic blood flow, PGE1 acts to maintain patency of the ductus arteriosus until definitive surgical treatment can be accomplished. Rarely, the patient with CHD may become progressively more unstable after the institution of PGE1 therapy, indicating a defect that has obstructed pulmonary venous flow, for example, total anomalous venous return with obstruction.

CYANOTIC CONGENITAL HEART DISEASE: DUCTAL-INDEPENDENT MIXING LESIONS

TRUNCUS ARTERIOSUS

Truncus arteriosus (Color Plate 9) is a rare form of cyanotic CHD that consists of a single arterial vessel arising from the base of the heart, which gives rise to the coronary, systemic, and pulmonary arteries. The number of valve leaflets varies from two to six, and the valve may be insufficient or stenotic. A ventricular septal defect (VSD) is always present. There is complete mixing of systemic and pulmonary venous blood in the truncal vessel. This lesion, along with other conotruncal anomalies (tetralogy of Fallot, interrupted aortic arch, VSD, isolated arch anomalies, and vascular rings), is frequently associated with 22q11 microdeletion (i.e., **DiGeorge syndrome**).

Clinical Manifestations

The clinical manifestations of truncus atteriosus varies depending on the amount of pulmonary blood flow. At birth, a nonspecific murmur and minimal symptoms may be present, due to limitation of pulmonary blood flow by higher neonatal pulmonary vascular resistance. Congestive heart failure develops in a matter of weeks as the pulmonary vascular resistance falls and pulmonary blood flow increases at the expense of systemic blood flow. On cardiac examination, a systolic ejection murmur is heard at the left sternal border, and there is usually a loud ejection click and a single second heart sound (S2). Pulse pressure is widened and bounding arterial pulses are palpated. A chest radiograph reveals mild cardiomegaly, increased pulmonary vascularity, and occasionally a right aortic arch (30% of the time). Seventy percent of children with truncus arteriosus have biventricular hypertrophy on ECG. Hypocalcemia and absence of the thymic shadow (on chest radiograph) may occur if the patient has DiGeorge syndrome in addition to truncus arteriosus.

Treatment

At most centers, surgical repair is performed in the neonatal period. This involves closing the VSD, separation of the pulmonary arteries from the truncal vessel (using the truncal valve and vessel as the neoaortic valve and neoaorta), and placing a conduit between the right ventricle and the pulmonary arteries to provide pulmonary blood flow.

D-TRANSPOSITION OF GREAT ARTERIES

D-transposition of great arteries (D-TGA) (Color Plate 10) accounts for 5% of congenital heart defects and is the most common form of cyanotic CHD presenting in the first 24 hours of life. There is a 3:1 male predominance. In this defect, the aorta arises anteriorly from the morphologic right ventricle, and the pulmonary artery arises posteriorly from the left ventricle. The pulmonary and systemic circuits thus are in parallel rather than in series; the systemic circuit (deoxygenated blood) is recirculated through the body, whereas the pulmonary circuit (oxygenated blood) recirculates through the lungs. An adequate-sized patent foramen ovale (PFO) is required to allow mixing of the systemic and pulmonary circulations and is necessary for survival. The three basic variants are D-TGA with intact ventricular septum (60%), D-TGA with VSD (30%), and D-TGA with VSD and pulmonic stenosis (10%).

Clinical Manifestations

Cyanosis is present from birth; the degree is dependent on the amount of mixing across the patent foramen ovale. The infant is often tachypneic. On cardiac examination, a loud, single S2 is appreciated. A systolic murmur indicates the presence of a VSD and/or pulmonic stenosis. The chest radiograph usually reveals mild cardiomegaly and increased pulmonary vascular markings. An "egg-shaped silhouette" is characteristic and results from the anterior aorta being superimposed on the posterior pulmonary artery, thereby narrowing the mediastinum (Fig. 7-1). The ECG generally reveals right-axis deviation and right ventricular hypertrophy.

Treatment

PGE1 administration is often necessary to increase aorta (deoxygenated) to pulmonary artery (oxygenated) shunting through the ductus arteriosus, which may further improve

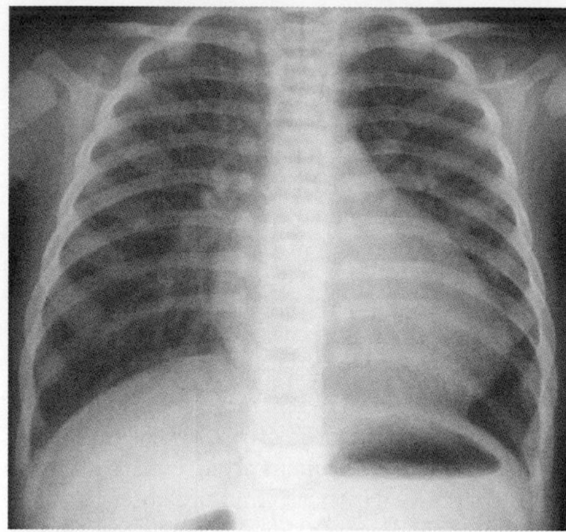

Figure 7-1 • Chest x-ray of transposition of the great arteries. (Image courtesy of Dr. Bradley Marino.)

mixing. A balloon atrial septostomy (Rashkind procedure) may need to be performed to enlarge the PFO and thereby increase atrial level mixing. The arterial switch procedure, which restores the left ventricle as the systemic ventricle, is generally performed during the first week of life.

TOTAL ANOMALOUS PULMONARY VENOUS CONNECTION

Total anomalous pulmonary venous connection (TAPVC) (Color Plate 11) is a rare lesion (1% to 2% of CHDs) in which the pulmonary veins are not connected to the left atrium. The pulmonary veins come to a confluence behind the left atrium, which then drains anomalously into the right atrium either directly or indirectly through other systemic venous pathways.

There are four variants:

- **Supracardiac** (50% of cases): Blood drains via a vertical vein into the innominate vein or directly into the superior vena cava.
- **Cardiac** (20% of cases): Blood drains into the coronary sinus or directly into the right atrium.
- **Infradiaphragmatic** (20% of cases): Blood drains via a vertical vein into the portal or hepatic veins.
- **Mixed** (10% of cases): Blood returns to the heart via a combination of the routes just described.

TAPVC can occur *with* or *without obstruction*. Pulmonary venous flow is obstructed when the anomalous vein enters a vessel at an acute angle or courses between or through other mediastinal structures. The presence or absence of obstruction determines whether there is pulmonary venous hypertension and severe cyanosis (obstruction) or increased pulmonary blood flow and mild cyanosis (no obstruction). Because there is no pulmonary venous return to the left side of the heart, shunting of blood from right to left (through an ASD or PFO) is necessary for blood flow to the systemic vascular bed.

Clinical Manifestations

The clinical presentation varies greatly depending on the pathway of pulmonary venous return and whether it is obstructed. The infant without obstruction may present with mild cyanosis at birth and progressive congestive heart failure due to excessive pulmonary blood flow. An active precordium will be present with a right ventricular heave, a wide and fixed split S_2 with a loud pulmonary component, and a systolic ejection murmur at the left upper sternal border. On chest radiograph, cardiomegaly is noted with increased pulmonary vascularity. The heart often has the characteristic contour of a "snowman," seen when the pulmonary veins drain via a vertical vein into the innominate vein and ultimately the right superior vena cava. On ECG, right-axis deviation and right ventricular hypertrophy are seen.

Infants with pulmonary venous obstruction display marked cyanosis and respiratory distress. A loud, single (or narrowly split) S_2 is heard on cardiac examination, and tachypnea with respiratory distress may be present. The chest radiograph generally shows normal heart size with markedly increased pulmonary vascular markings and diffuse pulmonary edema. Right ventricular hypertrophy is seen on ECG.

Treatment

Corrective surgery is performed emergently in the newborn period if pulmonary venous obstruction is present. If the anomalous pulmonary veins are unobstructed (more common in the supracardiac or cardiac subtypes), repair is elective and typically takes place during infancy.

CYANOTIC CONGENITAL HEART DISEASE: LESIONS WITH DUCTAL-DEPENDENT PULMONARY BLOOD FLOW

TRICUSPID ATRESIA

Tricuspid atresia (Color Plate 12) is a rare defect (<1% of CHD) that is characterized by complete atresia of the tricuspid valve. This lesion leads to severe hypoplasia or absence of the right ventricle. Tricuspid atresia can be divided into two types: tricuspid atresia with normally related great arteries (NRGA) or tricuspid atresia with transposition of the great arteries (TGA). Ninety percent of cases of tricuspid atresia have an associated VSD. In this anatomy, the systemic venous return is shunted from the right atrium to the left atrium through the PFO or an ASD, and the left atrium and left ventricle handle both systemic and pulmonary venous return. Oxygenated and deoxygenated blood is mixed in the left atrium. The VSD allows blood to pass from the left ventricle to the right ventricular outflow chamber and pulmonary arteries. The vast majority of patients with tricuspid atresia with NRGA have pulmonary stenosis. The amount of pulmonary blood flow (and therefore the degree of cyanosis) in these patients is dependent on the size of the VSD and degree of the pulmonary stenosis. In occasional patients, pulmonary stenosis is mild, pulmonary blood flow is adequate and cyanosis is minimal, but when pulmonary stenosis is significant, cyanosis may be severe. The latter patients may depend on patency of the ductus arteriosus to provide sufficient pulmonary blood flow.

In 30% of cases, transposition of the great vessels is also present, which results in blood passing from the left ventricle through the VSD to the right ventricular outflow and the ascending aorta. Tricuspid atresia with TGA is often associated with coarctation of the aorta and/or aortic arch hypoplasia. Unlike tricuspid atresia with NRGA, which has ductal-dependent pulmonary blood flow, tricuspid atresia with TGA will have ductal-dependent systemic blood flow.

Clinical Manifestations

The clinical features of tricuspid atresia are dependent on the degree of pulmonary stenosis present. Most commonly, neonates will have significant pulmonary stenosis or even pulmonary atresia. These infants present with progressive cyanosis during the first 2 weeks of life. If pulmonary atresia is present, severe cyanosis is noted when the ductus arteriosus becomes restrictive. Less commonly, infants may have minimal or no pulmonary stenosis. These infants may have normal or even increased pulmonary blood flow and may have no cardiac symptoms or symptoms of congestive heart failure. On cardiac examination, abnormalities include the holosystolic murmur of a ventricular septal defect at the left lower sternal border and (possibly) the continuous murmur of a PDA. On ECG, there is left-axis deviation, right-atrial enlargement, and left ventricular hypertrophy. Findings on chest radiograph include normal heart size and variable degrees of pulmonary vascularity.

Neonates with tricuspid atresia and TGA also present with cyanosis and possibly poor feeding. If severe arch hypoplasia or coarctation of the aorta is present, the patient may present with shock after closure of the ductus arteriosus. Clinical severity depends on the degree of arch obstruction. The chest radiograph may reveal cardiomegaly and increased pulmonary vascular markings as the pulmonary vascular resistance falls and the child's pulmonary blood flow increases, resulting in congestive heart failure.

Treatment

Treatment of tricuspid atresia is variable depending on the amount of pulmonary blood flow and the presence or absence of an aortic arch abnormality. A child with tricuspid atresia with NRGA and restriction to pulmonary blood flow should have PGE1 started to maintain ductal patency. Surgical management for tricuspid atresia with decreased pulmonary blood flow may involve placing a modified Blalock-Taussig shunt to maintain pulmonary blood flow. The modified Blalock-Taussig shunt is a Gore-Tex tube placed between the subclavian artery and the pulmonary artery. If the pulmonary blood flow is adequate, surgery will not be required during the neonatal period. Rarely, infants with increased pulmonary blood flow may require banding of the pulmonary artery to restrict flow. Regardless of the neonatal course, all infants with tricuspid atresia will undergo further surgeries to separate the pulmonary and systemic circulations. In infancy, a cavopulmonary anastomosis (anastamosis of the superior vena cava to the pulmonary artery, called a hemi-Fontan or bidirectional Glenn shunt) is performed to provide stable pulmonary blood flow. A final surgery is performed at 2 to 5 years of age. This procedure, the Fontan procedure, redirects the inferior vena cava and hepatic vein flow into the pulmonary circulation.

A child with tricuspid atresia with TGA should have PGE1 started to maintain ductal patency and systemic blood flow. Surgical management for tricuspid atresia with TGA depends on the degree of arch obstruction. Patients with hemodynamically significant arch obstruction will require a more extensive surgery with reconstruction of the aortic arch and placement of a reliable source of pulmonary blood flow.

TETRALOGY OF FALLOT

Tetralogy of Fallot (TOF) (Color Plate 13) is the most common CHD (10%) presenting in childhood. Fifteen percent of all patients with TOF have 22q11 microdeletion; 50% of patients with 22q11 microdeletion have TOF. The four components of TOF include an anterior malalignment VSD, which results in valvar and subvalvar pulmonary valve stenosis, right ventricular hypertrophy, and an "overriding" large ascending aorta (Fig. 7-2). Infants with TOF are cyanotic because of right-to-left shunting across the VSD. The degree of right ventricular outflow obstruction determines the timing and severity of the cyanosis. In neonates, blood shunted from the aorta to the pulmonary artery through the PDA provides additional pulmonary blood flow. Infants with severe obstruction and ductus-dependent blood

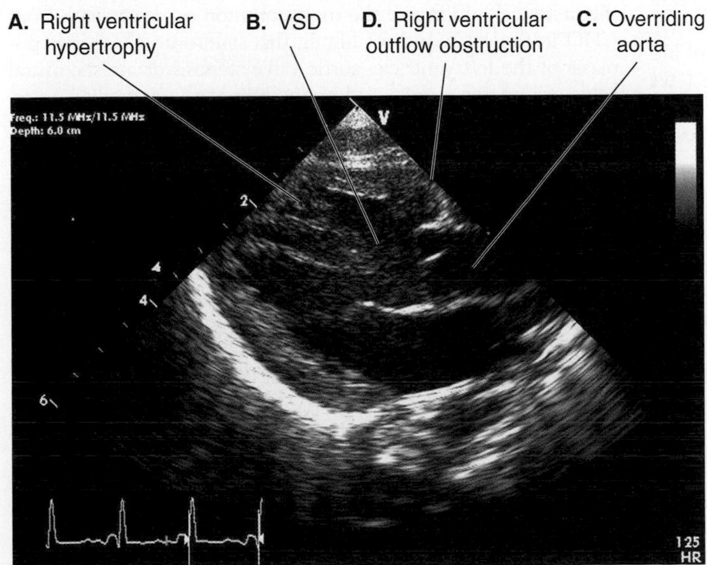

Figure 7-2 • Echocardiogram of tetralogy of Fallot. Characteristic features include **(A)** right ventricular hypertrophy; **(B)** ventricular septal defect; **(C)** overriding aorta; **(D)** right ventricular outflow tract obstruction (not visualized in this image).
(Image courtesy of Dr. Bradley Marino.)

flow present within hours of birth. Cyanosis may not develop in children with mild obstruction until later in the infant period. Associated lesions include additional VSDs, right aortic arch, left anterior descending (LAD) coronary artery from the right coronary artery coursing across the right ventricular outflow tract, and aortopulmonary collateral arteries.

Clinical Manifestations

Infants present with cyanosis and tachypnea of varying severity. They may have characteristic periodic episodes of cyanosis, rapid and deep breathing, and agitation known as "**tet spells**," caused by an increase in right ventricular outflow tract resistance, which leads to increased right-to-left shunting across the VSD. Such spells may last minutes to hours and may resolve spontaneously or lead to progressive hypoxia, metabolic acidosis, and death.

On cardiac examination, a right ventricular heave may be palpable, and a loud systolic ejection murmur is heard in the left upper sternal border. The heart size is generally normal on chest radiograph, with decreased pulmonary vascular markings. The right ventricular hypertrophy will lead to upturning of the apex on chest x-ray ("boot shaped" heart). Twenty-five percent of children with TOF have a right-sided aortic arch. The ECG reveals right-axis deviation and right ventricular hypertrophy.

Treatment

The treatment of "tet spells" is aimed at diminishing right-to-left shunting by increasing systemic vascular resistance, decreasing pulmonary vascular resistance, and/or increasing preload. The older child who has "tet spells" may squat to increase their venous return and improve their systemic perfusion. In the infant, initial measures include calming the patient and vagal maneuvers (holding the child in a knee–chest position), and the administration of supplemental oxygen and morphine sulfate to diminish the agitation and hyperpnea and minimize oxygen consumption. If these measures are not successful, volume expansion and vasoconstrictors may be given to increase systemic blood pressure and systemic vascular resistance and thereby "shunt" more blood through the restrictive right ventricular outflow tract and improve oxygen saturation. In addition, β-blockers may be given to decrease infundibular spasm, and sodium bicarbonate may be given to reduce acidosis and decrease pulmonary vascular resistance. In most institutions, elective surgical repair is performed during the first 3 to 6 months of life but urgent surgery is indicated if a hypercyanotic episode ("tet spell") occurs. Neonates with TOF with critical pulmonary valve stenosis are generally repaired at presentation. In some cases of TOF with associated anomalies (such as multiple VSDs, left anterior descending coronary artery from the right coronary artery coursing across the right ventricular outflow tract, or pulmonary atresia), a modified Blalock-Taussig shunt may be placed during the neonatal period prior to definitive repair later.

EBSTEIN ANOMALY

Ebstein anomaly (Color Plate 14) is a rare anomaly in which the septal leaflet of the tricuspid valve is displaced inferiorly into the right ventricular cavity and the anterior leaflet of the tricuspid valve is sail-like and redundant. This results in a portion of the right ventricle being incorporated into the right atrium. Functional hypoplasia of the right ventricle results, as well as tricuspid regurgitation. In severe cases of Ebstein anomaly, antegrade pulmonary blood flow from the right ventricle is limited by the severe tricuspid regurgitation so that the majority of the pulmonary blood flow comes from the PDA. A PFO is present in 80% of neonates with the anomaly, with resultant right-to-left shunt at the atrial level. The right atrium is massively dilated, which may result in atrial tachycardia. In addition, Wolff-Parkinson-White (WPW) syndrome occurs commonly with Ebstein anomaly. Ebstein anomaly can be associated with maternal lithium use.

Clinical Manifestations

Neonates with severe disease present with cyanosis and congestive heart failure in the first few days of life. The cardiac examination reveals a widely fixed split S_2 and a gallop rhythm. A blowing holosystolic murmur is heard at the left lower sternal border consistent with tricuspid regurgitation. Chest radiograph shows marked cardiomegaly with notable right atrial enlargement and decreased pulmonary vascular markings (Fig. 7-3). Characteristic ECG findings include right bundle branch block with right atrial enlargement. WPW syndrome is indicated by a delta wave and a short PR interval.

Children with milder forms of the disease may present later in childhood with fatigue, exercise intolerance, palpitations, and/or mild cyanosis with clubbing.

Treatment

Severely cyanotic newborns require PGE1 infusion to maintain pulmonary blood flow through the PDA.

In general, all attempts are made to avoid surgical intervention. Surgery on the abnormal tricuspid valve has yielded poor results. Patients with the most severe forms of Ebstein anomaly may require heart transplantation.

CYANOTIC CONGENITAL HEART DISEASE: LESIONS WITH DUCTAL-DEPENDENT SYSTEMIC BLOOD FLOW

HYPOPLASTIC LEFT HEART SYNDROME

Hypoplastic left heart syndrome (HLHS) (Color Plate 15) is the second most common congenital cardiac lesion presenting in the first week of life and the most common cause of death from CHD in the 1st month of life. In this syndrome, there is hypoplasia of the left ventricle, aortic valve stenosis or atresia, mitral valve stenosis or atresia, and hypoplasia of the ascending aorta.

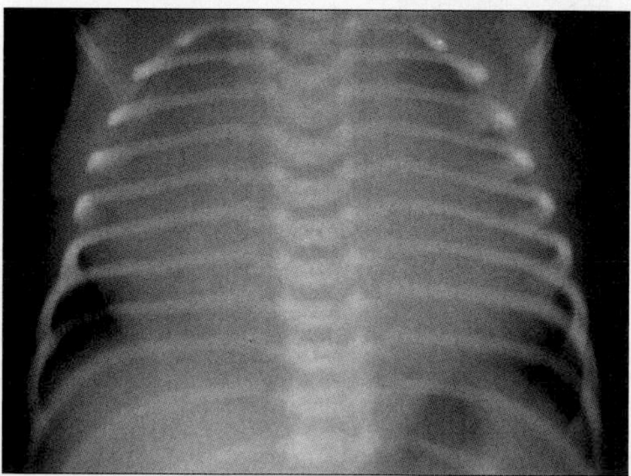

Figure 7-3 • Chest x-ray of Ebstein anomaly. (Image courtesy of Dr. Bradley Marino.)

These lesions reduce or eliminate blood flow through the left side of the heart. Oxygenated blood from the pulmonary veins is shunted left to right through an atrial septal defect. Right ventricular cardiac output goes to the pulmonary arteries and through the ductus arteriosus to the descending aorta. Systemic blood flow is completely ductal dependent, and coronary perfusion is retrograde when aortic atresia or critical aortic stenosis is present.

Clinical Manifestations

As the ductus arteriosus closes, neonates with HLHS will have severely diminished systemic blood flow and rapidly present in shock, with signs of poor systemic perfusion, tachycardia, and tachypnea. A right ventricular heave may be present. A single S_2 will be present and possibly a continuous murmur consistent with flow through the PDA. The chest radiograph reveals pulmonary edema and progressive cardiac enlargement. The ECG is consistent with right ventricular hypertrophy, and there is poor R wave progression across the precordial leads.

Treatment

PGE1 should be started to maintain ductal-dependent systemic blood flow. Only a palliative procedure is available; there is no corrective surgery for this lesion. The stage I (or Norwood) palliation is performed in the first week of life. The stage I procedure involves anastamosis of the pulmonary artery and aorta to provide unobstructed systemic blood flow, enlargement of the atrial communication with atrial septectomy, and placement of a modified Blalock-Taussig shunt or right ventricular to pulmonary artery conduit to provide a stable source of pulmonary blood flow. The second-stage procedure, a cavopulmonary anastomosis (bidirectional Glenn procedure or Hemi-Fontan) is performed at 3 to 6 months of age, and a modified Fontan completion procedure is generally performed between 2 to 5 years of age. Some centers do not perform the stage I surgical palliation and use a catheter based approach ("hybrid technique"), limiting pulmonary blood flow by placement of bilateral pulmonary artery bands, enlarging the atrial septal defect with balloon dilation, and stenting of the ductus arteriosus to maintain systemic blood flow. In these patients, surgical aortic arch reconstruction is performed at the time of the second stage of palliation.

INTERRUPTED AORTIC ARCH

Interrupted aortic arch is essentially an extreme form of coarctation of the aorta (Fig. 7-4). There are three types of interrupted aortic arch: Type A is interruption beyond the left subclavian artery, type B is interruption between the left subclavian and left common carotid arteries, and type C is interruption between the left common carotid and the brachiocephalic artery. Systemic blood flow depends on patency of the ductus arteriosus, which shunts blood from the pulmonary artery to the aorta. Interrupted aortic arch is often associated with a 22q11 microdeletion.

Clinical Manifestations

Neonates with interrupted aortic arch have ductal-dependent systemic blood flow and present with circulatory collapse as the ductus closes. The clinical presentation is similar to that of HLHS after the ductus arteriosus closes.

Treatment

PGE1 therapy should begin immediately to maintain systemic blood flow via right-to-left shunting at the PDA. Surgical

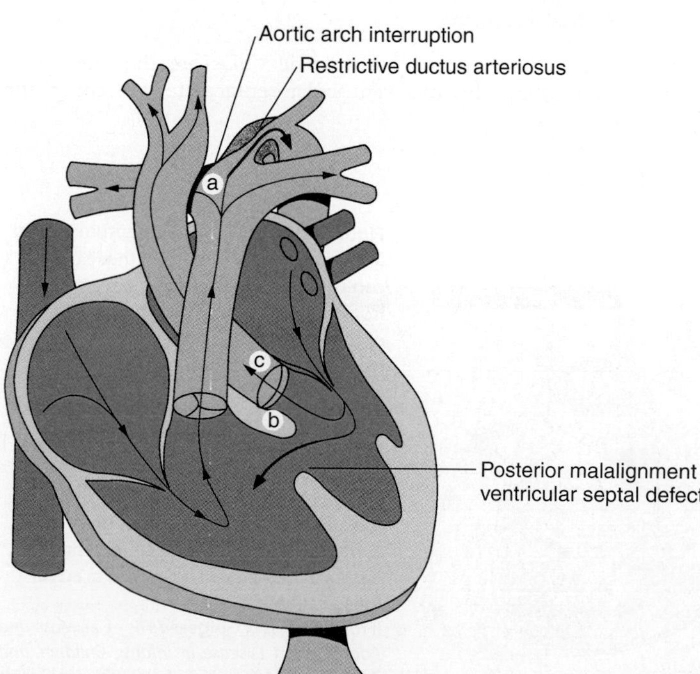

Figure 7-4 • Interrupted aortic arch with restrictive PDA. Typical anatomic findings include **(A)** atresia of a segment of the aortic arch between the left subclavian artery and the left common carotid (the most common type of interrupted aortic arch—"type B"); **(B)** posterior malalignment of the infundibular septum resulting in a large VSD and a narrow subaortic area; **(C)** a bicuspid aortic valve, which occurs in 60% of patients.

treatment involves an extended end-to-end anastomosis of the interrupted aortic segments.

ACYANOTIC CONGENITAL HEART DISEASE

Acyanotic cardiac defects that result in *increased pulmonary blood flow* (left-to-right shunts) include ASD, VSD, PDA, and common atrioventricular canal. Acyanotic lesions that result in *pulmonary venous hypertension* include coarctation of the aorta and aortic valve stenosis. The acyanotic structural anomaly that results in *normal or decreased pulmonary blood flow* is pulmonary valve stenosis.

ATRIAL SEPTAL DEFECTS

Atrial septal defects account for 8% of CHD and have a 2:1 female-to-male predominance. There are three types of atrial septal defects:

- Ostium secundum defect, seen in the midportion of the atrial septum
- Ostium primum defect, located in the lower portion of the atrial septum
- Sinus venosus defect, found at the junction of the right atrium and the superior or inferior vena cava. These defects are associated with anomalous drainage of the right pulmonary veins.

The degree of atrial shunting depends on the size of the ASD and the relative compliance of the ventricles in diastole. Because right ventricular diastolic compliance is usually greater than left ventricular diastolic compliance, left-to-right shunting occurs at the atrial level and results in right atrial and right ventricular enlargement and increased pulmonary blood flow.

Clinical Manifestations

Atrial septal defects are usually asymptomatic, although exercise intolerance may be noted in older children. Paradoxical embolism, leading to a stroke, may occur. Supraventricular tachycardia from atrial enlargement may also occur. On examination, a right ventricular heave is often present. A systolic ejection murmur in the pulmonic (left upper sternal border) area and a middiastolic rumble in the lower right sternal border reflect the increased flow across the pulmonary and tricuspid valves. S_1 is loud, and S_2 is widely split on both inspiration and expiration ("fixed" splitting). The chest radiograph reveals enlargement of the heart and main pulmonary artery with increased pulmonary vascularity. The ECG often shows right ventricular enlargement. Right-axis deviation is seen in secundum defects, whereas primum defects have characteristic extreme left-axis deviation.

Treatment

Spontaneous closure of small secundum ASDs (the most common type) often occurs in the first year of life. In both symptomatic and asymptomatic children with suitable secundum ASDs, transcatheter device closure may be undertaken after 2 years of age. Moderate- to large-size secundum ASDs that have not spontaneously closed and are not candidates for device closure must be addressed surgically. Ostium primum and sinus venosus ASDs will not close spontaneously and must be addressed surgically. Surgical closure involves pericardial patch or suture closure.

VENTRICULAR SEPTAL DEFECTS

The VSD is the most common congenital heart defect, accounting for 25% of all congenital heart defects. The five types of VSDs are as follows (as seen in Fig. 7-5):

- Muscular
- Inlet
- Conoseptal hypoplasia
- Conoventricular (also known as perimembranous)
- Malalignment

Muscular and conoventricular VSDs are the most common types. Muscular ventricular septal defects occur in the

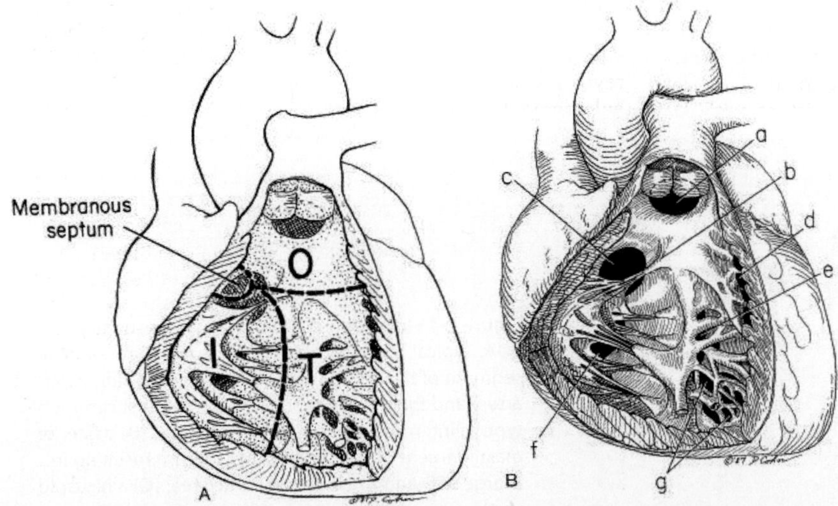

Figure 7-5 • **(A)** Ventricular septum viewed from right ventricular side is made of four components; I, inlet component extends from tricuspid annulus to attachments of tricuspid valve; T, trabecular septum extends from inlet out to apex and up to smooth-walled outlet; O, outlet septum or infundibular septum, which extends up to pulmonary valve, and membranous septum. **(B)** Anatomic position of defects: a, outlet defect; b, papillary muscle of the conus; c, perimembranous defect; d, marginal muscular defects; e, central muscular defects; f, inlet defect; g, apical muscular defects.
(From Allen HD, Gutgesell HP, et al. *Moss and Adams Heart Disease in Infants, Children, and Adolescents*, 6th ed. Philadelphia: Lippincott Williams & Wilkins, 2001.)

muscular portion of the septum and may be single or multiple and located in the posterior, apical, or anterior portion of the septum. The inlet VSD is an endocardial cushion defect and occurs in the inlet portion of the septum beneath the septal leaflet of the tricuspid valve. Conoseptal hypoplasia VSDs are positioned in the outflow tract of the right ventricle (RV) beneath the pulmonary valve. The conoventricular VSD occurs in the membranous portion of the ventricular septum. Malalignment VSDs result from malalignment of the infundibular septum. Anterior malalignment results in TOF, and posterior malalignment results in aortic stenosis or subaortic stenosis with arch hypoplasia or interruption.

When the VSD is small, shunt flow is left to right from the high-pressure LV to the lower pressure RV. Small shunts result in relatively normal pulmonary blood flow and pulmonary vascular resistance (PVR). When the VSD is large, LV and RV pressure become equal and PVR and systemic vascular resistance (SVR) determine shunt flow. When the PVR is less than the SVR (as is normal), the shunt flow is left to right. The amount of LV and left atrial dilatation is directly proportional to the size of the left-to-right shunt. Right ventricular hypertrophy occurs when PVR increases. If left untreated, the large VSD may result in elevated pulmonary arterial pressures and may lead to pulmonary vascular obstructive disease, pulmonary hypertension, and **Eisenmenger syndrome**. In severe cases of Eisenmenger syndrome, the VSD shunt reverses right to left when the PVR exceeds the SVR.

Clinical Manifestations

Clinical symptoms are related to the size of the shunt. A small shunt produces no symptoms, whereas a large shunt gives rise to signs of congestive heart failure and failure to thrive. The smaller the defect, the louder the harsh systolic murmur, heard best at the mid-to-lower left sternal border. As the PVR increases in patients with nonrestrictive VSDs, shunting from left-to-right decreases, the murmur shortens, and the pulmonary (late) component of S_2 increases in intensity. Eisenmenger syndrome results in a right ventricular heave, pulmonary valve ejection click, short systolic ejection murmur, diastolic murmur of pulmonary valve insufficiency, and a loud, single S_2.

Small VSDs have a normal chest radiograph and electrocardiogram. Moderate-size VSDs may show mild cardiomegaly and slightly increased pulmonary vascularity on chest radiograph. Large left-to-right shunts result in cardiomegaly, increased pulmonary vascularity, and enlargement of the left atrium and left ventricle. The ECG is consistent with left atrial, left ventricular, or biventricular hypertrophy. Right ventricular hypertrophy predominates when pulmonary vascular resistance is high.

Treatment

Most small VSDs close without intervention (40% by 3 years, 75% by 10 years); in cases which do not, surgery is often unnecessary. Muscular VSDs are the most likely to close spontaneously. The treatment for large VSDs, with significant left-to-right shunting and variable levels of congestive heart failure, is surgical closure before pulmonary vascular changes become irreversible. Surgical closure usually involves patch closure. In some cases, transcatheter device placement in the interventricular septum may be used for muscular VSD closure. Congestive heart failure may be treated with diuretics, and systemic afterload reduction with an angiotensin-converting enzyme (ACE) inhibitor. Growth failure may be improved with nasogastric enteral feeds to optimize caloric intake.

COMMON ATRIOVENTRICULAR CANAL DEFECT

The common atrioventricular canal defect (Fig. 7-6) is most commonly seen in children with Down syndrome. The lesion results from deficiency of the endocardial cushions and results in an ostium primum ASD and inlet VSD with lack of septation of the mitral and tricuspid valves (common atrioventricular valve [CAVV]). The various forms of atrioventricular canal defects account for 5% of all CHD. In an **incomplete atrioventricular canal defect**, the CAVV leaflets attach directly to the top of the muscular portion of the ventricular septum. As a result, there is no communication beneath the atrioventricular valves between the right and left ventricles. The communication at the atrial level is an ostium primum ASD. The mitral valve is cleft, and there may be some degree of mitral regurgitation. In **complete common atrioventricular canal**, there is a CAVV that is not attached to the muscular ventricular septum. As a result, there is a large inlet VSD located between the CAVV and the top of the muscular ventricular septum. In this defect, there is a left-to-right shunting at the ostium primum ASD and inlet VSD. Because of the increase in pulmonary blood flow, pulmonary hypertension and pulmonary vascular disease may develop over time. In untreated cases, Eisenmenger syndrome may develop.

Clinical Manifestations

The clinical manifestations and treatment of incomplete common atrioventricular canal are the same as those described for an ASD. There may be a blowing systolic murmur heard best at the left lower sternal border and apex, consistent with mitral regurgitation through the mitral valve cleft.

In complete common atrioventricular canal, the degree of congestive heart failure depends on the magnitude of the left-to-right shunting and the amount of CAVV regurgitation. If shunting or valve regurgitation is significant, congestive heart failure is seen early in infancy, with tachypnea, dyspnea, and failure to thrive. On examination, a blowing holosystolic murmur is heard at the left lower sternal border, and S_2 is widely split and fixed. Cardiac enlargement and increased pulmonary vascularity are visible on the chest radiograph. The ECG reveals a superior axis, characteristic of a canal defect, and enlargement of both right and left atria.

Treatment

Prior to surgical repair, congestive heart failure may be treated with, diuretics, and an ACE inhibitor. The symptomatic patient with complete common atrioventricular valve (CAVV) is generally repaired during infancy. The asymptomatic child with incomplete canal without pulmonary hypertension may undergo elective repair within the first few years of life. Infants with a large VSD component should be repaired by 6 months to decrease the risk of pulmonary artery hypertension and pulmonary vascular obstructive disease. The ASD and VSD portions are closed, and the CAVV is divided into left and right sides. Suture closure of the cleft leaflets of the septated left-sided atrioventricular inflow is performed to make the LV inflow as competent as possible. Complete heart block occurs

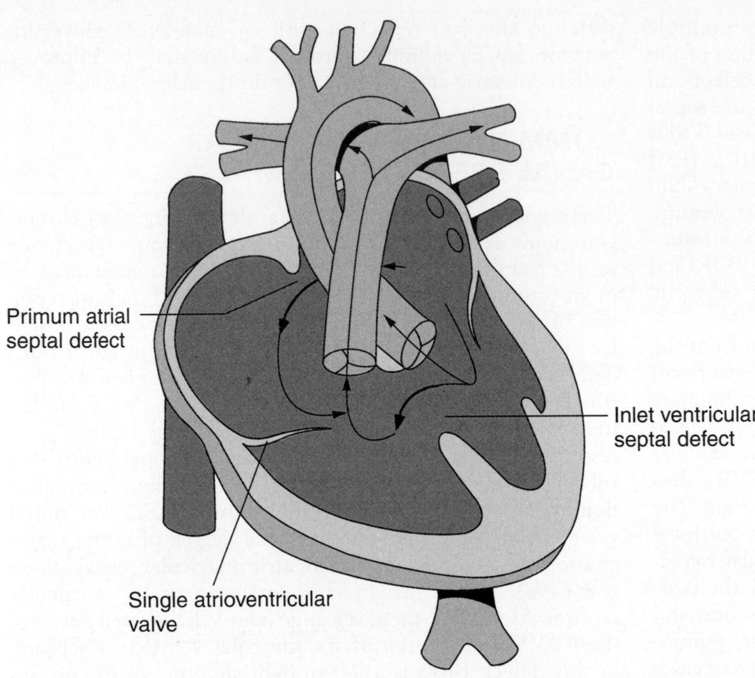

Figure 7-6 • Complete common atrioventricular canal. Typical anatomic findings include large atrial and ventricular septal defects of the endocardial cushion type; single atrio-ventricular valve; left-to-right shunting, which is noted at the atrial and ventricular level when pulmonary vascular resistance falls during the neonatal period.

in 5% of patients undergoing repair, and residual mitral insufficiency is not uncommon.

PATENT DUCTUS ARTERIOSUS

Persistent patency of the ductus arteriosus accounts for 10% of CHD. The incidence of PDA is higher in premature neonates. The ductus arteriosus connects the underside of the aorta and the left pulmonary artery just distal to the takeoff of the left subclavian artery from the aorta (Fig. 7-7). The direction of blood flow through a PDA depends on the relative resistances in the pulmonary and systemic circuits. In the nonrestrictive (large) PDA, a left-to-right shunt is present as long as the systemic vascular resistance is greater than the pulmonary vascular resistance. If pulmonary vascular resistance rises above systemic vascular resistance, a right-to-left shunt develops.

Clinical Manifestations

Symptoms are related to the *size* of the defect and the *direction* of flow. A small PDA causes no symptoms or abnormalities on chest radiograph or ECG. A large PDA with left-to-right shunting may result in congestive heart failure and failure to thrive. Bounding pulses are palpable. A continuous murmur begins after S_1, peaks at S_2, and trails off during diastole. The chest radiograph of a large patent ductus arteriosus shows cardiomegaly, increased pulmonary vascularity, and left atrial and ventricular enlargement. The ECG shows left or biventricular hypertrophy. If pulmonary vascular resistance rises above systemic resistance (pulmonary hypertension), flow at the PDA reverses, and cyanosis is noted.

Treatment

Indomethacin decreases PGE1 levels and is often effective in closing the ductus in the premature neonate but is associated with risk of renal insufficiency. A PDA usually closes in term infants in the first month of life. If the ductus remains patent, coil embolization or device closure in the cardiac catheterization laboratory or surgical ligation may be performed.

COARCTATION OF THE AORTA

Coarctation of the aorta (Color Plate 16) accounts for 8% of congenital heart defects and has a male-to-female predominance of 2:1. When coarctation of the aorta occurs in a female, **Turner syndrome** must be considered. The obstruction (narrowing) is usually located in the descending aorta at the insertion site of the ductus arteriosus. The coarctation results in obstruction to blood flow (between the proximal and distal aorta) and increased left ventricular afterload.

Clinical Manifestations

The degree of narrowing determines clinical severity. Infants may be asymptomatic or present with irritability, difficulty feeding, and failure to thrive. More than half of infants with coarctation will have no symptoms in infancy. Neonates with critical coarctation have ductal-dependent systemic blood flow and may present with circulatory collapse as the ductus closes, similar to HLHS and interrupted aortic arch. On examination, the femoral pulses are often weak and delayed or even absent, and there is upper extremity hypertension. On cardiac examination, there is a nonspecific ejection murmur at the heart apex. If the coarctation is associated with a bicuspid aortic valve, an apical ejection click will be heard. The chest radiograph and ECG are normal in mild lesions. In patients with more severe obstruction, the chest radiograph may reveal an enlarged aortic knob and cardiomegaly. Right ventricular hypertrophy is seen in the neonatal ECG; left ventricular hypertrophy is more common in the older patient.

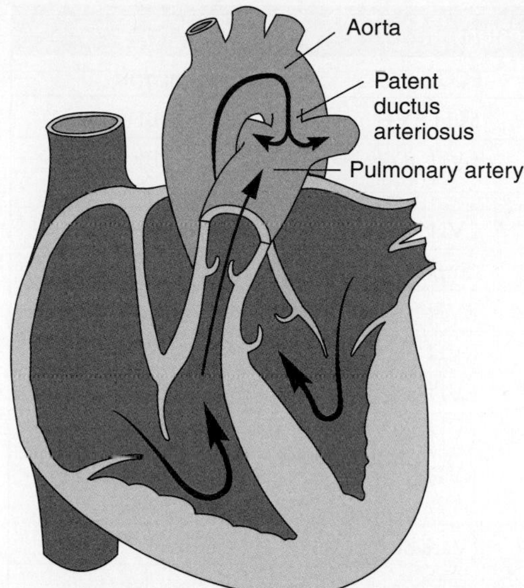

Figure 7-7 • Patent ductus arteriosus. The ductal arteriosus connects the underside of the aorta to the takeoff of the left pulmonary artery. When pulmonary vascular resistance falls, blood flows from left-to-right from aorta to pulmonary artery.
(From Pillitteri A. *Maternal and Child Nursing*, 4th ed. Philadelphia: Lippincott Williams & Wilkins, 2003.)

Treatment

In neonates with critical coarctation of the aorta, the child's systemic blood flow is ductal-dependent, and PGE1 should be started prior to surgical intervention. Treatment may be surgical, with end-to-end anastomosis or patch aortoplasty, or interventional, with balloon dilation angioplasty with or without stent placement. Timing and type of therapy depend on age at diagnosis, severity of illness, and related defects. Restenosis at the surgical repair site is not uncommon, especially in neonates. Persistent hypertension after intervention in the older child may require β-blocker therapy.

AORTIC STENOSIS

In aortic stenosis, the valvular tissue is thickened, rigid, and domes in systole. Commonly, the valve is bicuspid rather than tricuspid. The increased pressure generated in the left ventricle, as it attempts to direct blood flow across a stenotic valve, results in left ventricular hypertrophy and, over time, decreased compliance and ventricular performance.

Clinical Manifestations

The degree of symptoms is related to the severity of the stenosis and the level of ventricular function. Infants with minimal stenosis are asymptomatic (although with a murmur). The neonate with critical aortic stenosis has ductal-dependent systemic blood flow and may present with circulatory collapse if the ductus closes. The cardiac examination is characterized by a harsh systolic ejection murmur heard at the right upper sternal border that is preceded by an ejection click. In severe aortic stenosis, a thrill may be palpable. The more pronounced the stenosis, the louder the murmur. However, if ventricular function is highly compromised, only a soft murmur may be appreciated. The chest radiograph shows cardiomegaly. Pulmonary edema may be noted in cases with ventricular dysfunction. Left ventricular hypertrophy is seen on the ECG. In some cases, a strain pattern of ST depression and inverted T waves consistent with ischemia may be noted.

Treatment

In neonates with critical aortic stenosis, systemic blood flow is ductal-dependent, and PGE1 should be started prior to surgical or catheter-based intervention. If intervention is required, relief of the aortic valve narrowing is usually best accomplished by balloon valvuloplasty. Intervention does not create a normal valve and regurgitation and restenosis is common. These may progress over time with requirement for aortic valvuloplasty or aortic valve replacement with a mechanical, homograft, or autograft valve (Ross procedure).

PULMONIC STENOSIS

Pulmonic valve stenosis accounts for 5% to 8% of CHD. The valve is dysplastic with only a small central opening, and there is often poststenotic dilatation of the main pulmonary artery. Right ventricular hypertrophy occurs with time due to increased right ventricular afterload. In *critical pulmonic stenosis*, a decrease in the compliance of the right ventricle increases right atrial pressure and may open the foramen ovale, producing a right-to-left shunt.

Clinical Manifestations

Most patients are asymptomatic. Severe pulmonary stenosis may cause dyspnea on exertion and angina. Right-sided congestive heart failure is rare, except in infants with critical pulmonic stenosis who may have ductal-dependent pulmonary blood flow. Characteristically, the ejection click of pulmonic stenosis varies with inspiration, and a harsh systolic ejection murmur is heard at the left upper sternal border. In severe stenosis, a thrill and right ventricular heave are palpable. On chest radiograph, heart size and pulmonary vascularity are normal, but the pulmonary artery segment is enlarged. The degree of right ventricular hypertrophy and right-axis deviation present on ECG correlates with the degree of stenosis.

Treatment

In neonates with critical pulmonary stenosis, the child's pulmonary blood flow is ductal-dependent, and PGE1 should be started prior to surgical or catheter-based intervention. Catheter based intervention is performed most commonly, typically with excellent results.

Table 7-6 lists the findings for the ten most common congenital heart lesions.

ACQUIRED STRUCTURAL HEART DISEASE

RHEUMATIC HEART DISEASE

Acute rheumatic fever causes carditis in 50% to 80% of patients. Rheumatic heart disease results from single or multiple episodes of acute rheumatic fever. **Mitral regurgitation** is the most common valvular residual lesion of acute rheumatic carditis. Aortic insufficiency may also occur, with or without

TABLE 7-6 Findings for the Ten Most Common Congenital Heart Lesions

Lesion	Presentation	Physical Examination	ECG	Radiograph
Atrial septal defect	Murmur	Fixed split S_2	Mild RVH	±CE, ↑ PBF
Ventricular septal defect	Murmur, CHF	Holosystolic murmur	LVH, RVH	±CE, ↑ PBF
Patent ductus arteriosus	Murmur, ±CHF	Continuous murmur	LVH, ±RVH	±CE, ↑ PBF
AV canal defect	Murmur, ±CHF	Holosystolic murmur	"Superior" axis	±CE, ↑ PBF
Pulmonic stenosis	Murmur, ±cyanosis	Click, SEM	RVH	±CE, NL, or ↓ PBF
Tetralogy of Fallot	Murmur, ±cyanosis	SEM	RVH	±CE, ↓ PBF
Aortic stenosis	Murmur, ±CHF	Click, SEM	LVH	±CE, NL, PBF
Coarctation of the aorta	Hypertension	↓ Femoral pulses	LVH	±CE, NL, PBF
Transposition of the great arteries	Cyanosis	Marked cyanosis Loud S_2	RVH	±CE, NL, or ↑ PBF
Single ventricle	(Variable)	(Variable)	(Variable)	(Variable)

CE, cardiac enlargement; CHF, congestive heart failure; LVH, left ventricular hypertrophy; NL, normal; PBF, pulmonary blood flow; RVH, right ventricular hypertrophy; SEM, systolic ejection murmur.

mitral regurgitation. Late-stage disease may progress to mitral and/or aortic stenosis. Patients with severe valvular involvement manifest signs and symptoms of chronic congestive heart failure. Chapter 12 discusses acute rheumatic fever.

KAWASAKI DISEASE

Cardiac effects may include pericarditis, myocarditis, and coronary arteritis. It is the development of **coronary artery aneurysms**, with their potential for occlusion, however, that makes the disease life-threatening. Coronary artery aneurysms develop during the subacute phase (11th to 25th day) in approximately 25% of cases but regress in most patients. Early therapy with intravenous immunoglobulin decreases the incidence of coronary artery aneurysms to less than 10%. High-dose aspirin therapy given during the acute inflammatory period lessens the likelihood of aneurysm development. Low-dose aspirin is continued for 6 to 8 weeks (or indefinitely if the aneurysms do not resolve). An ECHO is used to assess ventricular function and detect and follow coronary artery aneurysms. Evidence of myocardial ischemia warrants a cardiac catheterization and in some cases may require coronary artery bypass surgery if obstruction exists. Chapter 11 offers a thorough discussion of Kawasaki disease.

ENDOCARDITIS

Pathogenesis

Bacterial endocarditis (BE) is a microbial infection of the endocardium. Although it may occur on normal valves, BE is more likely to occur where there is turbulent flow on congenitally abnormal valves, valves damaged by rheumatic fever, acquired valvular lesions (mitral valve prolapse), and prosthetic replacement valves. Factors that may precipitate BE include intravenous drug abuse, an indwelling central venous catheter, and/or prior cardiac surgery. In 2007, the American Heart Association's Endocarditis Committee, together with national and international experts on BE, extensively reviewed published studies in order to determine whether dental, gastrointestinal, or genitourinary tract procedures are possible causes of BE. These experts determined that there is no conclusive evidence that links dental, gastrointestinal, or genitourinary tract procedures with the development of BE. The prior practice of giving patients antibiotics prior to a dental procedure is no longer recommended **except** for patients with the highest risk of adverse outcomes resulting from BE:

- Prosthetic cardiac valve
- Previous endocarditis
- Congenital heart disease only in the following categories:
  - Unrepaired cyanotic congenital heart disease, including those with palliative shunts and conduits
  - Completely repaired congenital heart disease with prosthetic material or device, whether placed by surgery or catheter intervention, during the first 6 months after the procedure (Prophylaxis is recommended because endothelialization of prosthetic material occurs within 6 months after the procedure.)
  - Repaired congenital heart disease with residual defects at the site or adjacent to the site of a prosthetic patch or prosthetic device (which inhibits endothelialization)
- Cardiac transplantation recipients with cardiac valvular disease

In children, α-hemolytic streptococci (*Streptococcus viridans*) and *Staphylococcus aureus* are the most common etiologic agents. *S. viridans* accounts for approximately 67% of cases, whereas *S. aureus* is present in an estimated 20% of cases. When the infection is a complication of cardiac surgery, *Staphylococcus epidermidis* and fungi should be considered. Gram-negative organisms cause approximately 5% of cases of endocarditis in children and are more likely in neonates, immunocompromised patients, and intravenous drug abusers.

Clinical Manifestations

Fever is the most common finding in children with bacterial endocarditis. Often, a new or changing murmur is auscultated.

Children with endocarditis usually display nonspecific symptoms, including chest pain, dyspnea, arthralgia, myalgia, headache, and malaise. Embolic phenomena such as hematuria and strokes may occur. Other embolic phenomena (Roth spots, splinter hemorrhages, petechiae, Osler nodes, and Janeway lesions) are relatively rare in children with bacterial endocarditis.

Diagnostic Evaluation

Typical laboratory findings include elevation in white blood count, erythrocyte sedimentation rate (ESR), and C-reactive protein (CRP). Anemia is common. Hematuria may be seen on urinalysis. Multiple blood cultures increase the probability of discovering the pathogen. A transthoracic and/or transesophageal ECHO is used to define vegetations and/or thrombi in the heart. ECGs should be monitored on a serial basis to detect atrioventricular conduction abnormalities. Complete heart block can occur with severe endocarditis.

Treatment

Medical management consists of 6 to 8 weeks of intravenous antibiotics directed against the isolated pathogen. Surgery is indicated for endocarditis when medical treatment is unsuccessful, refractory congestive heart failure exists, serious embolic complications occur, myocardial abscesses develop, or when there is refractory infection of a prosthetic valve.

FUNCTIONAL HEART DISEASE

MYOCARDITIS

Most cases of myocarditis in the developed world result from viral infection of the myocardium, predominantly adenovirus, parvovirus, coxsackie A and B, echovirus, and HIV. It is unclear whether the myocardial damage results from direct viral invasion or an autoimmune antibody response.

Clinical Manifestations

If myocardial damage is mild, patients may be asymptomatic; the diagnosis may be made by finding ST- and T-wave changes on an ECG done for an unrelated reason. Severe myocardial damage presents with fulminant congestive heart failure and arrhythmia. Common symptoms include fever, dyspnea, fatigue, and abdominal pain. Tachycardia, evidence of hepatomegaly, and S3 ventricular gallop may be appreciated on examination. The ECG often reveals ST-segment depression, T-wave inversion, and low voltage. Arrhythmias and conduction defects may also be present. Heart size on chest radiograph varies from mild to markedly enlarged. The ECHO reveals ventricles that are dilated and/or poorly functioning. Pericardial effusion is common. Viral etiology should be investigated by polymerase chain reaction (PCR) from the throat, stool, and blood. Endomyocardial biopsy is indicated to confirm diagnosis.

Treatment

Therapy for patients with viral myocarditis is supportive to maintain perfusion and oxygen delivery. Ventricular arrhythmias, conduction abnormalities, and congestive heart failure are treated as indicated. Intravenous immunoglobulin is often given despite limited data, to minimize further damage to the myocardium. The prognosis for patients with myocarditis is directly related to the extent of myocardial damage. Although recovery may occur, heart failure may persist or worsen with late mortality or need for support with mechanical circulatory support and possibly cardiac transplantation.

CORONARY ARTERY DISEASE

Although coronary artery disease is rare in childhood, the atherosclerotic process appears to begin early in life. Evidence indicates that progression of atherosclerotic lesions is influenced by genetic factors (familial hypercholesteremia) and lifestyle (cigarette smoking; high-cholesterol diet, high-saturated-fat diet). Certain diseases place children at increased risk for hypercholesteremia (e.g., some storage and metabolic diseases, renal failure, diabetes, hepatitis, systemic lupus erythematosus). Because many lifetime habits are formed during childhood, the opportunity exists for prevention of coronary artery disease.

DILATED CARDIOMYOPATHY

Dilated cardiomyopathy (DCM) is characterized by myocardial dysfunction and ventricular dilation. In idiopathic cases (most common), the cause is theorized to be a prior undiagnosed episode of myocarditis. Dilated cardiomyopathy can also be associated with neuromuscular disease (Dystrophin abnormality) or drug toxicity (anthracyclines). In 25% to 48% of cases of DCM, there is genetic abnormality leading to cytoskeletal or sarcomeric protein abnormalities.

Clinical Manifestations

Signs and symptoms are related to the degree of myocardial dysfunction. Symptoms include feeding intolerance, abdominal pain, dyspnea, orthopnea, and paroxysmal nocturnal dyspnea. The cardiac examination reveals an S_3 gallop rhythm and often a murmur consistent with mitral regurgitation. As heart failure worsens, dependent edema, a right ventricular heave, and pulsus alternans (beat-to-beat variability in pulse magnitude) may be noted. The heart is enlarged on chest radiograph, often accompanied by pulmonary edema. The ECG is notable for broadening of the QRS complexes and nonspecific ST- and T-wave ischemic changes. Ventricular dilation and function is evaluated by ECHO. Cardiac MRI with delayed enhancement may be used to evaluate for the presence of fibrosis.

Treatment

Initial treatment of a child presenting with symptomatic heart failure, treatment includes diuretics (to reduce preload), vasodilators (decrease afterload), and if necessary inotropes (increase contractility). Ideally the child can be managed as an outpatient on oral medications, most commonly diuretics, an ACE inhibitor and possibly a β-blocker. If the child presents in cardiogenic shock, medical therapy with inotropes and positive pressure ventilation (decrease left ventricular afterload) are attempted, and if not successful at achieving adequate oxygen delivery and end organ support, the child may require mechanical circulatory support. Extracorporeal membrane oygenation (ECMO) or a ventricular assist device may be used as either a bridge to myocardial recovery or cardiac transplantation. Antiarrhythmic medications or placement of internal cardioverter-defibrillator (ICD) are reserved for treatment of potentially fatal ventricular arrhythmias.

HYPERTROPHIC OBSTRUCTIVE CARDIOMYOPATHY

Also known as idiopathic hypertrophic subaortic stenosis, hypertrophic cardiomyopathy is a disorder in which the ventricular septum is significantly thickened, resulting in variable degrees of left ventricular outflow tract obstruction. The thickened stiff left ventricle has compromised diastolic function and preserved systolic function. Abnormal motion of the mitral valve results in mitral insufficiency. Inheritance is autosomal dominant with incomplete penetrance.

Clinical Manifestations

Most cases are asymptomatic and discovered as a result of evaluation of a heart murmur. When present (generally in adolescence), symptoms include dyspnea on exertion, chest pain, and syncope. A systolic ejection murmur at the left lower sternal border and/or apex may be accompanied by the soft, holosystolic murmur of mitral regurgitation and an S_3 gallop. There may be a left ventricular heave and thrill. The chest radiograph shows normal vascularity and mild left ventricular enlargement. The ECG illustrates left-axis deviation, left ventricular hypertrophy, and possible ST- and T-wave changes consistent with ischemia or strain. The ECHO is diagnostic.

Unfortunately, hypertrophic cardiomyopathy may also present as sudden death during physical activity in an otherwise healthy, asymptomatic person with undiagnosed disease.

Treatment

Therapy is centered on preventing fatal ventricular arrhythmias and improving left ventricular filling by slowing the intrinsic heart rate. Medications that reduce the risk of arrhythmia and decrease chronotropy and inotropy include calcium channel blockers and β-adrenergic blocking agents. The avoidance of competitive sports is essential because sudden death during exertion is a significant risk (4% to 6% of affected patients a year).

ARRHYTHMIAS

Arrhythmias in children are much less common than in adults but can be just as life-threatening. Arrhythmias result from disorders of impulse formation, impulse conduction, or both, and they are generally classified as follows.

Bradyarrhythmias
- Sinus node dysfunction
- Conduction block

Tachyarrhythmias
- Narrow QRS
- Wide QRS

Premature beats
- Atrial
- Ventricular

Arrhythmias may result from congenital, functional, or acquired structural heart disease; electrolyte disturbances (potassium, calcium, and magnesium); drug toxicity; poisoning; or an acquired systemic disorder. Table 7-7 lists the etiologies predisposing children to arrhythmias.

TABLE 7-7 Factors Predisposing to Arrhythmiast

Congenital heart disease	Friedreich ataxia (atrial tachycardia or fibrillation)
Supraventricular arrhythmias	Muscular dystrophies (Duchenne, periodic paralysis)
Ebstein anomaly, atrial septal defects, atrial surgery, L-transposition of the great arteries, after Fontan operation	Glycogen storage diseases (Pompe disease)
Ventricular arrhythmias	Collagen vascular diseases (rheumatic carditis, systemic lupus erythematosus, periarteritis nodosa, dermatomyositis)
Aortic valve disease, pulmonary valve disease, after tetralogy of Fallot repair, anomalous left coronary artery, RV dysplasia	Endocrine disorders (hyperthyroidism, adrenal dysfunction)
Heart block (varying degrees)	Metabolic and electrolyte disturbances (hypomagnesemia, hyperkalemia, hypocalcemia, hypoxia)
After open-heart surgery (ventricular septal defect, Ebstein anomaly, L-transposition of the great arteries)	Lyme disease
Isolated conduction system disorders	Drug toxicity
Maternal lupus erythematosus	Chemotherapeutic agents
Prolonged QT-interval	Tricyclic antidepressants
Inherited syndromes (Romano-Ward, Jervell and Lange-Nielson)	Cocaine
Associated with systemic illness	Antiarrhythmia drugs (Digitalis, β-adrenergic blockers, calcium blockers)
Infectious myocarditis	Asthma medications (sympathomimetics)
Kawasaki disease	Blunt chest trauma (myocardial contusion)
Idiopathic dilated or hypertrophic cardiomyopathy	Increased intracranial pressure

RV, right ventricle.

BRADYARRHYTHMIAS

Bradyarrhythmias may result from depressed automaticity at the sinus node (sinus node dysfunction) or conduction block at the atrioventricular node or bundle of His (AV block). Bradyarrhythmias that may result from sinus node dysfunction include sinus bradycardia, junctional bradycardia, ectopic atrial bradycardia, and sinus pauses. Bradyarrhythmias that may result from AV block include first-degree heart block, second-degree heart block, and third-degree (complete) heart block.

Differential Diagnosis

Figure 7-8 shows the rhythm strips of various bradycardias. **Sinus bradycardia** is caused by a decreased rate of impulse generation at the sinus node. It may be associated with increased vagal tone, hypoxia, central nervous system disorders with increased intracranial pressure, hypothyroidism, hyperkalemia, hypothermia, drug intoxication (digoxin, β-blockers, calcium channel blockers), and prior atrial surgery. It is also a normal finding in healthy athletes. The ECG reveals a normal P wave with normal AV conduction at rates less than 100 beats per minute (bpm) in the neonate and 60 bpm in the older child. When sinus bradycardia becomes too slow, sinus pauses or escape rhythms (ectopic atrial bradycardia or ectopic atrial rhythm, junctional bradycardia or junctional rhythm, or a slow idioventricular ventricular rhythm) may occur. Patients with sinus bradycardia can increase their heart rate appropriately when stimulated.

First-degree heart block usually results from slowing of atrioventricular conduction at the level of the AV node. First-degree heart block is associated with increased vagal tone; medication administration (digoxin and β-blocker); infectious etiologies (viral myocarditis, Lyme disease); hypothermia; electrolyte abnormalities (hypo/hyperkalemia, hypo/hypercalcemia, and hypomagnesemia); CHD (ASD, atrioventricular canal defect, Ebstein anomaly, TAPVC, and L-transposition of the great arteries or "corrected transposition"); rheumatic fever; and cardiomyopathy. First-degree AV block is characterized on ECG by PR interval prolongation for age and rate. Otherwise, the rhythm is regular, originates in the sinus node, and has a normal QRS morphology.

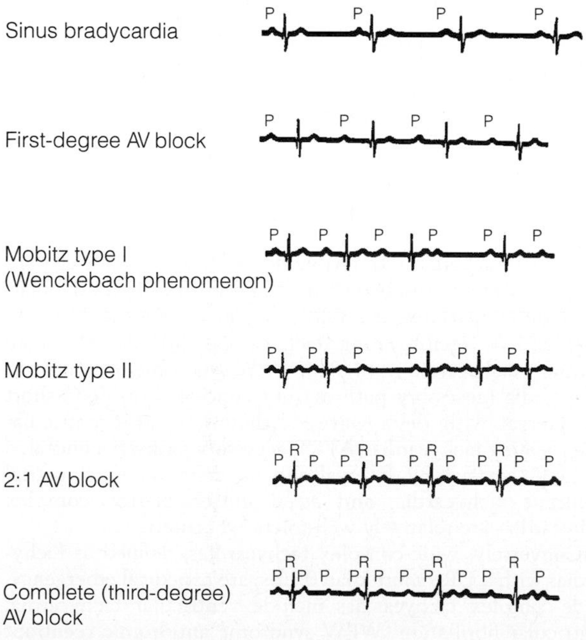

Second-degree heart block refers to episodic interruption of AV nodal conduction. Some P waves are followed by QRS complexes; others are not.

- **Mobitz type I** (Wenckebach) denotes progressive prolongation of the PR interval over several beats until a QRS is absent. This cycle repeats itself often, although the number of beats in a cycle may not be constant. The QRS configuration is normal. Etiologies for this rhythm are the same as those for first-degree heart block.
- **Mobitz type II** is caused by abrupt failure of atrioventricular conduction below the AV node in the bundle of His-Purkinje fiber system. It is a more serious bradycardia than first-degree heart block or Wenckebach because it can progress to complete heart block. On ECG, there is sudden AV conduction failure with a normal P wave without a QRS. No preceding PR interval prolongation is seen in normal conducted impulses.
- Fixed-ratio AV block is an arrhythmia in which the QRS complex follows only after every second (third or fourth) P wave, causing 2:1 (3:1 or 4:1) AV block. There is a normal PR interval in conducted beats. There is usually a normal or slightly prolonged QRS. Fixed-ratio block results from either AV node or His bundle injury, and intracardiac recordings are required to distinguish the site of injury. Patients may progress to complete heart block.

Third-degree heart block exists when no atrial impulses are conducted to the ventricles. The atrial rhythm and rate are normal for the patient's age, and the ventricular rate is slowed markedly (40 to 55 bpm). If an escape rhythm arises from the AV node (*junctional rhythm*), the QRS interval is of normal duration, but if an escape rhythm arises from the distal His bundle or Purkinje fibers, the QRS interval is prolonged (*idioventricular rhythm*). Congenital complete AV block can be an isolated abnormality or can be associated with L-transposition of the great arteries, atrioventricular canal defect, or maternal lupus erythematosus (particularly anti-Ro antibodies). Other causes include open-heart surgery (especially after large ventricular septal defect closure), cardiomyopathy, or Lyme disease. Fetuses or newborns with congenital complete heart block may present with hydrops fetalis.

Sinus bradycardia

First-degree AV block

Mobitz type I (Wenckebach phenomenon)

Mobitz type II

2:1 AV block

Complete (third-degree) AV block

Figure 7-8 • Bradyarrhythmias.

Treatment

No intervention is necessary for bradycardia if cardiac output is maintained. Figure 7-9 shows a management algorithm for bradycardia.

No treatment is necessary for first- or second-degree heart block (Mobitz type I). However, Mobitz type II, fixed-ratio AV block, and third-degree heart block all require pacemaker placement. In Mobitz type II and fixed-ratio AV block, prophylactic pacemaker insertion is essential to protect the patient should he or she progress to complete heart block with inadequate cardiac output away from medical care.

If the child with complete heart block is hemodynamically unstable, transcutaneous or transvenous pacing can be performed acutely and permanent transvenous or epicardial pacemaker placement can be performed later. Third-degree heart block is managed with either ventricular demand pacing or AV sequential pacing.

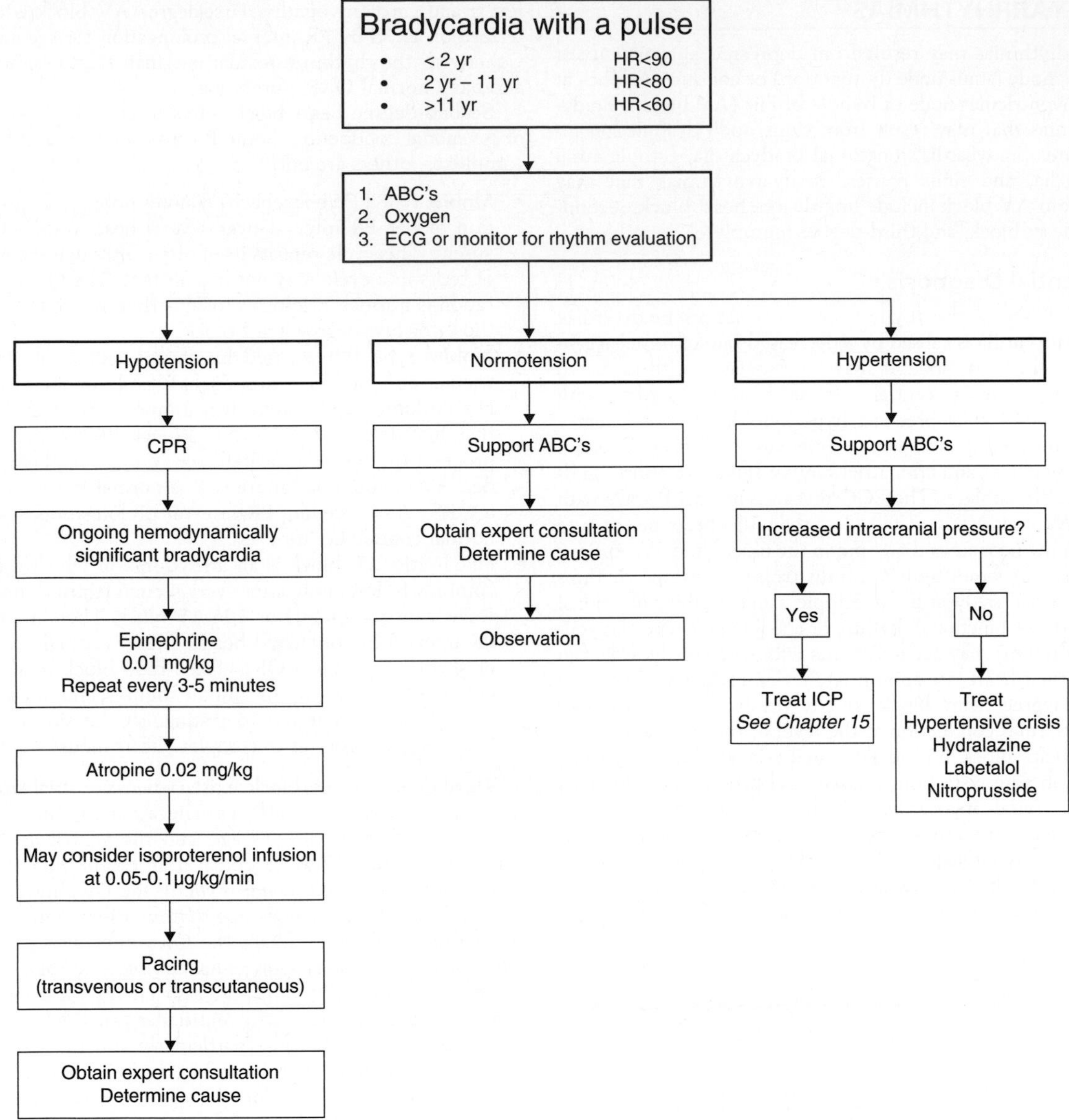

Figure 7-9 • Pediatric bradycardia management algorithm.

TACHYARRHYTHMIAS

Tachyarrhythmias arise from abnormal impulse formation caused by enhanced automaticity or a reentrant circuit. Narrow-complex tachycardias have a QRS morphology identical to that of normal sinus rhythm. Most SVTs are narrow-complex in appearance. Narrow-complex tachycardias may be caused by increased automaticity (e.g., sinus tachycardia, ectopic atrial tachycardia, junctional ectopic tachycardia, atrial fibrillation) or a reentrant circuit. Reentrant circuits are categorized into orthodromic reentrant tachycardia (ORT) or antidromic reentrant tachycardia (ART). In ORT, the SVT propagates down the AV node and up the bypass tract. Because the ventricles are depolarized in the normal fashion (down the AV node), the QRS *complex is narrow*. In ART, the SVT propagates down the bypass tract and up the AV node. Because the ventricles are depolarized down the bypass tract and the ventricles depolarize at different times, the QRS *complex is widened*. Narrow-complex AV reciprocating tachycardias include AV node reentrant tachycardia (AVNRT); WPW syndrome orthodromic tachycardia (accessory pathway not concealed on ECG-short PR interval with delta wave); orthodromic atrioventricular reciprocating tachycardia (AVRT; accessory pathway concealed on ECG; normal PR interval and no delta wave); sinoatrial reentrant tachycardia; and atrial flutter. Narrow-complex tachycardias are relatively well tolerated acutely.

Conversely, wide-complex tachycardias, defined as tachycardias with a QRS more than 0.12 s, are a medical emergency. Wide-complex tachycardias include ventricular tachycardia, ventricular fibrillation, WPW syndrome antidromic reentrant

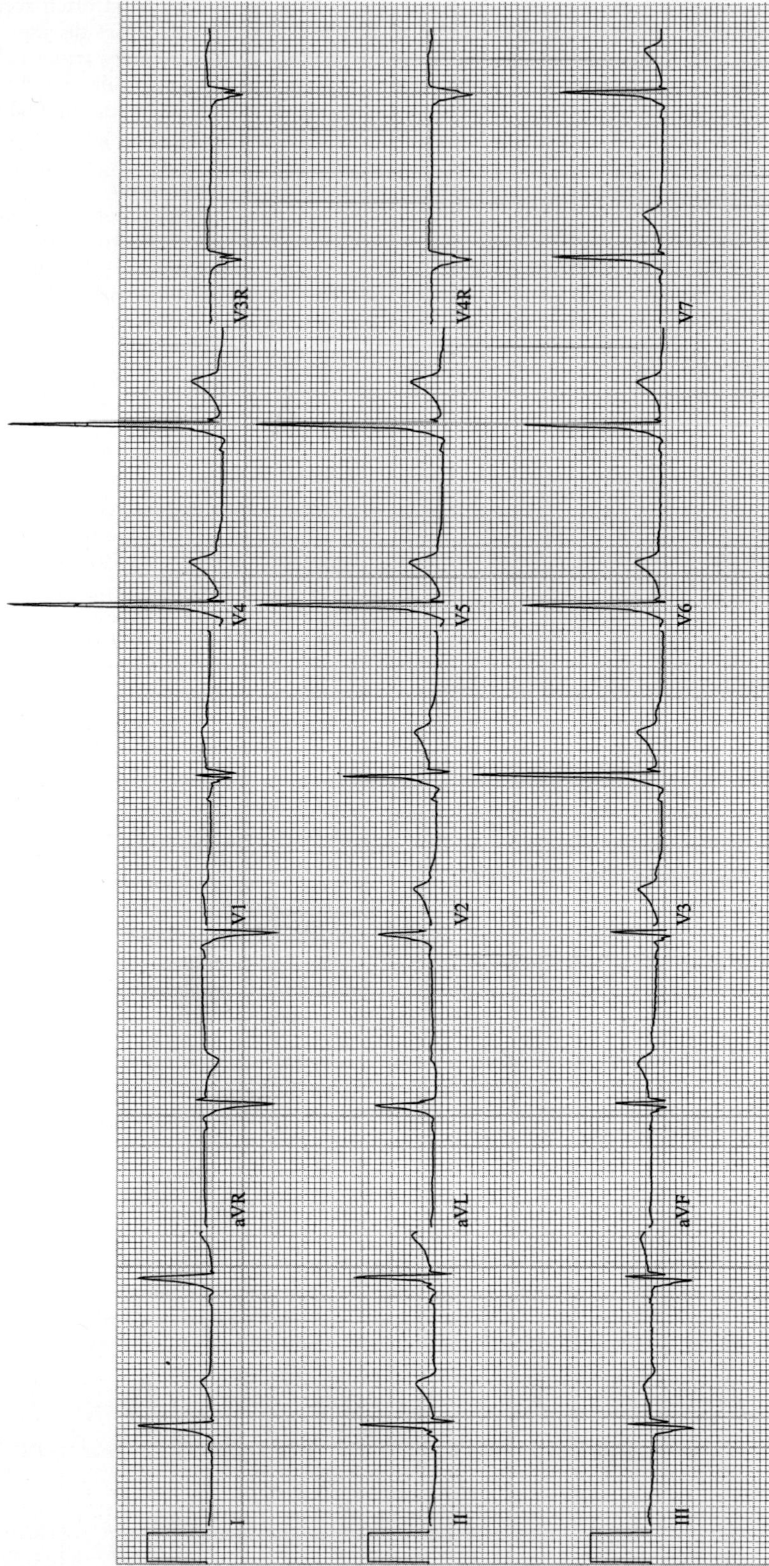

Figure 7-10 • Wolff-Parkinson-White ECG. Upslurring of QRS represents delta wave. Note short PR interval.

tachycardia, and orthodromic SVT with aberrancy. Note that patients with WPW syndrome may have antegrade impulse propagation through both the AV node and the accessory pathway. Characteristic findings on ECG include a short PR interval and delta wave (Fig. 7-10).

Differential Diagnosis

The causes of tachyarrhythmia are as follows:

Narrow-complex tachycardias

- *Sinus tachycardia*: Fever, stress, dehydration, hyperthyroidism, heart failure, and anemia.
- *ORT (most common nonsinus tachycardia SVT)*: Most cases result from a concealed bypass tract AV reentrant tachycardia (AVRT), WPW syndrome, Ebstein anomaly (associated with WPW syndrome), or L-transposition of the great arteries.
- *Atrial flutter*: Atrial surgery (such as D-TGA status post Mustard/Senning procedure, ASD status post repair, Hemi-Fontan, Fontan), myocarditis, structural heart disease with dilated atria (Ebstein anomaly, tricuspid atresia, rheumatic heart disease of the mitral valve), severe tricuspid regurgitation.

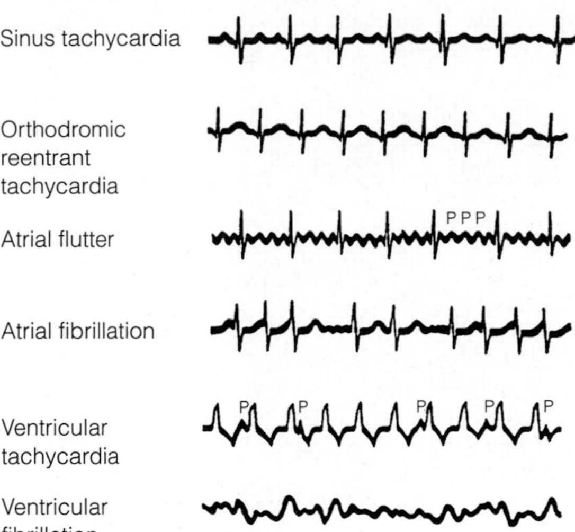

Figure 7-11 • Tachyarrhythmia.

- *Atrial fibrillation*: Most often seen with left atrial enlargement (rheumatic heart disease of the mitral valve, VSD, systemic to pulmonary artery palliative shunt placement); other causes that result in right atrial or biatrial enlargement include Ebstein anomaly, WPW syndrome, and myocarditis (Fig. 7-11).

Wide-complex tachycardia

- *Ven.tricular tachycardia*: Congenital or acquired heart disease resulting in ventricular dilatation or hypertrophy or ventricular suture line, drug ingestion, long QT syndrome, or WPW syndrome with ART.
- *Ventricular fibrillation*: Terminal rhythm that develops after hypoxia, ischemia, or high-voltage electrical injury; predisposing factors include WPW syndrome and long QT syndrome (Fig. 7-12).

Treatment

Narrow-Complex Tachycardia

Treatment of sinus tachycardia involves correcting the underlying cause of the tachycardia. Treatment for stable narrow-complex tachycardia progresses from vagal maneuvers to pharmacotherapy to cardioversion. Figure 7-13 outlines the management of pediatric supraventricular tachycardia. Vagal maneuvers (such as ice to face and carotid massage) enhance vagal tone to slow conduction in the AV node and often result in termination of the arrhythmia.

If vagal maneuvers are ineffective, adenosine may be given to block the AV node and break the reentrant SVT. Reentrant SVT, whose circuit involves the AV node (AV node reentrant tachycardia, WPW syndrome—type ORT, concealed bypass tract—type ORT), is likely to break with the administration of adenosine. Adenosine is ineffective on a narrow-complex tachycardia that results from increased automaticity or a reentrant mechanism that does not involve the AV node (sinus tachycardia, ectopic atrial tachycardia, junctional ectopic tachycardia, atrial flutter, or sinoatrial reentrant tachycardia). If adenosine returns the child to normal sinus rhythm and WPW is not suspected (no delta wave seen after conversion of tachycardia), the child may be started on digoxin to reduce the risk of future events. A β-blocker should be used if baseline ECG after conversion of tachycardia reveals WPW syndrome (short PR interval and delta wave). The use of digoxin in patients with WPW may slow the conduction across the AV node, leading to preferential depolarization down the accessory

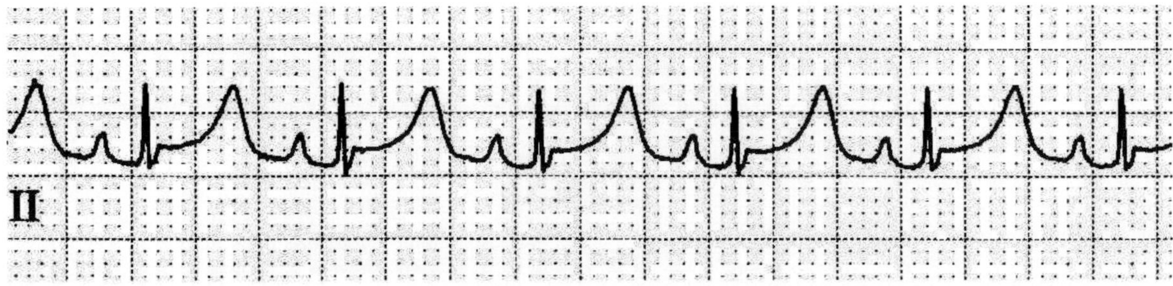

Figure 7-12 • Long QT syndrome ECG.
(Image courtesy of Dr. Bradley Marino.)

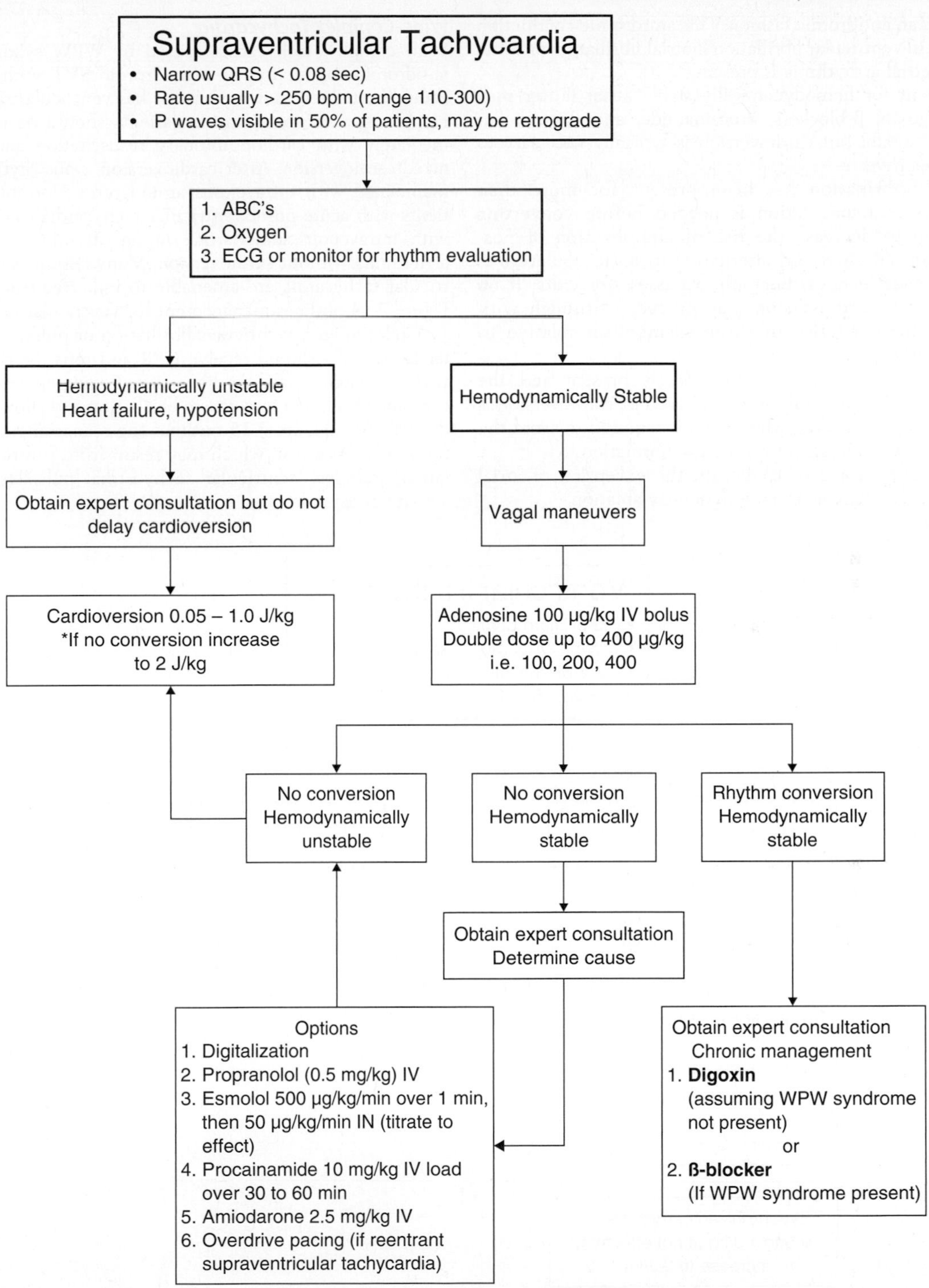

Figure 7-13 • Pediatric supraventricular tachycardia management algorithm.

pathway in an antidromic fashion. This antidromic conduction may result in ventricular fibrillation if atrial fibrillation or some other fast atrial arrhythmia is present.

Treatment for hemodynamically stable atrial flutter may include digoxin, β-blockers, procainamide, amiodarone, flecainide, or sotalol but cardioversion is typically necessary to restore sinus rhythm.

If atrial fibrillation has been present for more than a few days, anticoagulation is needed before converting the rhythm to decrease the risk of embolization of possible intra-atrial clots. An alternative to anticoagulation is transesophageal echocardiography to assess for clots. If no clots are seen, cardioversion may proceed, although with a slightly increased risk of thromboembolism relative to anticoagulation.

When narrow-complex tachycardia is present and the patient is hemodynamically unstable, prompt cardioversion is indicated. Synchronized cardioversion is required to avoid the inadvertent development of ventricular fibrillation.

Most chronic cases of SVT with the exception of atrial fibrillation are amenable to radiofrequency ablation.

Wide-Complex Tachycardia

Wide-complex tachycardia caused by WPW syndrome with antidromic conduction or orthodromic SVT with aberrancy should be treated as if the patient has ventricular tachycardia. Hypotensive or unresponsive patients should be treated immediately with cardiopulmonary resuscitation and synchronized cardioversion. After cardioversion, sinus rhythm can be maintained with intravenous amiodarone. Normotensive patients with acute-onset ventricular tachycardia can be treated with intravenous amiodarone in an attempt to break the arrhythmia without cardioversion. Many chronic cases of ventricular tachycardia are amenable to radiofrequency ablation. Figure 7-14 outlines management for ventricular tachycardia.

Children with ventricular fibrillation or pulseless ventricular tachycardia should receive CPR and must be defibrillated with nonsynchronized cardioversion. Giving epinephrine may turn fine fibrillation into coarse fibrillation and allow successful defibrillation. Figure 7-15 outlines the management algorithm for a pulseless arrest, which may result from ventricular fibrillation, pulseless ventricular tachycardia, pulseless electrical activity or asystole.

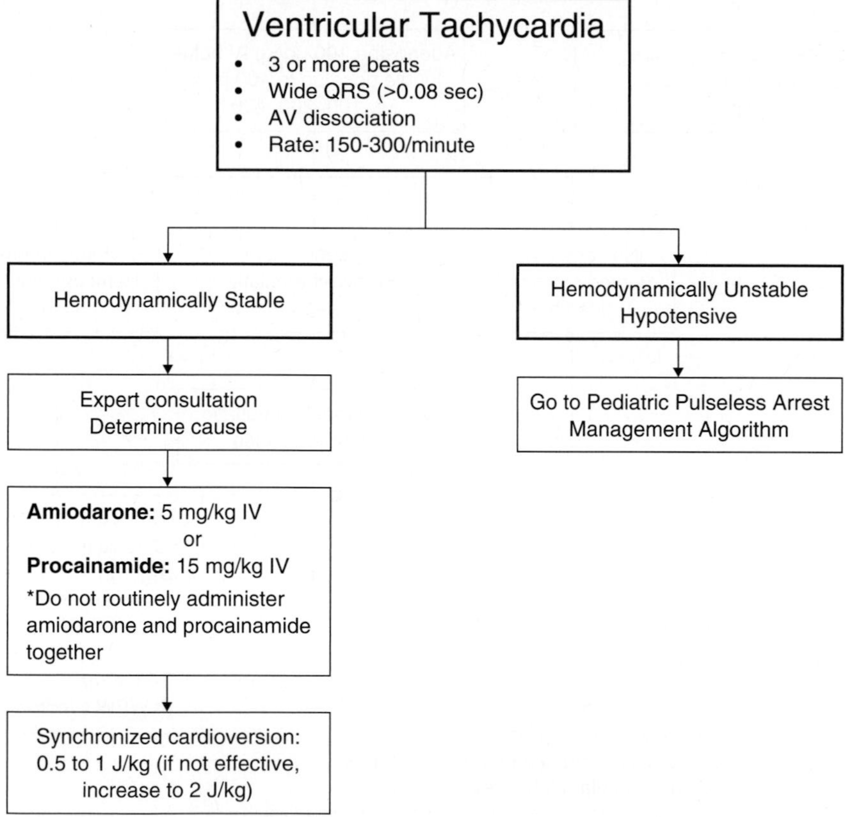

Figure 7-14 • Pediatric ventricular tachycardia management algorithm.

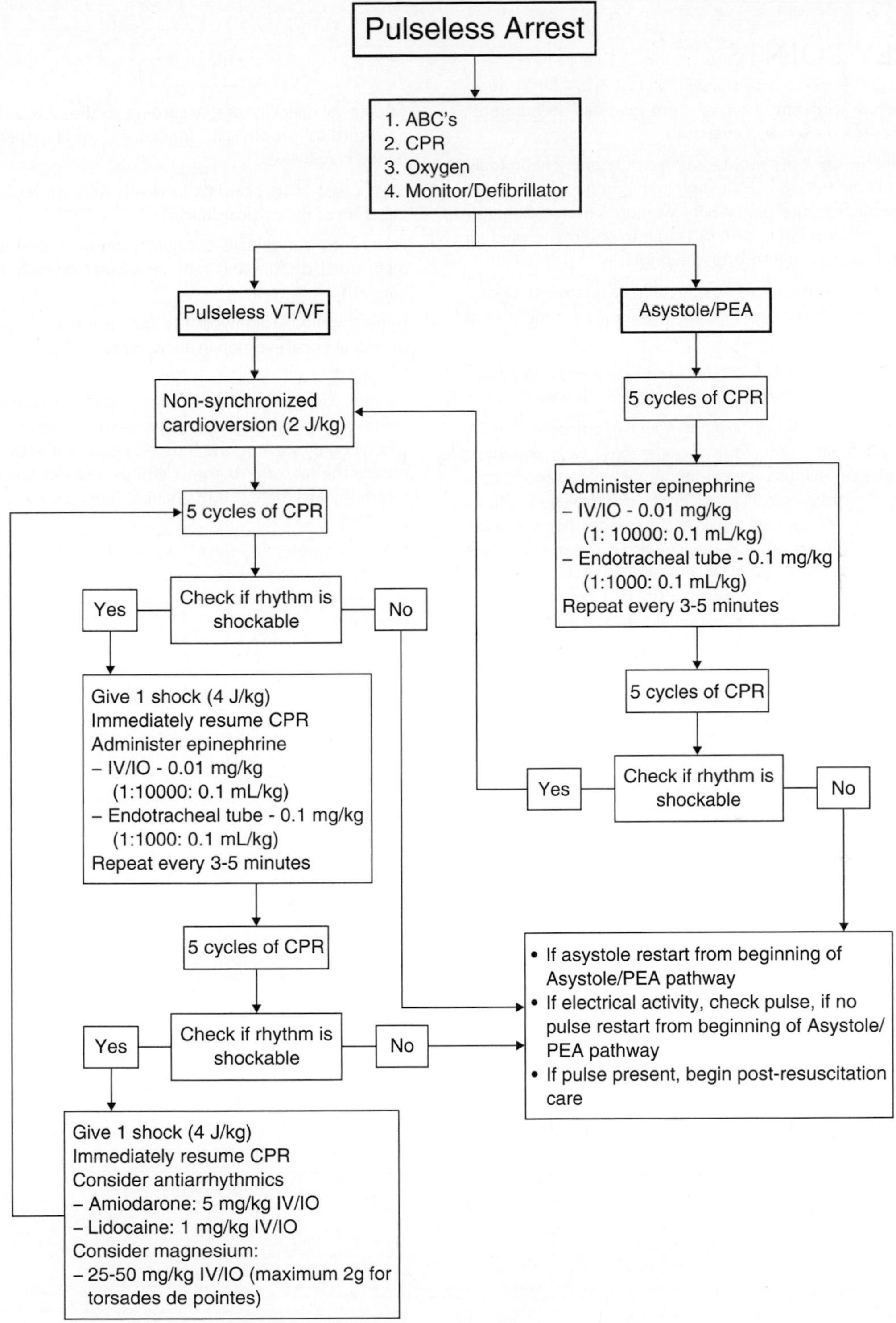

Figure 7-15 • Pediatric pulseless arrest management algorithm.

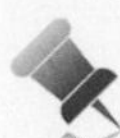

KEY POINTS

- The absolute concentration of deoxygenated hemoglobin determines the presence of cyanosis.
- Cyanosis in the newborn may be cardiac, pulmonary, neurologic, or hematologic in origin. Following stabilization of a cyanotic infant, the goal of the preliminary workup (chest radiograph, electrocardiogram, and hyperoxia test) is to determine whether the lesion is cardiac or noncardiac in origin.
- Comparison of preductal to postductal measurements of oxygen saturation allows the clinician to evaluate for differential cyanosis.
- Prostaglandin E1 (PGE1) therapy should be started in all unstable infants with suspected congenital heart disease (CHD).
- Patients with the highest risk of adverse outcomes resulting from bacterial endocarditis include those with prosthetic cardiac valves, previous endocarditis, unrepaired cyanotic congenital heart disease including those with palliative shunts and conduits, completely repaired congenital heart disease with prosthetic material or a device within 6 months of the procedure, repaired congenital heart disease with residual defects at the site or adjacent to the site of a prosthetic patch or prosthetic device, and cardiac transplantation recipients with cardiac valvular disease. According to the new 2007 bacterial endocarditis prophylaxis guidelines, these patients warrant dental prophylaxis.
- Most cases of myocarditis in North America result from viral infection of the myocardium.
- Dilated or congestive cardiomyopathy is characterized by myocardial dysfunction and ventricular dilation; it is usually idiopathic.
- Hypertrophic cardiomyopathy may present as sudden death during physical exertion in an asymptomatic, otherwise healthy individual.
- Therapy for hypertrophic cardiomyopathy is centered on preventing fatal ventricular arrhythmias and improving left ventricular filling by slowing the intrinsic heart rate. Medications that reduce the risk of arrhythmia and decrease chronotrophy and inotrophy include calcium channel blockers and β-adrenergic blocking agents.
- Narrow-complex tachycardias tend to be well tolerated acutely, whereas wide-complex tachycardias often result in hemodynamic instability and are considered a medical emergency.

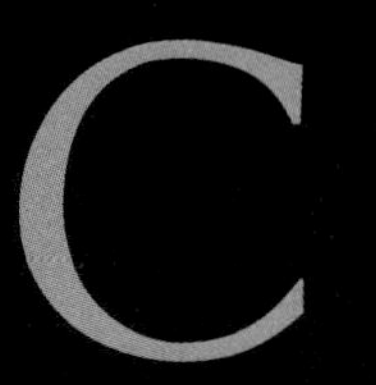

Clinical Vignettes

Vignette 1

A 7-day-old male infant presents to the ED with lethargy and grunting respirations. He was born at term after a normal pregnancy to a 34-year-old mother after an uncomplicated spontaneous vaginal delivery. His parents state that he has not eaten well over the last day and has been increasingly sleepy. His urine output has been normal until today. On examination, he appears pale and mottled with tachypnea and mild retractions. He is lethargic but responds appropriately to painful stimuli. His heart rate is 170 and respiratory rate 80. His lungs are clear to auscultation bilaterally. You are able to palpate a strong right brachial pulse but cannot palpate femoral pulses. Capillary refill in the legs is very prolonged.

1. Which of the following is the most likely diagnosis?
   - **a.** Neonatal sepsis
   - **b.** Dehydration
   - **c.** Coarctation of the aorta
   - **d.** Congenital adrenal hyperplasia
   - **e.** Transposition of the great arteries

2. The infant is endotracheally intubated and intravenous access is obtained. Which of the following is the most important diagnostic test to perform next?
   - **a.** Blood culture
   - **b.** Echocardiogram
   - **c.** Chest x-ray
   - **d.** Computed tomography of chest
   - **e.** 21-hydroxylase level

3. Which of the following treatments should be initiated next?
   - **a.** Normal saline bolus
   - **b.** Hydrocortisone
   - **c.** Nitroprusside infusion
   - **d.** Epinephrine infusion
   - **e.** Prostaglandin E1 infusion

4. Prostaglandin E-1 infusion is begun intravenously and the patient is stabilized. As you monitor the patient, which of the following is a common side effect of treatment with prostaglandin E1 infusion?
   - **a.** Dry mouth
   - **b.** Apnea
   - **c.** Hypotension
   - **d.** Vomiting
   - **e.** Rash

Vignette 2

A 5-year-old previously healthy boy presents to the emergency department with complaints of "chest feeling funny." His medical history is significant only for placement of bilateral ear tubes as a toddler. He has had normal growth and development and his parents report that he is very active, easily keeping up with peers. He has had no recent illnesses. His mother reports that he was playing in the house that morning, when he suddenly came to her complaining that his chest "felt funny, like butterflies." She felt his chest and reports that his heart felt like it was "beating fast." On examination, he is a well-developed child who is anxious but appears well. He is afebrile and is breathing comfortably. You are unable to count his heart rate by palpating his pulse so you connect him to a monitor which demonstrates that his heart rate is 220 and regular with a narrow complex. Blood pressure is 75/50 and respiratory rate is 24.

1. Which of the following is the most likely diagnosis?
   - **a.** Sinus tachycardia
   - **b.** Ventricular tachycardia
   - **c.** Supraventricular tachycardia
   - **d.** Complete heart block
   - **e.** Atrial fibrillation

2. You suspect that he has SVT. Which of the following tests is most likely to aid with the diagnosis?
   - **a.** Electrocardiogram
   - **b.** Echocardiogram
   - **c.** Chest x-ray
   - **d.** Telemetry
   - **e.** Cardiac catheterization

3. The EKG confirms a narrow complex tachycardia with a regular rhythm and a fixed rate of 220. P waves are not discernable. You ask the patient to try various vagal maneuvers (placing thumb in mouth and blowing, standing on head) without improvement. Which of the following is the next most appropriate therapy?
   - **a.** β-blocker
   - **b.** Amiodarone
   - **c.** Digoxin
   - **d.** Adenosine
   - **e.** Transcutaneous pacing

4. While placing an IV, the patient becomes unstable, with thready pulses. You are no longer able to obtain a blood pressure. He becomes unconscious. Which of the following is the next most appropriate therapy?
   a. Amiodarone
   b. Transcutaneous pacing
   c. Epinephrine
   d. β-blocker
   e. Synchronized cardioversion

Vignette 3

A 1-year-old male arrives in the ED with a 4-day history of vomiting and abdominal pain. His mother states that he has had low-grade fevers, decreased appetite and has been breathing "fast and hard." On examination, he is cool with delayed capillary refill. He is alert and answers questions appropriately. His heart rate is 150 bmp and respiratory rate 60 rpm. On abdominal exam his liver edge is 4 cm below the right subcostal margin. On cardiac auscultation, he has occasional irregularity and a gallop but no murmur is heard. He has mild subcostal retractions with coarse lung sounds throughout.

1. Which of the following is the most likely diagnosis?
   a. Pneumonia
   b. Viral gastroenteritis
   c. Aortic valve stenosis
   d. Dilated cardiomyopathy
   e. Dehydration

2. A chest x-ray is obtained which reveals a large heart with mild pulmonary edema. The vital signs remain stable and the child is neurologically appropriate. Which of the following is the most important diagnostic test to perform next?
   a. Blood culture
   b. Echocardiogram
   c. CBC with differential
   d. Computed tomography of chest
   e. B-type natriuretic peptide (BNP)

3. A bedside echocardiogram demonstrates severe systolic dysfunction with moderate mitral regurgitation. The child is breathing quickly but has a stable blood pressure, perfusion appears adequate, and he is interacting appropriately. What is the initial class of drugs to be prescribed?
   a. Diuretics
   b. Angiotensin converting inhibitors (ACEI)
   c. Anticoagulation
   d. Phenylephrine
   e. Narcotics

4. The toddler is transferred to the intensive care unit, and there he becomes extremely tachycardic and starts to act very agitated. His blood pressure is high but his perfusion is poor. What is the appropriate therapy for this patient who is now showing progressive evidence of poor cardiac output including changes in neurologic status?
   a. Phenylephrine
   b. β-blocker
   c. Benzodiazepine
   d. Intubation
   e. Narcotic

Vignette 4

A 1-day-old male infant is in the mother's delivery room and becomes increasingly cyanotic with agitation. The physician is called, and on examination he finds a comfortably tachypneic, well perfused but dusky newborn. There is no murmur auscultated but he detects a loud single S2. His lungs are clear to auscultation bilaterally. He has easily palpable, strong brachial and femoral pulses. He is taken back to the nursery and is placed on telemetry with a continuous pulse oximeter. His heart rate is 160 bmp and his saturation is 75% in the right upper extremity and 85% in the left lower extremity.

1. Which of the following is the most likely diagnosis?
   a. Neonatal sepsis
   b. Coarctation of the aorta
   c. Obstructed total anomalous pulmonary venous return (TAPVR)
   d. Transposition of the great arteries
   e. Anemia

2. The infant is transferred to an intensive care unit, and an echocardiogram is done, which confirms the diagnosis of transposition of the great arteries. As the echocardiogram is being done, the child is becoming more cyanotic. Which of the following pharmacologic intervention could be attempted to improve the saturations?
   a. Epinephrine infusion
   b. Prostaglandin E1 (PGE1) infusion
   c. Tylenol
   d. Hydrocortisone
   e. Antibiotics

3. The PGE1 is started and the child continues to have oxygen saturations in the 50%-to-60% range. The baby is becoming hypotensive and volume is being given. Which of the following interventional procedures should be attempted quickly?
   a. Arterial switch procedure
   b. Norwood procedure
   c. Atrial septostomy
   d. Pulmonary valve dilation
   e. Chest tube

4. What surgical intervention is required to correct this circulation?
   a. Arterial switch procedure
   b. Norwood procedure
   c. Bidirectional Glenn operation
   d. BT shunt
   e. Fontan operation

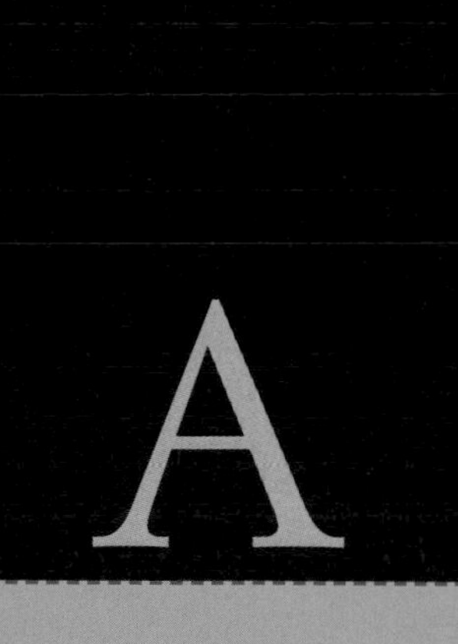

Answers

Vignette 1 Question 1

Answer C: Coarctation of the aorta accounts for 8% of congenital heart defects and has a male-to-female predominance of 2:1. The narrowing is usually located in the descending aorta at the insertion site of the ductus arteriosus and results in obstruction to blood flow and increased LV afterload. The degree of narrowing determines the clinical severity. A neonate with a critical coarctation (one where the narrowing is so severe that the ductus arteriosus is necessary to supply systemic blood flow) may present as in this vignette, with evidence of shock as the ductus arteriousus closes. On examination, pulses distal to the coarctation will be weak or absent but preductal pulses (right radial) may be preserved.

Late onset neonatal sepsis may present similarly, with nonspecific signs such as poor feeding, lethargy, and tachypnea, and can progress to shock. Dehydration may also occur commonly in this age group, due to insufficient intake, and can result in hypovolemic shock. Congenital adrenal hyperplasia is most commonly a result of 21-hydroxylase deficiency. Males born with this defect have no genital abnormalities and may present with poor feeding, failure to thrive, dehydration, and shock. Although physical exam findings may be similar and nonspecific in all of these scenarios, there should be no discrepancy between upper and lower extremity pulses. Transposition of the great arteries (TGA) is a common congenital heart defect in which the aorta arises from the right ventricle and pulmonary artery from the left ventricle so that the circuits are in parallel rather than in series. Infants with TGA typically present at birth with cyanosis, rather than shock.

Vignette 1 Question 2

Answer B: The diagnosis of coarctation of the aorta is made with echocardiogram, which can be done rapidly and at the bedside, allowing for further management. The echocardiogram may demonstrate the narrowing in the aorta, the presence or absence of the ductus arteriousus, the ventricular function and geometry, and presence of any associated lesions, such as bicuspid aortic valve.

A chest x-ray may demonstrate cardiomegaly but is typically nondiagnostic. A chest CT will provide diagnosis, but is not necessary in this scenario. Although a blood culture may be indicated in this child, it will not provide immediate diagnosis.

A bedside echocardiogram demonstrates a severe juxtaductal coarctation of the aorta with a tiny ductus arteriosus, decreased left ventricular function and a bicuspid aortic valve.

Vignette 1 Question 3

Answer E: The goal of early therapy in this scenario is reopening of the ductus arteriousus, which will restore perfusion distal to the coarctation. The ductus arteriousus is sensitive to prostaglandin. Prostaglandin E1 infusion has a very short half-life so must be given as a continuous intravenous infusion. In a stable infant, typical starting doses are 0.02 to 0.05 mcg/kg/min but in a patient in shock with a tiny or closed ductus, doses up to 0.1 mcg/kg/min may be necessary.

A normal saline bolus may be indicated in this child, who has been eating poorly and may have a degree of intravascular volume depletion. However, a fluid bolus will not restore distal perfusion since it will have no effect on the ductus arteriosus. Similarly, with decreased left ventricular function, epinephrine infusion may also be indicated. Ephinephrine is an excellent inotropic agent but at higher doses is associated with increased systemic vascular resistance, which may be detrimental to a failing ventricle. It will also not improve distal perfusion since that relies entirely on patency of the ductus arteriousus. Nitroprusside is a vasodilating agent which is used for hypertension and for heart failure, to decrease systemic afterload. Although the child in this scenario has heart failure, the increased afterload is due to a "fixed" obstruction (i.e., the coarctation) so administration of a vasodilator in this setting is contraindicated. Last, hydrocortisone is used in infants with glucocorticoid or mineralocorticoid deficiency but would have no role in this setting.

Vignette 1 Question 4

Answer B: The most concerning side effect of prostaglandin therapy is apnea, which occurs commonly with the institution of therapy and is dose dependent. Infants who are not intubated and ventilated prior to the start of prostaglandin infusion necessitate close monitoring and often require intubation. For this reason, when transferring a newborn on a prostaglandin infusion to a tertiary hospital, many centers will prophylactically intubate a newborn prior to the transfer.

Prostaglandin may cause systemic vasodilation, but significant hypotension is uncommon. The other side effects may be reported with many drugs, but in general prostaglandin infusion is well tolerated.

Vignette 2 Question 1

Answer C: Supraventricular tachycardia is the most common pathologic tachycardia that occurs in pediatric patients. Collectively, the term *supraventricular tachycardia* encompasses all tachycardia that originates above the ventricle. The characteristic features include abrupt onset and termination, fixed cycle length, normal

QRS complexes, and usually, lack of discernible p waves. In pediatric patients, two mechanisms, atrioventricular reentry tachycardia (AVRT) and atrioventricular nodal reentry tachycardia (AVNRT) predominate.

Sinus tachycardia occurs frequently in all ages and is the most common form of tachycardia. In this patient with absence of accompanying causes (such as fever), a heart rate above 200 points to a possible pathologic mechanism. Ventricular tachycardia is uncommon in the pediatric patient. The hallmark feature is a wide-QRS complex tachycardia. Although most ventricular tachycardias are unstable, a rare patient will present with a stable ventricular tachycardia. Complete heart block occurs when conduction does not occur across the AV node. This leads to bradycardia, typically with a junctional or ventricular escape rhythm. Atrial fibrillation can lead to tachycardia when there is rapid ventricular conduction. This arrhythmia, which is very uncommon in the pediatric population, is associated with an irregular rhythm.

Vignette 2 Question 2

Answer A: The diagnosis of SVT is made by electrocardiogram (EKG). The EKG will demonstrate a tachycardia with normal QRS duration. When P waves are evident, there is usually a 1:1 AV relationship. Rarely, the QRS may be wide, due to transient, rate-limited bundle branch block or in the setting of an unusual reentry tachycardia called antidromic SVT. Echocardiogram is useful for evaluating cardiac anatomy and function and may demonstrate that there is tachycardia but will not be diagnostic. Chest x-ray and cardiac catheterization are not indicated in this scenario. Telemetry may be useful but simple monitoring will not allow measurement of intervals or assessment of multiple leads.

Vignette 2 Question 3

Answer D: Rapid administration of adenosine causes transient block of the AV node and will result in prompt termination of most forms of SVT (those involving the AV node in the circuit). Adenosine must be delivered via rapid IV push since the half-life is extremely short. A β-blocker or digoxin may be prescribed for long term treatment/prevention of SVT but are unlikely to terminate an acute tachycardia. Amiodarone is an antiarrhythmic that may be useful for incessant SVT but should only be given under the supervision of a cardiologist. Transcutaneous pacing is not indicated.

Vignette 2 Question 4

Answer E: Patients with unstable hemodynamics and SVT should undergo immediate synchronized cardioversion (0.5-1 J/kg) without delay. Amiodarone, β-blocker therapy and transcutaneous pacing may have a role in stable incessant SVT. Epinephrine is an inotropic agent which is used for resuscitation and ventricular dysfunction.

Vignette 3 Question 1

Answer D: Cardiomyopathies are diseases of the heart muscle, characterized by abnormal findings of chamber size and wall thickness or functional abnormalities. Cardiomyopathies can be either primary (confined to heart muscle) or secondary (myocardial damage as a result of a systemic illness). The annual incidence of all case of pediatric cardiomyopathy is between 1.13 and 1.24 cases per 100,000 children. The most common cardiomyopathy in children is dilated cardiomyopathy (DCM) which is characterized by left ventricular systolic dysfunction with an increase in left ventricular size. Mitral regurgitation and ventricular arrhythmias can develop and be present at initial presentation.

Dilated cardiomyopathies can present with signs and symptoms of congestive heart failure-diaphoresis, breathlessness, abdominal pain, and pallor. Young children often present with abdominal pain, vomiting, and anorexia due to mesenteric ischemia. On examination, these patients may have sinus tachycardia with or without ectopy, a gallop rhythm, jugular venous distension, hepatomegaly, and a murmur that is consistent with mitral regurgitation.

Pneumonia can present similarly, with vomiting and increased work of breathing and if the infection is severe and leads to bacteremia the patient can present in septic shock. If the infection leads to lack of oral intake and fever leads to insensible fluid loss, the child could be dehydrated. The child in the above case has hepatomegaly out of proportion to symptoms and signs consistent with infection. The child also has a gallop rhythm and irregular heart beat due to ventricular ectopy, which is inconsistent with viral gastroenteritis or bacterial pneumonia.

A child with aortic valve stenosis would not present to the emergency department in shock. Aortic valve disease is usually detected on a routine examination when a care provider hears a systolic ejection murmur and click. It would not account for the many signs and symptoms of congestive heart failure that are present on this child's examination.

Vignette 3 Question 2

Answer B: The diagnosis of cardiomyopathy is dependent on patient history, physical examination, and echocardiographic features of dilated cardiomyopathy. The echocardiogram should be confirmatory and done quickly to assess the severity of the ventricular dilation and systolic dysfunction, but should not interrupt close surveillance and rapid initiation of additional therapy. On echocardiogram, the ventricular size will be measured, the ejection fraction calculated, and the presence and severity of mitral regurgitation will be determined. Patients presenting in this degree of failure often develop cardiogenic shock quickly after arrival and require rapid escalation of therapy. They are also at risk of life-threatening arrhythmias.

A computed tomography (CT) of the chest would show a large heart but would not be able to estimate the severity of the dysfunction. It would not be safe to place this child in a CT scanner until he is supported and well compensated.

The laboratory tests listed above may be done to guide future therapy but are not necessary for initial diagnosis or management. A BNP may help differentiate between myocardial disease and pneumonia, but it is not the sole test necessary to diagnosis a cardiomyopathy.

Vignette 3 Question 3

Answer A: Therapy of dilated cardiomyopathy is mainly directed at treatment of heart failure–related symptoms and prevention of disease-related complications. Treatment of decompensated heart failure is focused on diuresis with loop and thiazide diuretics for volume overload and afterload reduction.

This child's examination is concerning enough that starting an oral regimen with an ACEI would not be appropriate. Although anticoagulation will be important, eventually it is not the first class of drugs to use.

In decompensated heart failure, the systemic vascular resistance is elevated and initially the blood pressure will be maintained even if the overall cardiac output is poor. Further increasing the systemic vascular resistance will increase the afterload on the heart and lead to further decompensation.

Eventually, after initial resuscitation, the goal will be to optimize outpatient heart-failure management with an ACEI and a β-blocker.

In addition, the patient will require anticoagulation to prevent thrombus formation in the dilated left ventricle.

Vignette 3 Question 4

Answer D: Intubation and positive pressure ventilation will decrease the afterload on the left side of the heart. It will now be safe to sedate the child in order to decrease oxygen demand and allow for optimization of the child's cardiac output. Intubation in these children is not without risk and should be performed in a controlled manner with appropriate personal and resuscitation drugs close by. If perfusion does not increase with the initiation of positive pressure ventilation or the child becomes hypotensive, further therapy is warranted.

If the blood pressure is adequate but perfusion is poor, modulation of afterload should be attempted with vasodilator therapy such as nitroprusside or with Milrinone which will provide inotropic support and vasodilation. In children with heart failure and hypotension associated with hypoperfusion, continuous intravenous epinephrine should be considered.

Although sedation (benzodiazepines and narcotics) may decrease the oxygen demand and calm an agitated child, in patients' with heart failure it may blunt the catecholamine surge that is required to maintain cardiac output and lead to a rapid decline and cardiogenic shock.

Increasing afterload with phenylephrine, with no additional inotropic support, will lead to further deterioration.

Vignette 4 Question 1

Answer D: D-transposition of the great arteries (D-TGA) accounts for 5% to 8% of congenital heart defects and is the most common form of cyanotic congenital heart disease presenting in the first 24 hours of life. In this defect, the aorta arises anteriorly from the morphologic right ventricle and the pulmonary artery arises posteriorly from the left ventricle. The pulmonary and systemic circulations are therefore in parallel rather than series; the systemic circuit (deoxygenated blood) is recirculated through the body, whereas the pulmonary circuit (oxygenated blood) recirculates through the lungs. Associated lesions occur in one-third of infants, with ventricular septal defect being most common.

Only 25% of patients with D-transposition of the great arteries (D-TGA) are diagnosed in utero by ultrasound; most present after delivery with cyanosis. In the absence of apparent lung disease, cyanotic neonates usually have congenital heart disease. Children with transposition of the great arteries will usually present with "comfortable tachypnea." On examination, these newborns will have a loud, single S2 but most often do not have a murmur. Their oxygen saturations can range depending on the size of the intracardiac shunt. This patient has reverse differential cyanosis. This phenomenon is only seen in patients with transposition of the great arteries with pulmonary hypertension or an aortic coarctation.

Neonatal sepsis will not present with comfortable tachypnea. Children with sepsis may be cyanotic and tachypneic but will be working hard to breathe. Obstructed TAPVR presents with cyanosis, but these children will also have evidence of difficult breathing due to pulmonary edema from the venous obstruction.

Coarctation of the aorta also makes up 5% to 8% of all congenital heart disease. This illness usually presents later in the newborn period after the ductus arteriousus closes. These newborns do not present with cyanosis but usually with feeding intolerance.

Vignette 4 Question 2

Answer B: The goal of starting a PGE1 infusion is to reopen the ductus arteriousus, which will increase pulmonary blood flow and improve the oxygen saturations. The ductus arteriousus is sensitive to prostaglandin. The initiation of PGE1 can be quick and is relatively safe. The side effects of PGE1 include apnea, fever, and systemic vasodilation. Occasionally, a child will need to be intubated for frequent and/or persistent apneic events.

Epinephrine may increase cardiac output and may slightly improve oxygen saturations but not as reliably as reopening the ductus arteriousus.

Vignette 4 Question 3

Answer C: The definitive treatment of D-TGA is surgical but other management (pharmacologic and interventional) may be necessary urgently after delivery due to hypoxemia. This urgent, postdelivery treatment is directed toward the establishment of adequate tissue oxygen delivery, which is achieved via the mixing of the systemic and pulmonary circulations, thereby allowing oxygenated blood to reach the systemic circulation. The most important component to allow for adequate mixing is a large atrial septal defect. If the atrial communication is small, it must be enlarged to allow for adequate oxygenation. An atrial balloon septostomy can be done at the bedside with echocardiographic guidance, or it can be done in the cardiac catheterization laboratory with the guidance of fluoroscopy. Once an adequate intra-atrial communication is achieved, the child should have improved hemodynamics and often the PGE1 infusion can be discontinued. Once the atrial communication is adequate, the child should be able to wait safely for the corrective surgical intervention.

Vignette 4 Question 4

Answer A: After preoperative stabilization, arterial switch procedure is typically performed in the first week of life. The arterial switch operation establishes sequential circulations with concordant atrioventricular and ventriculo-arterial connections. Concurrent closure of intracardiac shunts (atrial or ventricular septal defects) is performed as well as ligation of the ductus arteriousus. Surgery for D-TGA generally occurs within the first week of life. In term infants, regardless of coronary artery pattern, mortality rates remain low for the arterial switch procedure (1.1%-6% in most centers).

The Norwood operation is the first-stage palliative operation that is performed for infants with hypoplastic left heart syndrome. The first operation consists of three components: an aortic arch reconstruction, atrial septectomy, and the institution of a stable source (Blalock-Taussig shunt or right-ventricle to pulmonary artery conduit) of pulmonary blood flow. At 3 to 6 months of age, the child will undergo a bidirectional Glenn or hemi-Fontan operation, a superior vena cava to pulmonary artery anastomosis. At 2–4 years of age, the child will have a Fontan procedure, an inferior vena cava to pulmonary artery anastomosis, thereby completing their single ventricle palliation.

Chapter

8 Pulmonology

Robert E. Wood • Katie S. Fine • Carolyn Kercsmar

Respiratory diseases are among the leading causes of death in young children worldwide, and respiratory symptoms are a complaint in the majority of pediatric sick visits. Although these symptoms are usually related to acute (most often viral) infection, they may be a consequence of congenital or acquired pulmonary disorders. Respiratory disorders specific to the newborn period (including bronchopulmonary dysplasia) are discussed in Chapter 2.

The primary function of the lungs is the exchange of oxygen and carbon dioxide between the blood and the atmosphere. Many abnormalities can affect this exchange adversely, including airway *obstruction*, *restrictive* lung disease (decreased compliance of the lungs and/or chest wall), ventilation-perfusion mismatch, and abnormal respiratory control. Effective respiration requires proper interaction between the respiratory, cardiovascular, and central nervous systems, with adequate support from the musculoskeletal system.

DIAGNOSTIC TECHNIQUES IN PEDIATRIC PULMONOLOGY

A standard **chest radiograph** is a vitally important tool in the evaluation of children with respiratory disorders. **Airway films** provide visualization of the trachea and nasopharyngeal airway. **Computed tomography** (CT) studies yield more detailed information and can be combined with vascular contrast. Radiation dosage should be considered before ordering a CT scan. The images obtained are influenced by body position and stage of inspiration or exhalation.

Pulmonary function testing measures lung volume and rates of airflow, permitting assessment of lung capacity and airway obstruction. Pulmonary function tests (PFTs) are generally performed only in patients old enough to cooperate (older than age 5 to 6 years). The data generated are dependent on patient effort and technique, and training of subjects is necessary before reproducible data are obtained.

In older children, **microscopic examination and culture** of expectorated sputum may yield important information, although the results are often somewhat equivocal due to contamination of the specimen with saliva or upper airway secretions.

Bronchoscopy—the direct visual examination of the airways—is a powerful diagnostic tool for evaluation of airway structure and dynamics, as well as to obtain definitive specimens from the lower airways. Rigid or flexible instruments of appropriate size may be used; in general, flexible instruments are best for evaluation of the bronchi (but not for extraction of aspirated foreign bodies) and airway dynamics; rigid instruments give a more detailed image, but result in some anatomic distortion because the rigid instrument does not follow the anatomic pathway (and it is necessary to extend the neck and lift the mandible/tongue base).

UPPER AIRWAY OBSTRUCTIVE DISEASE

The upper airway extends from the nostril to the thoracic inlet. In general, obstruction of the upper airway leads to *inspiratory* obstruction, while obstruction below the thoracic inlet results in *expiratory* obstruction.

UPPER AIRWAY OBSTRUCTION IN THE NEONATE/YOUNG INFANT

Choanal atresia or stenosis (narrowing of the nasal passages) can be life threatening in newborns, who are obligate nose breathers. Mandibular hypoplasia often results in posterior displacement of the tongue (glossoptosis); some children (typically, with trisomy 21) have large, obstructive tongues. Vocal cord paralysis can be unilateral or bilateral, and congenital or (more frequently) acquired. Laryngeal webs are uncommon congenital lesions that may produce respiratory distress in the delivery room and often disappear following intubation. **Laryngomalacia** due to large, floppy arytenoid cartilages or a floppy epiglottis is the most common cause of congenital stridor and usually resolves with growth over the first 1 to 3 years of life. Subglottic masses (hemangioma or cyst) may present in the first year of life; in the child with persistent stridor and a cutaneous hemangioma, a subglottic hemangioma should be suspected. Subglottic stenosis is rarely congenital; acquired stenosis should be considered in any child who has been intubated, even transiently. Children presenting in the first year of life with persistent stridor and/or hoarseness most likely have either vocal cord paralysis or laryngeal papillomatosis. Vascular compression of the trachea at the thoracic inlet by an anomalous vessel is a relatively common cause of upper airway obstruction in the first year of life.

Clinical Manifestations

Clinical manifestations of upper airway obstruction include noisy inspiration, increased work of breathing (nasal flaring, use of accessory muscles), and retractions (especially suprasternal). The character and intensity of the noise depend on the structures involved, the degree of muscle tone, and the rate of air flow. In general, obstruction in the subglottic space results in a high-pitched, monophonic stridor. Obstruction above the glottis produces a more variable, often fluttering stridor which typically varies considerably with position of the head and neck. Upper airway obstruction is often more pronounced during feeding, especially in neonates.

Diagnostic Evaluation

Diagnostic evaluation of upper airway obstruction involves assessment of the severity of the physiologic disturbance and identification of the etiology of the obstruction. Physiologic studies include **pulse oximetry** which measures oxygen saturation in peripheral blood, and **blood gas analysis,** which also measures blood pH and carbon dioxide level. During severe obstruction, oxygen saturation can remain within normal limits despite a significant rise in carbon dioxide levels. Patency of the nasal airway is confirmed by passage of a suction catheter through each nostril or by instillation of radiographic contrast material. Radiographs of the nasopharynx and neck can be helpful, but flexible bronchoscopy is often required to definitively evaluate the anatomy and dynamics of the upper airway. The sound of the cough can yield important clues—absence of a sharp "glottal stop" sound means that the vocal cords cannot close normally.

Treatment

Treatment of upper airway obstruction depends on the nature of the obstruction. Following definitive exclusion of more serious pathology, most infants with laryngomalacia or unilateral vocal cord paralysis need only be followed. If the airway obstruction is severe (e.g., hypoxemia, failure to thrive, feeding difficulties), provision of an artificial airway followed by surgical intervention may be warranted. In many patients, tracheostomy provides an effective and safe solution until more definitive treatment can be provided.

UPPER AIRWAY OBSTRUCTION IN THE OLDER CHILD

Children beyond the first year of life may have upper airway obstruction as a result of a congenital lesion, but acquired lesions are much more likely. Large adenoids and tonsils often result in inspiratory obstruction, with symptomatic exacerbations during periods of viral respiratory infection. Nasal obstruction can also be caused by a foreign body, polyps, or allergic rhinitis. There are many infectious causes of acute upper airway obstruction, such as acute laryngotracheitis and peritonsillar or retropharyngeal abscess.

OBSTRUCTIVE SLEEP APNEA

Many children have upper airway obstruction only during sleep, as a result of changes in upper airway muscle tone. Most have some degree of anatomic obstruction as well (i.e., large adenoids and/or tonsils, or tongue base [glossoptosis or lingual tonsillar hypertrophy]). Symptoms of obstructive sleep apnea (OSA) include restless sleep with frequent position changes, snoring that is irregular (especially with pauses and gasps), daytime somnolence, poor growth, behavioral problems, enuresis, and poor academic performance. OSA associated with marked obesity **(Pickwickian syndrome)** can lead to chronic hypoventilation with severe complications, including pulmonary hypertension and congestive heart failure.

Polysomnography is the diagnostic study of choice, measuring respiratory muscle activity, air flow, oxygenation, sleep stage, and heart rate. This test can define the degree and type of physiologic disturbance, whether central, obstructive, or mixed in nature. Treatment of OSA should be directed toward normalizing airway anatomy through the removal of enlarged tonsils and/or adenoids, if indicated. If initial interventions fail and the degree of disturbance is significant, then continuous positive airway pressure (CPAP) is indicated. Severe, untreated OSA may lead to **congestive heart failure** and even death.

LOWER AIRWAY OBSTRUCTIVE DISEASE

The intrathoracic airways narrow during exhalation; thus, any form of lower airway obstruction will be more apparent during exhalation. **Wheezing** is the sound of air squeezing past an intrathoracic obstruction of virtually any type. While most patients with asthma wheeze, *not all patients who wheeze have asthma*. There are two major lower airway obstructive diseases in childhood: asthma and cystic fibrosis. Primary ciliary dyskinesia, a rarer entity, is also primarily an obstructive disease.

ASTHMA

Asthma is a heterogeneous, chronic disorder of the airways characterized by *reversible airway obstruction*, inflammation, and bronchial hyperresponsiveness. The diagnosis is based on recurrence of symptoms and symptom responsiveness to bronchodilator and/or anti-inflammatory agents. Bronchospasm, which results from smooth muscle constriction, may occur in response to allergic, environmental, infectious, or emotional stimuli (the trigger). Common precipitants include upper respiratory infections, pet dander, dust mites, weather changes, exercise, cigarette smoke, and seasonal or food allergens. Cellular mediators of inflammation are recruited to the lower airway mucosa and submucosal structures, inciting mucus production and mucosal edema, and further increasing airway hyperresponsiveness. The inflammatory response typically involves both immediate and late-phase components; it is the latter that results in the prolonged nature of an asthma exacerbation.

Asthma **severity** is classified based on the degree of impairment prior to initiation of appropriate therapy (Tables 8-1 and 8-2). Following initiation of treatment, asthma **control** is monitored in two domains: impairment (current symptoms and lung function) and risk (future exacerbations and medication side effects) (Tables 8-3 and 8-4). Assessing and maintaining control is now considered more important than assigning severity classification. Additional information regarding the 2007 Expert Panel Report 3 Guidelines for the diagnosis and treatment of asthma can be found at www.nhlibi.nih.gov/guidelines/asthma/index.htm.

TABLE 8-1 Classifying Asthma Severity and Initiating Therapy in Children (Ages 0 to 11 Years)

Components of Severity		Intermittent		Persistent: Mild		Persistent: Moderate		Persistent: Severe	
		Ages 0 to 4	Ages 5 to 11	Ages 0 to 4	Ages 5 to 11	Ages 0 to 4	Ages 5 to 11	Ages 0 to 4	Ages 5 to 11
Impairment	Symptoms	≤2 days/week		>2 days/week but not daily		Daily		Throughout the day	
	Nighttime awakenings	0	≤2×/month	1 to 2×/month	3 to 4×/month	3 to 4×/ month	>1×/week but not nightly	>1×/week	Often 7×/week
	Short-acting beta$_2$-agonist use for symptom control	≤2 days/week		>2 days/week but not daily		Daily		Several times per day	
	Interference with normal activity	None		Minor limitation		Some limitation		Extremely limited	
	Lung function –FEV_1 (% predicted) or peak flow (personal best)	N/A	Normal FEV_1 between exacerbations >80% during exacerbation	N/A	>80%	N/A	60% to 80%	N/A	<50%
	–FEV_1/FVC		>85%		>80%		75% to 80%		<75%
Risk	Exacerbations requiring oral systemic corticosteroids (consider severity and interval since last exacerbation)	0 to 1×/year (see notes)	≥2 exacerbations in 6 months requiring oral systemic corticosteroids, or ≥4 wheezing episodes/1 year lasting > 1 day AND risk factors for persistent asthma	≥2×/year (see notes) Relative annual risk may be related to FEV_1					

Recommended Step for Initiating Therapy. (See "Stepwise Approach for Managing Asthma" for treatment steps.) The stepwise approach is meant to assist, not replace, the clinical decision making required to meet individual patient needs.	Step 1 (for both age groups)	Step 2 (for both age groups)	Step 3 and consider short course of oral systemic corticosteroids	Step 3: medium-dose ICS option and consider short course of oral systemic cortico-steroids	Step 3 and consider short course of oral systemic corticosteroids	Step 3: medium dose ICS option OR Step 4 and consider short course of oral systemic corti-costeroids
	In 2 to 6 weeks, depending on severity, evaluate level of asthma control that is achieved. Children 0 to 4 years old: If no clear benefit is observed in 4 to 6 weeks, stop treatment and consider alternative diagnoses or adjusting therapy. Children 5 to 11 years old: Adjust therapy accordingly.					

Level of severity is determined by both impairment and risk. Assess impairment domain by caregiver's recall of pervious 2 to 4 weeks. Again severity to the most severe category in which any feature occurs. Frequency and severity of exacerbation may fluctuate over time for patients in any severity category. At present, there are inadequate data to correspond frequencies of exacerbation with different levels of asthma severity. In general, more frequent and severe exacerbation (e.g., requiring urgent, unscheduled care, hospitalization, or ICU admission) indicate greater underlying disease severity. For treatment purposes, patients with ≥2 exacerbations described above may be considered the same as patients who have asthma, even in the absence of impairment levels consistent asthma.

FEV_1, forced expiratory volume in 1 second; FVC, forced vital capacity; ICS, inhaled corticosteroids; ICU, intensive care unit; N/A, not applicable.

Adapted from 2007 Expert Panel Report 3 Guidelines for the Diagnosis and Treatment of Asthma. Available online at http://www.nhlibi.nih.gov/guidelires/asthma/index.htm.

TABLE 8-2 Classifying Asthma Severity and Initiating Treatment (Ages ≥12 years)

Components of Severity		Classification of Asthma Severity ≥12 Years of age			
			Persistent		
		Intermittent	Mild	Moderate	Severe
Impairment	Symptoms	≤2 days/week	>2 days/week but not daily	Daily	Throughout the day
Normal FEV_1/FVC:	Nighttime awakenings	≤2×/month	3 to 4×/month	>1×/week but not nightly	Often 7×/week
8 to 19 yr 85% 20 to 39 yr 80% 40 to 59 yr 75% 60 to 80 yr 70%	Short-acting $beta_2$-agonist use for symptom control (not prevention of EIB)	≤2 days/week	>2 days/week but not daily, and not more than 1× on any day	Daily	Several times per day
	Interference with normal activity	None	Minor limitation	Some limitation	Extremely limited
	Lung function	- Normal FEV_1 between exacerbations - FEV_1 > 80% predicted - FEV_1/FVC normal	- FEV_1 >80% predicted - FEV_1/FVC normal	- FEV_1 >60% but <80% predicted - FEV_1/FVC reduced 5%	- FEV_1 < 60% predicted - FEV_1/FVC reduced >5%
Risk	Exacerbations requiring oral systemic corticosteroids	0 to 1×/year (see note)	≥2×/year (see note)		
		Consider severity and interval since last exacerbation. Frequency and severity may fluctuate over time for patients in any severity category. Relative annual risk of exacerbations may be related to FEV_1.			
Recommended Step for Initiating Treatment (See "Stepwise Approach for Managing Asthma" for treatment steps.)		Step 1	Step 2	Step 3 and consider short course of oral systemic corticosteroids	Step 4 or 5 and consider short course of oral systemic corticosteroids
		In 2 to 6 weeks, evaluate level of asthma control that is achieved and adjust therapy accordingly.			

The stepwise approach is meant to assist, not replace, the clinical decision making required to meet individual patient needs. Level of severity is determined by assessment of both impairment and risk. Assess impairment domain by patients/caregivers 2 to 4 weeks and spirometry. Assign severity to the most severe category in which any feature occurs. At present, there are inadequate data to correspond frequencies of exacerbations with different levels of asthma severity. In general, more frequent and intense exacerbations (e.g., requiring urgent, unscheduled care, hospitalization, or ICU admission) indicate greater underlying disease severity. For treatment purposes, patients who have had ≥ 2 exacerbations requiring oral systemic corticosteroids in the past year may be considered the same as patients who have persistent asthma, even in the absence of impairment levels consistent with persistent asthma.
EIB, exercise-induced bronchospasm; FEV_1, forced expiratory volume in 1 second; FVC, forced vital capacity; ICU, intensive care unit.
Adapted from 2007 Expert Panel Report 3 Guidelines for the Diagnosis and Treatment of Asthma. Available online at http://www.nhlibi.nih.gov/guidelines/asthma/index.htm.

TABLE 8-3 Assessing Asthma Control and Adjusting Therapy in Children (Ages 0 to 11)

Components of Control		Assessing Asthma Control and Adjusting Therapy in Children					
		Well Controlled		**Not Well Controlled**		**Very Poorly Controlled**	
		Ages 0 to 4	Ages 5 to 11	Ages 0 to 4	Ages 5 to 11	Ages 0 to 4	Ages 5 to 11
Impairment	Symptoms	≤2 days/week but not more than once on each day		>2 days/week or multiple times on ≤2 days/week		Throughout the day	
	Nighttime awakenings	≤1×/month		>1×/month	≥2×/month	>1×/week	≥2×/week
	Interference with normal activity	None		Some limitation		Extremely limited	
	Short-acting beta$_2$-agonist use for symptom control (not prevention of EIB)	≤2 days/week		>2 days/week		Several times per day	
	Lung function –FEV_1 (predicted) or peak flow personal best –FEV_1/FEV	N/A	>80% >80%	N/A	60% to 80% 75% to 80%	N/A	<60% <75%
Risk	Exacerbations requiring oral systemic	0 to 1×/year		2 to 3×/year	≥2×/year	>3×/year	≥2×/year
	Reduction in lung growth	N/A	Requires long-term follow-up	N/A		N/A	
	Treatment-related adverse effects	Medication side effects can vary in intensity from none to very troublesome and worrisome. The level of intensity does not correlate to specific levels of control but should be considered in the overall assessment of risk.					
Step for Initiating Therapy (See "Stepwise Approach for Managing Asthma" for treatment steps.)		- Maintain current step - Regular follow-up every 1 to 6 months		Step up 1 step	Step up at least 1 step	- Consider short course of oral systemic corticosteroids	
The stepwise approach is meant to assist, not replace, the clinical decision making required to meet individual patients needs		- Consider step down if well controlled for at least 3 months				- Step up 1 to 2 steps	
				- Before step up: Review adherence to medication, inhaler technique, and environment control. If alternative treatment was used, discontinue it and use preferred treatment for that step.			

(continues)

TABLE 8-3 Assessing Asthma Control and Adjusting Therapy in Children (Ages 0 to 11) *(continued)*

Components of Control	Assessing Asthma Control and Adjusting Therapy in Children					
	Well Controlled		Not Well Controlled		Very Poorly Controlled	
	Ages 0 to 4	Ages 5 to 11	Ages 0 to 4	Ages 5 to 11	Ages 0 to 4	Ages 5 to 11
			- Reevaluate the level of asthma control in 2 to 6 weeks to achieve control; every 1 to 6 months to maintain control. - Control 0 to 4 weeks, consider alternative diagnoses or adjusting therapy. - Children 5 to 11 years old: Adjust therapy accordingly. - For side effects, consider alternative treatment options.			

The level of control is based on the most severe impairment or risk category. Assess impairment domain by patient's or caregiver's recall of previous 2 to 4 weeks. Symptom assessment for longer periods should reflect a global assessment, such as whether the patient's asthma is better or worse since the last visit. At present, there are inadequate data to correspond frequencies of exacerbations with different levels of asthma control. In general, more frequent and intense exacerbations (e.g., requiring urgent, unscheduled care, hospitalization, or ICU admission) indicate poorer disease control.

EIB, exercise-induced bronchospasm; FEV_1, forced expiratory volume in 1 second; FVC, forced vital capacity; ICU, intensive care unit; N/A, not applicable.

Adapted from 2007 Expert Panel Report 3 Guidelines for the Diagnosis and Treatment of Asthma online at http://www.nhlibi.nih.gov/guidelines/asthma/index.htm.

Epidemiology

Asthma is the most frequently encountered pulmonary disease in children, and its prevalence is on the rise despite advances in therapy. As many as 15% to 20% of children in the United States will be diagnosed with asthma at some point in time; in some high risk populations (Black and Hispanics), the prevalence can reach 25%. It is among the most common reasons for hospitalization in pediatric practice. More than 50% of patients present before 6 years of age. Boys are affected more often than girls prior to adolescence; thereafter, the ratio is reversed.

Risk Factors

Risk factors for the development of asthma include genetic predisposition (parent[s] with asthma or allergy), atopy, cigarette smoke exposure, living in urban areas in poverty, and African American race and Puerto Rican ethnicity. Upper respiratory tract infections with certain viruses, including rhinovirus and respiratory syncytial virus, that occur in genetically susceptible children at certain critical times in early life are also thought to play a critical role.

Differential Diagnosis

When a child presents with wheezing and respiratory distress, the differential diagnosis includes intraluminal inflammation or failure to clear secretions (bronchiolitis, gastroesophageal reflux with aspiration, cystic fibrosis, tracheoesophageal fistula, primary ciliary dyskinesia); intraluminal mass effects (foreign body aspiration, tracheal or bronchial tumors or granulation tissue); dynamic airway collapse (tracheobronchomalacia); intrinsic narrowing of the airway (congenital or acquired stenosis); and extrinsic compression (vascular ring, mediastinal lymph nodes or masses). These diagnoses should also be considered in patients whose wheezing fails to respond to appropriate medical treatment. Anaphylaxis and angioneurotic edema may cause wheezing at any age. **Cough-variant asthma**, which is relatively uncommon, produces a chronic cough that may be triggered by exercise or noted primarily at night during sleep; wheezing may or may not be present. Improvement with treatment with inhaled corticosteroids helps confirm the diagnosis.

Clinical Manifestations

The presentations of asthma are varied. The history may be positive for wheezing and protracted cough with viral respiratory infections. Other possible signs and symptoms include prolonged respiratory infections, decreased exercise tolerance, and persistent day or nighttime coughing. Children with acute exacerbations present in respiratory distress with dyspnea, wheezing, subcostal retractions, nasal flaring, tracheal tugging, and a prolonged expiratory phase resulting from obstruction of airflow. Cyanosis is uncommon. The absence of wheezing, with poorly heard breath sounds, during an acute exacerbation is an ominous sign, indicating severe airway obstruction with very limited air movement. Mental status changes suggest significant hypercarbia and/or significant hypoxemia with impending respiratory failure.

Diagnostic Evaluation

Most children with asthma will have a normal physical examination when not in exacerbation. In children older than 6 years, pulmonary function tests (PFTs) can help delineate the degree of airflow obstruction at baseline and during exacerbations. However, most children with asthma will also have normal lung function when not acutely ill. An inhalation challenge test with an agent that induces bronchoconstriction in those with airway hyperreactivity (e.g., methacholine) can be useful in helping diagnose asthma. Patients with *persistent*

TABLE 8-4 Assessing Asthma Control and Adjusting Therapy (Ages ≥12 years)

Components of Control		Classification of Asthma Control (≥12 years of age)		
		Well Controlled	**Not Well Controlled**	**Very Poorly Controlled**
Impairment	Symptoms	≤2 days/week	>2 days/week	Throughout the day
	Nighttime awakenings	≤2×/month	1l to 3×/week	≥4×/week
	Interference with normal activity	Non	Some limitation	Extremely limited
	Short-acting beta$_2$-agonist use for symptom control (not prevention of EIB)	≤2 days/week	>2 days/week	Several times per day
	FEV$_1$ or peak flow	>80% predicted/personal best	60% to 80% predicted/personal best	<60% predicted/personal best
	Validated questionnaires	0	1 to 2	3 to 4
	ATAQ ACQ ACT	≤0.75[a] ≥20	≥1.5 16 to 19	N/A ≤15
Risk	Exacerbations requiring oral systemic corticosteroids	0 to 1×/year	≥2×/year (see note)	
		Consider severity and interval since last exacerbation		
	Progressive loss of lung function	Evaluation requires long-term follow-up care		
	Treatment-related adverse effects	Medication side effects can vary in intensity from none to very troublesome. The level of intensity does not correlate to specific levels of control but should be considered in the overall assessment of risk.		
Recommended Action for Treatment (See "Stepwise Approach for Managing Asthma" for treatment steps.)		- Maintain current step - Regular follow-up at every 1 to 6 months to maintain control - Consider step down if well controlled for at least 3 months	- Step up to 1 step - Reevaluate in 2 to 6 weeks - For side effects, consider alternative treatment options	- Consider short course of oral systemic corticosteroids - Step up 1 to 2 steps - Reevaluate in 2 weeks - For side effects, consider alternative treatment options

[a]ACQ values of 0.76 to 1.4 are indeterminate regarding well-controlled asthma.

The stepwise approach is meant to assist, not replace, the clinical decision making required to meet individual patient needs. The level of control is based on the most severe impairment or risk category. Assess impairment domain by patient's recall of previous 2 to 4 weeks by spirometry or peak flow measures. Symptom assessment for longer periods should reflect a global assessment, such as inquiring whether the patient's asthma is better or worse since the last visit. At present, there are inadequate data to correspond frequencies of exacerbations with different levels of asthma control. In general, more frequent and intense exacerbations (e.g., requiring urgent, unscheduled care, hospitalization, or ICU admission) indicate poorer disease control. For treatment purposes, patients who had ≥2 exacerbations requiring oral systemic corticosteroids in the past year may be considered the same as patients who have not-well-controlled asthma, even in the absence of impairment levels consistent with not-well-controlled asthma.

ATAQ, Asthma Therapy Assessment Questionnaire©; ACQ, Asthma Control Questionnaire©; ACT, Asthma Control Test™; Difference: 1.0 for the ATAQ; 0.5 for the ACQ; not determined for the ACT.

Before step up in therapy:

Review adherence to medication, inhaler technique, environmental control, and comorbid conditions.

If an alternative treatment option was used in a step, discontinue and use the preferred treatment for that step.

Adapted from 2007 Expert Panel Report 3 Guidelines for the Diagnosis and Treatment of Asthma. Available online at http://www.nhlibi.nih.gov/guidelines/asthma/index.htm.

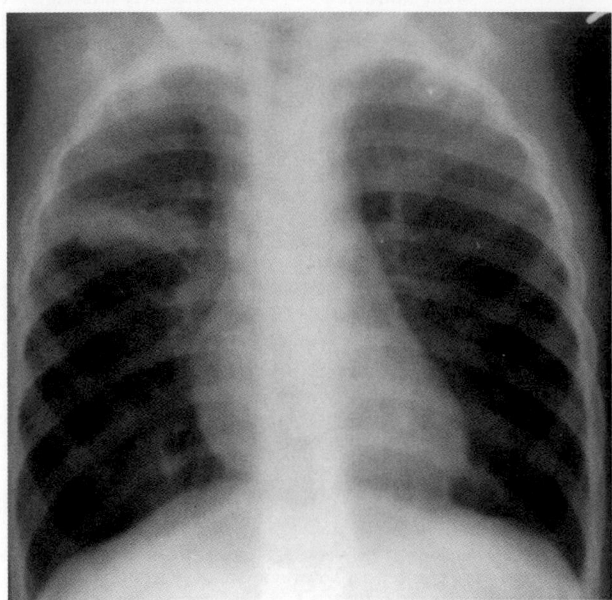

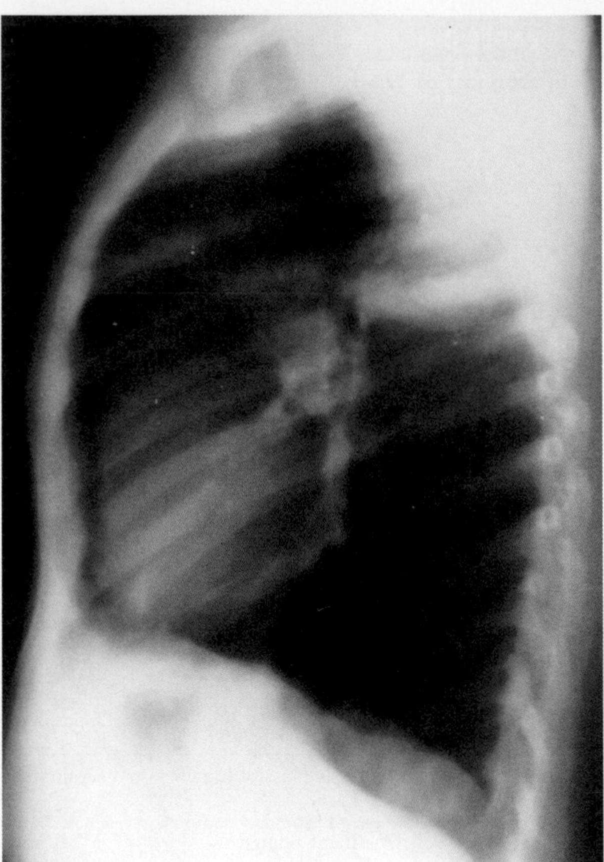

Figure 8-1 • Chest radiograph of a 3-year-old patient obtained during an asthma exacerbation test demonstrates severe hyperinflation, increased anteroposterior diameter of the chest, a depressed diaphragm, and several areas of atelectasis.

asthma should have PFT at least once a year in order to monitor for change and to help adjust therapy. Baseline chest radiographs typically show mild hyperinflation and/or increased bronchial markings. Peak flow (PF) monitoring may be useful for patients with moderate to severe asthma or those who poorly perceive their symptoms. PF meters are small, portable, and easy to use. They measure how fast a patient can forcibly expire air after a maximal inhalation; decreased readings indicate obstruction to airflow. Reductions to 50% to 80% of predicted values indicate mild to moderate disease exacerbation; readings less than 30% of predicted values are associated with severe obstruction. Unfortunately, peak flow meters are heavily dependent on technique and are therefore variably reliable.

During acute exacerbations, the chest radiograph demonstrates significant hyperinflation and occasionally focal or subsegmental atelectasis (Fig. 8-1). CO_2 retention can occur with fatigue and may be quite dramatic; hypoxemia is usually less pronounced.

Treatment

With appropriate therapy and good adherence, most patients with persistent asthma can remain symptom-free with few exacerbations. The most effective treatment involves removal of inciting agents (triggers) from the patient's environment and appropriate use of maintenance anti-inflammatory medication. Cigarette smoke should be strictly avoided. Limiting dust mite, mold, and pet exposure is beneficial to patients with an allergic component to their asthma. The National Institutes of Health has issued guidelines for the pharmacologic management of asthma based on disease severity and control (Tables 8-5 and 8-6).

The mainstays of medical maintenance therapy include **inhaled corticosteroids** (ICSs), β-2-adrenergic agonists, and **leukotriene receptor antagonists** (LTRAs). **β-2-agonists** such as albuterol reduce smooth muscle constriction and can be administered via nebulization or metered-dose inhalation. Longer-acting beta agonists (LABA) (salbutamol, formoterol) in combination with ICS, may be used in patients who fail to achieve good control with ICS therapy alone. In older children and adolescents, the additive effect of the LABA may allow for lower dosees of ICS. Long-acting β-agonists are not appropriate for monotherapy and should only be used in patients who cannot be controled on ICS alone or with the addition of other anti-inflammatory medications. Short-acting β-2-agonists are effective in preventing exercise-induced asthma if used 5 to 20 minutes before vigorous activity. The abuse of inhaled bronchodilators may result in some tolerance to their therapeutic effects.

TABLE 8-5 Stepwise Approach for Managing Asthma Long Term in Children (Ages 0 to 11 Years)

		Step 1	Step 2	Step 3	Step 4	Step 5	Step 6
		Intermittent Asthma		*Persistent Asthma: Daily Medication*[a]			
Children 0 to 4 years of age	Preferred	SABA PRN	Low-dose ICS	Medium-dose ICS	Medium-dose ICS + LABA or Montelukast	High-dose ICS + LABA or Montelukast	High-dose ICS + oral corticosteroids ICS + LABA or Montelukast
	Alternative		Cromolyn or Montelukast				
		Each step: Patient education and environmental control					
	Quick-relief medication	- SABA as needed for symptoms. Intensity of treatment depends on severity of symptoms. - With viral respiratory symptoms: SABA q 4 to 6 hours (longer with physician consult). Consider short course of oral systemic corticosteroids if exacerbation is severe or patient has history of previous severe exacerbations.					
		Intermittent Asthma		*Persistent Asthma: Daily Medication*[a]			
Children 5 to 11 years of age	Preferred	SABA PRN	Low-dose ICS	Lose-dose ICS + LABA, LTRA, or theophylline or medium-dose ICS	Medium-dose ICS + LABA	High-dose ICS + LABA	High-dose ICS + LABA + oral corticosteroids
	Alternative		Cromotyn, LTRA, nedocromil, or theophylline		Medium-dose ICS + LTRA or theophylline	High-dose ICS + LTRA or theophylline	High-dose ICA + LTRA or theophylline + oral corticosteroids
		Each step: Patient education, environmental control, and management of comorbidities Steps 2 to 4: Consider subcutaneous allergen immunotherapy for patients who have persistent, allergic asthma					
	Quick-relief medication	- SABA as needed for symptoms. Intensity of treatment depends on severity of symptoms: up to 3 treatments at 20-minute intervals as needed. Short course of oral systemic corticosteroids may be needed. Caution: Increasing use of SABA or use >2 days a week for symptom relief (not prevention of EIB) generally indicated inadequate control and the need to step up treatment.					

[a]Consult with asthma specialist if Step 3 care or higher is required. Consider consultation at Step 2.

Children 0 to 4 Years of Age

The stepwise approach is meant to assist, not replace, the clinical decision making required to meet individual patient needs.
If an alternative treatment is used and response is inadequate, discontinue it and use the preferred treatment before stepping up.
If clear benefit is not observed within 4 to 6 weeks, and patient's/family's medication technique and adherence are satisfactory, consider adjusting therapy or an alternative diagnosis.
Studies on children 0 to 4 years of age are limited. Most recommendations in this age group are based on expert opinion and extrapolation from studies in older children.

Children 5 to 11 Years of Age

The stepwise approach is meant to assist, not replace, the clinical decision making required to meet individual patient needs.
If an alternative treatment is used and response is inadequate, discontinue it and use the preferred treatment before stepping up.
Theophylline is a less desirable alternative due to the need to monitor serum concentration levels.
Rationale for recommendations in this age group is available at the NIH website.

Alphabetical listing is used when more than one treatment option is listed within either preferred or alternative therapy.

ICS, inhaled corticosteroid; LABA, inhaled long-acting beta$_2$-agonist; LTRA, leukotriene receptor antagonist; oral corticosteroids, oral systemic corticosteroids; SABA, inhaled short-acting beta$_2$-agonist.
Adapted from 2007 Expert Panel Report 3 Guidelines for the Diagnosis and Treatment of Asthma. Available online at http://www.nhlbi.nih.gov/guidelines/asthma/index.htm.

TABLE 8-6 Stepwise Approach for Managing Asthma (Ages ≥12 years)

Intermittent Asthma	**Persistent Asthma: Daily Medication** *Consult with asthma specialist if Step 4 care or higher is required. Consider consultation at Step 3*					
Step 1 Preferred: SABA PRN	Step 2 Preferred: Low-dose ICS Alternative: Cromolyn, LTRA, nedocromil, ortheophylline	Step 3 Preferred: Low-dose ICS + LABA or Medium-dose ICS Alternative: Low-dose ICS + either LTRA, theophy lline, or zileuton	Step 4 Preferred: Medium-dose ICS + LABA Alternative: Medium -dose ICS + either LTRA, theophylline, or zileuton	Step 5 Preferred: High-dose ICS + LABA and Consider Omalizuma for patients who have allergies	Step 6 Preferred: High-dose ICS + LABA + oral corticosteroid and consider Omalizu mab for patients who have allergies	Step up if needed (first, check adherence, environmental control, and comorbid conditions). Assess control. Step down if possible (and asthma is well controlled for at least 3 months)
Each step: Patient education, environmental control, and management of comorbidities Steps 2 to 4: Consider subcutaneous allergen immunotherapy for patients who have allergic asthma (see notes)						

The stepwise approach is meant to assist, not replace, the clinical decision making required to meet individual patient needs. If alternative treatment is used and response is inadequate, discontinue it and use the preferred treatment before stepping up. Zileuton is a less desirable alternative due to limited studies as adjunctive therapy and the need to monitor liver function. Theophylline requires monitoring of serum concentration levels. In Step 6, before oral corticosteroids are introduced, a trial of high-dose ICS + LABA + either LTRA, theophylline, or zileuton may be considered, although this approach has not been studied in clinical trials. Rationale for recommendations for preferred therapies in this age group is available at the NIH website: http://www.nhlbi.nih.gov/guidelines/archives/epr-2_upd/asthmafullrpt_archive.pdf

Alphabetical order is used when more than one treatment option is listed within either preferred or alternative therapy.

ICS, inhaled corticosteroid; LABA, long-acting beta$_2$-agonist; LTRA, leukotriene receptor antagonist; oral corticosteroids, oral systemic corticosteroids; SABA, inhaled short-acting beta$_2$-agonist.

Adapted from 2007 Expert Panel Report 3 Guidelines for the Diagnosis and Treatment of Asthma. Available online at http://www.nhlibi.nih.gov/guidelines/asthma/index.htm.

Inhaled corticosteroid therapy is the most effective treatment for chronic asthma and results in excellent control in the vast majority of patients. Topically active ICSs typically have very low systemic bioavailability and result in few systemic adverse effects. Options include beclomethasone, budesonide, fluticasone, and mometasone. Small measurable decreases in linear growth occur in children using daily inhaled corticosteroids; however, when budesonide and fluticasone are used at low doses, linear growth velocity declines initially but then rebounds, resulting in only a small reduction in final height (<1.5 cm). Short courses of oral steroids (3–7 days) are used for acute exacerbations; long-term use is reserved for severe, persistent, poorly controlled asthma.

LTRAs (montelukast, zafirlukast) are oral medications also recommended for the initial treatment of mild persistent asthma; they may be used as add-on medications to an ICS. They are most effective in younger patients and those with a shorter duration of asthma. LTRAs also provide some protection from exercise-induced symptoms.

The use of theophylline, once a commonly prescribed oral bronchodilator, has fallen out of favor as a first-line treatment option. Theophylline may be poorly tolerated, has significant interactions with multiple other medications, and requires drug-level monitoring. It is presently reserved for use as an add-on therapy in patients who do not respond to conventional medications and is sometimes used in the intensive care setting as adjunctive treatment for severe exacerbations. Patients (>12 years old) with severe allergic asthma that remains poorly controlled with use of inhaled corticosteroids, leukotriene receptor antagonists, and long-acting β-agonists may benefit from treatment with omalizumab, an injectable monoclonal antibody directed against IgE. This treatment is expensive and must be given every 2 to 4 weeks.

Mild to moderate exacerbations are managed by the addition of short-acting inhaled bronchodilators to maintenance regimens. Additional steps may include quadrupling the dosage of inhaled steroids for 7 to 10 days or initiating a 5-day pulse of oral steroids. Moderate to severe exacerbations usually require an emergency department visit, and in some cases, hospitalization.

Children who present to the emergency department in an acute asthma attack are initially assessed for airway patency, work of breathing, and ability to adequately oxygenate. Pulse oximetry is a simple, rapid screen for hypoxemia; patients with persistent hypoxemia (SaO_2 < 92%) after initial treatment with a short acting bronchodilator are likely to need more aggressive treatment and hospitalization. Patients in severe respiratory distress require blood gas measurements to assess for increasing $PaCO_2$, a sign of impending respiratory failure. A normal $PaCO_2$ in the face of tachypnea and fatigue is an equally ominous sign because the $PaCO_2$ should be well below 40 mm Hg in the patient with a rapid respiratory rate.

Nebulized bronchodilators are administered frequently (every 20 minutes or continuously) for severe episodes. Delivery of inhaled β-agonists using a metered dose inhaler (MDI) with a valved holding chamber is as equally effective as using a nebulizer. Ipratropium, an anticholinergic agent, may provide additive relief of symptoms in those patients with the most severe obstruction, as measured by PEF or spirometry. The drug is usually given simultaneously with albuterol. Subcutaneous epinephrine or terbutaline can rapidly decrease airway obstruction in severely affected patients who may be too fatigued or uncooperative to use inhaled albuterol. Corticosteroids, administered orally or intravenously, are indicated for treatment of acute exacerbations that fail to improve significantly after the first albuterol treatment in the emergency department. Children who do not respond with significant resolution of symptoms after several hours (i.e., children in status asthmaticus) and those who require ongoing oxygen therapy should be hospitalized for continued treatment and close observation.

Despite advances in therapy, some patients still die from asthma. However, the mortality rate for asthma in children is relatively low in developed countries and has stabilized in the past several years. Factors that increase the risk of death include noncompliance, poor recognition of symptoms, delay in treatment, history of intubation, African American race, and steroid dependence.

CYSTIC FIBROSIS

Pathogenesis

Cystic fibrosis (CF) is an inherited multisystem disease characterized by disordered exocrine gland function. The product of the **cystic fibrosis transmembrane regulator (CFTR) gene** is a cell membrane protein that functions as a cAMP-activated chloride channel on the apical surface of epithelial cells in the respiratory tract, pancreas, sweat and salivary glands, intestines, and reproductive system. This channel is nonfunctional in patients with CF, so chloride remains sequestered inside the cell. Sodium and water are drawn into the cell to maintain ionic and osmotic balance, resulting in relative dehydration at the apical surface of the cell. This in turn results in abnormally viscid secretions and impairment of mucociliary clearance in the respiratory tract.

Epidemiology

CF is acquired through autosomal recessive inheritance, with a disease frequency of ~1 in 3,500 Caucasian births (much lower in other races). More than 1,000 distinct gene mutations on chromosome 7 have been described; 70% of known mutant alleles involve a single nucleotide deletion (the ΔF508 mutation). The average life expectancy is currently in the mid- to late 30s in developed countries and has increased dramatically in the past 4 decades.

Clinical Manifestations

History and Physical Examination

Table 8-7 lists the most common presenting signs and symptoms of CF. All levels of the respiratory tract may be affected, including the nasal passages, sinuses, and lower airways. **Nasal polyps** in any pediatric patient should prompt further testing for CF. Sinusitis or radiographic opacification of the sinuses are extremely common. Mucus stasis and ineffective clearance lead to bacterial colonization and frequent pneumonias. Typical early childhood pathogens include *Staphylococcus aureus* and *Haemophilus influenzae*. This is generally followed by colonization with *Pseudomonas aeruginosa* in late childhood and early adolescence; more than 90% of patients eventually acquire

TABLE 8-7 Clinical Manifestations of Cystic Fibrosis

Chronic Sinopulmonary Disease
Persistent colonization/infection with pathogens typical of CF lung disease, including
Staphylococcus aureus
Pseudomonas aeruginosa (mucoid and nonmucoid)
Nontypeable *Haemophilus influenzae*
Burkholderia cepacia complex
Stenotrophomonas maltophilia
Endobronchial Disease Manifested by
Cough and sputum production
Wheezing and air trapping
Radiographic abnormalities
Evidence of obstruction on PFTs
Digital clubbing
Chronic sinus disease
Nasal polyps
Radiographic changes
Intestinal Abnormalities
Meconium ileus
Exocrine pancreatic insufficiency
Distal intestinal obstruction
Rectal prolapse
Recurrent pancreatitis
Chronic hepatobiliary disease manifested by clinical and/or laboratory evidence of
Focal biliary cirrhosis
Multilobular cirrhosis
Failure to thrive (protein-calorie malnutrition)
Hypoproteinemia-edema
Fat-soluble vitamin deficiencies
Genitourinary Abnormalities
Obstructive azoospermia in males
Reduced fertility in females
Metabolic Abnormalities
Salt-loss syndromes
Acute salt depletion
Chronic metabolic alkalosis

P. aeruginosa, and it is rarely eradicated. Colonization with *Burkholderia cepacia* is particularly ominous and may be associated with accelerated pulmonary deterioration and early death. Other pathogens, often with multiple antibiotic resistance, are becoming more common as the population of CF patients ages.

Gastrointestinal manifestations include pancreatic insufficiency, bowel obstruction and rectal prolapse, diabetes, and hepatic cirrhosis. Loss of pancreatic enzyme secretion leads to decreased fat absorption; parents may notice that the child's stools are large, bulky, and foul smelling. Later, stool becomes extremely dense, sometimes leading to distal intestinal obstruction. **Failure to thrive** is the most common manifestation of untreated CF in infants and children. **Meconium ileus** (neonatal intestinal obstruction in the absence of anatomic abnormalities) is virtually pathognomonic for CF.

Diagnostic Evaluation

The classic diagnostic findings in CF are related to the elevated sweat chloride concentration, pancreatic insufficiency, and chronic pulmonary disease. Recurrent lower airway infection results in bronchiectasis, fibrosis, parenchymal loss, and the characteristic bleb formation found on chest radiographs (Fig. 8-2). Pulmonary function tests demonstrate mostly obstructive and (later) some restrictive changes. The **sweat chloride test** is the initial diagnostic study of choice. A level greater than 60 mEq/L is generally considered abnormal, but both false positives and false negatives occur, and occasionally a borderline test is hard to interpret. Sweat testing, though simple in concept, is difficult in practice, and should only be performed in specialized centers with experience and expertise. Genetic and prenatal testing are now available; the finding of two mutations at the CFTR site, known to produce disease, is considered diagnostic of CF. Some mutations produce less CFTR dysfunction; if at least 10% of normal CFTR activity is present, the individual may remain symptom free. The availability of newborn screening has led to the identification of an increasing number of children with at least one mutation associated with CF but who do not meet the diagnostic criteria for CF otherwise; these children are said to have "cystic fibrosis metabolic syndrome"– unfortunately, we do not know how to predict whether these children will eventually develop some disease manifestation.

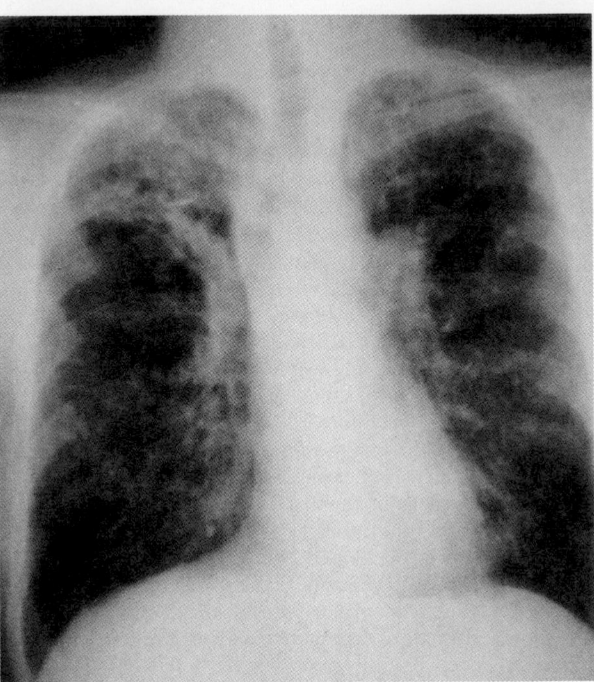

Figure 8-2 • Chest radiograph in this adolescent male with cystic fibrosis demonstrates marked chronic disease and bleb formation.

Treatment

The most fundamental aspect of CF therapy is the maintenance of effective airway clearance. Chest physical therapy, vigorous exercise, and frequent coughing are helpful in mobilizing secretions. Bronchodilators relax smooth muscle walls and increase mucociliary clearance. Antibiotics decrease the production of bacterial toxins, reduce inflammation, and curb tissue destruction. Recombinant human deoxyribonuclease, administered via nebulization, breaks down thick DNA complexes present in mucus as a result of cell destruction and bacterial colonization. Alternate months of regular inhaled tobramycin may be indicated for patients infected with *Pseudomonas*. More recently, azithromycin taken thrice weekly has been added as a possible immune/inflammatory modifier. Inhaled hypertonic saline may also improve airway clearance.

Acute disease exacerbations may be triggered by viral or bacterial infections and are treated by more aggressive chest physical therapy and antibiotics, which may be taken orally or by inhalation if the exacerbation is mild and the organisms are not resistant. Frequently, however, bacterial infections must be treated with intravenous antibiotics (often in combination), depending on organism susceptibilities. Research aimed at correcting the specific gene mutation is currently under way. Patients often improve in clinical status during hospital admission for reasons that are not entirely clear but may in part involve improved adherence to prescribed therapy and reduced exposure to allergens and other irritants.

Near-normal growth can often be achieved with pancreatic enzyme replacement, fat-soluble vitamin supplements, and high-calorie, high-protein diets. Nasogastric or gastrostomy tube feedings may be instituted if oral intake is inadequate. Maintenance of height and weight above the 25th percentile for age results in a better long-term prognosis. Many patients develop relative insulin deficiency and may benefit from insulin therapy, although type I diabetes is uncommon and ketoacidosis is rare.

Prognosis continues to improve with aggressive treatment of pulmonary exacerbations and optimal nutritional support. Respiratory complications remain the major contributors to morbidity and mortality in CF.

Hemoptysis is an alarming development that may occur in patients with severe bronchiectasis. Frequent coughing and inflammation lead to erosion of the walls of bronchial arteries in areas of bronchiectasis, and expectorated sputum becomes streaked with blood. Frank blood loss of more than 500 mL in 24 hours (or more than 300 mL/day for 3 days) is considered an emergency, often requiring bronchial arterial embolization.

Spontaneous pneumothorax is another potentially life-threatening complication of CF. It is usually manifest by the sudden onset of severe chest pain and difficulty breathing. Placement of a chest tube results in rapid reexpansion, but approximately half of pneumothoraces recur unless pleurodesis is performed. Pleurodesis is generally avoided if possible because lung transplantation becomes more difficult following this procedure.

Progressive airway obstruction and hypoxia in advanced disease can lead to **chronic pulmonary hypertension** and **cor pulmonale**. For CF patients with a predicted life expectancy limited to 1 to 2 years, lung transplantation is a potentially viable option. Survival postlung transplantation is currently on the order of 50% at 5 years.

PRIMARY CILIARY DYSKINESIA

Primary ciliary dyskinesia (PCD) is a group of recessive disorders of ciliary structure/function in which mucociliary clearance is markedly impaired because of ciliary dysfunction. Failure to clear secretions leads to bronchial obstruction, sinusitis, chronic otitis media, and recurrent respiratory infections. Respiratory symptoms may be similar to those of CF or asthma. The diagnosis is made by demonstration of abnormal ciliary beat under light microscopy or characteristic ultrastructural changes in samples of ciliated cells obtained from scrapings of the nasal or bronchial epithelium. A minority of patients have identifiable genetic mutations (*DNAI1* and *DNAH5*) that result in PCD. Treatment is similar to that of the pulmonary component of CF, although patients with PCD do not have the same propensity to infection with *P. aeruginosa*. Most patients with PCD develop bronchiectasis by the end of the second or third decade of life.

OTHER CAUSES OF AIRWAY OBSTRUCTION IN CHILDREN

Congenital abnormalities

Congenital tracheal stenosis is the result of tracheal cartilage rings that completely encircle the trachea and grow more slowly than the rest of the trachea. If the trachea is significantly narrowed, there may be a "washing machine" type inspiratory and expiratory noise, as well as hypoxemia, failure to thrive, and other symptoms. More than 90% of patients with complete tracheal rings will require surgical intervention (the most effective technique is the slide tracheoplasty), and these patients should be thoroughly investigated for other congenital anomalies (especially the heart and great vessels) prior to surgery. The trachea and/or main bronchi can be compressed by abnormal vascular structures (double aortic arch, aberrant left pulmonary artery, enlarged pulmonary arteries). A right aortic arch typically compresses the proximal right main bronchus. Children with these vascular anomalies may have wheezing or respiratory distress.

Tracheomalacia is a common cause of expiratory airway obstruction in children and is due to a widening of the posterior membranous portion of the trachea with dynamic collapse during exhalation (if severe) or coughing or forced exhalation (if not as severe). The process may extend down one or both main bronchi. These children typically have a harsh, brassy ("croupy") cough and are often misdiagnosed as having recurrent croup. Esophageal atresia with tracheoesophageal atresia is a common cause of tracheomalacia. Most children with tracheomalacia require no intervention, but there are surgical procedures that may help some children. Wheezing due to tracheomalacia is often made worse by treatment with a bronchodilator, as it makes the posterior tracheal membrane more flaccid, and thus more likely to collapse during exhalation. A paradoxical response to bronchodilator treatment should always raise the suspicion of tracheomalacia.

Bronchomalacia is the result of either poor cartilage (in central bronchi) or poor elastic recoil in the tissues surrounding the (more peripheral) bronchi, resulting in dynamic bronchial collapse on exhalation. These children typically have wheezing upon forced exhalation and fail to respond to bronchodilators or steroids (they are quite frequently misdiagnosed as having severe asthma).

Congenital and dynamic airway anomalies are most conveniently and definitively diagnosed by bronchoscopy. The bronchoscopic evaluation must be performed under conditions that allow the diagnosis (tracheomalacia or bronchomalacia may not be at all apparent if the bronchoscopy is performed with positive pressure ventilation or with very deep sedation/anesthesia).

RESTRICTIVE LUNG DISEASES

Restrictive lung diseases result from decreased compliance of the chest wall or of the lung itself. They cause a decrease in most measurements of lung volume, including functional residual capacity, tidal volume, and vital capacity. Restrictive lung disease is much less common in the pediatric population than obstructive pulmonary disorders.

Pectus excavatum refers to a depression in the sternum, and **pectus carinatum** refers to an outward deformity. Severe congenital forms of these malformations may result in restrictive lung disease as a result of mechanical interference with normal respiration, but typically these deformities are more cosmetic than functional. Severe scoliosis will usually have a greater effect, with restriction as well as airway compression. Marked obesity, in addition to being a risk for upper airway obstructive disease, may also be a cause of restrictive lung disease. **Neuromuscular disease** may result in restrictive lung disease as a consequence of insufficient respiratory muscle strength (Guillain-Barré syndrome, muscular dystrophy, spinal muscular atrophy).

Any lesion that occupies intrathoracic space, if large enough, will interfere with normal pulmonary expansion. Pleural effusion, pericardial effusion, chylothorax, hemothorax, pneumothorax, chest wall tumors, mediastinal masses, congenital lobar emphysema, cystic adenomatous malformations, diaphragmatic hernias, and pulmonary sequestrations may all compete with normal lung for thoracic space, resulting in restrictive pulmonary compromise.

Interstitial lung disease refers to disorders in which there is disease in the tissues of the lung outside the airways and alveoli. This usually results in decreased compliance and, therefore, restrictive physiology. A number of rare diseases can lead to interstitial changes, including chronic interstitial lung disease, desquamative interstitial pneumonitis, and sarcoidosis. Recurrent aspiration can also cause interstitial disease, as can acute chest syndrome in sickle cell disease (see Chapter 11).

Pulmonary hemosiderosis involves an abnormal accumulation of hemosiderin in the lungs as a result of diffuse alveolar hemorrhage. It may be idiopathic or the result of problems which produce repeated bleeding into the lung. Diagnosis is based on the presence of hemosiderin-laden macrophages (siderophages) in bronchial washings or gastric aspirates;

a specific cause of the bleeding should be sought. Clinical manifestations of pulmonary hemosiderosis may include hemoptysis/hematemesis and a microcytic hypochromic anemia with elevated reticulocyte counts. Many patients with hemosiderosis are mistakenly diagnosed clinically to have recurrent pneumonia.

Symptoms of restrictive lung disease typically reflect decreased pulmonary compliance, which may not become clinically apparent until the process is relatively advanced. Exercise intolerance, tachypnea, and eventually dyspnea at rest are common. Space-occupying lesions may or may not be detected by chest auscultation (noting decreased breath sounds over the affected area) and may be seen on chest radiographs or even an echocardiogram. The chronic nature of many restrictive lesions can put patients at risk for developing prolonged respiratory insufficiency. Pulmonary hypertension may develop; an accentuated pulmonic component of the second heart sound may be heard, but echocardiography is usually the diagnostic method of choice. Clubbing of fingers and toes may be noted.

ASPIRATION SYNDROMES

The primary purpose of the larynx is to protect the lower airways from aspiration of liquids and/or solids. Vocal cord closure and cough are both vitally important protective reflexes, and failure of either can result in aspiration. Aspiration of liquids (saliva, ingested liquids, or gastric contents resulting from reflux) leads to cough, bronchospasm, inflammation, infection, and, if persistent, to bronchiectasis and lung destruction. Decreased sensation, impaired vocal cord mobility, or structural defects (laryngoesophageal cleft, tracheoesophageal fistula) can result in aspiration. The acute, accidental aspiration of a solid object is surprisingly common in young children (prime age 1–4 years), and results in coughing, choking, perhaps respiratory distress. Witnessed aspiration events are not usually difficult diagnostic challenges, but most events are not witnessed, and the physician must be suspicious; sudden onset of symptoms such as wheezing or coughing out of context with the child's previous history should lead to suspicion. Radiographic studies are important but often not definitive (especially if the aspirated object is not radio-opaque); the radiologist should be made aware of the suspicion before the studies are done. Bronchoscopy may be necessary for definitive diagnosis or exclusion, and rigid bronchoscopy is indicated for removal of a known foreign body. Small foreign bodies can remain in the lower airways for years, causing persistent/recurrent pneumonia, atelectasis, chronic cough, and, eventually, bronchiectasis.

The diagnosis of recurrent aspiration can be supported by radiographic (video swallow) or endoscopic studies. There is no definitive marker for aspiration, unless the aspiration is

TABLE 8-8 Apnea of Infancy: Apparent Life-Threatening Events

Cause	Helpful Diagnostic Tests
Infectious	
Sepsis	CBC/Blood culture
Meningitis	LP
Pneumonia	Chest radiograph
Bronchiolitis (RSV)	RSV antigen test in season
Pertussis	PCR or fluorescent antibody staining
Neurologic	
Seizures	EEG
Central apnea	Polysomnography
Intraventricular hemorrhage	Cranial US
Respiratory	
Airway obstruction	Airway radiographs or bronchoscopy
Aspiration	Swallowing study
Cardiac	
Arrhythmias	ECG
Gastrointestinal	
Gastroesophageal reflux	Barium swallow or pH/impedance probe
Other	
Metabolic disorders	Tests for inborn errors of metabolism
Electrolyte disorders	Electrolyte panel/blood glucose
Abuse	Skeletal survey/fundoscopic exam

directly observed. Children with uncontrolled gastroesophageal reflux are at risk for aspiration and often have persistent/recurrent respiratory symptoms (cough, wheeze, recurrent pneumonias).

APNEA OF INFANCY

Apnea is defined as the cessation of breathing for longer than 20 seconds or pauses of any duration associated with color changes (cyanosis, pallor), hypotonia, decreased responsiveness, or bradycardia. It may be central (neurally mediated), obstructive, or mixed. Apnea is not a diagnosis but a potentially dangerous sign requiring aggressive evaluation to define the underlying cause. In contrast to apnea of prematurity, apnea of infancy occurs in full-term infants. Table 8-8 lists some of the more common potential causes.

Apnea of infancy may come to medical attention after an **apparent life-threatening event** (ALTE). ALTEs are very frightening to the caretaker; the infant either stops breathing or is found apneic and may be cyanotic or pale, hypotonic, difficult to rouse, or choking and gagging. The observer often believes that the child would have died without intervention (vigorous stimulation, cardiopulmonary resuscitation).

The goal of the diagnostic workup is to identify or rule out any treatable, life-threatening causes. Table 8-8 lists potential tests to be considered depending on the results of the history and physical examination. In approximately half the cases of apnea of infancy, no predisposing condition is ever found.

Management involves treating the underlying disorder. When no treatable cause can be found, the infant may be placed on a home monitor that senses chest movement (breathing) and heart rate and sounds an alarm when the child becomes apneic or bradycardic. Apnea of infancy does not raise an infant's risk of dying of sudden infant death syndrome (SIDS), which may be why **home monitors have never been proven to decrease the likelihood of SIDS.**

KEY POINTS

- Infants with bilateral choanal atresia often present with life-threatening respiratory distress in the delivery room, although oxygenation improves when the infant is crying.
- Severe obstructive sleep apnea can result in cor pulmonale which may be fatal.
- The three main components of asthma are reversible airway obstruction, increased airway responsiveness, and inflammation. Disease severity is classified before the onset of treatment as intermittent, mild persistent, moderate persistent, and severe persistent, although control of disease at any severity level is a more important concept.
- Inhaled bronchodilators are the treatment of choice in an acute asthma exacerbation. Inhaled corticosteroids are the treatment of choice for symptom control and avoidance of exacerbations for patients with persistent asthma.
- The disappearance of wheezing with increased respiratory distress signals increased obstruction rather than improvement.
- Cystic fibrosis (CF) is a disorder of exocrine gland function, affecting the lungs, sinuses, pancreas, sweat and salivary glands, intestines, and reproductive system. Failure to thrive, chronic cough, and malabsorptive stools are the most common presentations of CF in children. Meconium ileus in the neonate is virtually pathognomonic for CF.
- A diagnosis of CF is made by an elevated sweat chloride level in the presence of pulmonary disease/pancreatic insufficiency or by a genotype with two abnormal CFTR alleles known to cause disease.
- Apnea of infancy does not increase the risk of sudden infant death, and the use of home apnea monitors does not reduce the risk of SIDS.
- Persistent wheezing that does not respond to conventional medical treatment should raise strong suspicion of anatomic abnormalities or an aspirated foreign body.

C Clinical Vignettes

Vignette 1

A 4-year-old male with known asthma presents to the emergency department with a chief complaint of cough and shortness of breath. Physical examination reveals an afebrile child in mild distress with a respiratory rate of 40 breaths per minute, an occasional dry cough, and diffuse, symmetric wheezing on auscultation. He looks worried. There is no history of a choking episode prior to the onset of wheezing, and the child has no history of anaphylaxis.

1. Which of the following studies is most appropriate for initial assessment of the severity of this patient's acute episode?
   a. Chest radiograph
   b. Complete blood cell count
   c. Pulse oximetry
   d. Sputum culture
   e. Respiratory viral culture

2. Following one treatment with a short acting beta$_2$-agonist (albuterol), the patient has improved only slightly. The pulse oximetry reading is 92% while breathing room air, and the patient still has diffuse wheezing. Which of the following treatments is most likely to improve respiratory signs and symptoms within the next 30 minutes?
   a. Albuterol
   b. Albuterol plus ipratropium
   c. Oral theophylline
   d. Intravenous aminophylline
   e. Intramuscular epinephrine

3. After receiving the treatment above, the child improves somewhat clinically, but still has wheezing, subcostal retractions, and mild tachypnea. His respiratory rate has decreased to 26 breaths per minute, and he can talk in phrases and short sentences. His pulse oximetry reading on room air is now 96%. He is more alert and active. Which of the following interventions is indicated at this time, if not already administered?
   a. Oral corticosteroid (prednisone)
   b. Intravenous aminophylline
   c. Intramuscular ceftriaxone
   d. Supplemental oxygen
   e. Inhaled corticosteroid

Vignette 2

A 2-year-old male comes to your primary care office with the complaint of chronic cough, which has been present since the first few months of life. When he is very active physically, he sometimes wheezes. He has an uncle with asthma, and his parents have treated his wheezing with the uncle's bronchodilator inhaler without discernible improvement. He has two older siblings who are healthy. On physical examination, his height is at the 30th percentile for age, his weight is below the 5th percentile for age, and his chest is slightly hyperinflated. Auscultation of the chest is normal. His abdomen is protuberant, but no organs or masses are palpable. While in the examination room, he fills his diaper with stool, and the odor is extremely foul smelling. Your initial evaluation includes a chest radiograph, which reveals mild hyperinflation and bronchial thickening but is otherwise unremarkable.

1. Which of the following would be highest on your differential diagnosis list?
   a. Asthma
   b. Tracheoesophageal fistula
   c. Cystic fibrosis
   d. Primary ciliary dyskinesia
   e. Bronchiolitis

2. A person with PCD experiences chronic, recurrent infections in the lungs, ears, and sinuses due to the loss of ciliary activity in those areas. Faulty development of organ placement (aka "situs") may result in reversed organs or in other organ placement/development abnormalities. Reduced sperm motility means that most males with PCD are infertile (not sterile—the sperm are still viable, they just can't get where they need to be), and women with PCD may experience subfertility or increased risk for miscarriage or ectopic pregnancy. In very rare instances, PCD may be associated with hydrocephalus, a condition in which excess fluid in the ventricles of the brain causes them to be enlarged. Which of the following studies is most likely to support your suspected diagnosis?
   a. Chest computed tomography scan
   b. Sweat test
   c. Barium enema
   d. Complete blood count and quantitative serum immunoglobulin levels
   e. Genetics consultation

3. The sweat test result is 50 mEq/L, and the laboratory reports that the diagnostic value is >60 mEq/L. Which of the following is the most appropriate next response?
   a. Measure pancreatic enzyme concentration in a duodenal aspirate
   b. Send blood for CFTR genotyping
   c. Reassure the family that the sweat test is negative and the child does not have CF
   d. Repeat the sweat test
   e. Send the child to a research center for measurement of nasal mucosal electrical potential difference

Vignette 3

A 2-year-old male begins coughing and wheezing while at a birthday party. Physical examination reveals coarse wheezing but no other abnormalities. Breath sounds are equal. He has no personal history of asthma, but his father is described as a severe asthmatic. The child exhibited no symptoms of a respiratory infection prior to the party.

1. What is the most appropriate diagnostic technique in this situation?
   a. PA and lateral chest radiographs
   b. Administration of a bronchodilator aerosol, with subsequent reassessment of breath sounds
   c. Bilateral decubitus chest radiographs
   d. Magnetic resonance imaging scan of the chest
   e. Computed tomography scan of the chest

2. New history is now obtained that the child was seen with several peanuts in his hand just prior to the onset of wheezing. He has eaten peanut butter on multiple occasions in the past without incident. The decubitus film reveals failure of the left lung to empty when the child is lying on the left side. Given the positive results of the study, we now have a reasonably firm diagnosis of foreign body aspiration, most likely a peanut (or peanut fragment). Which of the following represents the most appropriate next step in diagnosis/management?
   a. Administration of bronchodilators and chest physiotherapy to help the child expectorate the putative peanut
   b. Admission to the hospital for observation while waiting for the foreign body to be coughed out spontaneously or to dissolve *in situ*
   c. Performance of flexible bronchoscopy as soon as possible
   d. Performance of rigid bronchoscopy as soon as possible
   e. Admission for observation, with NPO and IV fluids orders overnight, and schedule a rigid bronchoscopy for the next morning

3. The next morning, the child is taken to the operating room and a piece of peanut is removed via a rigid bronchoscopy. What is the most appropriate follow-up for this child?
   a. No follow-up is needed; the bronchoscopist removed the peanut
   b. Repeat chest radiograph in approximately 1 week
   c. Pulmonary function tests
   d. Chest CT scan

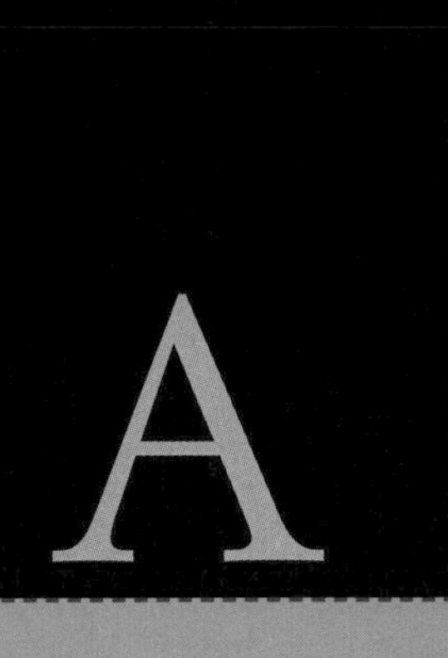

Answers

Vignette 1 Question 1

Answer C: Hypoxia, when present, indicates a severe episode of obstructive lung disease or the presence of a comorbid condition such as atelectasis or pneumonia. Hospital admission is indicated for hypoxemia that persists after initial treatment. In the absence of fever or localized physical findings on chest auscultation, a chest radiograph is of little diagnostic value in acute asthma. Complete blood cell count is also unlikely to yield any information relevant to management. Although sputum examination might provide information such as the presence of eosinophils, acute management is not likely to be affected. Moreover, most 4-year-olds cannot expectorate sputum. Although rhinovirus is a major cause of wheezing, treatment of the acute episode is not affected by knowledge of viral etiology unless this is the first documented episode of wheezing.

Vignette 1 Question 2

Answer B: Albuterol plus ipratropium is more effective than albuterol alone for patients who have more severe bronchospasm, such as those who fail to improve significantly after a single albuterol treatment. Oral theophylline or intravenous aminophylline, although often effective in cases of more severe, chronic asthma, is no longer recommended for acute treatment; albuterol is both more effective and safer. Although intramuscular epinephrine results in significant bronchodilation, its use is reserved for extremely severe bronchospasm, such as when a patient is unable to cooperate with administration of inhaled beta-agonist or is moving into respiratory failure/arrest.

Vignette 1 Question 3

Answer A: The efficacy of inhaled corticosteroids in acute asthma has been studied, but systemic administration is the preferred and more effective route. As indicated previously, aminophylline has been replaced by the more effective inhaled beta$_2$-agonists. In the absence of clinical infection, antibiotics have no role in the treatment of acute asthma. Supplemental oxygen can act as a weak bronchodilator, but this patient's pulse oxygenation measurement, respiratory rate, work of breathing, and mental status have improved, so oxygen is no longer indicated.

Vignette 2 Question 1

Answer C: The correct choice is cystic fibrosis (CF). A major clue is the failure to thrive and the foul-smelling stools, which accompany maldigestion and malabsorption. Asthma can cause cough and wheezing but should not result in failure to thrive or foul smelling stools, and the wheezing would be expected to respond to bronchodilators. A tracheoesophageal fistula will lead to chronic cough, typically associated with feedings, and possibly recurrent pneumonias, but not impaired digestion. Primary ciliary dyskinesia (PCD), discussed in detail below, is also not associated with malabsorption. Bronchiolitis is an acute process which should resolve within a week or two.

Vignette 2 Question 2

Answer B: The correct choice is sweat test. This is the conventional diagnostic test for cystic fibrosis. A chest scan may be indicated later in the disease process if the diagnosis is confirmed, given the association of long-standing CF with pulmonary hemorrhaging and bronchiectasis. Since the underlying disorder is not associated with an intestinal anatomic anomaly, a barium enema would not yield any additional information. The complete blood count and immunoglobulin levels would be normal unless the patient was acutely infected. A genetics consultation may be indicated if the diagnosis is confirmed, as the results will assist the parents in decisions regarding future pregnancies.

Vignette 2 Question 3

Answer D: The correct choice is repetition of the sweat test. Even if the sweat test result is positive, the test should be repeated on a separate date. The diagnosis of CF is a life-changing event, and the practitioner needs to be quite confident of the diagnosis. A significant proportion of children with cystic fibrosis have false negative sweat test results, so it is also important that the sweat testing be performed in a center with significant experience and expertise with the technique. A sweat test result of 50 should *always* be repeated, and the child should be studied *very* carefully.

Measurement of pancreatic enzyme concentrations in duodenal fluid is a useful (although difficult) test of pancreatic function, but is rarely necessary for clinical purposes. CFTR genotyping can be done, even as a primary diagnostic tool, but is more expensive and takes longer than sweat testing.

Genotyping can provide some useful additional information. There are some genotypes with mild clinical presentation, and newer drugs are capable of specifically reversing the defect in patients with certain genotypes.

In patients with CF, there is an elevated electrical potential difference across the respiratory mucosa (nose and airways) that is a reflection of the inherent abnormality in electrolyte transfer. This is sometimes a useful adjunctive diagnostic tool in patients with atypical presentations, but not until all other reasonable approaches have been utilized.

Vignette 3 Question 1

Answer C: The correct choice is bilateral decubitus chest radiographs. The most likely diagnosis, and the one which is most urgent in terms of immediate therapeutic intervention, is foreign body aspiration. Most aspiration events in toddlers are unwitnessed. In the context of a party, with many children and often chaotic activities, the potential for aspiration of a small (food) object is higher than usual, especially since many well-meaning adults will put out candies, peanuts, and other small objects. The decubitus films will reveal air trapping as the result of the foreign body blocking egress of air from one lung, even when the obstruction is not complete and inspiration sounds normal (the central wheezing may be difficult to lateralize with a stethoscope). The dependent lung, if the main bronchus is blocked, will not deflate, thus revealing the presence of the obstruction. On the other hand, PA and lateral radiographs are snapped at full inspiration and will often appear normal.

It would not be unreasonable to administer a bronchodilator, but this can often give a false sense of security. Foreign objects in the airways may also move from one to another location, especially in the first hours after the aspiration event, and auscultation is not a reliable indicator of foreign body aspiration.

MRI and CT scans are unlikely to reveal a small foreign body, and both are much more expensive than plain films.

Vignette 3 Question 2

Answer E: This child has just been at a party, and his stomach surely contains a fair amount of food, which places him at significant risk when undergoing anesthesia induction. Only if there is significant respiratory distress and a high risk of complete airway obstruction should such a child be taken directly to the operating room for general anesthesia, unless it can be ascertained that he has been NPO for at least several hours.

The use of chest physiotherapy to help expectorate a foreign body is contraindicated unless there is definitive evidence that the foreign body is quite small and cannot be extracted with a bronchoscope. Many children have died from complete airway obstruction when a foreign body had lodged in the larynx after being coughed up from a more peripheral location.

It is appropriate to admit the child to the hospital for observation while awaiting safe transport to another facility where rigid bronchoscopy can be performed (if not at the initial facility), but allowing the child to cough up the foreign body (presumed in this case to be a peanut) places the child at grave risk. Most foreign bodies will not disintegrate, and many will swell as they absorb moisture, thus producing more airway obstruction. Granulation tissue often forms around a foreign body that has been in place for more than a day or so.

Flexible bronchoscopy is a very important and useful procedure for the diagnosis of a foreign body aspiration and could be used as a first step in this patient, but not without the ability (and preparation) to proceed immediately to rigid bronchoscopy. Flexible bronchoscopes do not permit safe and effective removal of most foreign bodies and should not be used for this purpose except in very specific situations.

Vignette 3 Question 3

Answer B: Nuts are sometimes aspirated whole, but more often they are aspirated in multiple fragments. It is not at all uncommon to find more than one significant fragment of an aspirated nut in the airways, and most bronchoscopists know to look for them on the first procedure. However, small fragments may lodge out of sight of the bronchoscopist and produce problems later in smaller airways. Such fragments will most often lead to the formation of granulation tissue, bronchial obstruction, and atelectasis, which usually become evident on subsequent chest films.

Pulmonary function testing is not suitable for 2-year-olds, as children this age are developmentally unlikely to understand the verbal instructions. A chest CT scan is even less likely to find a small fragment of nut than a large one.

Chapter

9 Gastroenterology

Mitchell Cohen • Morissa Ladinsky • Bradley S. Marino

ABDOMINAL PAIN

Abdominal pain is a common pediatric problem encountered by primary care physicians and medical and surgical subspecialists. Chronic abdominal pain is defined as at least three bouts of pain severe enough to affect activities over a period of at least 3 months. Although the exact prevalence of chronic abdominal pain in children is not known, it appears to account for 2% to 4% of all pediatric office visits; approximately 15% of middle school and high school students experience weekly abdominal pain. In children with typical symptoms and without objective evidence of an underlying organic disorder, chronic abdominal pain is most frequently functional.

DIFFERENTIAL DIAGNOSIS

Functional abdominal pain is now classified as a pain-related functional gastrointestinal disorder (FGID). It is a specific diagnosis that needs to be distinguished from anatomic, infectious, inflammatory, or metabolic causes of abdominal pain. There is growing evidence to suggest that FGIDs may be associated with visceral hyperalgesia, that is, a decreased threshold for pain in response to changes in intraluminal pressure. Functional abdominal pain may be categorized as functional dyspepsia (discomfort in the upper abdomen), irritable bowel syndrome or IBS (pain associated with changes in bowel habits, either diarrhea, constipation, or both), abdominal migraine (paroxysmal abdominal pain associated with anorexia, nausea, and/or vomiting), or functional abdominal pain syndrome (functional pain without the features of dyspepsia, irritable bowel syndrome, or abdominal migraine), or a combination of these. Although these entities may have discrete definitions, the symptoms of one may often overlap with another and none has a clearly distinct etiology. In addition to FGIDs, functional constipation is among the most common causes of abdominal pain. Lactase deficiency may cause recurrent pain with exposure to milk sugar in dairy food. Inflammatory bowel disease (ulcerative colitis and Crohn's disease) are chronic conditions often associated with diarrhea, anemia, and poor growth in which pain is a major symptom. Celiac disease may present with abdominal pain, although anemia and poor growth without pain are also common manifestations. A less frequent cause of intestinal inflammation is an eosinophilic gastrointestinal disorder of the small intestine or colon.

Infectious conditions (including bacterial and viral gastroenteritis) are a common cause of *acute* abdominal pain. Mesenteric lymphadenitis may cause persistent pain following an infection. Extraintestinal infections may also cause abdominal pain. These include group A streptococcal infections, urinary tract infections, and lower lobe pneumonias. Pelvic inflammatory disease (PID) is an important consideration in adolescent females. Infectious mononucleosis is one of several systemic infections that can cause abdominal pain.

Gall bladder diseases, including cholecystitis, choledocolithiasis and biliary colic, pancreatitis, gastritis, and peptic ulcer disease, are less common in children but warrant consideration, especially when the pain is localized to the right upper quadrant or epigastrium and is worsened by meals. *Helicobacter pylori* is a cause of gastritis and ulcer disease. Abdominal pain is a primary feature in Henoch-Schonlein purpura (HSP), but may also be seen in other vasculitides, including Kawasaki disease, polyarteritis nodosa, and lupus erythematosus, and can also be a manifestation of sickle cell crisis.

Crohn's appendicitis is the most common surgical cause of abdominal pain. Intussusception is an important pediatric disease that presents with intermittent but severe pain and may also manifest with striking lethargy. Incarcerated hernia, volvulus, bowel obstruction, and testicular torsion represent surgical emergencies. Trauma can lead to significant intra-abdominal injury and pain.

Urologic obstruction at any level is an important consideration. Ureteropelvic junction obstruction, hydronephrosis, and renal stones can cause significant pain. Gynecologic causes are an important part of the differential diagnosis in adolescent girls. Pregnancy should always be considered, especially if symptoms are consistent with an ectopic pregnancy. Dysmenorrhea, ovarian cysts, mittelschmerz, pelvic inflammatory disease, cervicitis, endometriosis, and ovarian or adnexal torsion are all potential problems in this population and one may consider a pelvic examination warranted.

Psychiatric causes of abdominal pain are uncommon in children. True malingering is unusual, as are conversion disorders. However, many children do experience abdominal pain in the setting of stress, especially in the context of school, and abdominal pain also can be seen in children with depression.

Although children with chronic abdominal pain and their parents are more often anxious or depressed, the presence of anxiety, depression, behavior problems, or recent negative life events are not useful in distinguishing between functional and organic abdominal pain. Nonetheless, inquiry into recent social changes in the family unit or at school may provide great insight into the etiology of the pain.

CLINICAL MANIFESTATIONS

History

The history should localize the pain and determine its quality, temporal characteristics, and exacerbating and alleviating factors. With "inflammatory" pain, the child tends to lie still, whereas with "colicky" pain, the child cannot remain still. Colicky pain usually results from obstruction of a hollow viscus. It is important to ascertain whether the child has had previous abdominal surgery; with a history of previous laparotomy, small bowel obstruction becomes more likely. Pain may be accompanied by anorexia, nausea, emesis, diarrhea, or constipation. If the pain wakes the child at night, an organic cause is more likely, but night time pain does not exclude functional disorders. Both bilious emesis and nonbilious emesis may be seen in small bowel obstruction. The presence of alarm symptoms or signs including, but not limited to, involuntary weight loss, deceleration of linear growth, gastrointestinal blood loss, significant vomiting, chronic severe diarrhea, persistent right upper or right lower quadrant pain, unexplained fever, and/or family history of IBD is generally an indication to pursue further diagnostic testing.

Physical Examination

One goal of the abdominal examination is to ascertain whether the child has an abdominal process that requires surgical intervention. Watching the child walk, climb onto the examination table, and interact with both parents and staff before formally examining the child's abdomen helps one to gain an appreciation for the degree of incapacitation or emotional overlay that may be present. The abdomen should be inspected, auscultated, and palpated. Peritoneal signs include rebound tenderness, guarding, psoas or obturator signs, and rigidity of the abdominal wall. Right lower quadrant tenderness requires the consideration of appendicitis. Rectal skin tags or fistulae may suggest the diagnosis of Crohn's disease. Unless the diagnosis is thought to be uncomplicated viral gastroenteritis, a rectal examination is most often indicated to detect tenderness or hard stool and to obtain stool for occult blood testing. If the patient is an adolescent female, a pelvic examination is often indicated as part of the appropriate evaluation. Cervical motion tenderness is consistent with PID.

The examination of children with functional abdominal pain is often devoid of positive physical findings. Alarm signs on abdominal examination include localized tenderness in the right upper or right lower quadrants, a localized fullness or mass effect, hepatomegaly, splenomegaly, costovertebral angle tenderness, tenderness over the spine, and perianal abnormalities.

DIAGNOSTIC EVALUATION

The diagnostic test strategy is dictated by the history and findings on the physical examination. Surgical consultation should be sought if there is concern for appendicitis, volvulus, testicular torsion, or other conditions requiring urgent surgery. A complete blood count with differential, serum electrolytes and chemistries, amylase, lipase, stool hemoccult examination, urinalysis, and radiographic studies should be performed if there has been abdominal trauma or an acute surgical condition is suspected. Blood should also be typed for possible transfusion. A computed tomography (CT) scan may be useful when appendicitis is being considered. When uncomplicated viral gastroenteritis is the most likely cause and the child is well hydrated, no studies need be performed, but if bacterial enterocolitis is being considered because of the presence of blood, travel history or ill contacts, stool should be obtained for culture. Group A streptococcal pharyngitis and PID require appropriate cultures. To diagnose a urinary tract infection, a urinalysis and urine culture should be performed. Celiac disease is best diagnosed with serologic screening studies, for example, tissue transglutaminase (IgA) or antiendomysial antibodies (IgA). Screening for IBD is best performed by history and physical examination, but a CBC and ESR or CRP may be helpful screening tools. Increasingly fecal calprotectin is being used as a screening test for intestinal inflammation, especially when diarrhea is present, but this test too is neither perfectly sensitive nor specific for IBD. Higher specificity for IBD is achieved when the level is >250 µg/gm. In many cases, especially when functional pain is thought to be the cause of the pain, less diagnostic testing may be more helpful than more testing. This will enable the focus to remain on appropriate treatment strategies.

TREATMENT

Treatment is directed at the underlying cause of the pain. Infections may require antimicrobial therapy. Lactase deficiency and celiac disease improve with specific dietary intervention. Constipation is well treated with polyethylene glycol and a bowel rehabilitation plan. Diagnostic trials of histamine-2 receptor antagonists or proton pump inhibitor therapy may be very helpful when esophagitis, gastritis, duodenitis, or nonulcer dyspepsia is suggested. Functional abdominal pain is best treated with a biopsychosocial model. Medical treatment might include acid reduction therapy for pain associated with dyspepsia, antispasmodic agents, or low dosages of tricyclic psychotropic agents for pain, or nonstimulating laxatives or antidiarrheals for pain associated with altered bowel pattern.

APPENDICITIS

Appendicitis is the most common indication for abdominal surgery in childhood. Appendicitis results from bacterial invasion of the appendix, which is more likely when the lumen is obstructed by a fecalith, parasite, or lymph node. Appendicitis occurs most frequently in children between 10 and 15 years of age. Less than 10% of patients are younger than 5 years.

CLINICAL MANIFESTATIONS

Classically, fever, emesis, anorexia, and diffuse periumbilical pain develop. Subsequently, pain and abdominal tenderness localize to the right lower quadrant as the parietal peritoneum becomes inflamed. Guarding, rebound tenderness, and obturator and psoas signs are commonly found. The appendix tends to perforate approximately 36 hours after pain begins. The incidence of perforation and diffuse peritonitis is higher in children younger than 2 years, when diagnosis may be delayed. Atypical presentations are common in childhood, especially with retrocecal appendicitis, which may present with periumbilical pain and diarrhea. Retrocecal appendicitis usually does not induce right lower quadrant pain until after perforation. Bacterial enterocolitis caused by *Campylobacter* and *Yersinia* species may mimic appendicitis because both can result in right lower quadrant abdominal pain and tenderness. Diagnosis of appendicitis is established clinically by history and by physical examination, which should include a rectal examination to detect tenderness or a mass? A moderately elevated white blood cell count with a left shift is often seen in appendicitis. A plain film of the abdomen may demonstrate a fecalith. An inflamed appendix may be noted on ultrasound or CT, which is often used to evaluate patients with suspicion of acute appendicitis.

TREATMENT

Laparotomy and appendectomy should be performed before perforation. When appendicitis results in perforation, the patient may be given broad spectrum antibiotics, for example, ampicillin, gentamicin, and metronidazole or piperacillin/tazobactam monotherapy to treat peritonitis from intestinal flora. The mortality rate rises significantly with perforation.

INTUSSUSCEPTION

Intussusception results from telescoping of one part of the intestine into another. Intussusception causes impaired venous return, bowel edema and ischemia, necrosis, and perforation. It is one of the most common causes of intestinal obstruction in infancy. Most intussusceptions are ileocolic; the ileum invaginates into the colon at the ileocecal valve. Previous viral or bacterial enteritis may cause hypertrophy of the Peyer patches or mesenteric nodes, which are hypothesized to act as the lead point in intussusception. A specific lead point is identified in only 5% of cases but should be sought in neonates or in children older than 5 years. Recognizable lead points in intussusception include Meckel diverticulum, an intestinal polyp, lymphoma, or a foreign body. Intussusception has also been associated with HSP, but in this setting is usually ileo-ileal. It can be very difficult to distinguish HSP complicated by intussusception from the inflammatory abdominal pain seen in simple HSP.

CLINICAL MANIFESTATIONS

Violent episodes of irritability, colicky pain, and emesis are interspersed with relatively normal periods. Rectal bleeding occurs in 80% of patients but less commonly in the form of the classic "currant jelly" stools (stools containing bright red blood and mucus). The degree of lethargy shown by the child may be striking. A tubular mass is palpable in approximately 80% of patients. A plain abdominal film may show a paucity of gas in the right lower quadrant or evidence of obstruction with air fluid levels. An ultrasound examination may be very helpful as a screening tool. A contrast enema or air enema, which often proves therapeutic as well as diagnostic, demonstrates a characteristic coiled spring appearance to the bowel.

TREATMENT

Fluid resuscitation with normal saline or lactated Ringer solution is usually necessary. Hydrostatic reduction with a contrast enema or pneumatic reduction with an air enema is successful in 75% of cases if performed in the first 48 hours. Peritoneal signs are an absolute contraindication to this procedure. Laparotomy and direct reduction is indicated when reduction by enema is either unsuccessful or contraindicated. The immediate recurrence rate is approximately 15%. When a specific lead point is identified, the recurrence rate is higher.

EMESIS

Vomiting is one of the most common presenting symptoms in pediatrics and can be caused by both gastrointestinal (GI) and non-GI pathologies. Complications of severe, persistent emesis include dehydration and hypochloremic, and hypokalemic metabolic alkalosis. Forceful emesis can result in a Mallory-Weiss tear of the esophagus at the gastroesophageal junction or erosion of the gastric cardia; chronic emesis can result in distal esophagitis.

DIFFERENTIAL DIAGNOSIS

Table 9-1 lists the most common causes of vomiting in infants and children.

CLINICAL MANIFESTATIONS

History

In infants, the history should differentiate between true vomiting (forceful expulsion of gastric contents) and effortless regurgitation ("spitting up"). The latter is often due to gastroesophageal reflux. Frequency, appearance (bloody or bilious), amount, and timing of the emesis are important. Emesis shortly after feeding in the infant is probably gastroesophageal reflux. If the emesis is projectile and the child is 1 to 3 months of age, pyloric stenosis must be considered. Poor weight gain and emesis may indicate pyloric stenosis or a metabolic disorder. Macrolide antibiotics are known to cause emesis and diarrhea; chemotherapeutic agents and some toxic ingestions cause emesis. If the child has a ventriculo-peritoneal shunt, vomiting may be a sign of shunt obstruction and increased intracranial pressure. Emesis with seizure, or headache, or both may indicate an intracranial process. Diarrhea, emesis, and fever are seen with gastroenteritis. Fever, abdominal pain, and emesis are typical for appendicitis, whereas bilious emesis and abdominal pain are seen with intestinal obstruction. Emesis and syncope may result from pregnancy.

Physical Examination

On physical examination, the initial assessment should focus on the child's vital signs and hydration status. Chapter 7 discusses signs and symptoms of dehydration. A bulging fontanelle or papilledema implicates increased intracranial pressure as the cause of the emesis. Emesis is common in infectious pharyngitis. The lung fields should be auscultated for crackles or an asymmetric examination to rule out pneumonia. Emesis and vaginal discharge in the female adolescent warrant a pelvic examination to evaluate for PID. The abdominal examination should focus on bowel sounds and the presence of distention, tenderness, or masses. Hypoactive bowel sounds may indicate ileus or obstruction, whereas hyperactive bowel sounds suggest gastroenteritis. Abdominal mass with emesis may indicate intussusception or malignancy. Tenderness on examination is suggestive of appendicitis, pancreatitis, cholecystitis, peritonitis, or PID.

DIAGNOSTIC EVALUATION

Specific laboratory studies depend on the suspected cause. Appropriate cultures, a complete blood count, and serum electrolytes may help determine the cause of vomiting and the metabolic complications secondary to vomiting. A chest radiograph will help rule out pneumonia. If a surgical process within the abdomen is considered, upright and supine abdominal films should be obtained, along with a complete blood count and electrolyte and chemistry panels. Amylase and lipase should be elevated in pancreatitis. If vomiting is prolonged or the patient is significantly dehydrated, electrolytes will help guide replacement therapy. An ammonia level, serum amino acids, and urine organic acids should be sent if metabolic disease is suspected. Urinalysis and urine culture should be obtained to assess the degree of dehydration and rule out urinary tract infection.

TREATMENT

If the cause appears to be a self-limited nonsurgical infectious process (viral gastroenteritis or bacterial enterocolitis) and the patient is not significantly dehydrated, outpatient therapy is indicated. Oral rehydration therapy (ORT), discussed in Chapter 7, is recommended for dehydrated infants. For older children, fluids should be encouraged, with advancement to a regular diet as tolerated. Children who are severely dehydrated or unable to effectively hydrate themselves orally should be admitted to the hospital. A surgical consultation should be obtained if indicated. If ventriculo-peritoneal shunt malfunction is a possibility, the standard of care dictates that a CT of the head and a shunt series be obtained in tandem with a neurosurgical consultation.

PYLORIC STENOSIS

Pyloric stenosis is an important cause of gastric outlet obstruction and vomiting in the first 2 to 3 months of life. The most common age of presentation is 2 to 4 weeks of life, with an incidence of 1 in 500 infants. Male infants are affected 4:1 over female infants, and pyloric stenosis occurs more frequently in infants with a family history of the condition. Current evidence suggests that erythromycin therapy may precipitate pyloric stenosis.

CLINICAL MANIFESTATIONS

Projectile nonbilious vomiting is the cardinal feature of the disorder. Physical findings vary with the severity of the obstruction. Dehydration and poor weight gain are common when the diagnosis is delayed. Hypokalemic, hypochloremic metabolic alkalosis with dehydration is seen secondary to persistent emesis in the most severe cases. The classic finding of an olive-sized, muscular, mobile, nontender mass in the epigastric area occurs in most cases but may be difficult to palpate. Visible gastric peristaltic waves may be seen. Ultrasonography reveals the hypertrophic pylorus. Upper GI study may show the classic "string sign."

TREATMENT

Initial treatment involves nasogastric tube placement to decompress the stomach, and correction of dehydration, alkalosis, and electrolyte abnormalities. Pyloromyotomy should take place after the metabolic anomalies are corrected.

MALROTATION AND VOLVULUS

Malrotation occurs when the small intestines rotate abnormally *in utero*, resulting in malposition in the abdomen and abnormal posterior fixation of the mesentery. When the intestine attaches improperly to the mesentery, it is at risk for twisting on its vascular supply; the twisting phenomenon is called volvulus. This condition has its most common presentation in the newborn period and is a surgical emergency.

CLINICAL MANIFESTATIONS

The history almost always includes bilious emesis and in older children, a history of past attacks of bilious emesis is occasionally elicited. Physical examination may reveal abdominal distention or shock. Blood-stained emesis or stool may be noted. Abdominal radiographs typically show gas in the stomach with a paucity of air in the intestine. An upper GI series with small bowel follow-through confirms the diagnosis by illustrating the abnormal position of the ligament of Treitz and the cecum. A positive stool test for blood may indicate significant bowel ischemia. Unexplained lactic acidosis may be an important sign of intestinal ischemia.

TREATMENT

Operative correction of the malrotation and the volvulus should be undertaken as soon as possible because bowel ischemia, metabolic acidosis, and sepsis can progress quickly to death.

GASTROESOPHAGEAL REFLUX

Gastroesophageal reflux (GER), defined as the passage of gastric contents into the esophagus, and GER disease (GERD), defined as symptoms or complications of GER, are common pediatric problems. Clinical manifestations of GERD in children include regurgitation, poor weight gain, dysphagia, abdominal or substernal pain, esophagitis and respiratory disorders.

DIFFERENTIAL DIAGNOSIS

If the infant is having forceful emesis, projectile vomiting, or retching, then simple reflux is not the most likely cause, and the differential diagnosis for emesis should be broadened (see Table 9-1). In the infant with recurrent regurgitation, a thorough history and physical examination, with attention to warning signals, is generally sufficient to allow the clinician to establish a diagnosis of uncomplicated GER (the "happy spitter").

CLINICAL MANIFESTATIONS

History

The diagnosis of GER is often clinical, based upon typical symptoms and the lack of signs and symptoms of other disorders. Infants typically have effortless regurgitation as opposed to retching and vomiting. Adolescents are more likely to have

TABLE 9-1 Differential Diagnosis of Vomiting in Children

Infectious	***Gastrointestinal: Infant***
Viral gastroenteritis, e.g., Rotavirus and Norovirus	Gastroesophageal reflux
Bacterial enteroscolitis/sepsis	Cow or soy milk protein intolerance
Hepatitis	Bowel obstruction[a]
Food poisoning	Duodenal atresia
Pelvic inflammatory disease	Pyloric stenosis
Peritonitis	Malrotation with or without volvulus
Pharyngitis/tonsillitis	Incarcerated hernia
Pneumonia	Intussusception
Otitis media	Meckel diverticulum with torsion
Urinary tract infection	Hirschsprung disease
Metabolic	***Gastrointestinal: Child***
Diabetic ketoacidosis	Appendicitis
Inborn errors of metabolism	Eosinophilic gastroenteritis
Addisonian crisis/adrenal insufficiency	Pancreatitis
Reye syndrome	Hepatitis
Other	Cholecystitis
Renal failure	Bowel obstruction
Hepatic failure	Malrotation
Congestive heart failure or pericarditis	Incarcerated hernia
Lead poisoning	Intussusception
Munchausen syndrome and Munchausen syndrome by proxy	Meckel diverticulum with torsion
Central Nervous System	Adhesions
Increased intracranial pressure	Superior Mesenteric Artery Syndrome
Ventricular-peritoneal shunt malfunction	Posttraumatic obstruction[b]
Meningitis	***Respiratory***
Encephalitis	Posttussive emesis
Labyrinthitis	Reactive airway syndrome
Migraine	***Medications***
Seizure	Chemotherapeutic agents
Tumor	Cancer chemotherapy
Gynecologic	Digoxin and other cardiac drugs
Pregnancy	Antibiotics, e.g., erythromycin
	Theophylline
	Caustic agents
	Ipecac
	Emotional/Behavioral
	Psychogenic
	Bulimia
	Rumination

[a]Malrotation with or without volvulus is much more likely in an infant than in a child.
[b]From duodenal hematomoa, ruptured viscus.

typical heartburn than young children and infants. Upper airway symptoms may occur although there is limited data to link reflux to hoarseness, chronic cough, sinusitis, otitis media, and erythema/"cobblestoning" of the larynx. Reflux is not a common cause of irritability, unexplained crying, or distress in otherwise healthy infants, and treatment with histamine type-2 receptor antagonists or proton pump inhibitors will not improve these symptoms despite raising the gastric pH. Most apparent life-threatening events (ALTE) are not related to GERD

Physical Examination

In most cases, the physical examination of the child with GER is normal. In severe cases, infants present with poor weight gain or failure to thrive.

DIAGNOSTIC EVALUATION

In most infants with vomiting, and in most older children with regurgitation and heartburn, a history and physical examination is sufficient to reliably diagnose GER, recognize complications, and initiate management. The upper gastrointestinal (GI) series is neither sensitive nor specific for the diagnosis of GER, but impedance manometry with esophageal pH monitoring is useful to establish the presence of abnormal acid reflux, determine if there is a temporal association between acid reflux and frequently occurring symptoms, and assess the adequacy of therapy in patients who do not respond to treatment with acid suppression. Endoscopy with biopsy can assess the presence and severity of esophagitis, strictures, and Barrett esophagus, as well as exclude other disorders such as Crohn's disease and eosinophilic or infectious esophagitis in older children. Eosinophilic esophagitis (EoE) does not respond to antacid therapy and may be a cause of poorly responsive reflux symptoms. A characteristic endoscopic appearance with furrowing, and white exudate and biopsy with >15 eosinophils/high-power field is diagnostic for EoE. A normal appearance of the esophagus during endoscopy does not exclude GER. A trial of time-limited medical therapy for GER is useful for determining if GER is causing a specific symptom.

TREATMENT

Diet and Lifestyle Changes

Esophageal pH monitoring has demonstrated that infants have significantly less GER when placed in the prone position than in the supine position. However, prone positioning is associated with a higher rate of sudden infant death syndrome (SIDS). In infants from birth to 6 months of age with GERD, the risk of SIDS generally outweighs the potential benefits of prone sleeping. In children older than 1 year it is likely that there is a benefit to left side positioning during sleep and elevation of the head of the bed. There is evidence to support a 1 to 2 week trial of a hypoallergenic formula in formula fed infants with regurgitation. Milk-thickening agents do not improve reflux index scores by pH monitoring but do decrease the number of episodes of vomiting. Children and adolescents with GERD should avoid identified food triggers. While these may be individualized based on history, caffeine, spicy foods, and high fat foods that delay gastric emptying may provoke symptoms. Obesity, exposure to tobacco smoke, and alcohol are also associated with GERD.

Medications

Histamine type-2 receptor antagonists (H 2 RAs) produce relief of symptoms and mucosal healing in older children and adults. Proton pump inhibitors (PPIs), the most effective acid suppressant medications, are superior to H 2 RAs in relieving symptoms and healing esophagitis in children and adults. While a brief therapeutic trial may be indicated, in infants with GER, it is not evident that treatment with either H 2 RA or PPI therapy results in symptomatic improvement and may increase the risk of pneumonia and some gastrointestinal infections. Chronic antacid therapy is generally not recommended since more convenient and safe alternatives (H 2 RAs and PPIs) are available.

Surgical Therapy

Case series indicate that surgical therapy generally results in favorable outcomes but this intervention should be restricted to patients who fail failure of medical therapy, have intractable pain, neurological impairment, recurrent bleeding, or aspiration. The potential risks, benefits, and costs of successful prolonged medical therapy versus fundoplication have not been well studied in infants or children in various symptom presentations.

DIARRHEA

Diarrhea is defined as an increase in the frequency and the water content of stools. Viral gastroenteritis is the most common cause of acute diarrheal illness throughout the world. The complications of acute diarrhea includes dehydration, electrolyte and acid–base disturbances, bacteremia and sepsis, and malnutrition in chronic cases. Enteritis refers to small bowel inflammation, whereas colitis refers to large bowel inflammation.

DIFFERENTIAL DIAGNOSIS

Table 9-2 lists the most common causes of diarrhea in the pediatric population in developed countries.

CLINICAL MANIFESTATIONS

History

The history should ascertain whether the diarrhea is acute or chronic/recurrent and establish the frequency and appearance of the stools (bloody with mucopus, or watery). Dietary indiscretions and manipulations may result in diarrhea. Small infants have diarrhea when they are fed concentrated formula and certain fruit juices, for example, apple and pear may cause toddler's diarrhea. Weight loss or lack of weight gain in association with diarrhea indicates more severe disease. Certain medications, especially antibiotics and chemotherapeutic agents, may cause diarrhea. Viral and bacterial gastroenteritis are both highly contagious, so sick contacts are likely. C. *difficile* infection was previously almost always associated with antibiotic therapy, especially in hospitalized patients. Community acquired C. *difficile* infection without antecedent antibiotic therapy is now recognized as common. Unfortunately, relapses of C. *difficile* infection are common, occurring in 15% to 30% of patients. Test of cure is not indicated but symptomatic illness within 14 days of completion of treatment is often indicative of a recurrence and should be reinvestigated. Recurrence requires

TABLE 9-2 Differential Diagnosis of Diarrhea in Children

Acute Diarrhea	Infectious
Intestinal infections	*Clostridium difficile*
Viral, e.g., Rotavirus, Norovirus, Adenovirus, Astrovirus	Parasites, e.g., *Giardia*, *Cryptosporidium*
Bacterial, e.g., *Shigella*, *Salmonella*, *Campylobacter*, diarrheagenic *Escherichia coli* (*E. coli* O157:H7, enteroaggregative, and others), *Yersinia*, *Clostridium difficile*, *Vibrio* spp, e.g., *V. cholerae*, possibly *Aeromonas* spp, *Plesiomonas* spp	***Gastrointestinal***
	Cow/soy milk intolerance
	Ulcerative colitis
Parasitic, e.g., *Giardia*, *Cryptosporidium*, *Entamoeba histolytica*	Crohn's disease
Noninfectious	Lactase or sucrase deficiency
Intussusception	Irritable bowel syndrome
Appendicitis	Encopresis with overflow incontinence
Osmotic diarrhea, i.e., hyperconcentrated infant formula, medications, dissacharidase deficiency (acute)	Excessive fructose or sorbitol intake
	Pancreatic insufficiency, e.g., cystic fibrosis
Toxic ingestion: Iron, mercury, lead, fluoride ingestion	Celiac disease
Antibiotics, chemotherapeutic agents	Neuroendocrine tumor
Chronic Diarrhea	***Allergy***
Immunodeficiency	Food allergies
Acquired immunodeficiency	Eosinophilic gastrointestinal disorders
Congenital immunodeficiency	***Vasculitis***
	Henoch-Schönlein purpura

either retreatment or a change in therapeutic approach with prolonged treatment (taper therapy), pulse therapy, probiotics, intravenous immunoglobulin therapy or fecal transplantation.

Physical Examination

Chapter 5 discusses signs and symptoms of dehydration, which are critical in the evaluation of a patient with diarrhea. An attempt should be made to determine the degree of dehydration to guide therapy. The abdominal examination focuses on bowel sounds and the presence of distention, tenderness, or masses. Hypoactive bowel sounds point to intestinal obstruction. Hyperactive sounds are consistent with gastroenteritis. Abdominal mass with diarrhea could indicate intussusception or malignancy.

DIAGNOSTIC EVALUATION

When evaluating a child with diarrhea, inspecting the stool is critical to evaluation and formulation of a treatment plan. If there is a history of blood and/or mucous in the stool, if the child needs hospitalization, or the child is younger than 3 months of age, bacterial cultures should be obtained. Rapid tests for rotavirus and norovirus are available; however, laboratory tests need not be routinely performed in children with signs and symptoms of acute gastroenteritis. Serum electrolytes are sometimes useful in assessing children with moderate to severe dehydration who require intravenous (IV) or nasogastric (NG) fluids. A normal bicarbonate concentration may be useful in ruling out or characterizing dehydration. For persistent diarrhea, the diagnostic evaluation should proceed in a stepwise fashion, including a complete blood count and stool tests for bacterial pathogens (including C. *difficile*, and common parasitic pathogens, i.e., giardia and cryptosporidium). Subsequent evaluation for chronic diarrhea may include tests for immunodeficiency, pancreatic insufficiency and celiac disease, and the like, as appropriate. Persistent diarrhea may complicate acute diarrhea in infants, especially when there is preexisting undernutrition.

TREATMENT

Acute gastroenteritis (AGE) is often self-limited and most often results in inconvenience and expense to the family in terms of work lost. However, the goals of treatment are primarily prevention and/or management of dehydration and secondarily improvement of symptoms, the latter being an appropriate concern of the family. Immunization with rotavirus vaccine is an important approach to limit severe diarrhea, prevent dehydration, and reduce the likelihood of hospitalization when rotaviral illness occurs. When a child has mild to moderate diarrhea, continued use of the child's preferred, usual, and age appropriate diet should be encouraged to prevent or limit dehydration. Regular diets are generally more effective than restricted and progressive diets, and in numerous trials have consistently produced a reduction in the duration of diarrhea. The historical BRAT diet (consisting of bananas, rice, applesauce, and toast) is unnecessarily restrictive, but may be offered as part of the child's usual diet. Clear liquids are not recommended as a substitute for oral rehydration solutions (ORS) or regular diets in the prevention or therapy of dehydration. The vast majority of patients with mild to moderate AGE do not develop clinically important lactose intolerance and do not need to be milk restricted. In selected patients with documented, persistent clinical lactose intolerance, lactose-free formulas are recommended. The vomiting child should be offered frequent small feedings (every 10 to 60 minutes) of any tolerated foods or ORS. Dehydration should be treated with ORS, for a period of 4 to 6 hours or until an adequate degree of rehydration is achieved. When the care provider is unable to replace the estimated fluid deficit and keep up with ongoing losses using oral feedings alone, or the child is severely dehydrated with an obtunded mental status, IV fluids or NG ORS should be given for a period of 4 to 6 hours or until adequate rehydration is achieved. It is appropriate to involve the family in the decision regarding the method of fluid replacement. Refeeding of the usual diet should be started at the earliest opportunity after an adequate degree of rehydration is achieved. Following rehydration therapy in the child with mild to moderate dehydration, regular diets may be supplemented with ORS containing at least 45 mEq Na^+/L, and targeted to deliver 10 mL/kg for each stool or emesis. It is important to reassess hydration status by phone or in the office when a child refuses ORS. This can be a sign of severe illness or refusal may indicate an absence of salt craving, and, as such, resolution of dehydration. Antidiarrheal agents and antiemetics are not recommended for the routine management of children with AGE. Certain probiotics, in particular Lactobacillus GG, have been shown to decrease the duration of rotaviral and nonrotaviral diarrhea. Ondansetron may decrease vomiting and hospitalization rates in those patients who require IV or NG fluids. It is recommended that antimicrobial therapies be used only for selected children with AGE who present with special risks or evidence of a serious bacterial infection. The infant with salmonellosis represents just such a special case. If the stool culture is positive for salmonella and the infant is afebrile and does not appear toxic, the infant can be reexamined and observed at home. If the stool culture is positive and the infant is febrile, the infant's age determines therapy:

- The infant younger than 3 months should be admitted to the hospital; a blood culture is obtained, and intravenous antibiotics started. A lumbar puncture and urinalysis should also be considered in this age group.
- The infant older than 3 months should be admitted to the hospital; a blood culture should be sent, but antibiotics may be withheld pending the results of the blood culture.
- Any infant with a positive stool culture who looks toxic or has a positive blood culture should be admitted for intravenous antibiotics and evaluation for pyelonephritis, meningitis, pneumonia, and osteomyelitis.

Treatment for C. *difficile* involves enteral therapy with metronidazole or vancomycin. Vancomycin may be somewhat more effective but is much more expensive. Fidaxomicin is another treatment option. Giardia lamblia and Cryptosporidium are also common causes of persistent diarrhea and, if found, treatment is available with metronidazole or nitazoxanide.

CONSTIPATION

Constipation is defined as the infrequent passage of hard stools. Constipated infants fail to empty the colon completely with bowel movements and over time stretch the smooth muscle of the colon, resulting in a functional ileus. In contrast to constipation, obstipation is the absence of bowel movements. Beyond the neonatal period, the most common cause (90%–95%) of constipation is voluntary withholding or "functional" constipation. Intentional withholding is often noted from the very beginning of toilet training. A family history of similar problems is often obtained. Stool retention may be caused by conflicts in toilet training but is usually caused by pain on defecation, which creates a fear of defecation and further retention. Voluntary withholding of stool increases distention of the rectum, which decreases rectal sensation, necessitating an even greater fecal mass to initiate the urge to defecate. Complications of stool retention include impaction, abdominal pain, overflow diarrhea resulting from leakage around the fecal mass, anal fissure, rectal bleeding, and urinary tract infection caused by extrinsic pressure on the urethra. Encopresis, which is daytime or nighttime soiling by formed stools in children beyond the age of expected toilet training (3 to 5 years), is another complication of constipation. In older children, it is important to ask specifically about soiling, because such information may not be expressed because of embarrassment. These children are unable to sense the need to defecate because of stretching of the internal sphincter by the retained fecal mass. Organic causes of failure to defecate include decreased peristalsis, decreased expulsion, and anatomic malformation. Nonorganic and organic etiologies are delineated in the following section.

DIFFERENTIAL DIAGNOSIS

Nonorganic

- Functional constipation (intentional withholding)
- Dysfunctional toilet training

Organic

- Dietary: Low-fiber diet, inadequate fluid intake
- GI: Functional ileus, Hirschsprung disease, anal stenosis, rectal abscess or fissure, stricture following necrotizing enterocolitis (NEC), collagen vascular disease
- Drugs or toxins: Lead, narcotics, phenothiazines, vincristine, anticholinergics
- Neuromuscular: Meningomyelocele, tethered spinal cord, infant botulism, absent abdominal
- muscles (prune belly syndrome)
- Metabolic: Cystic fibrosis, hypokalemia, hypercalcemia
- Endocrine: Hypothyroidism

CLINICAL MANIFESTATIONS

History and Physical Examination

Abdominal pain caused by constipation is often diffuse and constant. The pain may be accompanied by nausea, but vomiting is unusual. Stools are hard, difficult to pass, and infrequent. Discussion of withholding behavior (potty dance) can be helpful in identifying functional etiologies of constipation. An organic cause of constipation (cystic fibrosis, Hirschsprung disease) is more likely in a patient who did not pass meconium in the first 24 to 48 hours of life. Findings that suggest concern for an organic etiology of constipation include: failure to grow, pilonidal dimple covered with a tuft of hair, absent anal wink, tight empty rectum in the presence of a palpable fecal mass, anteriorly displaced anus, and decreased lower extremity tone or strength.

DIAGNOSTIC EVALUATION

Most often no diagnostic studies are needed. If the diagnosis is unclear, a plain abdominal film can be helpful because a colon full of feces makes the diagnosis of constipation. Thyroid studies, including free T4 and TSH levels are indicated if hypothyroidism is suspected. If hypokalemia or hypocalcemia is a potential cause, an electrolyte and chemistry panel may be obtained. A rectal mucosal biopsy is required to make the diagnosis of Hirschsprung disease. An elevated lead level implicates plumbism as the cause of constipation.

TREATMENT

The general approach to the child with functional constipation includes the following steps: determine whether fecal impaction is present, treat the impaction if present, initiate treatment with oral medication, provide patient and family education and follow-up, and adjust medications as necessary. Polyethylene glycol (PEG) 3350 is efficacious for colonic clean out in children. When daily medication is necessary in the treatment of constipation, PEG 3350 also appears to be superior to other osmotic agents in palatability and acceptance by children. The goal is to achieve a soft (mashed potato or pudding consistency stool) on a daily or more frequent basis. Data in children under a year of age indicate that PEG 3350 is safe and effective in this age group as well. There is extensive experience with other therapies including mineral oil, magnesium hydroxide, and lactulose or sorbitol. Long-term studies show that these therapies are effective and safe. Because mineral oil, magnesium hydroxide, lactulose, and sorbitol seem to be equally efficacious, the choice among these is based on safety, cost, the child's preference, ease of administration, and the practitioner's experience. A behavioral program of daily sit downs and positive reinforcement is often helpful in structuring the approach for the family.

While dietary changes are anticipated by families as part of the treatment plan, no randomized controlled studies have demonstrated an effect on stools of increasing intake of fluids, nonabsorbable carbohydrates, or dietary fiber in children. Forceful implementation of diet is undesirable. The education of the family and the demystification of constipation, including an explanation of the pathogenesis of constipation, are important steps in treatment. Providing hope to a frustrated family is key. If fecal soiling is present, an important goal for both the child and the parent is to remove negative attributions. It is especially important for parents to understand that soiling from overflow incontinence is not a willful and defiant maneuver.

HIRSCHSPRUNG DISEASE

Hirschsprung disease, or congenital aganglionic megacolon, occurs in 1 in 5,000 children and results from the failure of the ganglion cells of the myenteric plexus to migrate down the developing colon. As a result, the abnormally innervated distal colon remains tonically contracted and obstructs the flow of feces. Hirschsprung disease is three times more common among boys and accounts for 20% of cases of neonatal intestinal obstruction. In 75% of cases, the aganglionic segment is limited to the rectosigmoid colon, whereas 15% extend beyond the splenic flexure.

CLINICAL MANIFESTATIONS

The diagnosis should be suspected in any infant who fails to pass meconium within the first 24 to 48 hours of life or who requires repeated rectal simulation to induce bowel movements. In the first month of life, the neonate develops evidence of obstruction with poor feeding, bilious vomiting, and abdominal distention. In some cases, particularly those with short segment (less than 5 cm) involvement, the diagnosis goes undetected into childhood. In the older child, failure to grow may be seen, as well as intermittent bouts of intestinal obstruction, enterocolitis with bloody diarrhea, and, occasionally, bowel perforation, sepsis, and shock. Stool that is palpable throughout the abdomen and an empty rectum on digital examination are most suggestive of the disease. Abdominal radiographs show distention of the proximal bowel and no gas or feces in the rectum. Contrast enema may demonstrate a transition zone between the narrowed abnormal distal segment and the dilated normal proximal bowel. However, a normal contrast enema does not rule out the diagnosis. Anal manometry demonstrates failure of the internal sphincter to relax with balloon distention of the rectum. Rectal biopsy reveals absence of ganglion cells, an abnormal pattern of acetylcholinesterase staining, and hypertrophied nerve trunks and is the diagnostic study of choice.

TREATMENT

Hirschsprung disease is often treated surgically in two stages. The first stage involves the creation of a diverting colostomy with the bowel that contains ganglion cells, thus permitting decompression of the ganglion-containing bowel segment. In the second stage, the aganglionic segment is removed and the ganglionic segment is anastomosed to the rectum. This procedure is often postponed until the infant is 12 months of age or delayed for 3 to 6 months when the disease has been diagnosed in an older child. The mortality rate for this disorder is low in the absence of enterocolitis; major complications include anal stenosis and incontinence.

GASTROINTESTINAL BLEEDING

GI bleeding may be acute or chronic, gross or microscopic, and may manifest as hematemesis, hematochezia, or melena. A plethora of disorders in childhood can cause GI bleeding. Hematemesis refers to the emesis of fresh or old blood from the GI tract. Fresh blood becomes chemically altered to a ground-coffee appearance within 5 minutes of exposure to gastric acid. Hematochezia is the passage of fresh (bright red) or dark maroon blood from the rectum. The source is usually the colon, although upper GI tract bleeding that has a rapid transit time can also result in hematochezia. Melena describes shiny, jet black, tarry stools that are positive for occult blood. It usually results from upper GI bleeding and the color and consistency results from the blood being chemically altered during passage through the gut.

DIFFERENTIAL DIAGNOSIS

The differential diagnosis for GI bleeding is generally divided into upper and lower GI tract etiologies. Upper GI bleeding occurs at a site proximal to the ligament of Treitz, whereas lower GI bleeding occurs at a site distal to this ligament. Although hematemesis from upper GI bleeding can be seen in critically ill children from esophagitis or gastritis, or in children with portal hypertension from esophageal varices, most GI bleeding in children is from the lower tract and manifests as rectal bleeding. Table 9-3 lists the most common causes of rectal bleeding by age. Minor bleeding presents as stool streaked with blood and is usually caused by an anal fissure or polyp. Inflammatory diseases, such as IBD or infectious enterocolitis, result in diarrheal stool mixed with blood. In contrast, Meckel diverticulum typically results in a significant amount of bleeding without diarrhea. Table 9-4 lists the associated signs and symptoms of the major causes of GI bleeding.

CLINICAL MANIFESTATIONS

History

It is important to define the onset and duration of bleeding, color (bright red vs. dark maroon vs. tarry black), rate (brisk vs. gradual), and type of bleeding (hematochezia, hematemesis, melena, blood-streaked stool). For upper GI bleeding, questions about forceful vomiting, ingestion of ulcerogenic drugs (salicylates, nonsteroidal anti-inflammatory drugs, steroids), and a history of liver disease or peptic ulcer disease are helpful. For lower GI tract bleeding, inquire about diarrhea, or

TABLE 9-3 Causes of Rectal Bleeding by Age of Patient

Newborn	Infant to 2 Yr	2 Yr to Preschool	Preschool to Adolescence
Most frequent causes			
Vitamin K deficiency	Anal fissure	Infectious diarrhea	Infectious diarrhea
Ingested maternal blood	Cow/soy milk enterocolitis	Polyp	Polyp
Cow/soy milk enterocolitis	Infectious diarrhea	Anal fissure	IBD
Necrotizing enterocolitis	Intussusception	Meckel diverticulum	HSP
Hirschsprung disease	Meckel diverticulum		
Less frequent causes			
Volvulus	Duplication cyst	IBD	Anal fissure
Duplication cyst	Vascular malformation	Vascular malformation	Vascular malformation
Upper GI tract bleeding	Upper GI tract bleeding with rapid transit	Upper GI tract bleeding with rapid transit	Hemorrhoid

TABLE 9-4 Diagnosis of Gastrointestinal Bleeding

Site	Cause	Signs and Symptoms
Upper	Medication	Ingestion of NSAIDs
	Varices	Splenomegaly or evidence of liver disease
	Esophagitis	Dysphagia, vomiting, dyspepsis
	PUD	Epigastric pain, meal related
Lower	Fissure	Bright red blood on surface of the stool
	Chronic polyps	Painless rectal bleeding on the surface of stool; may have some mucus admixed
	Cow's milk–soy enterocolitis	Blood mixed with stool; may have diarrhea, hypoalbuminemia, and edema
	Meckel diverticulum	Painless, often a large amount of blood
	IBD	Diarrhea, fever, abdominal pain, poor growth, associated systemic signs and symptoms
	Bacterial colitis	Diarrhea, abdominal pain, antecedent watery diarrhea, e.g., *E. coli* O157:H7 or antibiotic exposure, e.g., C. *difficile*
	HSP	Joint pain, abdominal pain, purpura
	Intussusception	Intermittent abdominal pain, pallor, currant jelly stools, right-sided abdominal mass

HSP, Henoch-Schönlein purpura; IBD, inflammatory bowel disease; NSAID, nonsteroidal anti-inflammatory drug; PUD, peptic ulcer disease.

constipation with large or hard stools and difficult or painful defecation. Emesis of red fluid may not be blood and can be due to vomiting of ingested fluids or foods (sugared children's drinks, beets, red gelatin, acetaminophen elixir). Black stool is not always caused by blood in the stool; it can occur in children who have ingested iron, bismuth, or blackberries.

Physical Examination

The immediate priority when examining a child with GI bleeding is to determine if hypovolemia exists from an acute bleed. Vital signs should be examined for orthostatic changes or for evidence of shock (tachycardia, tachypnea, hypotension). The earliest sign of significant GI bleeding is a raised resting heart rate. A drop in blood pressure is not seen until at least 40% of the intravascular volume is depleted. Dermatologic abnormalities such as petechiae and purpura indicate coagulopathy, whereas cool or clammy skin with pallor is suggestive of shock or anemia. On abdominal examination, masses (e.g., in the right lower quadrant mass may be caused by Crohn's disease or intussusception) and tenderness (e.g., in the epigastrium) suggest peptic ulcer disease, and splenomegaly or hepatosplenomegaly and *caput medusae* suggest evidence of portal hypertension and risk of varices.

Capillary refill (thenar eminence in neonates and infants) should be assessed on the extremity examination. On rectal examination, the clinician may assess for anal fissure, which is best seen by spreading the buttocks and everting the anal canal (most fissures are located at the 6- and 12-o'clock positions), perform a stool test for occult blood, feel for hard stool, and look for a dilated rectum in children with chronic constipation or anal fissure.

DIAGNOSTIC EVALUATION

Unless the source of bleeding is clearly the nasopharynx, an anal fissure, or hemorrhoids, a complete blood count with differential and platelet count and usually coagulation studies should be sent. Hemodynamically significant GI bleeding is a medical emergency and requires careful monitoring, often in an intensive care unit with blood available for transfusion. If the bleeding source is unclear and the patient is unstable, gastric lavage determines whether the bleeding is from the upper GI tract proximal to the ligament of Treitz. The stomach is lavaged with room-temperature normal saline. Esophageal varices are not an absolute contraindication to the placement of a nasogastric or orogastric tube. Return of clear lavage fluid makes the diagnosis of upper GI bleeding unlikely, although occasionally duodenal ulcers may bleed only distally. Return of bright red blood or "coffee grounds" that eventually clear indicates upper GI bleeding that has remitted. Persistent return of bright red blood indicates active bleeding and mandates aggressive intravenous fluid management and monitoring. A pediatric gastroenterologist should be consulted. A surgical consultation is often indicated although it is now uncommon to require surgery for an upper GI bleed in children. In the stable patient, a thorough history and physical examination with consideration of the age-related causes usually leads to diagnosis. Gastric lavage is unnecessary in children with minor or nonacute GI bleeding. The precise diagnosis is often made by upper or lower endoscopy. If there is bloody diarrhea, stool should be sent for culture. Bloody diarrhea following several days of nonbloody diarrhea is commonly seen in infection with *E. coli* O157:H7 which in 10% to 15% of patients can lead to hemolytic uremic syndrome. In the hospitalized neonate with bloody stool, necrotizing enterocolitis must be considered, and an abdominal film and evaluation for sepsis should be performed. When swallowed maternal blood is suspected as the cause of GI bleeding, the Apt red blood cell fragility test is performed on the child's stool or emesis to differentiate maternal blood from the blood of the neonate. A Meckel diverticulum should be considered when there is a large amount of painless rectal bleeding.

TREATMENT

The unstable child with severe bleeding or hypovolemia is evaluated by primary and secondary surveys as outlined in Chapter 1. A normal hemoglobin or hematocrit does not rule out severe acute bleeding; full hemodilution takes up to 12 hours in the acutely bleeding patient. Intravenous normal saline or Ringer lactate at 20 mL per kg boluses should be given until the vital signs are sufficiently improved. Type O-negative whole blood should be reserved for the unstable patient with acute bleeding that cannot quickly be brought under control. The most common error in management of the child with severe GI bleeding is inadequate volume replacement. Hypotension is a late finding; fluid resuscitation should be governed by the level of tachycardia. The stable child without heavy bleeding or signs of hypovolemia should be evaluated and treated according to the particular diagnosis. Figure 9-1 illustrates a useful algorithm for the evaluation and management of GI bleeding. Three common causes of GI bleeding—Meckel diverticulum, ulcerative colitis, and Crohn's disease—are discussed in the following sections.

MECKEL DIVERTICULUM

Meckel diverticulum, the vestigial remnant of the omphalomesenteric duct, is the most common anomaly of the GI tract. It is present in 2% to 3% of the population and is located within 100 cm of the ileocecal valve in the small intestine. The peak incidence of bleeding from the diverticulum is at 2 years of age. Heterotopic tissue, usually gastric, is ten times more common in symptomatic cases because of acid secretion and ulceration of nearby ileal mucosa.

CLINICAL MANIFESTATIONS

The most common presentation of Meckel diverticulum is painless rectal bleeding. Eighty-five percent of patients with Meckel diverticulum have hematochezia, 10% develop intestinal obstruction from intussusception or volvulus, and 5% suffer from painful diverticulitis mimicking appendicitis. The diagnosis is made by performing a Meckel scan. The technetium-99 pertechnetate scan, preceded by prepentagastrin stimulation or an H2 RA, identifies the ectopic acid-secreting cells that mediate the hemorrhage.

TREATMENT

Definitive treatment is surgical resection.

INFLAMMATORY BOWEL DISEASE

IBD is a generic term for Crohn's disease and ulcerative colitis, which are chronic inflammatory disorders of the intestines.

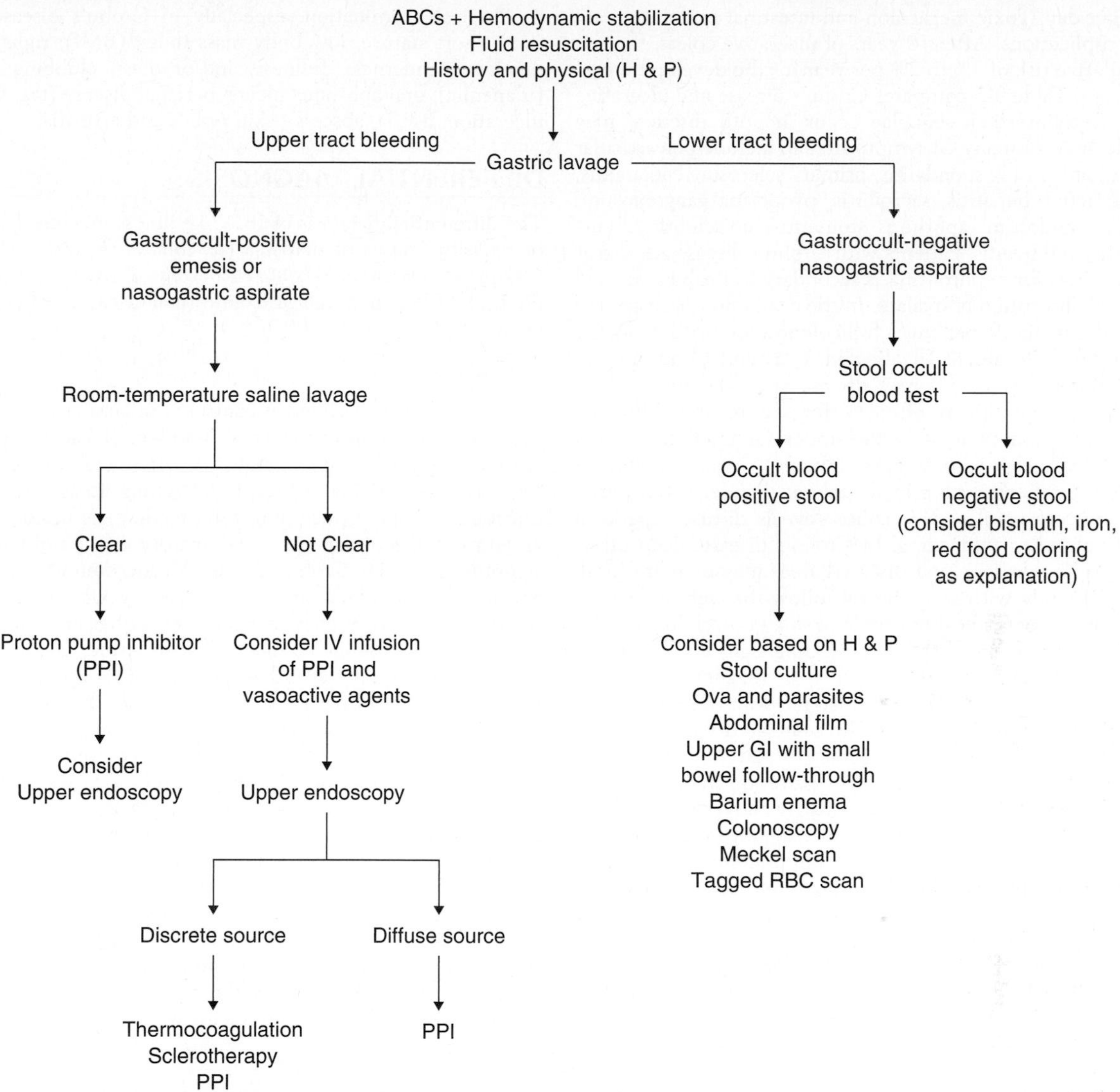

Figure 9-1 • Algorithm for evaluation and management of GI tract bleeding.

Ulcerative colitis produces diffuse superficial colonic ulceration and crypt abscesses. It involves the rectum in 95% of patients, with or without contiguous extension higher in the colon. Ulcerative colitis does not affect the small intestine. The pathology of Crohn's disease involves transmural inflammation often in a discontinuous pattern, which results in skip lesions. Crohn's disease may involve any part of the GI tract (mouth to anus). In pediatric patients, the process is ileocolonic in 40% of cases, involves the small intestine alone in approximately 30% of cases, and is isolated to the colon in only 20% of cases. Crohn's disease may result in transmural inflammation with fistula formation, or perforation, or fibrostenotic disease with stricture formation. Although the exact etiology of these disorders is not known, a combination of genetic, immunologic, and environmental mechanisms is implicated. Most pediatric patients are adolescents, but both diseases are seen in infancy and in preschool children.

CLINICAL MANIFESTATIONS

Crampy abdominal pain, recurrent fever, and weight loss are common manifestations in Crohn's disease. Although diarrhea is common, it is not universal. Rectal bleeding is noted in only 35% of cases of Crohn's disease. Abdominal pain tends to be more severe in Crohn's disease than in ulcerative colitis; it may be diffuse, and is frequently worse in the right lower quadrant. Perianal disease may produce skin tags, fissures, fistulas, or abscesses. Anorexia, poor weight gain, and delayed growth occur in 40% of patients. Most children with ulcerative colitis exhibit bloody diarrhea with mucopus (100%), abdominal pain (95%), and tenesmus (75%). Ninety percent of patients exhibit mild to moderate disease. Severe disease may be fulminant, with high fever, abdominal tenderness, distention, tachycardia, leukocytosis, hemorrhage, severe anemia, and more than eight stools per day. Toxic megacolon and intestinal perforation are rare complications. After 10 years of ulcerative colitis, there is a cumulative risk of 1% to 2% per year for the development of carcinoma. Table 9-5 compares Crohn's disease and ulcerative colitis. Extraintestinal sequelae occur in both diseases, may precede or accompany GI symptoms, and include polyarticular arthritis, ankylosing spondylitis, primary sclerosing cholangitis, chronic active hepatitis, sacroiliitis, pyoderma gangrenosum, erythema nodosum, aphthous stomatitis, episcleritis, recurrent iritis, and uveitis. Patients with Crohn's disease are also at increased risk for nephrolithiasis secondary to ileal disease and abnormal absorption of oxalate. In the evaluation of suspected IBD in the pediatric patient, a full colonoscopy with ileoscopy is indicated to evaluate all affected areas and to attempt to differentiate between Crohn's disease and ulcerative colitis. An upper endoscopy is often performed to assess for any microscopic inflammation in the upper GI tract. Even with a full evaluation, it is sometimes difficult to make a definitive diagnosis in patients with primary colonic disease. Visualization of the mucosa in ulcerative colitis reveals diffuse superficial ulceration and easy bleeding. In Crohn's disease, deep ulcerations may be present, and diseased areas may be more focal. Upper GI study with small bowel follow-through in Crohn's disease often reveals ileal or proximal small bowel disease with segmental narrowing of the ileum (string sign) and longitudinal ulcers. A capsule endoscopy test or magnetic resonance enterography may help identify small intestinal lesions in IBD.

Anemia is common and usually associated with iron deficiency. Megaloblastic anemia secondary to folate and vitamin B12 deficiency may also be present. An elevation in the erythrocyte sedimentation rate and the CRP is common but severe inflammation can be present without significant elevation of these inflammatory markers. Hypoalbuminemia can be seen with malnutrition or a protein losing enteropathy in Crohn's disease. Serum aminotransferase levels are increased if hepatic inflammation is a complicating feature. Stool examination reveals blood and fecal leukocytes with a negative stool culture and there is frequent elevation of fecal calprotectin which can be used to monitor disease activity.

Physical examination, especially in Crohn's disease may show short stature, low body mass index (BMI); right lower quadrant tenderness, fullness, and/or mass; clubbing; pallor (if anemic); oral aphthous ulcers; perianal disease (tag, fissure, ulceration, fistula, abscess); skin rashes and arthritis.

DIFFERENTIAL DIAGNOSIS

The differential diagnosis of IBD like illness includes bacterial or parasitic causes of diarrhea (*C. difficile*, *E. coli O157:H7*, *Campylobacter jejuni*, *Yersinia enterocolitica*, amebiasis), appendicitis, HSP, eosinophilic gastrointestinal disease, and radiation enterocolitis.

Treatment

Treatment of IBD is aimed at control of inflammation and suppression of the immune system. 5-aminosalicylic compounds are a mainstay of anti-inflammatory treatment. Antibiotics have a role as anti-inflammatory agents in Crohn's disease. Aggressive nutritional support (including tube feeding) is important for growth but also has an anti-inflammatory effect and improves symptom control in Crohn's disease. Corticosteroids have both anti-inflammatory and immunosuppressive effects, and they remain a mainstay of early management. Other immunomodulatory treatments including mercaptopurine, azathioprine, and methotrexate are useful as steroid sparing agents. Biologic therapy with antitumor necrosis factor antibody is increasingly used for moderate and severe disease. Because anorexia and increased nutrient losses in the stool are common in children with IBD, adequate calories and protein are essential. Oral supplements, nasogastric tube feedings, and, in some severe cases, central venous hyperalimentation are necessary. Vitamin and mineral supplementation, especially with iron, folate and B12, may be required. Patients with ulcerative colitis for more than 10 years need annual colonoscopy and biopsy because of the high risk of colon cancer development. Studies have shown that patients with long-standing Crohn's colitis are also at an increased risk for development of neoplasia. Surgery is eventually needed in 25% of patients with ulcerative colitis and

TABLE 9-5 Comparison of Crohn's Disease and Ulcerative Colitis

Feature	Crohn's Disease	Ulcerative Colitis
Malaise, fever, weight loss	Common	Sometimes
Rectal bleeding	Sometimes	Nearly always
Abdominal pain	Common	Common
Abdominal mass	Common	Rare
Perianal disease	Common	Rare
Ileal involvement	Common	Rare (backwash ileitis)
Stricture	Sometimes	Not seen
Fistula	Sometimes	Not seen
Skip lesions	Common	Rare
Transmural inflammation	Common	Not seen
Granulomas	Sometimes	Not seen
Long-term risk of cancer	Increased	Greatly increased

50% to 70% of children with Crohn's disease. Surgery is indicated in ulcerative colitis when there is fulminant colitis with severe blood loss or toxic megacolon, intractable disease with a high-dosage steroid requirement, steroid toxicity, growth failure, or colonic dysplasia. Because ulcerative colitis is restricted to the colon, colectomy is curative. Surgery is performed in Crohn's disease when inflammation is not controlled with medical therapy, or when hemorrhage, obstruction, perforation, or severe fistula formation is present. In general, conservative management is warranted because removal of the diseased bowel is not curative in Crohn's disease. Recurrence rates of up to 50% have been reported after segmental resection.

LIVER DISEASE

Hyperbilirubinemia and biliary atresia are discussed in Chapter 2 and infectious hepatitis is reviewed in Chapter 10. In this section, we will review elevation of aminotransferases, acute liver failure, Wilson disease, Alagille syndrome and nonalcoholic fatty liver disease.

ELEVATION OF AMINOTRANSFERASES

AST (aspartate aminotransferase) and ALT (alanine aminotransferase) are released from damaged hepatocytes, indicating liver injury. ALT is more specific for liver disease, due to its presence in low concentrations in other tissues. The degree of elevation of aminotransferases may give a clue as to the etiology. The differential diagnosis of mild to moderately elevated aminotransferases (<1,000) includes, α1-antitrypsin deficiency, autoimmune hepatitis, chronic viral hepatitis (B, C, and D), hemochromatosis, medications and toxins, steatosis and steatohepatitis, Wilson's disease, celiac disease, and hyperthyroidism. More dramatic elevation of aminotransferases, ALT > AST (>1,000 U/L) suggests acute bile ducts obstruction, acute Budd-Chiari syndrome, acute viral hepatitis, autoimmune hepatitis, ischemic hepatitis (shock), and medications/toxins. In alcohol-related liver injury, there may be very elevated transaminases with AST > ALT.

ACUTE LIVER FAILURE

Acute liver failure is defined as biochemical evidence of liver injury, no history of known chronic liver disease, coagulopathy not corrected by vitamin K with our without mental status changes. A specific etiology cannot be identified in about 50% of pediatric cases. However, among identifiable causes, toxins and medications including acetaminophen, anticonvulsants (phenytoin, carbamazepine, and valproic acid) and autoimmune hepatitis predominate. Other causes include mushroom poisoning, other drugs, Wilson disease, other metabolic conditions often presenting in the first 3 years of life (galactosemia, hereditary fructose intolerance, tyrosinemia, urea cycle defects, fatty acid oxidation defects, mitochondrial disorders, and neonatal hemochromatosis). Hematophagocytic lymphohistiocytosis (HLH) can also present with acute liver failure. Hepatitis A and E are important causes of acute liver failure in endemic areas.

WILSON DISEASE

Wilson disease, also known as hepatolenticular degeneration, is a rare autosomal-recessive disease of copper metabolism with a prevalence of 1:30,000. The abnormal gene (ATP7B) found in chromosome 13, encodes for a P-type ATPase expressed mainly in hepatocytes, which transports copper into bile and incorporates it into ceruloplasmin. Absent or reduced function of this protein leads to decreased hepatocellular excretion of copper into bile resulting in copper accumulation in the liver and decreased ceruloplasmin As liver copper levels increase, copper is released in the circulation and deposits in other organs, brain, kidneys, and cornea. Wilson disease usually manifests as liver disease in children and teenagers; and as neuropsychiatric illness in adults. It should be considered in any child or teenager with chronic liver disease because it can be well treated and can be fatal if missed. The classic criteria are liver disease, decreased ceruloplasmin and Kaiser-Fleischer rings. Dramatically increased hepatic copper is the best evidence for Wilson disease. Treatment includes chelating agents (D-penicillamine, trientine, and tetrathiomolybdate), zinc which interferes with uptake of copper and induces an endogenous chelator, and avoidance of food with high copper content.

ALAGILLE SYNDROME

Alagille syndrome (AGS) or arteriohepatic dysplasia, is an autosomal-dominant disorder. The traditional clinical diagnosis of AGS follows the guidelines of bile duct paucity plus 3 of 5 clinical criteria including cholestasis, cardiac murmur or heart disease, skeletal anomalies, ocular findings, and characteristic facial features. Mutations in the JAG1 gene, which encodes a ligand in the Notch signaling pathway, cause AGS. JAG1 and the Notch signaling pathway are crucial for the development of the liver, bile ducts, heart, vasculature, kidneys, and other organs affected in this multisystem disorder.

Clinical Features

The clinical features of AGS include neonatal cholestasis, hypercholesterolemia with the appearance of skin xanthomas, and pruritis. A minority of AGS patients develop progressive liver disease leading to cirrhosis and portal hypertension although 20% to 40% of AGS patients will eventually require liver transplantation. Cardiac murmurs occur in 85% to 98% of affected individuals with the most common abnormality being stenosis at some level in the pulmonary arterial system. Vertebral arch defects, the typical finding of butterfly vertebrae, and other minor skeletal defects can be seen. However, unexplained recurrent and poorly healing bone fractures in AGS patients is a significant source of morbidity and may be an indication for liver transplantation in severe cases. The most common ocular features of AGS are hypertelorism and bilateral posterior embryotoxon visible by indirect opthalmoscopy. During childhood, the facies are typically described as triangular, with a broad forehead, deeply set eyes, a pointed chin and a straight nose with a bulbous tip. Renal anomalies occur in 40% to 50% of AGS patients, and renal involvement is now considered one of the major criteria for the diagnosis. Structural abnormalities include solitary kidney, ectopic kidney, bifid renal pelvis, and multicystic or dysplastic kidneys. Functional abnormalities include renal tubular acidosis, neonatal renal insufficiency, nephronophthisis, lipidosis of the glomeruli, and tubulointerstitial nephropathy. Vascular anomalies in AGS involve the aorta, renal arteries, and cerebral vessels; intracranial vessel aneurysms; internal carotid artery aneurysms; and moya moya disease, which occurs in up to

9% of AGS patients. Growth failure is multifactorial in etiology, including a genetic contribution, chronic cholestasis, fat malabsorption, congenital heart disease, and limited oral intake.

Management

Adequate nutrition is crucial and a high-calorie diet with a high proportion of fat from medium-chain triglycerides is recommended in the neonatal period. Ursodeoxycholic acid is recommended to enhance bile flow, and supplemental fat-soluble vitamins treatment is required to prevent deficiencies. Biliary diversion may relieve pruritus and slow the progression of the disease. Liver transplantation is indicated in patients with decompensated cirrhosis or failed diversion with incapacitating pruritus.

NONALCOHOLIC FATTY LIVER DISEASE AND STEATOHEPATITIS (NAFLD/NASH)

Nonalcoholic fatty liver disease (NAFLD) is the most common cause of liver disease in childhood and adolescence. NAFLD includes macrovesicular fat accumulation within hepatocytes, without inflammation, whereas nonalcoholic steatohepatitis (NASH), includes fat accumulation associated with inflammation and/or evidence of cellular injury. NAFLD in children and adults predisposes to Type 2 diabetes, hypertension, and dyslipidemia. The most common factor associated with NAFLD is obesity. Other predisposing factors include: male sex, Hispanic ethnicity, and Asian race (especially those of Chinese or Filipino descent). The pathophysiology of NAFLD is thought to be multifactorial with hyperinsulinemia and hepatic insulin resistance important in development of fatty liver.

Clinical Features

Clinically, most children are asymptomatic. Acanthosis nigricans is found in >50% of patients with NAFLD. Laboratory findings that may indicate NAFLD include elevated serum aminotransferases with ALT > AST, elevated GGT and alkaline phosphatase, low HDL, and elevated fasting triglycerides. Ultrasound and MRI may be used for diagnosis. Ultrasound is readily available and inexpensive, but this technique is less sensitive and cannot quantify the degree of hepatic steatosis, fibrosis, or inflammation. Liver biopsy and histological examination are helpful for definitive diagnosis.

Management

The treatment goal is weight loss through lifestyle modification including diet change and increased exercise. The amount of weight loss required to induce a significant change in NAFLD is unknown. Pharmacological treatments are still undergoing trials.

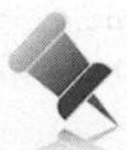

KEY POINTS

- The history and physical examination help to determine whether abdominal pain is acute or chronic/recurrent and whether a medical, surgical, or nonorganic disorder is most likely. In the adolescent female, genitourinary pathology must be considered, and a pelvic examination should be performed.
- Appendicitis is the most common surgical indication for abdominal pain in childhood.
- Most intussusception results from invagination of the ileum into the colon of the ileocecal valve, which results in periodic episodes of irritability, colicky pain, and emesis.
- Most cases of emesis are caused by gastroesophageal reflux, acute gastroenteritis, or non-GI infectious disorders such as tonsillitis, otitis media, or urinary tract infection. However, intestinal obstruction, neurologic, metabolic, and drug-induced etiologies and nondigestive organ failure are important causes not to miss.
- Pyloric stenosis is an important cause of gastric outlet obstruction and emesis in the first 2 months of life.
- In most infants and older children with emesis, reflux, and heartburn, a history and physical examination are sufficient to reliably diagnose GERD, recognize complications, and initiate management.
- The most common cause of diarrhea in children is viral gastroenteritis.
- Most children with uncomplicated viral gastroenteritis or bacterial enterocolitis can be rehydrated orally; antidiarrheal medications are not indicated in children with acute diarrhea.
- Infants with diarrhea should be fed as close to their normal diet as possible. Recovery is faster than if a restricted diet is used.
- Constipation resulting from organic causes may be caused by decreased peristalsis, decreased expulsion, and anatomic malformation.
- Constipation is commonly associated with anal fissure in infancy and voluntary withholding or functional constipation in children and adolescents.
- Hirschsprung disease should be suspected in any infant who fails to pass meconium within the first 24 to 48 hours of life or who requires repeated rectal stimulation to induce bowel movements, or has poor feeding, bilious vomiting, and abdominal distention in the first month of life.
- The earliest sign of significant GI bleeding is a raised resting heart rate. A drop in blood pressure is not seen until at least 40% of the intravascular volume is depleted. Hemodynamically significant GI bleeding is a medical emergency and requires careful monitoring, often in an intensive care unit and blood available for transfusion.
- Meckel diverticulum is the most common anomaly of the GI tract, and presents with painless rectal bleeding.
- Ulcerative colitis produces diffuse superficial colonic ulceration and crypt abscesses. It involves the rectum in 95% of patients, with or without contiguous extension higher in the colon. Ulcerative colitis does not affect the small intestine.
- The pathology of Crohn disease involves transmural inflammation in a discontinuous pattern, which results in skip lesions. Crohn disease may involve any part of the GI tract (mouth to anus).
- Therapy for IBD is aimed at achieving maximum symptom control with minimum side effects.

C Clinical Vignettes

Vignette 1

A 14-year-old girl presents to her primary care provider with a 3-to-4-month history of abdominal pain. Several mornings each week, the patient awakens with epigastric and periumbilical pain and she does not want to eat breakfast. Eating makes her pain worse and she does have some nausea. She does not have diarrhea, constipation, or blood in her stool. She has not gained weight since her last visit 6 months ago. On physical examination, she is a healthy-appearing, Tanner Stage IV adolescent whose weight and height are at the 50th percentile for age. Her abdomen is soft but mildly tender throughout. There is no perianal disease, and the stool in her rectum is hemoccult negative.

1. You suspect that she has functional abdominal pain (functional dyspepsia). Which of these tests would be helpful to obtain to exclude other likely causes of her pain?
   a. ESR, CBC, Antitissue transglutaminase IgA
   b. Upper gastrointestinal endoscopy
   c. Breath test for *Helicobacter pylori*
   d. Upper GI series (x-ray)
   e. RAST testing for food allergies

2. Which of the following additional items in the history would support your suspicion of functional abdominal pain?
   a. Unexplained fever
   b. Intermittent diarrhea
   c. Family history of inflammatory bowel disease (IBD)
   d. Weight loss
   e. Perianal disease

3. Which of the following are appropriate options for treatment?
   a. Narcotic therapy for the pain
   b. Polyethylene glycol 3350
   c. Food elimination diet
   d. Emphasis on maintaining daily functioning despite pain
   e. Cholecystectomy

Vignette 2

A 4-month-old girl presents to the hospital with a 2-day history of watery, nonbloody diarrhea and fever. The infant was reported to have had 10 watery stools over the previous 24 hours. There was no history of vomiting. Her birth history was unrevealing and she was fed exclusively on milk-based formula from birth. One month ago, she weighed 5.5 kg. On the day of presentation, physical examination revealed an alert but irritable and ill-appearing infant with a weight of 5.1 kg, a temperature of 38.9°C, heart rate between 170 and 190 beats/min, respiratory rate between 40 and 80 breaths/min, and blood pressure of 102/55 mmHg. The anterior fontanel is flat. The skin was pale; she had dry lips and dry buccal mucosa, reduced tears, and a capillary refill time of 3 seconds.

1. Which of the following is the most likely etiology of her illness?
   a. Salmonella
   b. Giardia
   c. Rotavirus
   d. *Clostridium difficile*
   e. Pneumonia

2. What is the most appropriate treatment for this patient?
   a. Intravenous or oral rehydration followed by a clear liquid diet
   b. Intravenous antibiotics
   c. Oral rehydration and antidiarrheal medications
   d. Intravenous or oral hydration followed by a cow's milk based or soy milk diet
   e. Oral rehydration and ondansetron

3. Which of the following is the most likely explanation for this persistent diarrhea?
   a. Celiac disease
   b. Giardia
   c. Pancreatic insufficiency
   d. Postviral enteritis
   e. Congenital diarrhea

Vignette 3

An otherwise healthy 14-year-old girl presents with 2 weeks of daily abdominal cramping, nausea, 1 to 2 episodes of nonbilious emesis, and worsening malaise. She felt too unwell to attend school the past 2 days. Low-grade fever to a max of 100°F has been recorded on several days. Though she noted a decreased appetite, there has been no notable weight loss. Each of the past 5 days, she notes 2 to 3 episodes of nonbloody but "really nasty" diarrhea. She is a quiet, cooperative, nontoxic teen. Vital signs are normal with no orthostatic changes noted. Her physical exam is normal excepting a diffusely tender abdomen more so on the right side with no rebound, guarding, or pain with jumping.

1. Which diagnostic plan would best guide management at this juncture?
   a. CBC, ESR, fecal calprotectin
   b. Stool for culture, ova and parasites (O&P), *Clostridium difficile* testing
   c. Serum electrolytes
   d. Watchful waiting, review of bland diet
   e. Serum amylase, lipase, and liver panel

2. What is the optimal treatment plan for this particular patient?
   a. Oral metronidazole
   b. IV metronidazole
   c. Oral vancomycin
   d. IV vancomycin
   e. Azithromycin for 5 days

3. Which of the following should be included in further surveillance?
   a. Repeating stool testing for *C. difficile* at the completion of her antibiotic course to document eradication
   b. Repeating stool testing for *C. difficile* in 4 weeks
   c. Repeating stool testing for *C. difficile* only if her symptoms should return
   d. Repeating stool testing for *C. difficile* following any future antibiotic course
   e. Testing family members for *C. difficile*

Vignette 4

An 11-year-old boy presents with a 3-month history of intermittent bloody diarrhea and weight loss. He has perianal skin tags and fullness in the right lower quadrant on examination. He has a microcytic anemia and an elevated sedimentation rate. There is a family history of ulcerative colitis in an uncle.

1. Which of the following is the most likely diagnosis?
   a. Ulcerative colitis
   b. Crohn's disease
   c. Infectious colitis
   d. *C. difficile* infection
   e. Immunodeficiency syndrome

2. What is the most useful next step in the evaluation of this patient?
   a. Upper GI x-ray series
   b. Fecal calprotectin
   c. Upper endoscopy (esophagogastroduodenoscopy) and colonoscopy
   d. Abdominal ultrasound
   e. Serologic IBD panel

3. What is the most likely intervention in his future?
   a. Varicella vaccine
   b. Medication to reduce stress
   c. Endocrine referral for growth failure/growth hormone consideration
   d. Restriction of milk
   e. Surgery

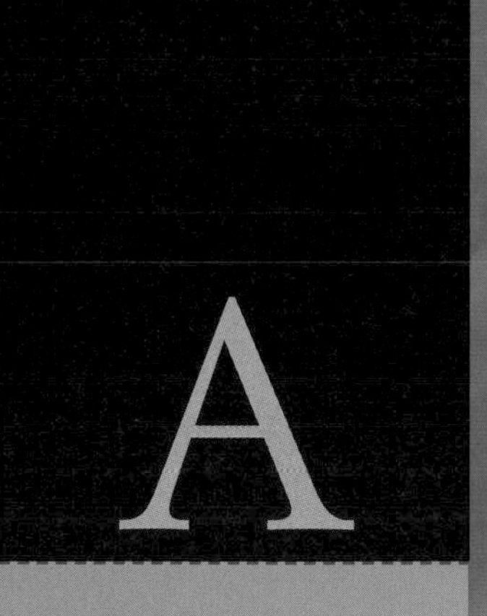

Answers

Vignette 1 Question 1

Answer A: A series of relatively low-cost tests can exclude common causes of abdominal pain resulting from inflammation (ESR, CBC), celiac disease (antitissue transglutaminase IgA), gall bladder disease or liver disease (serum aminotransferase, alkaline phosphatase, and bilirubin), and urinary tract disease (urinalysis). An ulcer is less likely without a history of pain relieved by eating, and it is more likely to cause acute and daily pain rather than intermittent pain lasting 3 to 4 months. Upper gastrointestinal endoscopy is somewhat insensitive for ulcer disease. *H. pylori* infection is a cause of symptomatic peptic ulcer disease and gastritis but is not more common is children with functional abdominal pain symptoms. Food allergies usually trigger symptoms temporally related to the time of food ingestion, that is, within 1 to 2 hours. Eosinophilic gastroenteritis, which is not IgE mediated, is not likely to demonstrate positive RAST testing.

Vignette 1 Question 2

Answer B: Diarrhea without blood, but sometimes with mucus, can be seen in functional gastrointestinal disorders (FGIDs). Although functional dyspepsia is distinct from irritable bowel syndrome, there is a great deal of overlap in this spectrum of disorders. The presence of alarm symptoms or signs suggests a higher possibility of organic disease and may justify the performance of additional diagnostic tests. Alarm symptoms or signs include but are not limited to involuntary weight loss, deceleration of linear growth, gastrointestinal blood loss, significant vomiting, chronic severe diarrhea, persistent right upper or right lower quadrant pain, unexplained fever, and family history of inflammatory bowel disease. A family history of IBD, especially in first-degree family members, increases the likelihood of IBD and at a minimum increases the concern on the part of the patient and family. While weight loss may occur in FGIDs, is it unusual and minimal. Perianal disease is a hallmark of IBD and physical examination for abdominal pain should therefore include perianal inspection if not a rectal examination. All of the tests return normal and you continue the counseling you began at the first office visit.

Vignette 1 Question 3

Answer D: Improvement in symptoms will require cooperation of the patient and family. Patients currently missing school should be encouraged to return to school. School attendance is not part of the problem and in fact is part of the solution. Distraction from pain is a useful strategy and normal daily activities fulfill this role. Use of acid-reducing medications may improve pain even when not due to gastritis or ulcer disease, but the lowest effective dose should be used and the medication discontinued if not effective. Low doses of antidepressant drugs, which inhibit serotonin uptake and facilitate endogenous endorphin release, may benefit children with pain predominant FGIDs. Biofeedback, hypnosis, and other cognitive behavioral treatments have been beneficial in many conditions associated with chronic pain, including childhood FGIDs. Narcotic therapy will simply create a second problem, that is, dependency, and is better reserved for acute severe pain rather than chronic pain. Polyethylene glycol 3350 is extremely helpful for constipation, but is not helpful for FGIDs without this symptom. A food elimination diet is difficult and there is no evidence that it helps in FGIDs or evidence in this patient's history for food allergy. This patient did not have evidence of gallstones; moreover, gallstones in the absence of specific signs and symptoms are rarely the cause of vague abdominal pain. A gall bladder emptying scan was not done, but this too, even when abnormal, has poor predictive value for gall bladder pain.

Vignette 2 Question 1

Answer C: Rotavirus is the most common cause of severe diarrhea among infants and young children and is one of several viruses that cause similar infections. Although the incidence and severity of rotaviral illness is decreasing with increasing immunization against rotavirus, it is still a major cause of illness, especially in unimmunized patients. Salmonella is much less common but in a child this ill, it is reasonable to obtain a bacterial stool culture to exclude salmonellosis. Salmonella infection can but does not always have bloody diarrhea. The irritability of this child is a concern and could be due to dehydration (compensated shock) and acidosis. However, the irritability seen with salmonellosis always raises a concern in a young infant for sepsis or meningitis. The flat fontanel and the child's mental status should be reassessed after hydration to ensure that the fontanel is not bulging and the irritability is improved. Giardia is less common in a child who is not ambulatory. It does not cause fever and usually does not cause this degree of dehydration. *C. difficile* is uncommon as a cause of diarrhea in children below 1 year of age and does not cause this degree of dehydration. Pneumonia can cause fever and tachypnea and even be associated with mild diarrhea but not this degree of dehydration.

Vignette 2 Question 2

Answer D: Oral rehydration is the mainstay of treatment to resolve the dehydration. This child is close to 10% dehydrated. There has been a 400 g weight loss since the last measured weight. Assuming the child had continued to grow at the 50th percentile, she would weigh approximately 6.1 kg but is actually 600 g less. Intravenous rehydration is also appropriate if the child refuses to drink or there is concern about decompensated shock. Most commonly, after a period of rehydration, a normal diet can be resumed with additional oral rehydration solution to compensate for ongoing losses. Because this child is young and the diarrhea severe, there is a higher chance that she will have temporary lactose intolerance and a soy milk based formula is also a reasonable option for a short time, for example, 7 to 10 days. Probiotics may also shorten the course of the diarrheal illness. A clear liquid diet will not provide adequate energy and will not shorten the duration of diarrhea. Intravenous antibiotics would be appropriate if this child appears septic but antibiotics are not useful to treat viral diarrhea. Antidiarrheal medications, for example, loperamide may cause a sense of false security with decreased diarrhea due to pooling of intestinal secretions in the intestinal lumen, the so-called third spacing. They do not decrease loss of fluid from the intravascular space. Loperamide is not indicated in this age group as it may cross the blood–brain barrier with resultant lethargy and respiratory depression. Ondansetron is a useful adjunct if vomiting is present from uncomplicated gastroenteritis. However, it has not been studied for this purpose in infants below 6 months. The acute dehydration resolves with treatment but the diarrhea persists for more than 14 days.

Vignette 2 Question 3

Answer D: Diarrhea lasting more than 14 days is considered to be chronic or persistent. Postinfectious enteritis diarrhea may result from incomplete repair of the intestinal mucosa, a process that is normally complete in a week or less. Use of probiotics and temporary removal of lactose from the infant's diet can accelerate resolution. In developed countries, severe, persistent diarrhea has become far less common. Persistent diarrhea is associated with undernutrition, both before and after the illness. Shigella and Cryptosporidium infection are also risk factors but persistent diarrhea can occur after acute viral gastroenteritis. Immunodeficiency is a concern and should also be evaluated in an infant with persistent diarrhea. Celiac disease is not symptomatic until there has been activation of the immune-mediated mechanism through consumption of gluten, which should not be present in cow's milk (or soy)–based formula. Giardia infection can cause persistent diarrhea, but is uncommon in an infant who is not ambulatory. Pancreatic insufficiency is most commonly due to cystic fibrosis and is present in 85% of patients with cystic fibrosis at birth. It does not present as an acute, febrile diarrheal illness at 4 months of age that does not improve. Congenital diarrhea, for example, structural enterocyte disorders such as microvillus inclusion disease, congenital sodium or chloride diarrhea, or autoimmune diarrhea would generally present with watery diarrhea and growth failure before 3 to 4 months of age.

Vignette 3 Question 1

Answer B: Stool culture, testing for O&P and *C. difficile* is most appropriate. The duration of symptoms exceeds the allotted maximum of 10 to 14 days seen in a self-limited viral gastroenteritis. The presence of fever suggests an infectious and also, but less likely, an inflammatory process. While inflammatory bowel disease can present with a similar symptom constellation, the duration is usually longer and course more indolent. Weight loss is often present. Should stool studies remain normal and symptoms persist, the screening labs in choice A are worthy of consideration. Electrolytes are helpful when the clinical picture warrants oral or IV fluid to rehydrate or correct imbalances. Our patient had neither high output losses nor clinical concern for dehydration. Though acute pancreatitis and biliary disease in this age could present with abdominal pain, the location, presence of diarrhea, and fever speak against this. Stool testing was positive for the detection of toxin producing *Clostridium difficile* by PCR. Culture and ova, and parasite testing were negative.

Vignette 3 Question 2

Answer A: *Clostridium difficile* is now a fairly common infection seen in community settings. Normal children who have had neither recent inpatient hospital stay nor antibiotic regimen are experiencing clinically significant disease. More virulent strains may be contributing to the increased incidence. In this patient who is tolerating oral fluids and solids, is nontoxic, and is otherwise healthy, oral metronidazole is the drug of choice. Oral vancomycin is extremely effective however, its formidable cost and limited accessibility on prescription benefit plans, encourage limiting use to more ill patients and medically fragile children. IV therapy for *C. difficile*, which is more invasive and not as effective, is not preferred unless there is an ileus. Colonic concentrations of vancomycin are negligible following intravenous administration, and there is little support for this therapeutic option. In the absence of diarrhea, stool levels of metronidazole after oral intake are low because of absorption in the small bowel. However, in the presence of diarrhea, stool concentrations are therapeutic. Azithromycin is not an effective antibiotic for *C. difficile.* Fidaxomicin is a new oral antibiotic which is effective. Our patient recovers uneventfully with resolution of her cramping, nausea, and diarrhea over a few days.

Vignette 3 Question 3

Answer C: Recurrence of *C. difficile* infection typically develops 1 to 2 weeks after stopping metronidazole or vancomycin, but can be delayed for up to 12 weeks. Recurrence rates following treatment with metronidazole or vancomycin are similar at 15% to 30%. Indeed, recurrent disease is so common that all patients should be forewarned that this complication can occur after their course of therapy is complete, thereby facilitating prompt diagnosis (retesting) and retreatment. Despite the risk of recurrent infection, test of cure is not recommended because there are no data that persistent positive tests at the end of treatment put the patient at greater risk for disease recurrence. Symptomatic patients should be retested but not asymptomatic patients. Repeat testing following future antibiotic courses is similarly not indicated, although minimizing future antibiotic exposure is indicated. Risk factors for recurrent *C. difficile* infection include a history of prior recurrence and use of additional antimicrobials. Although good hand washing is always important, and nosocomial spread of *C. difficile* is a major route of infection, intrafamilal spread of *C. difficile* is low enough as to not warrant surveillance, anticipatory treatment, or other interventions.

Vignette 4 Question 1

Answer B: The family history of IBD and the duration of symptoms with weight loss are suggestive of IBD. Crohn's disease is the most common inflammatory bowel disease in children. The perianal skin tags and fullness in the right lower quadrant suggest transmural inflammation and ileitis, respectively, which are both associated with Crohn's disease. Ulcerative colitis would also have bloody diarrhea but not skin tags and less likely fullness in the right lower quadrant. A family history of ulcerative colitis raises concern for either Crohn's disease or ulcerative colitis. Infectious colitis is usually more self-limited, except for *C. difficile* infection. Although he should be tested for enteric pathogens including *C. difficile*, there would still be a high degree of suspicion for IBD if an infection is present, suggesting this infection might be a comorbidity or a presenting feature of the chronic illness. When immunodeficiency syndromes present as colitis, this occurs in younger children, that is, infantile (<2 years old) or very early onset (<10 years old) inflammatory bowel disease.

Vignette 4 Question 2

Answer C: In the evaluation of suspected IBD in the pediatric patient, a full colonoscopy with ileoscopy is indicated to evaluate all affected areas and to attempt to differentiate between Crohn's disease and ulcerative colitis. An upper endoscopy is often performed to assess for any microscopic inflammation in the upper GI tract. This would be much more typical of Crohn's disease. Only endoscopy and biopsy can provide a tissue diagnosis which is the gold standard. Upper GI study with small bowel follow-through in Crohn's disease often reveals ileal or proximal small bowel disease with segmental narrowing of the ileum (string sign) and longitudinal ulcers. However, a tissue diagnosis would still be lacking. Fecal calprotectin is helpful to decide whether to perform an endoscopy in a patient with equivocal signs or symptoms or to follow a patient who has a diagnosis but may have mild symptoms. This patient would likely have a colonoscopy even with a normal fecal calprotectin. Abdominal ultrasound can be useful for evaluation of an abdominal abscess or appendicitis but is less useful for identifying mucosal disease. Again, a tissue diagnosis would still be lacking. Although a serologic panel for IBD can be helpful, especially to add to the information which helps distinguish Crohn's disease from ulcerative colitis, it is not a sensitive or specific way of screening a general population. A diagnosis of Crohn's disease was made and treatment initiated. The patient returns to the PCP for well child care while being followed by a pediatric gastroenterologist.

Vignette 4 Question 3

Answer E: Children with Crohn's disease are likely to have surgery in their future, to treat penetrating disease (fistulas, perforation) or strictures. In the first 5 years of diagnosis, about 50% of children will need surgery. Varicella titers should be checked at diagnosis. Most children who received a varicella vaccination on schedule will be immune. However, patients on steroids or other immunosuppressive medications have a contraindication to live virus vaccination. Most patients with IBD are not treated with stress relieving medication. There is no evidence that IBD is caused by stress. However, living with a chronic illness can be stressful, and stress can make a child with IBD feel less well or even contribute to a flare-up. It is important to address normal as well as special case stressors that may be affecting the patient's ability to cope with chronic illness. Growth failure is not expected in children with adequately treated IBD. In some patients with growth stunting, catch-up growth may be achieved with adequate suppression of inflammation, nutritional supplementation, and, rarely and in addition, growth hormone therapy. Lactase deficiency may occur transiently at the time of diagnosis if there is extensive small bowel disease. Otherwise, lactose restriction is not needed as part of routine management of IBD.

Chapter

10 Infectious Disease

Rebecca C. Brady • Katie S. Fine

Remarkable advances in the diagnosis, management, and prevention of infectious diseases have occurred during the past century. Specific treatment of bacterial illnesses began with the introduction of sulfonamides in the 1930s and penicillin in the 1940s. Newer classes of antibacterial agents include semisynthetic penicillins, tetracyclines, macrolides, fluoroquinolones, aminoglycosides, carbapenems, and four generations of cephalosporins. Antifungal, antiviral, and antiparasitic agents have also been developed. Other anti-infective agents include specific antibodies, intravenous immunoglobulin, phagocyte-stimulating factors, and interferons. Vaccines have led to a dramatic decline in certain infectious diseases. Smallpox was eradicated worldwide in 1977, and indigenous poliomyelitis was eliminated from the United States in 1979. The annual incidence of measles, mumps, rubella, diphtheria, and *Haemophilus influenzae* type b meningitis has decreased by more than 98% because of vaccine use in the United States. However, measles in particular is now making a comeback due to widespread geographic pockets with high rates of parental vaccine refusal.

Unfortunately, new pathogens continue to emerge. Severe acute respiratory syndrome (SARS) appeared early in the new millennium, caused by a previously unknown coronavirus. In 2009, a novel H1N1 strain of influenza emerged and spread rapidly throughout the world. Equally disconcerting is the rapid emergence of resistance to known antibiotics (e.g., methicillin-resistant *Staphylococcus aureus* and penicillin-resistant *Streptococcus pneumoniae*). Thus, after 100 years of progress against infectious diseases, the current challenges are every bit as formidable as at the beginning of the last century.

FEVER OF UNKNOWN ORIGIN

The phrase *fever of unknown origin* (FUO) implies fever of prolonged duration (≥14 days), documented temperature greater than 38.3°C (101°F) on multiple occasions, and uncertain etiology.

DIFFERENTIAL DIAGNOSIS

FUO in the pediatric population is usually a common disorder presenting in an uncommon manner. Overall, infectious etiologies are more common than rheumatologic ones, which are more common than oncologic illnesses as a source for FUO. Diagnostic considerations include the following:

- **Infection:** Sinusitis, hepatitis, cytomegalovirus (CMV), Epstein–Barr virus (EBV), cat-scratch disease, Rocky Mountain spotted fever (RMSF), endocarditis, septic arthritis, osteomyelitis, intra-abdominal abscess, enteric fever, tuberculosis, HIV, opportunistic infection
- **Connective tissue disease:** Systemic juvenile idiopathic arthritis, systemic lupus erythematosus
- **Malignancy:** Leukemia, lymphoma, neuroblastoma
- **Other:** Inflammatory bowel disease, Kawasaki disease, drug fever, thyrotoxicosis, sarcoidosis, and factitious fever

CLINICAL MANIFESTATIONS

History

The age and gender of the patient narrow the differential diagnosis. Inflammatory bowel disease and connective tissue disorders are uncommon in younger children. Autoimmune disorders occur more frequently in girls. Sexual history, travel history, current medications, exposure to animals, tick bites, antecedent illness, trauma, associated symptoms, and family history are important areas of inquiry. Different fever patterns (constant, recurrent, cyclical) occasionally suggest particular diagnoses. A thorough history and physical examination (usually after repeated encounters) will reveal the diagnosis in more than half of the children in whom a cause of the fever is found.

Physical Examination

Conjunctivitis, lymphadenopathy, joint tenderness, oral ulcers, thrush, heart murmurs, organomegaly, masses, abdominal tenderness, rashes, joint findings, and mental status changes may suggest a specific cause and guide further evaluation.

DIAGNOSTIC EVALUATION

The initial evaluation can be performed in the outpatient setting in older, well-appearing children. Neonates and ill-appearing children require hospitalization.

Screening laboratory tests include complete blood count (CBC) and differential, serum electrolytes, blood urea nitrogen (BUN) and creatinine levels, liver function tests (LFTs), alkaline phosphatase, and urinalysis (UA). Bacterial cultures should be obtained from specimens of blood, urine, stool, and possibly cerebrospinal fluid (CSF). Additional tests to consider include ESR, C-reactive protein, and specific serologic tests such as antibody studies for cat-scratch disease and EBV. A chest radiograph and skin testing for tuberculosis are often performed. More expensive and invasive studies may be warranted based on screening results. Usually, children recover without sequelae even if no etiology is determined.

BACTEREMIA AND SEPSIS

Bacteremia is the presence of bacteria in the blood. Bacteremia is further described as **occult** if it occurs in a well-appearing child without any obvious source of infection. The risk of occult bacteremia is highest (1.5% to 2.5%) in children between 2 and 24 months of age with a fever greater than 39.0°C and leukocytosis. Most episodes are caused by *Streptococcus pneumoniae* and resolve spontaneously. Rarely, localized infection (e.g., meningitis, pneumonia) occurs. Since 2000, when a conjugated seven-valent pneumococcal vaccine (PCV7) was recommended for routine use in infants, the incidence of all invasive pneumococcal infections has decreased by approximately 80% for children younger than 24 months of age. A 13-valent pneumococcal vaccine introduced in 2010 has replaced PCV7 for universal administration in the United States.

In contrast, **sepsis** implies bacteremia with evidence of a systemic response (tachypnea, tachycardia, etc.) and altered organ perfusion. Affected children appear quite toxic and may develop shock. The cause of sepsis varies by age. In neonates, group B streptococci, enteric gram-negative bacilli, and *Listeria monocytogenes* are most prevalent. In older children up to 5 years of age, *S. pneumoniae* predominates, followed by *Neisseria meningitidis*. *Staphylococcus aureus* is a common pathogen in children ≥5 years of age. Less common causes include *Salmonella* species, *Pseudomonas aeruginosa*, and viridans streptococci.

The evaluation of the child with suspected sepsis includes cultures from the blood, urine, and CSF (if meningitis is a concern). A chest radiograph is obtained if respiratory signs or symptoms are present. Initial empiric antimicrobial therapy is selected based on the age of the child, the likely etiologic agents, and any identified foci of infection.

ACUTE OTITIS MEDIA

Pathogenesis

Color Plate XX(1) demonstrates a normal tympanic membrane with pertinent anatomic areas labeled. Suspected or confirmed acute infection of the middle ear accounts for more physician visits than any other pediatric illness. The middle ear is normally sterile; a patent but collapsible Eustachian tube allows fluid drainage from the middle ear into the nasopharynx but normally prevents the retrograde entry of upper respiratory flora. In children, the angle of entry, short length, and (in some patients) decreased tone of the tube (eustachian tube dysfunction) increase susceptibility to infection. When the Eustachian tube is further narrowed by edema from a concurrent viral upper respiratory infection (URI), a relative vacuum is created, drawing secretions (and bacteria) from the nasopharynx into the middle ear.

Epidemiology

Acute otitis media (AOM) is most common in children 6 to 24 months of age. By 2 years of age, 90% of all children in the United States have had at least one episode of otitis media (OM), and 50% have had at least three episodes. Viruses (respiratory syncytial virus, parainfluenza virus, and influenza viruses) are a common cause of AOM, which may be complicated by bacterial superinfection. Common bacterial causes include *S. pneumoniae* (40%), nontypeable *Haemophilus influenzae* (25%), and *Moraxella catarrhalis* (10%). Unfortunately, approximately 50% of *S. pneumoniae* isolates are resistant to penicillin and many species of *H. influenzae* and almost all *M. catarrhalis* exhibit beta-lactamase activity.

Risk Factors

Caretaker smoking, bottle feeding, day-care attendance, allergic disease, craniofacial anomalies, immunodeficiency, genetic tendencies, and pacifier use all predispose children to AOM.

CLINICAL MANIFESTATIONS

History and Physical Examination

Children may have local or systemic complaints or both, including ear pain, fever, and fussiness. AOM is frequently preceded by symptoms of URI (cough, rhinorrhea, congestion). On physical examination, the affected tympanic membrane appears bulging, opaque, and erythematous with an aberrant light reflex. Pneumatic otoscopy reveals decreased tympanic membrane mobility. The diagnosis of AOM should only be made when there is an acute history of symptoms and a bulging, poorly or nonmobile tympanic membrane is noted in the presence of signs of local or systemic inflammation (Color Plate XX2).

Differential Diagnosis

Otitis media with effusion (OME) is diagnosed when there is apparent fluid behind the tympanic membrane (reduced mobility on pneumatic otoscopy) but no evidence of inflammation (tympanic membrane translucent/gray, no fever, no evidence of ear pain). **Myringitis** is inflammation of the eardrum accompanied by normal mobility. This condition often accompanies a viral URI. Neither OME nor myringitis respond to antibiotic treatment. **Otitis externa** (inflammation of the external ear canal) also causes ear pain; however, the tympanic membranes should appear normal on physical examination. The pain of otitis externa is exacerbated by manipulation of the external ear, and the ear canal appears erythematous, often with patchy areas of purulence. Otitis externa, often called swimmer's ear, is treated with topical antibiotic drops. A tympanic membrane that is erythematous without any other signs of disease may be caused by vigorous crying and should not be considered AOM.

Treatment

Because more antibiotics are prescribed for AOM than any other pediatric condition, and because antibiotic resistance is a growing concern, the Centers for Disease Control has issued consensus recommendations relating to the treatment of AOM. Patients younger than 24 months of age, patients thought to be at risk for poor follow-up, ill-appearing patients, and any patients with chronic illnesses (including immunodeficiencies) or recurrent, severe, or perforated AOM should be prescribed antibiotics. High-dose amoxicillin is the recommended first-line treatment. Patients who have been treated with antibiotics within the last month and those who have not improved within 48 hours are eligible for second-line therapy with amoxicillin/clavulanic acid, an oral second- or third-generation cephalosporin, or IM ceftriaxone. Children older than 24 months with less severe disease may be offered the choice of immediate antibiotic therapy versus pain control and watchful waiting. Those children who initially have antibiotics withheld should receive a prescription to fill 48 hours later if there has been no improvement. Patients with perforated tympanic membranes in addition to AOM should receive oral (and possibly topical) antibiotics at initial diagnosis. Most spontaneous perforations caused by AOM resolve within 24 to 72 hours.

The most common complication of AOM is OME, which follows virtually all cases of AOM and takes a variable amount of time to resolve. Children with OME that persists longer than 3 months should be referred for a hearing evaluation. Chronic OME increases the risk of hearing loss and delay of language acquisition. Children who have normal hearing despite persistent OME should be reevaluted every 3 to 6 months. Those who develop moderate hearing loss may be referred for possible tympanostomy tube placement. Tympanostomy tubes may also be considered for children with at least 3 episodes of AOM within 6 months or 4 episodes within 12 months. Complications of frequent episodes of AOM include excessive scarring (tympanosclerosis), cholesteatoma formation, and chronic suppurative OM.

Mastoiditis (infection of the mastoid bone of the skull) is a potentially severe but uncommon complication of AOM characterized clinically by high fever, tenderness of the mastoid bone, and anterior displacement of the external ear. Mastoiditis is treated with intravenous antibiotics; surgical drainage may also be required.

SINUSITIS

The maxillary and ethmoid sinuses are present at birth; the sphenoid and frontal sinuses develop later in childhood. The spectrum of pathogens responsible for sinusitis is virtually identical to that for OM. Sinusitis is often difficult to diagnose in a young child because the classic symptoms of headache, facial pain, and sinus tenderness may be absent or difficult to articulate. Acute bacterial sinusitis has two common clinical presentations: (a) persistent respiratory symptoms (>10 to 14 days) without improvement, including either nasal discharge (clear or purulent) or a daytime cough and (b) severe symptoms including high fever and purulent nasal discharge for at least 3 days. The differential diagnosis includes viral URIs, allergic rhinitis, and nasal foreign body. Sinusitis is primarily a clinical diagnosis. Radiologic studies of the sinuses may be useful in older children when there is a poor response to therapy and the diagnosis is in doubt. Sinus aspiration may be needed for recurrent or recalcitrant disease. Antibiotic coverage is similar to that for AOM, although treatment should continue longer (14 to 21 days). Complications are uncommon but include bony erosion, orbital cellulitis, and intracranial extension. Children with recurrent or chronic sinusitis should be evaluated for cystic fibrosis, ciliary dyskinesia, or primary immune deficiency.

HERPANGINA

Herpangina is a symptom complex caused by enteroviruses (including groups A and B coxsackieviruses and other enterovirus serotypes). It is typically diagnosed during the summer and fall in younger children. Initially, the patient develops a high fever and very sore throat. On examination, characteristic vesicular lesions that progress to ulcers are scattered over the soft palate, tonsils, and pharynx. Primary herpetic gingivostomatitis (caused by herpes simplex virus [HSV]) presents in a similar manner, although the lesions are generally more widespread over the gums, lips, and mucosa. Herpangina is self-limited (5 to 7 days) and requires no specific therapy. When similar lesions are noted on the palms and soles (and occasionally on the buttocks), the more inclusive name **hand-foot-and-mouth disease** is used.

STREPTOCOCCAL PHARYNGITIS

Pathogenesis

Group A beta-hemolytic streptococci (group A *Streptococcus* [GAS]; *Streptococcus pyogenes*) are the most important cause of bacterial infection of the throat. Antimicrobial therapy for streptococcal disease is recommended because of the frequency of **suppurative (peritonsillar abscess, retropharyngeal abscess)** and **nonsuppurative (rheumatic fever, poststreptococcal glomerulonephritis)** complications.

Epidemiology

Strep throat most commonly afflicts school-aged children and adolescents. The organism is spread person to person through infected oral secretions. At any one point in time, approximately 10% to 15% of well children carry GAS as part of their normal oral flora.

CLINICAL MANIFESTATIONS

History and Physical Examination

Classic symptoms include sore throat, fever, headache, malaise, nausea, and occasionally abdominal pain. Physical examination reveals enlarged, erythematous, exudative tonsils, and tender anterior cervical lymphadenopathy. Petechiae may be present on the soft palate. Rhinorrhea, hoarseness, and coughing, the hallmarks of viral URIs, are notably absent. The diagnosis of **scarlet fever** is made when a characteristic erythematous, "sandpaper-like" rash accompanies the fever and pharyngitis. The rash commonly begins on the neck, axillae, and groin, spreads to the extremities, and may desquamate 10 to 14 days later.

Differential Diagnosis

Differentiating viral pharyngitis and infectious mononucleosis from streptococcal pharyngitis may be impossible based on clinical symptoms; definitive diagnosis requires either throat culture or antigen detection test for GAS.

Diagnostic Evaluation

Therapeutic decisions should be based on throat culture or rapid antigen-detection test results. The specificity of most rapid antigen tests is greater than 95% (compared with throat culture), so false positive test results are rare. The sensitivity of rapid antigen tests is more variable and is highly dependent on the quality of the throat swab specimen. Therefore, a negative rapid antigen test should be confirmed by a throat culture.

Treatment

Patients with documented group A streptococcal pharyngitis should receive a 10-day course of oral penicillin (or a single dose of IM benzathine penicillin G) to hasten symptom resolution, decrease transmissibility, and prevent acute rheumatic fever. A clinical isolate of GAS resistant to penicillin never has been documented. Erythromycin, azithromycin, and clindamycin are acceptable alternatives for children allergic to penicillin. The treatment of scarlet fever is identical to that for streptococcal pharyngitis.

Acute rheumatic fever (ARF) occurs about 3 weeks after streptococcal pharyngitis in a small percentage of untreated patients. ARF is an inflammatory condition involving connective tissues of the heart (carditis, valvular destruction), joints (migratory polyarthritis), and CNS (transient chorea). Diagnosis rests on fulfilling the Jones criteria (Table 10-1). Initially, fever, dyspnea, chest pain, cardiac murmur, and arthritis predominate; long-term morbidity results from valvular destruction with consequent mitral or aortic valve insufficiency or stenosis. Acute episodes respond favorably to antibiotics, anti-inflammatory drugs, and cardiac management. ARF may recur after the initial episode; thus, individuals diagnosed with ARF should receive prophylactic penicillin therapy to prevent recurrent ARF.

Acute poststreptococcal glomerulonephritis may follow either group A streptococcal pharyngitis or skin infection (cellulitis) and is not prevented by timely antibiotic therapy. Clinical manifestations follow infection by approximately 10 days and include hematuria, edema, oliguria, and hypertension. Complement (C3) levels are low. Treatment consists of penicillin therapy and diuretics; steroids are rarely indicated. In contrast to affected adults, the majority of affected children recover without renal sequelae.

INFECTIOUS MONONUCLEOSIS

Pathogenesis

Infectious mononucleosis (IM) is a disease that occurs in older children and adolescents when they develop a primary EBV infection. Other pathogens, notably cytomegalovirus and *Toxoplasma gondii*, can result in a similar clinical picture.

Epidemiology

Transmission occurs by mucosal contact with infected saliva (hence the term *kissing disease*) or possibly genital fluids. A majority of people are infected with EBV and seroconvert in early childhood. Such early infections are generally asymptomatic or mild in immunocompetent hosts, although the mononucleosis syndrome can occur in younger children as well.

CLINICAL MANIFESTATIONS

History and Physical Examination

The predominant symptom is usually a severe, exudative pharyngitis. Fever, generalized lymphadenopathy, and profound fatigue occur. Although the pharyngitis usually resolves within 1 to 2 weeks, the malaise may persist for several weeks. Other manifestations include hepatosplenomegaly, palatal petechiae, jaundice, and rash. Patients infected with EBV who are misdiagnosed with a bacterial infection and receive amoxicillin or ampicillin are much more likely to manifest the rash, which involves the face and trunk and is generally maculopapular.

Differential Diagnosis

Classic mononucleosis caused by EBV accounts for most cases. Other infectious agents that cause similar symptoms include CMV, *Toxoplasma gondii*, human herpesvirus 6, adenovirus, and HIV. Pharyngitis caused by GAS is difficult to distinguish from that of viruses without laboratory studies. Pancytopenia in the presence of the clinical manifestations listed previously suggests malignancy.

Diagnostic Evaluation

Leukocytosis or leukopenia may be present; lymphocytes account for more than 50% of leukocytes, and usually at least 10% are **atypical lymphocytes**. A heterophile antibody (or monospot) test allows rapid detection of EBV-associated mononucleosis in the outpatient setting; however, it has limited sensitivity in younger patients (<4 years of age) because they do not typically produce detectable heterophile antibodies. Specific serologic

TABLE 10-1 Revised Jones Criteria for the Diagnosis of Acute Rheumatic Fever

Manifestations	Minor Manifestations	Supporting Evidence of Major Antecedent GAS Infection
Carditis	***Clinical***	Positive throat culture for GAS or
Polyarthritis	Fever	Positive rapid antigen test or
Sydenham chorea	Arthralgia	Increased streptococcal antibody titer[a]
Erythema marginatum	***Laboratory***	
Subcutaneous nodules	Elevated ESR or	
	C-reactive protein	
	Prolonged P-R interval on ECG	

Diagnosis of acute rheumatic fever requires two major or one major and two minor criteria plus supporting evidence of antecedent group A streptococcal infection.
[a]Antibody tests include antistreptolysin-O (ASO), anti-DNase B, antihyaluronidase, or antistreptokinase.

antibody testing is available for EBV (Fig. 10-1) and CMV. Other laboratory findings may include thrombocytopenia and elevated hepatic transaminase levels.

Treatment

The disorder is typically self-limited, requiring only supportive care. Activity restrictions (i.e., no contact sports) are advised until any associated splenomegaly resolves because of the possibility of splenic rupture.

Rare but serious complications include upper airway obstruction (treated with corticosteroids), splenic rupture, and meningoencephalitis. Immunocompromised individuals are at risk for severe disseminated disease and lymphoproliferative disorders.

CROUP

Acute laryngotracheobronchitis, commonly called **croup**, refers to virus-induced inflammation of the laryngotracheal tissues, resulting in a syndrome of upper airway obstruction. Croup usually is caused by a paramyxovirus but can also result from other viruses, such as influenza and respiratory syncytial virus (RSV). It is most pronounced in young children (6 to 36 months of age) because of the narrow caliber of the airway below the vocal cords (subglottic region). Incidence peaks during the late fall and winter. At its most severe, the disease progresses to partial or total airway obstruction.

CLINICAL MANIFESTATIONS

History and Physical Examination

Children typically experience the sudden onset of a hoarse voice, barky (seal-like) cough, and inspiratory stridor, which may progress to respiratory distress. There is often a prodrome consisting of low-grade fever and rhinorrhea 12 to 24 hours prior to the onset of stridor. Respiratory compromise varies from minimal stridor with agitation to severe distress with tachypnea, hypoxia, nasal flaring, retractions, and impending airway obstruction.

Diagnostic Evaluation

The diagnosis usually is made on the basis of clinical findings. If obtained, anteroposterior neck and chest radiographs may reveal a tapered, narrow subglottic airway (steeple sign; Fig. 10-2). However, this finding is present in less than 50% of cases and does not correlate with disease severity.

Differential Diagnosis

The differential diagnosis of upper airway obstruction (Chapter 8) includes epiglottitis, bacterial tracheitis, foreign body aspiration, anaphylaxis, and angioneurotic edema. **Epiglottitis** consists of inflammation and edema of the epiglottis and aryepiglottic folds. It is considered a life-threatening emergency because of the propensity of the swollen tissues to result in sudden and irreversible airway occlusion. Most cases occur during the winter months in children 3 to 5 years of age. Fever, sore throat, hoarseness, and progressive stridor develop over 1 to 2 days. On examination, the child appears toxic, drools, and leans forward with chin extended to maximize airway patency. Lateral neck radiographs show "thumbprinting" of the epiglottis (Fig. 10-3). Although radiographs may aid in diagnosis, they are not recommended because they delay appropriate care. The child with suspected epiglottitis requires timely transport to the operating room and emergent endotracheal intubation. Emergency cricothyroidotomy may be performed if an endotracheal airway cannot be secured in the face of rapidly progressive obstruction. Intravenous ampicillin-sulbactam or a third-generation cephalosporin provides appropriate empirical coverage until the organism is identified by culture

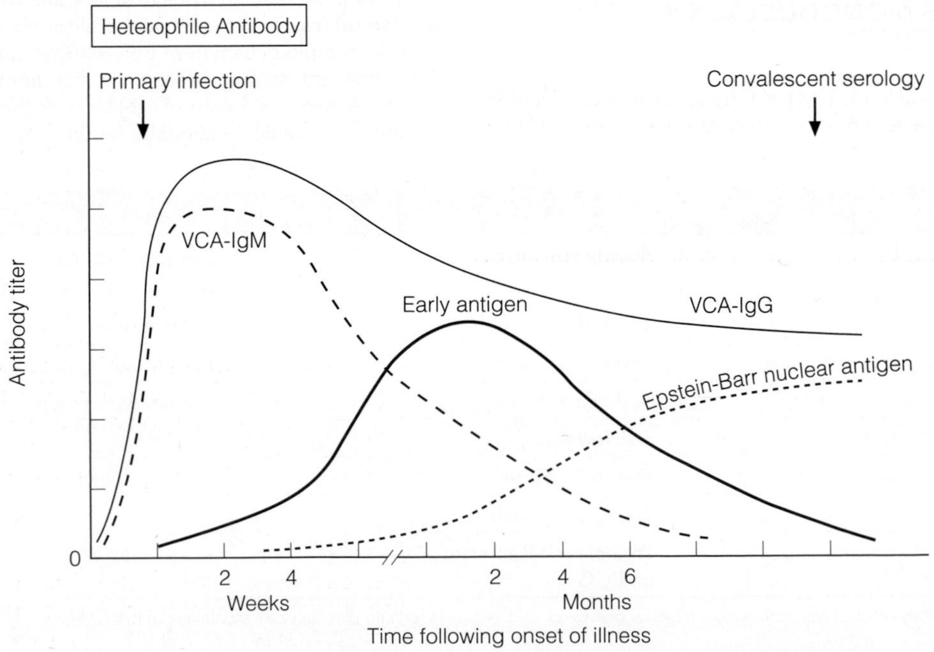

Figure 10-1 • Appearance of antibodies during EBV infection. (VCA: EBV-Viral Capsid Antigen)

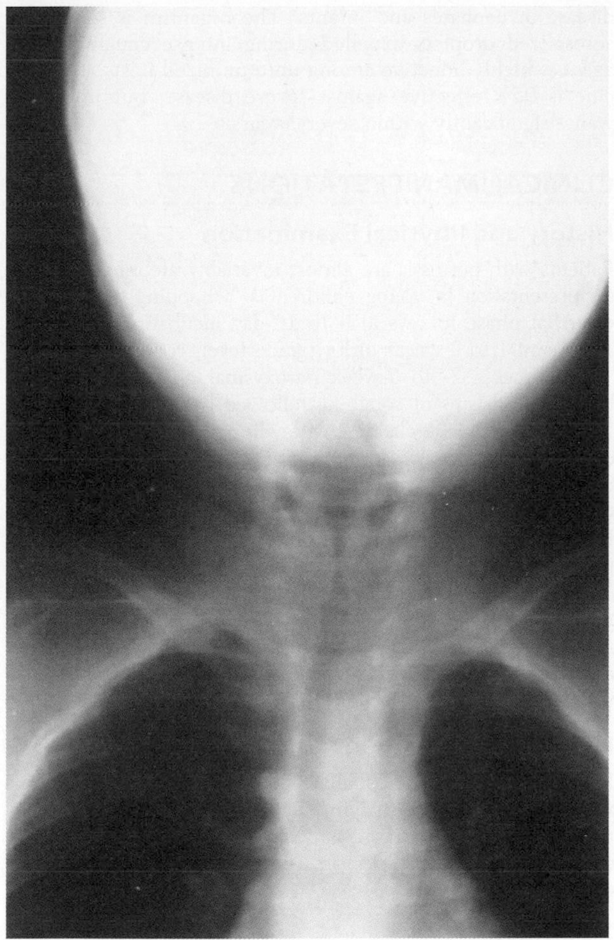

Figure 10-2 • Croup in a 3-year-old child. Note the "steeple sign" indicative of subglottic narrowing.

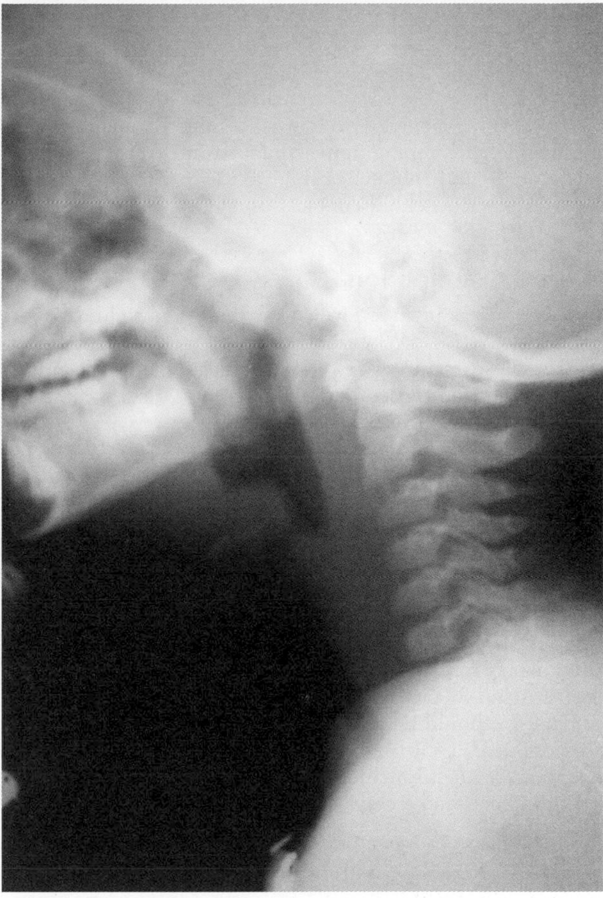

Figure 10-3 • Epiglottitis in a 4-year-old child with massive edema of the epiglottis, thickened aryepiglottic folds, and effacement of the valleculae.

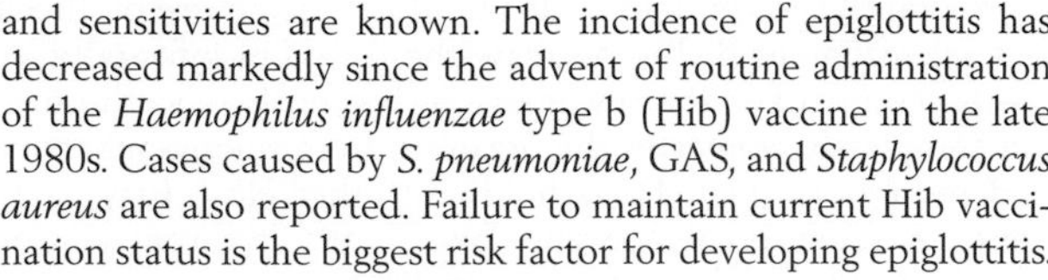

and sensitivities are known. The incidence of epiglottitis has decreased markedly since the advent of routine administration of the *Haemophilus influenzae* type b (Hib) vaccine in the late 1980s. Cases caused by *S. pneumoniae*, GAS, and *Staphylococcus aureus* are also reported. Failure to maintain current Hib vaccination status is the biggest risk factor for developing epiglottitis.

Treatment

Most children with croup never become symptomatic enough to prompt a visit to the pediatrician. Cough and stridor respond well to cool night air or humidity, and the disease resolves over 4 to 7 days. In the emergency department, stridulous infants receive cool mist, nebulized racemic epinephrine, and oral, intravenous, or intramuscular corticosteroids. Impending respiratory failure and airway obstruction constitute medical emergencies and are addressed accordingly (Chapter 20).

BRONCHIOLITIS

Pathogenesis

Bronchiolitis is an acute viral lower respiratory tract infection that results in inflammatory obstruction of the peripheral airways. There is a predominantly lymphocytic infiltrate into the peribronchial and peribronchiolar epithelium that promotes submucosal edema. Intraluminal mucous plugs and cellular debris accumulate because of impaired mucociliary clearance.

Epidemiology

Respiratory syncytial virus (RSV) causes the majority of cases; parainfluenza, influenza, human metapneumovirus, and adenovirus are also responsible viruses. Bronchiolitis typically occurs between November and April. At least half of all children are infected with RSV before 1 year of age, and recurrent infections throughout life are common. About 3% of infants in the first 12 months of life are hospitalized with bronchiolitis.

Risk Factors

Children with chronic lung disease, congenital heart disease, and congenital or acquired immunodeficiencies are more susceptible to severe disease. Hospitalization rates peak between 2 and 5 months of age. Predictors of severe illness include a respiratory rate greater than 70 per minute, hypoxia, atelectasis on chest radiograph, and a history of preterm birth.

CLINICAL MANIFESTATIONS

History

The acute illness lasts for 5 to 10 days, followed by gradual recovery over the next 1 to 2 weeks. Infected neonates may develop life-threatening **apnea**. Infants initially present with fever, cough, and rhinorrhea followed by progressive respiratory distress. Household contacts usually have upper respiratory symptoms.

Physical Examination

Physical findings include fever, tachypnea, and mild to severe respiratory distress. Wheezing, rhonchi, crackles, and accessory muscle use during respiration (tugging) may be noted. Ill infants may be restless or lethargic. Hypoxia is common in severely affected patients.

Differential Diagnosis

The wheezing associated with bronchiolitis may be difficult to distinguish from asthma or airway foreign body in older infants. Causes of recurrent episodes of wheezing include vascular rings, cystic fibrosis, and ciliary dyskinesia.

Diagnostic Evaluation

Rapid assays from nasal secretion samples exist for RSV, influenza A and B, and many other respiratory pathogens. Chest radiographs should be obtained for ill or hypoxic patients and for those with recurrent or unexplained wheezing. Findings consistent with bronchiolitis include lung hyperinflation, peri-bronchial thickening ("cuffing"), and increased interstitial markings.

Treatment

Hypoxic or ill-appearing children require hospitalization. Children with oxygen saturations greater than 94%, minimal respiratory distress, good fluid intake, reliable caretakers, and good follow-up may be treated as outpatients.

Most hospitalized infants require only supportive care (oxygen, fluid support) for their self-limited illness. Corticosteroids are not effective and are not indicated. Beta-adrenergic agents are not recommended for routine care of first-time wheezing associated with bronchiolitis. **Palivizumab**, an intramuscular RSV monoclonal antibody, provides passive prophylaxis and is recommended during the winter months for selected patients younger than 2 years of age who are at risk for severe disease. These patients include those with hemodynamically significant congenital heart disease or with chronic lung disease of prematurity requiring medical therapy within the 6 months prior to the start of the RSV season. Palivizumab is also recommended for select infants born prematurely (<35 weeks' gestation).

The mortality rate for hospitalized patients with RSV is less than 1%. Children with congenital heart defects, chronic lung disease, and immunodeficiency fare particularly poorly. Patients with documented RSV bronchiolitis may have more airway hyperresponsiveness later in life than the general population.

PERTUSSIS

Infection with *Bordetella pertussis* causes a URI and persistent cough in adults but may result in life-threatening respiratory disease in neonates and infants. The organism is spread via aerosolized droplets expelled during intense coughing. The agent is highly infective among unimmunized hosts. The vaccine is 95% effective against severe disease, but immunity wanes significantly within several years.

CLINICAL MANIFESTATIONS

History and Physical Examination

Patients with pertussis are almost invariably afebrile. The classic presentation in young children is "whooping cough." The **catarrhal phase** follows a 7- to 10-day incubation period and consists of 1 to 2 weeks of low-grade fever, cough, and coryza. Then comes a 2- to 6-week **paroxysmal phase** characterized by intense spasms of coughing followed by sudden inhalation, which produces the characteristic whoop. Posttussive emesis is common. Facial petechiae and scleral hemorrhages often develop due to forceful coughing. Most symptoms remit during the **convalescent phase**, but the cough may persist for 2 to 8 weeks. Infants with severe disease may present with apnea or the typical paroxysmal cough followed by choking and progressive cyanosis. The characteristic whoop is absent in very young infants because they cannot generate sufficient negative inspiratory force.

Adolescents and adults can also be infected with pertussis and usually present with nonspecific upper respiratory symptoms and a protracted cough.

Diagnostic Evaluation

Laboratory evaluation usually reveals significant leukocytosis with a predominance of lymphocytes. Nasopharyngeal secretions contain the organism, which may be detected by PCR or culture. The chest radiograph usually is normal, but nonspecific infiltrates may be seen.

Treatment

Young infants with severe disease should be hospitalized to manage apnea, cyanosis, hypoxia, and feeding difficulties. Erythromycin estolate or azithromycin shortens the duration of illness *if given early in the catarrhal phase*. After the coughing paroxysms begin, antibiotics do not affect the course of illness but are recommended to decrease the period of infectivity. A 14-day course of erythromycin or a 5-day course of azithromycin completely eradicates the organism from the nasopharynx and respiratory tract. Household and other close (day care) contacts require chemoprophylaxis with erythromycin or azithromycin regardless of immunization status.

PNEUMONIA

Pathogenesis

Pneumonia refers to an acute inflammatory process occurring in the lungs. It may be infectious or noninfectious. Inflammation can occur in the alveolar space (lobar pneumonia), the alveolar walls (interstitial pneumonia), and/or the bronchi.

Epidemiology

The age of an immunocompetent child suggests an etiologic organism (Table 10-2). Viruses are the most common cause of pneumonia in young children. *Chlamydia trachomatis* pneumonia manifests at 2 to 3 months of age in infants born to women with untreated genital C. *trachomatis* infection.

TABLE 10-2 Causes of Infectious Pneumonia by Age

<1 Month	1 to 6 Months	6 Months to 5 Years	School Age/Adolescent
Group B streptococci	*Streptococcus pneumoniae*[a]	*Streptococcus pneumoniae*[a]	*Mycoplasma pneumoniae*
Escherichia coli/gram-negative enteric bacilli	*Staphylococcus aureus*	*Moraxella catarrhalis*	*Chlamydophila pneumoniae*
Haemophilus influenza	*Moraxella catarrhalis*	*Haemophilus influenzae*	*Streptococcus pneumoniae*[a]
Streptococcus pneumonia	*H. influenzae*	*Staphylococcus aureus*	*H. influenzae*
Group D streptococci	*Bordetella pertussis*	*Neisseria meningitidis*	*S. aureus*
Listeria monocytogenes	*Chlamydia trachomatis*[b]	*Mycoplasma pneumoniae*	*Mycobacterium tuberculosis*
Anaerobes	*Ureaplasma urealyticum*[b]	Group A streptococci	Viruses[c]
Cytomegalovirus	Cytomegalovirus[b]	*Mycobacterium tuberculosis*	
Herpes simplex virus	Viruses[c]	Viruses[c]	
Ureaplasma urealyticum			
Staphylococcus aureus			

[a]Most common cause of bacterial pneumonia in this age group.
[b]Although acquired perinatally, these infections often do not present as pneumonia until after 1 month of age.
[c]Including respiratory syncytial virus, influenza, parainfluenza, and adenovirus.

S. pneumoniae should be considered in any community-acquired lower respiratory tract infection. *Mycoplasma pneumoniae* pneumonia is uncommon in children younger than 5 years but, along with *Chlamydophila* (formerly *Chlamydia*) *pneumoniae*, becomes a more frequent and important pathogen in school-age children and adolescents. Less common bacterial causes include nontypeable *H. influenzae*, *M. catarrhalis*, *S. aureus*, *N. meningitidis*, and GAS.

Risk Factors

Conditions associated with an increased risk of bacterial pneumonia include the following:

- Chronic lung disease, including cystic fibrosis and asthma
- Neurologic impairment (swallowing dysfunction or neuromuscular disease)
- Gastroesophageal reflux with aspiration of gastric contents
- Upper airway anatomic defects (tracheoesophageal fistula, cleft palate)
- Hemoglobinopathies (including sickle cell anemia)
- Immunodeficiency or immunosuppressive therapy

CLINICAL MANIFESTATIONS

History

Viral pneumonia develops gradually over 2 to 4 days. It is usually preceded by upper respiratory symptoms such as cough, rhinorrhea, postnasal drip, coryza, and low-grade fever. Infants with pneumonia caused by *C. trachomatis* are afebrile and have conjunctivitis and a staccato cough. Infants and young children with bacterial pneumonia may present with nonspecific constitutional complaints, including fever, irritability, poor feeding, vomiting, abdominal pain, and lethargy. Abrupt onset of fever, chills, dyspnea, and chest pain is typical. Productive cough is more common in older patients. *M. pneumoniae* and *C. pneumoniae* pneumonia present initially with fever, headache, and myalgia. These symptoms gradually subside over 5 to 7 days, whereas coughing increases and persists for 2 weeks or more.

Physical Examination

Any indication of respiratory distress can signal pneumonia, although tachypnea and dyspnea are most common. Tachypnea out of proportion to fever is an important clue to pneumonia in the young child. Diffuse wheezing and crackles suggest involvement of multiple areas of the lung, characteristic of viral or atypical (*M. pneumoniae*, *C. pneumoniae*, *C. trachomatis*) pneumonia. Focal findings such as focal crackles or decreased breath sounds, dullness to percussion, egophony, and bronchophony suggest pneumonia of bacterial origin. Pneumonia can also present with only fever and tachypnea in the absence of chest findings.

Cyanosis is uncommon except in severe disease. Approximately 10% of patients with *M. pneumoniae* infection develop a rash, usually macular and erythematous or urticarial; erythema multiforme has also been reported.

Differential Diagnosis

Pneumonia is much more common in the pediatric population than are other conditions with similar presentations, including congestive heart failure (CHF), chemical pneumonitis, pulmonary embolism, sarcoidosis, and primary or metastatic malignancy.

Diagnostic Evaluation

A thorough history and physical examination usually suggest the diagnosis. Sputum culture is not likely to be helpful because pediatric patients typically do not produce adequate sputum samples. Chest radiograph remains an excellent test for defining the extent and pattern of involvement and assessing related complications (i.e., pleural effusion, pneumatocele). Bacterial pneumonia usually causes lobar consolidation. Diffuse interstitial infiltrates suggest viral or atypical pneumonia, although children with *Mycoplasma* pneumonia may have lobar consolidation. Aspiration pneumonia is typically located in the right middle or right upper lobe.

In selected children with pneumonia, laboratory evaluations are indicated to try to identify a specific pathogen. When a large pleural effusion is present, the pleural fluid should be drained and sent for cell counts, Gram stain, and culture. When a child with a high fever is hospitalized with pneumonia, a blood culture should be considered. When influenza is circulating locally, rapid influenza testing is helpful in guiding decisions about antiviral therapies. *C. trachomatis* pneumonia is diagnosed by direct fluorescent antibody, PCR testing or tissue culture of conjunctival or nasopharyngeal specimens. *M. pneumoniae* can be noted by PCR of specimens obtained by nasopharyngeal swab or by specific antimycoplasmal IgM antibody determination. However, these IgM antibodies persist in serum for several months and may not represent current infection. Cold-agglutinin titers are elevated not only in *M. pneumoniae* infections but also in many cases of viral (and some cases of bacterial) pneumonia.

Treatment

Therapy depends on the most likely pathogen. In the outpatient setting, high-dose amoxicillin or amoxicillin/clavulanic acid is appropriate for most cases of bacterial pneumonia when antibiotics are thought to be necessary. Erythromycin, azithromycin, or clarithromycin is recommended for so-called "walking pneumonia" caused by *M. pneumoniae* or *C. pneumoniae*. Azithromcyin or erythromycin is used to treat infants with pneumonia caused by *C. trachomatis*.

Any child with persistent hypoxia (which necessitates oxygen therapy), moderate to severe respiratory distress, and/or hemodynamic instability requires hospitalization. Intravenous antibiotic options for bacterial pneumonia include ampicillin/sulbactam, clindamycin, cefuroxime, ceftriaxone, azithromycin, and vancomycin depending on the suspected pathogens and community susceptibility patterns. Neonates with suspected bacterial pneumonia receive additional workup (lumbar puncture) and are started on ampicillin and cefotaxime (or gentamicin if the CSF is sterile). Most viral infections are self-limited. Patients with severe disease (bacterial or viral) may require supportive therapy and intubation.

The most frequent complication is development of a pleural effusion large enough to compromise respiratory effort. Empyema results when purulent fluid from an adjacent lung infection drains into the pleural space. Although virtually any infectious agent can cause an effusion, large effusions are much more likely to result from *S. aureus*. Community-acquired, methicillin-resistant *S. aureus* is increasingly being recognized as a cause of complicated pneumonia and empyema. Pleurocentesis (with possible chest tube placement) provides rapid relief. Lung abscesses may complicate anaerobic infections.

MENINGITIS

Pathogenesis

Almost any pathogen can infect the leptomeninges and CSF. Viral meningitis is typically an acute, self-limited illness; bacterial meningitis is a life-threatening condition associated with substantial morbidity and mortality. The term **aseptic meningitis** refers to meningeal inflammation caused by an antigenic stimulus other than pyogenic bacteria (e.g., enterovirus or Lyme disease).

Epidemiology

The likely etiology of meningitis depends on age (Table 10-3). Beyond the neonatal period, viral meningitis is much more common than bacterial meningitis. Both infants and older children are at risk for meningitis caused by enteroviruses (the most common cause of viral meningitis). Enteroviruses primarily circulate in the late summer and early fall. Overall, *S. pneumoniae* and *N. meningitidis* are the most common bacterial pathogens. Neonates and children younger than 3 years are at highest risk for bacterial meningitis. The Hib vaccine has nearly eliminated *H. influenzae* type b meningitis in the United States. Lyme meningitis, caused by *Borrelia burgdorferi*, usually affects school-age children and adolescents. Rare causes of meningitis and meningoencephalitis include EBV, *Bartonella henselae* (cat-scratch disease), *M. tuberculosis*, and *Cryptococcus neoformans*.

Risk Factors

Risk factors for bacterial meningitis are the same as those for sepsis, because most cases result from hematogenous seeding. Direct invasion occurs as a result of trauma, mastoiditis, sinusitis,

TABLE 10-3 Causes of Meningitis by Age

<1 Month	1 to 2 Months	2 Months to 6 Years	School Age/Adolescent
Group B streptococci	*Escherichia coli*	*Streptococcus pneumoniae*	*S. pneumoniae*
Escherichia coli	*S. pneumoniae*	*Neisseria meningitidis*	*N. meningitidis*
Other gram-negative bacilli	Enteroviruses	Enteroviruses	Enteroviruses
Herpes simplex virus	*Haemophilus influenzae* type b[a]	*Borrelia burgdorferi*	*B. burgdorferi*
Listeria monocytogenes	Group B streptococci	*H. influenzae* type b[a]	
Streptococcus pneumonia			

[a]Rare in immunized populations.

and anatomic defects in the scalp or skull. In the neonate, low birth weight, prolonged rupture of membranes, and chorioamnionitis predispose to septicemia and meningitis; myelomeningocele also increases the risk.

CLINICAL MANIFESTATIONS

History

Classic symptoms of meningitis include nausea, vomiting, photophobia, irritability, lethargy, headache, and stiff neck. Viral meningitis is preceded by a nonspecific prodrome of fever, malaise, sore throat, and myalgias. Unless complicated by encephalitis, symptoms of most viral CNS infections generally resolve over 2 to 4 days and may improve after LP. In bacterial meningitis, the prodromal phase is absent and the fever is generally quite high. Mental status changes, focal neurologic signs, ataxia, seizures, and shock are not uncommon. Lyme meningitis is characterized by low-grade fever, headache, stiff neck, and photophobia developing over the course of 1 to 2 weeks. Cranial nerve palsies may occur.

Physical Examination

Patients with bacterial meningitis often appear toxic and may be hypertensive, bradycardic, and even apneic. In older children, signs of increased intracranial pressure include cranial nerve palsies and papilledema. Nuchal rigidity and positive **Kernig** (flexion of the leg at the hip with subsequent pain on knee extension) and **Brudzinski** (involuntary leg flexion on passive neck flexion) **signs** are markers for meningeal irritation. These findings are rarely present in children younger than 1 year. Infants may present with a bulging fontanelle. A rash is often present with *N. meningitidis* (petechial or purpuric) and Lyme (erythema migrans) CNS infections.

Differential Diagnosis

The differential diagnosis includes encephalitis, which may develop concurrently or subsequently (Chapter 15). Other conditions that may present with a similar clinical picture include drug intoxication or side effects, recent anoxia or hypoxia, primary or metastatic CNS malignancy, bacterial endocarditis with septic embolism, intracranial hemorrhage/hematoma, malignant hypertension, and demyelination disorders.

Diagnostic Evaluation

CSF analysis is diagnostic. Tests include cell counts and differential, Gram stain, glucose and protein levels, and culture. Bacteria are detected on Gram stain in approximately 80% of cases of bacterial meningitis. PCR assays for CSF HSV and enteroviruses are available and are highly sensitive and specific. Table 10-4 describes CSF findings that suggest a specific etiology. Because of the potential for brainstem herniation, LP should not be attempted in a child with focal neurologic deficits and/or increased intracranial pressure until an expanding mass lesion is excluded by CT or MRI. Other contraindications include cardiopulmonary instability and skin infection overlying the LP site.

Treatment

When the diagnosis of uncomplicated viral meningitis is unequivocal, hospitalization is generally not necessary. If bacterial meningitis cannot be excluded, the patient should be hospitalized for intravenous antibiotic therapy.

Vancomycin plus a third-generation cephalosporin (cefotaxime or ceftriaxone) achieves therapeutic levels in the CSF and provides broad-spectrum coverage of the most likely pathogens in infants and older children. Neonates should be treated with ampicillin to other group B streptococci and *L. monocytogenes*; cefotaxime is added to cover gram-negative pathogens. Once an organism and its susceptibility pattern are known, antibiotic coverage may be adjusted. The course of therapy for bacterial meningitis is usually 10 to 14 days. Exceptions include meningococcal meningitis (5 to 7 days), Lyme meningitis (14 to 28 days), and neonatal meningitis (14 to 21 days).

The current mortality rate for bacterial meningitis is up to 30% for neonates and less than 10% for infants and older children. However, 10% to 20% of patients experience some persistent neurologic deficit, most commonly hearing loss, developmental delay, motor incoordination, seizures, and hydrocephalus.

GASTROENTERITIS

Pathogens cause diarrhea by a variety of mechanisms. For example, some bacteria invade intestinal tissue directly, whereas others secrete injurious toxins before or after ingestion. Viruses, parasites, and protozoa also are capable of inflicting disease. Excessive stooling causes dehydration, inadequate nutrition, and electrolyte abnormalities, all of which are poorly tolerated in infants and small children.

CLINICAL MANIFESTATIONS

History

The history should include information about symptoms in other family members, recent travel, medication use, immune

TABLE 10-4 Cerebrospinal Fluid Findings Suggesting a Specific Etiology for Meningitis in Childhood

CSF Parameter	Bacterial	Viral	Lyme
White blood cells (per mm^3)	>1,000	<500	<100
Neutrophils	>75%	<50%[a]	<30%
Protein	↑↑	Normal or ↑	Normal or ↑
Glucose	↓ or ↓↓	Normal	Normal

[a]Neutrophils may predominate early in the course of viral meningitis; mononuclear cells usually predominate in Lyme meningitis.
↑, mild increase; ↑↑, moderate or severe increase; ↓, mild decrease; ↓↓, moderate or severe decrease.

status, day care attendance, source of drinking water, contact with animals, duration of symptoms, fever, and number, color, and character of stools.

The most common bacterial causes of gastroenteritis include *Salmonella* species, *Shigella* species, *Escherichia coli*, *Yersinia enterocolitica*, and *Campylobacter jejuni*; *Vibrio cholerae* may be acquired during travel to developing nations and from eating undercooked Gulf Coast shellfish. Patients with bacterial diarrhea present with fever, significant abdominal cramping, malaise, and tenesmus; vomiting is less common. The stools contain mucus and may be guaiac positive or streaked with blood. Occasionally, children with shigellosis present with **neurologic** manifestations (lethargy, seizures, mental status changes). *Salmonella* species are capable of invading the bloodstream and causing extraintestinal disease, including meningitis and osteomyelitis (particularly in children with sickle cell anemia). *Shigella dysenteriae* and *E. coli* O157:H7 produce an enterotoxin (Shiga or Shigalike toxin) associated with **hemolytic uremic syndrome**, a serious complication consisting of microangiopathic hemolytic anemia, nephropathy, and thrombocytopenia. Up to 30% of individuals infected with *Y. enterocolitica* develop subsequent **erythema nodosum**. In some patients, particularly those with *Yersinia*, severe pain localizes to the right lower quadrant, creating a "pseudoappendicitis" picture.

In cholera, the stools quickly become colorless and flecked with mucus, termed "rice-water" stools. Severe diarrhea leading to hypovolemic shock may develop in hours to a few days.

Clostridium difficile produces toxins that cause antibiotic-associated diarrhea and pseudomembranous colitis. Colonization by toxin-producing strains without symptoms is common in infants younger than 1 year of age.

Rotavirus is the major cause of nonbacterial gastroenteritis in infants and toddlers throughout the world. Infections peak in the cooler months. Complaints include profuse diarrhea, vomiting, and low-grade fever. Severe diarrhea may lead to significant dehydration, acidosis, and electrolyte disturbances. **Noroviruses** cause similar episodic outbreaks of vomiting and watery diarrhea in all age groups.

Giardiasis is the most commonly reported intestinal parasitic disease in the United States. More water-related outbreaks of diarrhea are caused by *Giardia lamblia* than any other organism. The illness presents with frequent, foul-smelling, watery stools that rarely contain blood or mucus; abdominal pain, nausea, vomiting, anorexia, and flatulence often accompany the diarrhea. Symptoms generally resolve within 5 to 7 days, although some cases linger for more than a month. Patients with chronic giardiasis are at risk for failure to thrive resulting from ongoing malabsorption.

Physical Examination

The main goals of the physical examination are estimating the degree of dehydration (Chapter 5), judging the stability of the patient's condition, identifying findings that may point to a specific infectious or noninfectious etiology, and ruling out a surgical condition.

Differential Diagnosis

Acute diarrhea in childhood is usually caused by infection. Other conditions associated with diarrhea include malabsorption, celiac disease, antibiotic use, cystic fibrosis, and inflammatory bowel disease.

Diagnostic Evaluation

Electrolyte and renal function studies ($Na+$, $K+$, Cl^-, HCO_3^-, BUN, creatinine) guide replacement therapy in significantly dehydrated children (Chapter 5). Abdominal radiographs, if obtained, are generally normal or nonspecific. Blood, mucus, and fecal leukocytes suggest a bacterial origin for the illness. Blood culture should be performed at the time of initial evaluation if bacterial disease is suspected. Bacterial stool culture results take several days but are helpful in determining the need for antibiotics. If there is a history of antibiotic use, stool should be tested for *Clostridium difficile* toxins A and B. Rapid antigen testing is available for rotavirus. If *G. lamblia* infection is suspected, multiple stool samples from different times should be examined for cysts. Immunofluorescent antibody detection in stool can also be used to diagnose *G. lamblia* infection. Endoscopic biopsy may be indicated if the diarrhea becomes chronic and no etiology has been identified.

Treatment

Treatment incorporates oral rehydration whenever possible; aggressive parenteral therapy may be required in severe cases. Antidiarrheal agents are to be avoided in children.

Unless the patient is a febrile infant younger than 3 months or appears toxic, antibiotics should generally be withheld pending culture results. Antibiotic therapy prolongs *Salmonella* shedding and should be reserved for bacteremia or extraintestinal dissemination and for high-risk patients with noninvasive gastroenteritis, including infants less than 3 months of age and immunocompromised persons. Antibiotics may enhance the likelihood of development of hemolytic uremic syndrome among patients with diarrhea caused by *E. coli* O157:H7. Trimethoprim-sulfamethoxazole or azithromycin is often effective in treating shigellosis. Erythromycin or azithromycin is the treatment of choice for *C. jejuni*. Patients with *C. difficile* enterocolitis usually improve with suspension of antibiotic therapy, but if treatment is warranted, metronidazole is the medication of choice for initial treatment. Patients with giardiasis are also treated with oral metronidazole.

As long as the patient does not develop hypovolemic shock, prognosis for full recovery is excellent. Even in life-threatening cases, appropriate management often prevents permanent sequelae.

PINWORM INFECTION

The roundworm *Enterobius vermicularis* causes pinworm infection. Preschool- and school-aged children have the highest rates of pinworm infection. Itching in the perianal and vulvar regions is a common presenting symptom. Examination may be normal. Diagnosis can be established by touching the perianal skin with transparent adhesive tape to collect any eggs; the tape is then applied to a glass slide and examined under a low-power microscopic lens. Very few ova are present in stool; therefore, stool ova and parasite examinations are not recommended. The drugs of choice are mebendazole, pyrantel pamoate, or albendazole, given in a single dose and repeated in 2 weeks. Pinworm infections may cluster in families, and therefore all household members are often treated as a group. Reinfections are common and may be treated in the same manner as the first infection. Hand washing is the most effective method of preventing pinworm infection.

HEPATITIS

Pathogenesis

Acute hepatic inflammation in children can be caused by a large number of infectious and noninfectious etiologies. Primary hepatotropic viruses include hepatitis A virus (HAV), hepatitis B virus (HBV), hepatitis C virus (HCV), hepatitis D virus (HDV, formerly delta hepatitis), and hepatitis E virus (HEV). Table 10-5 compares features of HAV, HBV, and HCV, the three most common pathogens.

Epidemiology

HAV and HEV are acquired via fecal–oral transmission. The incidence of hepatitis A infection among United States children is decreasing because of the addition of routine vaccination against hepatitis A in infancy. HBV, HCV, and HDV are transmitted by percutaneous or mucosal exposure to infectious body fluids and by vertical transmission from an infected mother to her infant. HDV, or delta antigen, consists of single-stranded RNA. It is a "defective" virus in that it requires the presence of an active HBV infection to replicate. HBV and HCV can persist for many years following acute infection. This "carrier state" is associated with development of hepatocellular carcinoma. The incidence of hepatitis B infection is low in the pediatric population because of routine vaccination against hepatitis B in infancy.

Risk Factors

Intravenous drug users and those who have unprotected sex with multiple partners are at increased risk of contracting HBV, HCV, and HDV. Transmission by transfusion of contaminated blood or blood products is rare in the United States. Risk factors for HAV and HEV include foreign travel, poor sanitation, and contact with other children in day care.

CLINICAL MANIFESTATIONS

History

Perinatally infected infants are usually asymptomatic. Clinical signs of acute hepatitis include anorexia, nausea, malaise, vomiting, jaundice, dark urine, abdominal pain, and low-grade fever. Children with HAV and HEV may also have diarrhea. However, a wide range of severity exists, and as many as 30% to 70% of infected children are asymptomatic. HBV and HCV infection are usually silent, in that the patient complains of no symptoms unless chronic infection has caused significant hepatic damage.

Physical Examination

Scleral icterus and jaundice may or may not be present. Other possible signs and symptoms include hepatomegaly and right upper-quadrant tenderness. A benign-appearing rash may appear early in the course of hepatitis B.

Differential Diagnosis

EBV, CMV, enterovirus, and other viral infections can also cause hepatitis, but other organ systems are usually involved. Jaundice may also result from autoimmune hepatitis, metabolic liver disease, biliary tract disorders, and drug ingestions.

Diagnostic Evaluation

Liver enzymes are uniformly elevated in hepatitis. Because the clinical manifestations are so similar, specific serologic tests are indispensable for securing an accurate diagnosis. The presence of anti-HAV IgM antibody confirms HAV infection (Fig. 10-4). Tests are also available to detect antibodies to the delta antigen.

Three different particles may be found in the serum of patients infected with HBV. The Dane particle is the largest, made up of a core antigen (HBcAg) and envelope antigen (HBeAg) surrounded by a spherical shell of HBsAg ("surface") particles. Figure 10-5 and Table 10-6 present the clinical course and serologic markers important in diagnosing HBV disease stage. Anti-HBs heralds resolution of the illness and confers lifelong immunity.

HCV antibody is present in both acute and chronic infection. HCV RNA can be detected by PCR within 1 week of infection, whereas the "window period" from infection to antibody response for HCV may be as long as 12 weeks. Therefore, the presence of HCV RNA in the absence of an antibody response indicates acute infection. Recovery is characterized by the disappearance of HCV RNA from the blood.

TABLE 10-5 Viruses Responsible for Hepatitis: Comparison and Summary

Feature	Hepatitis A	Hepatitis B	Hepatitis C
Virus type	RNA	DNA	RNA
Incubation (days)	15 to 45	45 to 180	14 to 180
Period of infectivity	Late incubation to early symptomatic state	When HBsAg seropositive	Unknown
Fulminant hepatitis	<1%	1% to 3%	1%
Chronic hepatitis	No	5% to 10% of adults; 25% to 50% of infants; 90% of neonates whose mothers are HBeAg positive	50%
Diagnostic evaluation	Anti-HAV IgM	HBsAg, HBeAg, anti-HBs, anti-HBc, anti-HBe	Anti-HCV antibody, HCV PCR

anti-HBc, total antibody to hepatitis B core antigen; anti-HBe, total antibody to hepatitis B e antigen; anti-HBs, total antibody to hepatitis B surface antigen; HAV, hepatitis A virus; HBeAg, hepatitis B e antigen; HBsAg, hepatitis B surface antigen; HCV, hepatitis C virus.

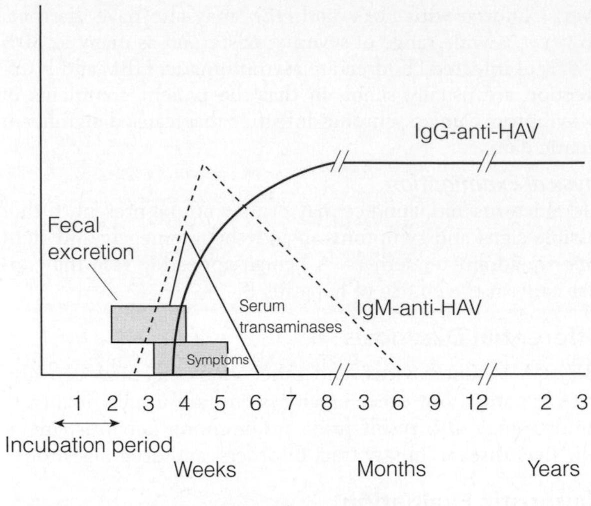

Figure 10-4 • Typical course of acute hepatitis A.

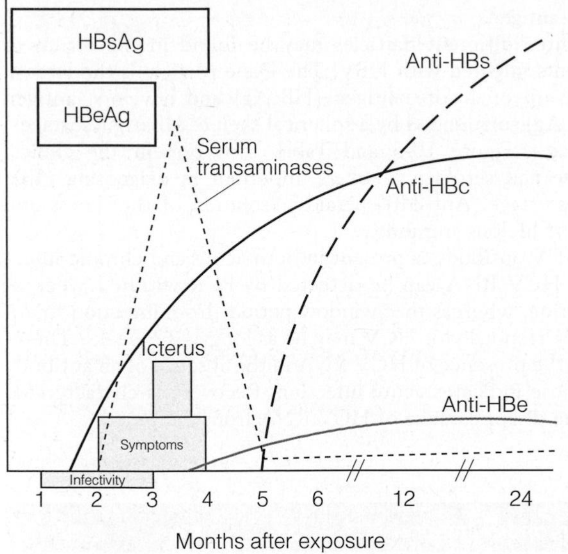

Figure 10-5 • The course of acute hepatitis B.

Prevention

Both active and passive forms of immunization are available, depending on the source of infection. HAV immunization is recommended for all infants in the United States. Immune globulin prevents hepatitis A clinical disease when administered within 14 days of exposure. The HBV vaccine series is also recommended for all infants in the United States. Infants of infected mothers should receive both the vaccine and the HBV immunoglobulin at delivery to prevent the disease and development of the carrier state.

Prognosis

The prognosis for patients with hepatitis depends on the virus responsible.

- HAV: Very few patients develop fulminant hepatitis, but the mortality rate among those who do is almost 50%.
- HBV: HBV may persist as chronic hepatitis, and the course may be relatively benign or more severe. Chronic persistent hepatitis B is characterized by little cellular inflammation and usually resolves within 1 year. Chronic active hepatitis is more aggressive, progressing to cirrhosis and increasing the risk of hepatocellular carcinoma. Chronic infection is more likely among infected children than adults.
- HDV: When HDV and HBV are acquired simultaneously, the recipient is at greater risk for more severe chronic hepatitis B and fulminant hepatitis associated with a higher mortality rate. When an individual is infected with HDV on top of preexisting HBV, acute exacerbation and an accelerated course result. The risk of progressing to cirrhotic liver disease is also increased when HDV is present.
- HCV: Half of those infected with HCV develop chronic hepatitis, with an increased risk for cirrhosis.
- HEV: HEV does not appear to result in chronic hepatitis.

SYPHILIS

Pathogenesis

Syphilis is primarily a sexually transmitted disease (STD) resulting from infection with the spirochete *Treponema pallidum*.

Epidemiology

Syphilis in the pediatric population may be acquired transplacentally (congenital syphilis) or through sexual contact. The incidence of syphilis has increased sharply over the past few decades. Coinfection with other STDs is common.

TABLE 10-6 Comparisons of Disease States in Hepatitis B Virus

Test	Acute HBV	Resolved HBV	Chronic HBV
HBsAg	+	–	+
Anti-HBs	–	+	–
Anti-HBc	+	+	+
HBeAg	±	–	±
Anti-HBe	–	+	±

anti-HBc, total antibody to hepatitis B core antigen; anti-HBe, total antibody to hepatitis B e antigen; anti-HBs, total antibody to hepatitis B surface antigen; HBeAg, hepatitis B e antigen; HBsAg, hepatitis B surface antigen; HBV, hepatitis B virus.

Risk Factors

Neonates born to mothers with untreated infections are at risk for congenital syphilis. Adolescents and adults who have unprotected sex with an infected partner or multiple partners are at risk for primary syphilis.

CLINICAL MANIFESTATIONS

History and Physical Examination

Approximately half of infants with congenital syphilis die shortly before or after birth. Those who survive are often asymptomatic at birth but develop symptoms within 1 month if untreated. Infants with congenital syphilis may have hepatomegaly, splenomegaly, mucocutaneous lesions, jaundice, lymphadenopathy, and the characteristic **snuffles** (a bloody, mucopurulent nasal discharge). Long-term sequelae include deafness and mental retardation.

Syphilis acquired through sexual contact progresses through three stages. After a 2- to 4-week incubation period, infected individuals enter the **primary** stage of syphilis, characterized by the classic **chancre** at the inoculation site: a well-demarcated, firm, painless genital ulcer with an indurated base (Color Plate 17). Because the lesion heals spontaneously within 3 to 6 weeks, patients with primary syphilis often do not seek medical attention.

Untreated patients may develop **secondary** syphilis, manifested by widespread dermatologic involvement coinciding with dissemination of the spirochete throughout the body. Onset follows the primary stage directly, often while the chancre is still present. The typical rash consists of generalized (including the soles and palms) erythematous macules (3 to 10 mm) that progress to papules (Color Plate 18). Some patients also develop systemic symptoms including fever, malaise, pharyngitis, mucosal ulcerations, and generalized lymphadenopathy; patchy alopecia and thinning of the lateral third of the eyebrow are also associated with secondary syphilis. Symptoms of secondary syphilis resolve in 1 to 3 months.

About one-third of untreated patients develop late manifestations or **tertiary** syphilis years after primary exposure. Tertiary syphilis is rare in the pediatric population. Granulomatous lesions called **gummas** destroy surrounding tissues, especially in the skin, bone, heart, and CNS. Unfortunately, tertiary syphilis may occur without any previous primary or secondary manifestations.

Differential Diagnosis

Syphilis is one of the great masqueraders, a disease with a wide spectrum of presentations. The presence of the rash, if characteristic, greatly aids in diagnosis.

Diagnostic Evaluation

Chancre scrapings (and mucosal secretions in infected neonates) demonstrate rapidly mobile organisms moving in a corkscrew-like motion under dark-field microscopy. Aspiration of enlarged lymph nodes may also yield the organism. Both the VDRL (developed by the Venereal Disease Research Laboratory of the U.S. Public Health Service) and the RPR (Rapid Plasma Reagin) are excellent blood screening tests for high-risk populations, providing rapid, inexpensive, quantitative results. Both are nontreponemal tests for antibodies to a lipoidal molecule rather than the organism itself. Both are considered highly sensitive when titers are high or when the test is complemented by historical or physical evidence of the disease. However, infectious mononucleosis, connective tissue disease, endocarditis, and tuberculosis may all result in false positive VDRL and RPR results. By contrast, treponemal tests, such as the fluorescent treponemal antibody absorption (FTA-ABS) and *Treponema pallidum* particle agglutination (TP-PA) are much less likely to produce false positives. A positive screening VDRL or RPR coupled with a positive FTA-ABS or TP-PA in a newborn or sexually active adolescent is virtually diagnostic of untreated syphilis. Nontreponemal tests may become negative after treatment, whereas treponemal studies remain positive for life.

Neonates with suspected congenital syphilis require lumbar puncture. CSF pleocytosis and elevated protein suggest neurosyphilis. A positive CSF VDRL is diagnostic. Untreated infants may develop anemia, thrombocytopenia, and radiographic abnormalities of the long bones.

Treatment

Parenteral penicillin G (IM or intravenous) remains the treatment of choice for any stage of infection and fully eradicates the organism from the body.

GENITAL HSV INFECTION

Genital herpes usually results from infection with HSV type 2. However, HSV type 1 may also cause genital lesions. Small mucosal tears or skin cracks are inoculated with the virus during sexual activity. Herpes is one of the most common sexually acquired diseases; about 20% of adults have a history suggestive of prior genital herpes infection. Transmission of HSV from mother to infant at the time of birth may result in devastating infection in the newborn.

Clinical Manifestations

History and Physical Examination

After a variable incubation period (5 to 14 days), genital burning and itching progress to vesicular, often pustular, lesions. These burst to form painful shallow ulcers that heal without scarring (Color Plate 19). Fever, pharyngitis, headache, and malaise may accompany the primary episode. After acquisition, the virus ascends peripheral nerves to dorsal root ganglia, where it may lie latent or recur periodically. Recurrences have fewer symptoms than the primary episode, and asymptomatic shedding occurs. Individuals with genital herpes should be counseled that HSV can potentially be spread to their sexual partners even when genital lesions are not present.

Diagnostic Evaluation

Giant multinucleated cells with intranuclear inclusions are found in scrapings from the ulcer base (Tzanck testing). HSV may be cultured from the active lesions in 1 to 4 days; direct fluorescent antibody staining and PCR testing are also available. Serum tests for HSV (type-common and type-specific) IgG antibodies are not routinely recommended. They may be negative early in primary infection. However, if positive, HSV type 2-specific IgG is useful in confirming a clinical diagnosis of genital herpes.

Treatment

Oral antiviral agents (including acyclovir) diminish the length of both symptoms and shedding but do not eradicate HSV. They have limited efficacy in recurrent episodes. Continued prophylactic use of oral acyclovir prevents or reduces the frequency of recurrences. Patients should be counseled regarding potential to spread HSV to others even without active or visible genital lesions.

OTHER SEXUALLY TRANSMITTED INFECTIONS

Infections with *Neisseria gonorrhoeae* (gonorrhea), *Chlamydia trachomatis*, *Trichomonas vaginalis*, and human papillomaviruses are covered in Chapter 3.

PELVIC INFLAMMATORY DISEASE

Pathogenesis

Pelvic inflammatory disease (PID) is a constellation of symptoms and signs related to the ascending spread of pathogenic organisms from the lower female genital tract (vagina, cervix) to the endometrium, fallopian tubes, and contiguous structures.

Epidemiology

PID is generally polymicrobial, with *Chlamydia trachomatis* and *Neisseria gonorrhoeae* the most commonly isolated organisms. Other potential causes of PID include anaerobes and enteric gram-negative bacilli. Barrier contraceptive methods provide some protection. *N. gonorrhoeae* or genital *C. trachomatis* infection in a prepubertal child strongly suggests sexual abuse.

Risk Factors

Adolescence is a period of increased risk for development of PID because of the presence of cervical ectopy (the extension of columnar cells that line the endocervical canal onto the external cervix) and the increased incidence of high-risk behavior during the teenage years. Risk factors also include sexual intercourse with multiple partners, unprotected intercourse, and a preexisting mucosal sexually transmitted infection (STI).

Clinical Manifestations

The clinical diagnosis of PID is based on the presence of at least one of the two **minimum criteria. Additional criteria** are often used to support the diagnosis of PID.

Minimum criteria:

- cervical motion tenderness
- uterine or adnexal tenderness

Additional criteria:

- Oral temperature greater than 38.3°C (101°F)
- Elevated ESR and/or C-reactive protein
- Presence of WBCs on saline microscopy of vaginal secretions
- Mucopurulent cervical or vaginal discharge
- Laboratory evidence of cervical infection with *N. gonorrhoeae* or *C. trachomatis*

History and Physical Examination

Other symptoms include cramping, vaginal discharge or bleeding, nausea/vomiting, and malaise. The physical examination may be positive for peritoneal signs if the disease is severe.

Diagnostic Evaluation (NAATs)

Nucleic acid amplification tests are sensitive and specific for both gonorrhea and chlamydia. If a patient is suspected of having PID, she should be offered testing for syphilis, HIV, and other STI. Often, a specific pathogen responsible for PID is not identified because PID is an upper genital tract disease whereas samples are routinely obtained from the lower tract.

Differential Diagnosis

Other gynecologic conditions and intra-abdominal pathology are included in the differential diagnosis:

- Gynecologic: mucopurulent cervicitis, ectopic pregnancy, ruptured ovarian cyst, septic abortion, endometriosis
- Nongynecologic: appendicitis, pyelonephritis, inflammatory bowel disease

Patients with suspected PID should always receive a pregnancy test because treatment may need to be altered and because ectopic pregnancy is a life-threatening condition that must be ruled out.

Treatment

Patients with clinical PID should be treated for both *N. gonorrhoeae* and *C. trachomatis*. Coverage against anaerobes (such as metronidazole and clindamycin) and other gram-negative organisms is often added.

Patients with mild to moderate PID may receive outpatient therapy. A single dose of a long-acting parenteral third-generation cephalosporin, such as ceftriaxone, combined with a 14-day course of oral doxycycline (100 mg twice daily) is recommended to eradicate both *N. gonorrhoeae* and *C. trachomatis*. The duration of doxycycline therapy (14 days) is longer for patients with PID than for those with uncomplicated gonorrhea or chlamydial infections (7 days). Oral metronidazole (500 mg twice daily) may be added to this dual therapy regimen. All patients who are released for outpatient treatment should return for a follow-up visit within 72 hours. Sexual contacts need to be treated to avoid reinfection.

Indications for hospitalization include severe illness, vomiting, pregnancy, blood pressure instability, or a possible surgical condition. These patients should receive intravenous antibiotics, including cefotetan or cefoxitin plus doxycycline. An alternative regimen consists of clindamycin and gentamicin. Within 24 to 48 hours of clinical improvement, these patients may be transitioned to oral therapy.

Women with repeated episodes of PID may have problems with fertility. Other gynecologic complications include increased risks for ectopic pregnancy, dyspareunia, chronic pelvic pain, and adhesions.

N. gonorrhoeae is capable of invading the bloodstream and thus any organ system. Joint involvement is most common. The arthritis may affect only one joint or may be polyarticular and migratory with associated tenosynovitis and skin lesions. Although *C. trachomatis* seldom causes systemic illness, untreated individuals may go on to develop **Reiter syndrome** (a constellation of urethritis, conjunctivitis, and arthritis). **Fitz-Hugh-Curtis syndrome**, a form of perihepatitis, is a known complication of infection with either organism.

VULVOVAGINAL INFECTIONS

Bacterial vaginosis and *Candida* vaginitis are bothersome but relatively benign vaginal infections manifested by changes in the amount and character of vaginal secretions. *Trichomonas vaginalis*, a sexually transmitted pathogen, also causes vulvovaginal infection. All three are easily diagnosed during the office visit by examination of vaginal fluid samples.

Clinical Manifestations and Treatment

Trichomoniasis

Trichomoniasis results from sexually transmitted *Trichomonas vaginalis*, a mobile flagellated protozoan. Most infected individuals remain asymptomatic. Typical symptoms in women include a malodorous, frothy gray discharge and vaginal discomfort. Some patients also develop dysuria and vague lower abdominal pain. The cervix and vaginal mucosa may be either normal or visibly irritated and inflamed. A fresh wet preparation of the vaginal fluid reveals polymorphonuclear leukocytes and the characteristic motile trichomonads. Male partners may have penile discharge. Oral metronidazole twice daily for 7 days is the treatment of choice for adolescent patients and their sexual partners.

Bacterial Vaginosis

Bacterial vaginosis, long thought to be harmless, is now known to increase the risks of PID, chorioamnionitis, and premature birth. Its microbiologic cause has not been clearly delineated, but concentrations of *Gardnerella vaginalis*, *Mycoplasma hominis*, and various anaerobic organisms are increased in the vagina. In contrast, concentrations of *Lactobacillus* species are decreased. The epidemiology of the disease suggests sexual transmission. Infection is usually asymptomatic except for a thin, white, foul-smelling discharge that emits a fishy odor when mixed with potassium hydroxide. The clinical diagnosis is based on patient history (much more common in sexually active females), the appearance and odor of discharge, a vaginal pH greater than 4.5, and characteristic clue cells on the wet prep (squamous epithelial cells with smudged borders caused by adherent bacteria). Oral metronidazole twice daily for 7 days effectively cures the infection. Concurrent antibiotic treatment of male partners seems to have no effect on recurrence rates.

Vaginal Candidiasis

Vulvovaginal candidiasis is not an STD. All women are colonized with *Candida*; however, factors such as antibiotic use, pregnancy, diabetes, immunosuppression, and oral contraceptive use predispose women to candidal overgrowth (moniliasis). Signs and symptoms include a thick white vaginal discharge with vaginal itching and burning. Yeast and pseudohyphae are evident on wet preparation treated with potassium hydroxide. Over-the-counter topical antifungal creams are safe and generally effective. A single dose of oral fluconazole is an alternative.

URETHRITIS

Urethritis is inflammation of the urethra caused by infection with an STD. It occurs much more commonly in adolescent males than females. *N. gonorrhoeae* and *C. trachomatis* are the most important pathogens. *Mycoplasma genitalium* and *Trichomonas vaginalis* also cause urethritis. Symptoms include urethral discharge, itching, dysuria, and urinary frequency. Asymptomatic infections are common. The disease is diagnosed by notation of at least one of the following: mucoid or purulent urethral discharge; positive leukocyte esterase test or WBCs on microscopic examination of a first-void urine; or gram-negative intracellular diplococci on Gram stain. Patients with suspected urethritis should be offered testing for other STDS including syphilis and HIV. If available, specific diagnostic testing for *N. gonorrhoeae* and *Chlaymdia trachomatis* (e.g., nucleic acid amplification tests on urine or urethral swabs) is recommended. Treatment for gonococcal urethritis is dual therapy with 250 mg IM ceftriaxone AND either 1 dose of oral azithromycin OR 7 days of oral doxycycline. If gonorrhea has been ruled out, then the patient may be treated with 1 dose of oral azithromycin or 7 days of oral doxycycline. Azithromycin is preferred because it provides better coverage for *Mycoplasma genitalium*. Trichomoniasis is treated with oral metronidazole. Complications are rare.

HIV AND AIDS

Pathogenesis

HIV is a retrovirus that infects CD4+ T-lymphocytes. HIV produces a wide range of clinical manifestations in children, the most severe of which is AIDS. A child is defined as having AIDS when an AIDS-defining illness occurs (see later) or when the CD4+ lymphocyte count is less than a defined number for age (e.g., <200 per mm^3 for children older than 12 years).

Epidemiology

The disease is more common in urban populations, lower socioeconomic classes, and racial minorities. Most infections in children are acquired in utero or perinatally (>90%). The risk of HIV transmission from an untreated seropositive mother to her fetus is approximately 25%. Treatment of infected pregnant women with zidovudine (AZT; a reverse transcriptase inhibitor) alone or in combination with other antiretrovirals during the second and third trimesters, followed by treatment of the infant for the first 6 weeks of life, reduces the vertical transmission rate to approximately 2%. Asymptomatic HIV-positive women may not realize they are infected, and therefore they often do not receive therapy.

As a group, the adolescent population has the most rapidly increasing rate of HIV infection in the United States.

Risk Factors

Risk factors include birth to an HIV-positive mother, birth to a woman who uses intravenous drugs and shares needles, and birth to a woman with multiple sexual partners who does not practice safe sex. Other groups at risk include patients who received multiple units of blood products (e.g., hemophiliacs) before 1985, victims of sexual abuse, and adolescents who engage in high-risk behaviors (intravenous drug use or unprotected sexual activity with multiple partners).

Clinical Manifestations

History and Physical Examination

HIV may present in infants and children with any one or several of the following signs and symptoms: generalized lymphadenopathy, hepatomegaly, splenomegaly, failure to thrive, recurrent or chronic diarrhea, oral candidiasis, parotitis, and developmental delay. Respiratory manifestations include lymphoid interstitial pneumonia (LIP) and *Pneumocystis jiroveci* pneumonia (PCP). Regression in developmental milestones and progressive encephalopathy may occur. Recurrent, often severe, bacterial and opportunistic (fungal, disseminated HSV or CMV, and *Mycobacterium avium*) infections are the hallmark of the acquired helper T-lymphocyte immunodeficiency.

A significant percentage of infected adolescents presents with a mononucleosis-type syndrome within 6 weeks of HIV acquisition. Symptoms and signs include sore throat, fatigue, fever, rash, and cervical or diffuse lymphadenopathy.

PCP and LIP are two of several AIDS-defining illnesses in the pediatric population. When any of these conditions occurs, the child is considered to have AIDS regardless of the absolute CD4+ T-lymphocyte count.

Differential Diagnosis

HIV has become known as a "great masquerader" because of its variable presentation; the virus can affect any organ system, and symptoms are often nonspecific. A high degree of suspicion is required to diagnose the disease at an early stage when it is most easily contained.

Diagnostic Evaluation

Infants born to HIV-positive mothers are seropositive for maternally derived IgG antibodies to the virus (i.e., ELISA and Western blot testing are positive); these tests are not helpful in children younger than 18 months. If the mother is HIV positive, HIV DNA PCR of the infant's blood should be performed at birth. If this test is positive on two separate occasions, the infant is considered HIV positive. Negative tests should be repeated at regular intervals (1 and 4 months of age). Almost all HIV-infected infants have positive HIV DNA PCR results by 1 month of age.

Treatment

The standard of care consists of nucleoside analogue reverse transcriptase inhibitor drugs such as AZT and 3TC (lamivudine), nonnucleoside analogue reverse transcriptase inhibitors (NNRTIs), and protease inhibitors. Trimethoprim-sulfamethoxazole provides prophylaxis against PCP, the most common opportunistic infection. New pharmacologic therapies have drastically improved the chances of converting HIV infection from a disease of near-certain death to a chronic lifelong condition.

VIRAL INFECTIONS OF CHILDHOOD

Viral infections are quite common in the infant and young child but decrease with age due to acquired immunity. Table 10-7 describes the typical presentations and complications of some viral illnesses in children.

Measles, mumps, rubella, and varicella (chickenpox) have all decreased because live attenuated vaccines are routinely administered to prevent them. Measles, rubella, and chickenpox present with characteristic rashes that permit reliable clinical diagnosis. Chickenpox is discussed further in Chapter 6. Mumps does not have a rash but may be considered when a child or adolescent presents with parotid gland swelling (parotitis). However, in fully immunized patients, parotitis is more often caused by other viruses (i.e., parainfluenza viruses, influenza A virus, HIV), *Staphylococcus aureus*, or salivary duct stones.

Roseola and erythema infectiosum are generally benign in children. The peak of roseola is between 6 and 24 months of age. Infants and children with roseola may present with 3 to 7 days of high fever >39.0°C (103.0°F). The rash initially appears on the trunk as the fever resolves, establishing the clinical diagnosis. Erythema infectiosum is caused by human parvovirus B19, which infects red blood cell precursors. In a child with hemoglobinopathy, a transient aplastic crisis precedes the onset of the "slapped cheeks" rash. Arthritis is observed more often in adult women than in children.

TABLE 10-7 Presentations and Complications of Childhood Viral Illnesses

Virus	Exanthem	Other Features	Complications
Measles	Confluent, erythematous maculopapular rash that starts on head and progresses caudally (Color Plate 20)	Coryza, cough, conjunctivitis, Koplik spots (on buccal mucosa early in disease)	Pneumonia, myocarditis, encephalitis; rare: subacute sclerosing panencephalitis
Mumps	None	Swollen salivary glands, especially parotid glands	Orchitis, pancreatitis; rare: meningitis, encephalitis
Rubella	Similar to measles but does not coalesce	Suboccipital and posterior auricular lymphadenopathy	Polyarticular arthritis or arthralgias; rare: encephalitis
Roseola (human herpesvirus 6)	Maculopapular (Color Plate 21)	High fever resolves as rash appears	Febrile seizures; rare: meningoencephalitis
Erythema infectiosum (fifth disease; parvovirus B19)	Facial erythema giving "slapped cheeks" appearance followed by spread to extremities in reticular pattern (Color Plate 22)	Transient aplastic crisis in child with hemoglobinopathy	Arthritis; rare: encephalitis
Chickenpox (varicella)	Pruritic, erythematous macules evolve to vesicles and then crust over; begins on face and spreads to extremities (Color Plate 23)	As initial lesions resolve, new crops form so that lesions in different stages are observed simultaneously	Secondary bacterial infection; rare: pneumonia, cerebellar ataxia, encephalitis, hepatitis

ROCKY MOUNTAIN SPOTTED FEVER (RMSF)

Pathogenesis

RMSF is a tick-borne disease caused by *Rickettsia rickettsii*, a gram-negative intracellular bacterium. Rickettsiae are introduced into the skin by a tick bite and subsequently spread via the lymphatics and blood vessels. They invade and multiply within the endothelial cells of blood vessels, causing thrombosis and increasing vascular permeability (vasculitis).

Epidemiology

RMSF occurs more often between April and September in tick-infested areas of the south Atlantic states (but has been reported year round). Despite the name, none of the top 10 states reporting RMSF is near the Rocky Mountains. Tick vectors include the wood tick, dog tick, and lone star tick.

Risk Factor

The most significant risk factor is residence in or travel to an endemic area during times of the year when ticks are most active.

Clinical Manifestations

History and Physical Examination

The classic presentation of RMSF includes fever, headache, and rash. Symptoms develop approximately 7 days after a tick bite. Initial symptoms often are nonspecific and include fever, chills, headache, malaise, nausea, vomiting, and myalgias. The rash begins on the 2nd to 5th day and consists of blanching, erythematous, macular lesions that progress to form petechiae or purpura (Color Plate 24). It characteristically appears initially on the wrists and ankles and spreads proximally to involve the trunk and head over several hours. Typically, the palms and soles are involved as well. The rash is absent in up to 20% of patients. Children may have some impairment of mental status.

Diagnostic Evaluation

Although immunofluorescent staining of skin biopsies taken from rash sites may demonstrate the organism, there is no reliable diagnostic test that becomes positive early enough in the course of the disease to guide therapy. Thus, the clinician must maintain a high suspicion for the disease. Antibodies to confirm the clinical diagnosis are detectable approximately 10 days after symptom onset. Key laboratory features include thrombocytopenia and hyponatremia; however, these are present in only a minority of patients.

Differential Diagnosis

RMSF is essentially indistinguishable from ehrlichiosis (another tick-borne illness) and meningococcemia. Because approximately half of patients with RMSF and ehrlichiosis do not remember being bitten by a tick, initial antibiotic therapy for patients with these suspected illnesses and no tick history should include coverage for *N. meningitidis* as well. Atypical measles may present in a similar fashion; knowledge of a local outbreak should clarify this diagnosis.

Treatment

Treatment with doxycycline is effective in all age groups. Cefotaxime or ceftriaxone should be added if meningococcemia is a possibility. If RMSF is suspected, antibiotics must not be withheld pending laboratory results. Mortality is higher when treatment is delayed.

LYME DISEASE

Pathogenesis

Lyme disease is a tick-borne illness resulting from infection with the spirochete bacterium *Borrelia burgdorferi*. The pathogen lives in deer ticks (eastern United States) and western black-legged ticks (Pacific states).

Epidemiology

Although cases have been reported across the country, most occur in southern New England, southeastern New York, New Jersey, eastern Pennsylvania, Maryland, Delaware, Minnesota, and Wisconsin. The incidence of Lyme disease is highest among children 5 to 9 years of age. Most cases occur between April and October.

Risk Factors

Individuals with increased occupational or recreational exposure to tick-infested woodlands in endemic areas are at highest risk of Lyme disease. An infected tick must feed for more than 48 hours to transmit *B. burgdorferi*.

Clinical Manifestations

History

Most patients do not recall a tick bite. The clinical manifestations depend on the stage of the disease: early localized, early disseminated, or late. **Erythema migrans**, the manifestation of **early localized** disease, appears at the site of the tick bite 3 to 30 days after the bite. The rash begins as a red macule or papule and progressively enlarges to form a large, annular, erythematous lesion with central clearing (resembling a bull's eye) up to 10 cm in diameter. The skin lesion often is accompanied by fever, malaise, headache, arthralgias, and myalgias. **Early disseminated** Lyme disease (days to weeks after the tick bite) may manifest as multiple erythema migrans lesions (Color Plate 25), cranial nerve palsy, meningitis, and carditis (heart block). The most common manifestation of **late** Lyme disease (>6 weeks after tick bite) is arthritis, usually involving the knee.

Physical Examination

Children with early disseminated Lyme disease may have multiple erythema migrans lesions, facial nerve palsy, or signs of meningitis. Late disease may present with swollen and tender joints.

Differential Diagnosis

The differential diagnosis depends on the presentation. When the rash is atypical, it may be confused with erythema multiforme or erythema marginatum (seen in acute rheumatic fever). The differential diagnosis of arthritis also includes juvenile idiopathic arthritis, reactive arthritis, and Reiter syndrome. The differential diagnosis of Lyme meningitis includes other causes of aseptic meningitis.

Diagnostic Evaluation

Testing for Lyme disease in the presence of vague or nonspecific complaints is not helpful; false-positive test results can occur, especially with ELISA (enzyme-linked immunosorbent assay) or immunofluorescent antibody testing. For the most part, early localized Lyme disease is a clinical diagnosis, based on suggestive history and the characteristic rash on physical examination. Lyme IgM titer is elevated several weeks after the tick bite. Antibodies to *B. burgdorferi* cross-react with other infectious agents, particularly other spirochetes (including syphilis). The VDRL and RPR tests remain negative in patients with Lyme disease. The Western blot is specific for antibodies to *B. burgdorferi* but does not usually become positive early enough in the course of disease to guide therapy. Cardiac involvement, usually in the form of conduction abnormalities, is rare but can be diagnosed by ECG in conjunction with supporting history and antibody studies.

Treatment

Treatment of early localized Lyme disease prevents early disseminated and late disease, including meningitis and arthritis. Younger children can be treated with oral amoxicillin or cefuroxime. Children older than 8 years should receive oral doxycycline. Patients with vomiting, persistent arthritis, cardiac disease, or neurologic involvement warrant parenteral therapy with high-dose penicillin G or ceftriaxone. A small minority of patients continues to experience low-grade, chronic symptoms despite appropriate therapy; long-term antibiotic treatment is not helpful in this population.

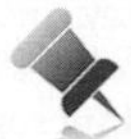

KEY POINTS

- The three most common bacteria implicated in acute otitis media (AOM) are *S. pneumoniae*, nontypeable *H. influenzae*, and *M. catarrhalis*. In AOM, the tympanic membrane is bulging, opaque, and erythematous, with diminished mobility. Symptom onset is acute. High-dose amoxicillin is the appropriate first-line treatment for most cases of AOM. Tympanostomy tubes should be considered for children with recurrent episodes of AOM. Chronic effusions and recurrent infection predispose to permanent conductive hearing loss and language delay.
- Children with pharyngitis should not be treated with antibiotics empirically because most episodes are caused by viruses. Therapeutic decisions should be based on throat culture or rapid antigen detection test results. Penicillin is the antibiotic of choice for GAS pharyngitis.
- Classic infectious mononucleosis is caused by EBV. Clinical manifestations include exudative pharyngitis, generalized lymphadenopathy, fever, and profound fatigue. Helpful laboratory findings include lymphocytosis with a high percentage (10%) of atypical lymphocytes and a positive heterophile antibody test.
- Children with croup develop a hoarse voice, barky ("seal-like") cough, and stridor, which may progress to respiratory distress. Infants with severe stridor are treated with corticosteroids and nebulized epinephrine. The typical patient with epiglottitis, a life-threatening emergency, has a toxic appearance, with drooling and severe, progressive respiratory distress. When epiglottitis is suspected, the child should be transported to the operating room for endotracheal intubation and direct visualization of the epigloths under general anesthesia.
- The classic presentation of bronchiolitis includes fever, wheezing, tachypnea, rhinorrhea, and respiratory distress. Apnea is a frequent presentation in neonates. Prophylactic administration of palivizumab, an intramuscular RSV monoclonal antibody, is indicated during the winter months for selected patients younger than 24 months who were born prematurely (<35 weeks' gestation), or who have hemodynamically significant congenital heart disease, or who have chronic lung disease of prematurity requiring medical therapy within the 6 months prior to the start of the RSV season.
- *S. pneumoniae* is the most common cause of bacterial pneumonia in most age groups. *M. pneumoniae* and *C. pneumoniae* should be considered in older children and adolescents. The majority of large pleural effusions complicating pneumonia are caused by *S. aureus* pneumonia.
- Meningitis may be septic (bacterial) or aseptic. LP is invaluable in the diagnosis and development of a treatment strategy for meningitis. Appropriate empirical antibiotic choices for presumed bacterial meningitis are ampicillin and cefotaxime (in the neonate) and vancomycin and a third-generation cephalosporin (in the child).
- Infectious diarrhea may be bacterial, viral, parasitic, or toxin-mediated. Children with shigellosis may present with mental status changes. *S. dysenteriae* and *E. coli* O157:H7 are associated with hemolytic uremic syndrome.
- Clinical signs of acute hepatitis include anorexia, nausea, malaise, vomiting, jaundice, dark urine, abdominal pain, and low-grade fever. However, a wide range of severity exists, and as many as 30% to 70% of infected children are asymptomatic. HAV and HEV are spread via fecal-oral transmission. HBV, HCV, and HDV are transmitted through infected bodily fluids. Liver enzymes are uniformly elevated in hepatitis. Because the clinical manifestations are so similar, specific serologic tests are indispensable for securing an accurate diagnosis.
- Syphilis may be transmitted transplacentally or sexually. Neonates with congenital syphilis present with snuffles, hepatosplenomegaly, mucocutaneous lesions, jaundice, and lymphadenopathy. The VDRL and RPR are excellent screening tests but may produce false positives. Parenteral penicillin G is the treatment of choice.
- The diagnosis of PID is clinical, based on history, physical examination, and supporting laboratory results. *C. trachomatis* and *N. gonorrhoeae* are the most commonly isolated organisms in PID. A single dose of a parenteral cephalosporin (for *N. gonorrhoeae*) and 14 days of oral doxycycline (for *C. trachomatis*) are appropriate outpatient therapy for mild PID.
- Most HIV infections in children are acquired in utero or perinatally. Infants born to HIV-positive mothers are seropositive for maternally derived IgG antibodies to HIV; thus, the ELISA and Western blot are not helpful in children younger than 18 months. The HIV DNA PCR should be used in this population.
- The classic presentation of RMSF includes fever, headache, and rash. The disease is rapidly progressive, and there is no laboratory test that becomes abnormal soon enough in the disease process to guide therapy. Treatment (doxycycline) should be started based on clinical suspicion alone.
- The classic rash of Lyme disease is erythema migrans. Lyme disease is treated with oral amoxicillin in children younger than 8 years and with oral doxycycline in older children. Lyme meningitis requires intravenous ceftriaxone.

C Clinical Vignettes

Vignette 1

An 8-year-old boy presents to your office with a 3-day history of fevers, sore throat, and headache. His mother also states that he occasionally has been complaining that his abdomen hurts. This morning, the boy's mother noticed that he has developed a red, bumpy rash on his neck and under his arms. On physical exam, he is nontoxic but uncomfortable appearing. His tonsils are erythematous and enlarged with visible exudates, and he has several petechiae on the soft palate. He has a few tender anterior cervical lymph nodes and an erythematous, papular rash most prominent on the neck and in his axilla. His cardiopulmonary exam is normal and his abdomen is nontender and benign. You suspect scarlet fever and perform a rapid antigen test in the office.

1. While waiting for the test results, you explain to the patient's mother that the organism which is most likely responsible for this infection, if bacterial, is which of the following?
   a. Group A streptococcus (*Streptococcus pyogenes*)
   b. Group B streptococcus (*Streptococcus agalactiae*)
   c. *Streptococcus pneumoniae*
   d. *Staphylococcus aureus*
   e. Viridans streptococcus group (*Streptococcus viridans*)

2. Within a few minutes, the patient's rapid test returns and is read as negative. The following day, the patient's throat culture returns positive for Group A streptococcal infection. You call the boy's mother to discuss prescribing antibiotics to treat the infection. Which of the following is the most important diagnostic test to perform next?
   a. Throat culture
   b. Anti-streptolysin O (ASO) titer
   c. Blood culture
   d. Monospot test
   e. No further testing is recommended.

3. If the child is treated appropriately, which of the following is the least likely to be affected?
   a. Duration of symptoms
   b. Development of acute rheumatic fever
   c. Risk of transmission
   d. Development of poststreptococcal glomerulonephritis
   e. Abscess formation

Vignette 2

A 3-year-old boy presents to your office with 3 days of nonproductive cough, malaise, and fevers. His mother says his cough is infrequent and wet sounding. He has not been going to day care during this illness and today developed some brief periods of shortness of breath. Findings on physical examination include a temperature of 38.5°C, respiratory rate of 30 breaths/min, pulse of 110 beats/min, and blood pressure of 100/60 mm Hg. He has an oxygen saturation of 100% on room air. On lung auscultation, he has rhonchi prominently over the right lower lung field. He has no significant past medical history and has not been ill in the recent past. He has no allergies to medications and is up-to-date on his vaccinations.

1. Which of the following organisms is most likely to be the cause of the child's illness?
   a. *Streptococcus pneumoniae*
   b. *Mycoplasma pneumoniae*
   c. *Bordetella pertussis*
   d. *Pneumocystis jirovecii*
   e. Nontypable *Haemophilus influenzae*

2. Which antibiotic would be the best choice to treat this child's condition?
   a. Azithromycin
   b. Doxycycline
   c. Amoxicillin
   d. Ceftriaxone
   e. Ciprofloxacin

3. Two days later, the child presents to the emergency department with worsened respiratory distress. He has taken his antibiotics as prescribed but has developed higher fevers and progressive respiratory symptoms since he was last seen. On examination, he has a temperature of 39.8°C, a respiratory rate of 35, heart rate of 110 bpm and a blood pressure of 100/65 mmHg. His oxygen saturation is 98% on room air. He has moderate retractions and decreased lung sounds over his right lower lung fields. A chest x-ray is obtained which shows a large right-sided pleural effusion and underlying consolidation. In addition to administering empiric intravenous antibiotics, which of the following is the most important next step in management?
   a. Administer oxygen.
   b. Perform a thoracentesis to obtain fluid for cell count, culture, and gram stain.

c. Administer albuterol and intravenous/oral steroids.
d. Obtain a CBC, ESR, and CRP.
e. Obtain a blood culture.

Vignette 3

You are an intern seeing a 16-year-old female in the emergency department presenting with a chief complaint of lower abdominal pain. She has been ill for the past 4 to 5 days with worsening of her pain and fevers to 102°F since yesterday. The pain is described as sharp, constant, and present "all over" her lower abdomen. She denies back pain. She has had little appetite and has vomited twice since the pain started. She has also had a foul-smelling, white vaginal discharge for the past week and burning with urination. Prior to this illness, she has been healthy. She is sexually active with one partner, takes oral contraceptive pills, and uses condoms "most of the time." Her last menstrual period was 2 weeks ago. On your examination, she is mildly dehydrated and uncomfortable appearing. Her cardiac and pulmonary exams are normal. She has tenderness to palpation diffusely over her lower abdomen without guarding.

1. Which of the following tests is most likely to confirm the probable cause of this patient's condition?
   a. Urinalysis
   b. Right lower-quadrant ultrasound
   c. Bimanual pelvic examination
   d. Pregnancy test
   e. Stool culture

2. You perform the remainder of your evaluation and confirm the diagnosis of pelvic inflammatory disease. What is the most likely organism responsible for the patient's illness?
   a. Herpes simplex virus (HSV)
   b. *Neisseria gonorrhoeae*
   c. *Treponema pallidum*
   d. *Trichomonas vaginalis*
   e. *Chlamydia trachomatis*
   f. A and/or C
   g. B and/or D
   h. B and/or E

3. As part of your evaluation, you recommend that she undergo testing for other sexually transmitted infections (STIs) including HIV. Although nervous, she agrees to be tested. You try to quell her fears over the testing process by providing her with counseling about HIV infection and the screening process for this infection. Which of the following statements about HIV testing or infection is FALSE?
   a. An HIV screening test may be falsely negative in a patient with a recently acquired infection.
   b. The prevalence of HIV-1 infection is higher than that of HIV-2.
   c. Most HIV infections in children are acquired in the perinatal period.
   d. The confirmatory test most commonly used following a positive screening test is an HIV enzyme-linked immunosorbent assay (ELISA).
   e. Transmission of HIV in a teenager is more likely to occur through sexual contact than IV drug use.

Vignette 4

It is July and you are working in the emergency department. You evaluate a 13-year-old boy who presents with 2 days of fever and headache. He has been vomiting today and, according to his parents, he has been lying around and complaining of feeling very tired. They report no respiratory symptoms. His vital signs in the emergency department are: temperature, 39.7°C; heart rate, 105 bpm; BP, 112/80 mmHg; respiratory rate, 16 breaths per minute. On examination, you notice an ill-appearing and somnolent young man. He has strong distal pulses and his capillary refill is normal. He has no focal neurologic deficits but mild nuchal rigidity is present. He has a blanching, macular rash on his distal extremities, which is notably absent from his head and trunk.

1. Which of the following would be the least important to include in your initial management of this patient?
   a. Establish intravenous access.
   b. Obtain an immunization history.
   c. Perform a lumbar puncture.
   d. Perform a head CT.
   e. Start empiric antibiotics.

2. You obtain some additional historical details from the child's parents. They tell you that the boy was previously healthy. Recently, the family vacationed in North Carolina and had gone camping. When asked about tick exposures, they do not recall any specific bites but they do remember seeing them on his clothing. Given this information, you become concerned about the potential for Rocky Mountain spotted fever (RMSF). Which is the best choice of antimicrobial to specifically cover the organism responsible for RMSF?
   a. Doxycycline
   b. Cefotaxime
   c. Vancomycin
   d. Gentamicin
   e. Acyclovir

3. The child is admitted to the hospital and his condition gradually improves while on broad-spectrum antibiotics. The following day, his cerebrospinal fluid (CSF) returns positive for *Neisseria meningitidis*. The parents tell you that he has not been around anyone sick but that he shares a room at home with his 8-year-old brother. You decide that chemoprophylaxis of the family is warranted. What is the drug of choice to use as prophylaxis for close contacts exposed to invasive meningococcal infection?
   a. Doxycycline
   b. Rifampin
   c. Amoxicillin-clavulanate
   d. Nitrofurantoin
   e. Amoxicillin

A Answers

Vignette 1 Question 1

Answer A: *Streptococcus pyogenes*, or group A beta-hemolytic streptococci (GAS), is responsible for "strep throat" (streptococcal pharyngitis) and scarlet fever. Acute pharyngotonsillitis is the most common manifestation of acute infection, followed by skin infections (impetigo or pyoderma). Both suppurative (peritonsillar and retropharyngeal abscesses, adenitis, otitis media, and sinusitis) and nonsuppurative (rheumatic fever and glomerulonephritis) complications may be seen following strep pharyngitis, particularly if untreated. *Streptococcus agalactiae*, or group B streptococci, are a major cause of invasive perinatal bacterial infections such as meningitis, bacteremia, or pneumonia. *Streptococcus pneumoniae* (pneumococcus) is a major cause of bacterial illness in children. Although its prevalence has decreased due to widespread vaccination, it is frequently responsible for otitis media, sinusitis, community-acquired pneumonia, and less commonly bacteremia or meningitis. Pneumococcus infection is extremely unlikely to be associated with rash. *Staphylococcus aureus* is a ubiquitous organism that is most frequently responsible for skin and soft tissue infections. It can cause a variety of invasive suppurative infections and toxin-mediated infections as well. *Streptococcus viridans* is a group of non-A and non-B streptococcal bacteria which may cause a variety of clinical infections in children. Most often, viridans streptococcus group are associated with endocarditis in children with congenital heart disease or artificial heart valves.

Vignette 1 Question 2

Answer E: Several rapid diagnostic tests are available for practitioners and are frequently implemented in the office setting. While these tests have a high specificity (few false positive results), their sensitivity is variable. These tests are also highly dependent on proper collection of the sample to accurately identify infection. Thus, throat culture is used as the gold standard for confirmation of the diagnosis of streptococcal pharyngitis and should be obtained on all children who have a negative rapid streptococcal antigen test. This patient's sample was cultural for GAS and was reported as positive. An anti–streptolysin O titer may be useful in the diagnosis of recent or past GAS infections. However, it is not commonly used in the acute setting and is often more helpful to confirm recent infection in the setting of a negative throat culture, or when potential systemic complications of GAS infection, such as glomerulonephritis, are present. Bacteremia is rare in scarlet fever; therefore, the yield of blood cultures is low. A blood culture would not be indicated in this case. A monospot test is used to assess for the diagnosis of mononucleosis caused by EBV. While it may be helpful to distinguish strep pharyngitis from mononucleosis, it would not be recommended in this case. Despite a negative rapid antigen test, GAS would be more likely than EBV given the patient's age and clinical presentation. While the clinical presentation in this case is consistent with scarlet fever caused by group A beta-hemolytic streptococci, it can be difficult to distinguish streptococcal pharyngitis infection from viral pharyngitis or infectious mononucleosis. Therefore, laboratory confirmation of GAS pharyngitis via culture was warranted, but no additional testing is required.

Vignette 1 Question 3

Answer D: Antibiotic use impacts the development of several potentially serious complications. However, it does not affect a child's likelihood of developing poststreptococcal glomerulonephritis. This potential complication may occur following GAS pharyngitis or skin infection regardless of antibiotic administration. Families should be counseled on signs of this complication (hematuria, edema, hypertension, etc.), as additional therapies may be needed if they occur. Treatment of GAS pharyngitis decreases the likelihood of development of many poststreptococcal complications including suppurative sequelae (such as retropharyngeal or paratonsillar abscess formation) and acute rheumatic fever. Treatment with oral penicillin, or a one-time intramuscular dose of penicillin G, is highly effective and will also shorten the clinical course and decrease transmissibility.

Vignette 2 Question 1

Answer A: *Streptococcus pneumoniae* is a bacterial pathogen responsible for pneumonia and a variety of other sinopulmonary infections including otitis media and sinusitis. It is the most common cause of bacterial pneumonia in young children, although its frequency is declining given universal pneumococcal vaccination. In a young child, such as in this case, it is a more common cause than atypical pathogens. This child presents with classic findings suggestive of community-acquired pneumonia including fever, tachypnea, and cough. In children, the most sensitive sign of pneumonia is tachypnea. Other features suggestive of this condition include dyspnea and pleuritic chest pain. The most likely organisms responsible for pneumonia vary by age and the underlying health of the child. In school-aged children, atypical pneumonias, caused by organisms such as *Mycoplasma pneumoniae* or *Chlamydophila* (formerly *Chlamydia*) *pneumonia* are more common than bacterial pathogens. Based on the child's age and focal lung findings on examination, an atypical pneumonia would be a less likely diagnosis in this case. *Bordetella* *pertussis* is the organism responsible for pertussis, or whooping cough. It begins with upper respiratory symptoms and is followed by a prolonged period of cough. Fever is uncommon in this illness. The characteristic inspiratory whoop which follows a paroxysm of coughing may be absent in an older child or adolescent. The clinical scenario described in the vignette would not be consistent with a child with pertussis. *Pneumocystis jirovecii*, also known as *Pneumocystis carinii*, is an organism which causes subacute diffuse pneumonitis or pneumonia. Symptoms of infection include dyspnea, tachypnea, fever, nonproductive cough, and hypoxia. Classically, these features are present without findings on examination to suggest pneumonia. It is uncommon for this organism to cause clinically significant illness in an immunocompetent child. However, in immunocompromised individuals, such as those who have undergone organ transplantation or have HIV, it should be suspected when significant respiratory symptoms develop. Nontypable strains of *Haemophilus influenzae* can cause sinopulmonary infections including conjunctivitis, otitis media, sinusitis, and pneumonia. Pneumonia caused by this organism would present similarly to other causes of bacterial pneumonia, but would be a less common cause of pneumonia in this age group.

Vignette 2 Question 2

Answer C: Amoxicillin is a first-line antibiotic choice directed against certain bacterial causes of pneumonia. It would be the drug of choice for outpatient management of community-acquired pneumonia in younger children (nonschool aged) or in a child with physical examination or radiologic findings suggestive of a focal lung process. Given the child's age in the vignette, amoxicillin would be the best first choice. High dosing (80–90 mg/kg/day divided bid) is typically used. Azithromycin is a macrolide antibiotic and is the drug of choice for treatment of pneumonia in school-aged children due to its efficacy against atypical agents and ease of administration (once daily for 5 days). Doxycycline is an appropriate choice for treating atypical pneumonia in an older child. However, due to increased frequency of dosing (twice daily), longer duration of therapy (7 days), and increased likelihood of side effects (GI upset and photosensitivity most commonly), it would not be the best first option in this age. It is also not used in children less than 8 years of age. Ceftriaxone is a drug used to treat a variety of bacterial infections including pneumonia. However, it is administered intravenously or intramuscularly and is therefore not typically used first-line in the office setting. Ciprofloxacin is a fluoroquinolone antibiotic which is sometimes effective against *S. pneumoniae*. Respiratory quinolones such as levofloxacin are a better choice for treatment of pneumonia. Regardless, quinolones are not approved as first-line agents in children less than 18 years of age due to an increased risk of arthropathy and tendon rupture.

Vignette 2 Question 3

Answer B: In a stable child with a clinically significant pleural effusion, the ideal plan of action would be to obtain pleural fluid for analysis prior to initiating antibiotic therapy. It can be assumed that amoxicillin did not adequately treat the organism responsible for his underlying pneumonia, either because the responsible organism was not susceptible to amoxicillin or because the amoxicillin did not penetrate well into the consolidated lung and pleural space. Accurate identification of the organism responsible for the child's pneumonia will allow for more directed therapy and ensure appropriate antibiotic coverage. Thoracentesis also may provide symptomatic relief for the patient. Oxygen is not indicated in this case. The child is in mild/moderate distress, but is stable and has a normal oxygen saturation. Oxygen will be of little benefit. His work of breathing is likely due to both the sizable lung infiltrate and the presence of an effusion. Drainage of fluid would provide more symptomatic relief than oxygen. Albuterol and systemic steroid use would be indicated if the child had bronchospasm such as is seen in an asthma exacerbation. There is no evidence to suggest that bronchodilators and steroids are beneficial in alleviating respiratory symptoms due to pneumonia. It is expected that the child's white blood cell count and inflammatory markers (ESR, CRP) will be elevated in this case considering that he has clinically worsened. Following these labs over time can be useful to indicate improvement or worsening of an underlying infectious process in circumstances where clinical changes are subtle. Although routinely collected in cases such as this, these labs should not take precedence over performing a thoracentesis for culture. A blood culture may be useful in this scenario and should be performed if the child is ill-appearing. However, the diagnostic yield of a blood culture compared to a pleural fluid culture will be considerably less. Therefore, obtaining a blood culture is not the most important next step.

Vignette 3 Question 1

Answer C: The most likely diagnosis in this case is pelvic inflammatory disease (PID). PID is due to ascending infection of the female genital tract and refers to infection of the uterus, fallopian tubes, or any portion of the female reproductive organs. It should be considered in any sexually active female with a history of abdominal pain. History of fever, vaginal discharge, dysuria, dyspareunia, irregular vaginal bleeding, and lower abdominal pain are all suggestive features, many of which are present in this case. Bimanual pelvic examination is necessary to confirm the diagnosis by detecting the presence of cervical motion tenderness or uterine or adnexal tenderness. Pyelonephritis is an ascending urinary tract infection which involves the kidney. Common historical details suggestive of this type of infection include dysuria, fever, flank pain, abdominal or pelvic pain, or costovertebral angle tenderness. Diagnosis is suggested based on history and urinalysis. However, urinary tract infections, including pyelonephritis, can only be confirmed by urine culture. In this scenario, pyelonephritis should be considered and urinalysis and urine culture should be performed. However, it is less likely than PID given the history. Appendicitis is inflammation of the appendix. It is frequently caused by obstruction of the appendix and will classically present as right lower-quadrant pain. Right lower-quadrant ultrasound is often the first imaging test used to confirm this diagnosis because it avoids the radiation exposure encountered in a CT scan. Early in the disease process, abdominal pain may be generalized or periumbilical. While this etiology must be considered in any child presenting with lower abdominal pain, the history and exam findings described would be more suggestive of PID. Pregnancy must be considered in the workup of any sexually active female presenting with abdominal pain. In practice, pregnancy testing should be performed on any female of child-bearing age presenting with abdominal pain, vaginal bleeding, or any concerning pelvic or abdominal complaints. Given her recent menses, pregnancy would be less likely. Acute gastroenteritis (AGE) may be due to a number of bacterial, viral, or parasitic agents. Stool culture is used to identify bacterial agents responsible for AGE. A history of diarrhea is the key historical detail and is absent in this case. AGE may also be associated with vomiting or abdominal pain, but these are less commonly seen. Some causes of AGE may be associated with crampy abdominal pain, but constant and severe abdominal pain would be rare. Given the history provided, acute gastroenteritis would be unlikely.

Vignette 3 Question 2

Answer H: Pelvic inflammatory disease is usually a polymicrobial infection. *Chlamydia trachomatis* and *Neisseria gonorrhoeae* are the most commonly isolated organisms from testing associated with this infection. *Neisseria gonorrhoeae* can cause a number of genital tract infections including vaginitis, urethritis, cervicitis, or salpingitis. *Chlamydia trachomatis* is the most common reportable STI in the United States, with prevalence ranging from 2% to 20% among adolescent females, and would be the most likely organism responsible for the patient's infection among those listed. Any patient with PID should be treated for both gonococcal and chlamydial infections while awaiting test results since coinfection is common. Human papillomavirus (HPV) infections are the most common STIs of any type, but are not reportable and do not cause PID. HSV can be transmitted through sexual contact. Genital infections may be characterized by vesicular lesions but often times go unnoticed. While HSV can cause painful genital lesions, it not responsible for PID. *Treponema pallidum* is the organism responsible for syphilis. Although all sexually active adolescents should be screened for syphilis, especially those with other STIs, it does not cause PID. Primary disease is characterized by painless ulcers (chancres) at the site of inoculation. Secondary syphilis consists of a maculopapular rash, mucocutaneous lesions, and generalized symptoms such as lymphadenopathy, fever, and malaise. Tertiary syphilis occurs many years later, if untreated, and involves gumma formation of the skin, bones, and internal organs. *Trichomonas vaginalis* is responsible for trichomoniasis and is often asymptomatic. When symptoms develop in females, vaginal discharge, itching, and irritation are present. It is the second most common STI in the United States, and coinfection with chlamydial and gonoccocal infections is common.

Vignette 3 Question 3

Answer D: An HIV ELISA test is a screening test. A patient's serum is combined with HIV antigens. If antibodies to HIV are present in the patient's blood, they will combine with the antigens and yield a positive result upon analysis. This test has a high sensitivity (few false negative results) and is therefore a good screening test. The test used most often to confirm a positive screening test is a Western blot. It is used to confirm the presence of antibodies to HIV in a patient's serum. In a several step process, antibodies in the patient's serum bind to specific HIV viral proteins indicating a true positive result. Most screening tests performed detect the presence of antibodies to HIV in a patient's serum. Therefore, there is a period of time after contraction of HIV, prior to the development of detectable antibodies, when a screening test will be falsely negative. This period is commonly referred to as the "window period" and may be anywhere from 6 weeks to several months, depending on the type of screening test used. Many experts recommend retesting a patient for HIV several months later if a false negative is suspected due to testing which took place in a window period. HIV-1 and HIV-2 are the two types of HIV present in humans. HIV-1 is much more prevalent than HIV-2, which tends to be a more indolent virus and exists predominantly in West Africa. Approximately 90% of HIV transmissions in children occur in the perinatal period. There is a high risk of transmission of HIV to a fetus or newborn baby by infected mothers who are untreated. With treatment of the mother, this risk is greatly reduced. However, perinatal infection still far outnumbers those cases in which HIV is acquired through sexual contact, IV drug use, or exposure to contaminated body fluids by other means. Adolescents have the most rapidly increasing rate of HIV infection in the United States, but still represent a minority of total cases. For these teenagers, the most likely route of exposure is through unprotected sexual contact with an HIV-positive individual. Although sharing needles with an HIV-infected person would carry the single greatest risk for transmission, this practice is relatively uncommon compared to exposure from sexual contact.

Vignette 4 Question 1

Answer D: Based on the described examination, the patient has no focal deficits. His presentation (both history and physical examination) suggests an infectious process rather than a traumatic one. Since the patient has no focal neurologic deficits but does have a fever, it is unlikely that he has enlarged ventricles or an intracranial bleed, two conditions which would be evident on head CT. Isolated meningitis is associated with a normal head CT. In the vignette, the child has evidence of possible meningitis. Establishing intravenous access is critical, both for administering parenteral medications and for rehydration, which is likely to be necessary in this case based on the patient's history of vomiting and fever. Moreover, the patient's condition could change quickly, so establishing IV access will be important. Asking the parents about the child's immunization history is also essential. Given that meningitis is a concern, knowing whether the child has received all age-appropriate vaccines will impact the likelihood that certain organisms are responsible for his condition. Specifically, a 13-year-old child should have received immunizations against *Haemophilus influenzae* type b, *Streptococcus pneumoniae,* and *Neisseria meningitidis* groups A, C, Y, and W-135. Obtaining CSF for analysis is crucial in the diagnosis of meningitis. Cell count and differential, protein, glucose, and culture are all necessary diagnostic tests to perform in this case. In addition, given the time of year, viral PCR may be useful to confirm a viral source of infection. While it is not certain that the child's illness is due to a bacterial source, starting empiric antibiotics is imperative. Bacterial meningitis is a life-threatening condition and antibiotics should not be withheld while awaiting test or culture results. It is recommended that blood and CSF cultures be obtained prior to starting antibiotics, if possible, to optimize their diagnostic yield.

Vignette 4 Question 2

Answer A: RMSF is caused by *Rickettsia rickettsii*, a bacterium carried by dog ticks. This illness classically presents as fever, headache, and a centrally spreading rash. The rash initially begins as erythematous macules, which develop into petechiae and purpura as the illness progresses. Doxycycline is the drug of choice, even for young children in whom this medication would ordinarily be contraindicated. If RMSF is suspected based on history, doxycycline should be given promptly. None of the other medications listed would effectively treat RMSF. While their use may be indicated as part of empiric coverage for the above-described child, these antibiotics would not be used to specifically treat this rickettsial illness. Cefotaxime is a third-generation cephalosporin and is generally a good choice for empiric coverage of suspected meningitis. It provides good gram-negative and some gram-positive coverage as well. Vancomycin is typically used in the setting of potential serious infections where gram-positive bacteria are suspected. It provides excellent gram-positive coverage and is the agent of choice for empiric treatment of methicillin-resistant *Staphylococcus aureus* (MRSA). Vancomycin does not penetrate the blood–brain barrier when used alone; therefore it should be given with a third-generation cephalosporin (e.g., ceftriaxone, cefotaxime) in these cases. Gentamicin offers broad gram-negative coverage. It is not a great antibiotic choice for management of meningitis as it does not penetrate the blood–brain barrier well. Acyclovir is an antiviral that provides therapy for several viruses including HSV. It is often used empirically in the setting of meningitis since HSV meningoencephalitis is a devastating illness when not treated promptly.

Vignette 4 Question 3

Answer B: Rifampin is the drug of choice for prophylaxis of all close contacts. Two days of therapy is advised, with the dose depending on the individual's age. Other options for chemoprophylaxis include a single intramuscular dose of ceftriaxone or a single dose of ciprofloxacin for adults. Anyone who has had contact with the child's oral secretions or who lives in the same household as the child should be treated. Generally, health care workers do not require prophylaxis unless they have had significant exposure to the child's respiratory secretions. The other answers given in the question would not provide adequate protection against the development of disease and therefore should not be given.

Chapter

11 Hematology

Charles T. Quinn • Franklin O. Smith • Bradley S. Marino

This chapter reviews the common, nonmalignant blood disorders of children. It is divided into four main sections: (1) anemia, (2) disorders of white blood cells, (3) disorders of hemostasis, and (4) transfusion of blood products. This is not an exhaustive review of all blood disorders, rather it focuses on the commonly encountered hematologic issues (normal and abnormal) and diseases in children. Some conditions span multiple pathophysiologic categories, but are only discussed in one section of this chapter.

ANEMIA

Anemia is defined physiologically as a hemoglobin concentration that is too low to deliver enough oxygen to meet cellular metabolic demands. Anemia is defined practically as a hemoglobin concentration two or more standard deviations below the mean value for age and sex. The normal hemoglobin concentration is relatively high in newborns, but declines with age reaching a nadir known as the **physiologic anemia** of infancy. This nadir occurs at 6 to 8 weeks of age in premature infants and 2 to 3 months of age in term infants. Thereafter, the hemoglobin concentration rises gradually throughout childhood, reaching adult values after puberty. The sex difference in hemoglobin concentration, males higher than females, becomes increasingly prominent during puberty. Anemia is not one condition, or a "disease" in and of itself. Anemia has many causes, and it may occur in isolation or as part of a broader pathophysiologic state.

DIFFERENTIAL DIAGNOSIS

There are three mechanisms of anemia: decreased red cell production, increased red cell destruction (hemolysis), and blood loss or sequestration. Decreased red cell production may be caused by nutritional deficiencies (e.g., iron), suppression or inhibition of the bone marrow (by drugs, infections, autoimmune processes, toxins, inflammation, and other medical conditions such as renal or liver disease), bone marrow replacement (e.g., leukemia, metastatic disease), or bone marrow failure syndromes, either acquired (severe aplastic anemia) or congenital (e.g., Diamond-Blackfan anemia, Fanconi anemia). Hemolysis is synonymous with increased red blood cell destruction and is defined as a shortened red cell lifespan. Hemolysis may be caused by extrinsic (extracorpuscular) forces, like autoantibodies, or intrinsic (intracorpuscular) defects like enzyme deficiencies. Blood may be lost from the body acutely or chronically, or it may be sequestered from the circulation in certain disease states (e.g., acute splenic sequestration of sickle cell disease). Anemia is sometimes the result of a combination of two or more of these three basic mechanisms. Table 11-1 outlines the common causes of anemia in children.

CLINICAL MANIFESTATIONS

History

A birth history should elicit risk factors for the development of childhood anemia, such as prematurity, low birth weight, hemorrhagic obstetrical or perinatal complications, and, if known, the occurrence of twin–twin, feto-maternal, or feto-placental transfusion. For the young child, it is critical to obtain a dietary history with attention to excessive consumption of cow's milk or prolonged exclusive breastfeeding, both of which may cause iron-deficiency anemia. It is also important to ask about pica, which is a neurobehavioral manifestation of iron deficiency, as it can lead to lead poisoning if there is lead in the child's environment. One should ask about overt bleeding from any site, including the gastrointestinal tract (melena, hematochezia), genitourinary tract (hematuria, menorrhagia), and other mucocutaneous sites (epistaxis, oral bleeding). The patient's race or ancestry and a family history of splenectomy or cholecystectomy may suggest an inherited hemolytic anemia. Poor weight gain should prompt consideration of a systemic disease or malabsorption. A history of recurrent acute or chronic inflammation, such as recurrent otitis media, may suggest anemia of inflammation. Medications can cause either decreased red cell production or hemolysis. One should also inquire about fever, bone pain, weight loss, bruising, jaundice, fatigue, rash, and cough that might suggest other systemic causes of anemia.

Physical Examination

A careful examination can reveal the presence and severity of anemia by the degree of pallor (skin, conjunctivae, mucosae) and loss of palmar crease pigmentation. The skin of severely

TABLE 11-1 Common Types of Anemia Classified by Cell Size (MCV) and Mechanism of Anemia

Classification	Examples
Microcytic	Iron deficiency
	Thalassemia
	Anemia of inflammation[a]
Normocytic	
Blood loss or sequestration	Acute blood loss
	Splenic sequestration
Decreased RBC production	Anemia of inflammation[a]
	Transient erythroblastopenia of childhood
	Chronic renal disease
	Malignant infiltration of the bone marrow[b]
	Parvovirus-associated transient aplastic crisis
	Myelosuppressive drug toxicity[b]
Increased RBC destruction	
Intrinsic defects	Abnormal hemoglobins
	Sickle cell disease
	Unstable hemoglobins
	Red blood cell enzyme disorders
	G6PD deficiency
	Pyruvate kinase deficiency
	Red blood cell membrane disorders
	Hereditary spherocytosis
	Hereditary elliptocytosis
Extrinsic insults	Immune hemolytic anemia
	Autoimmune
	Neonatal alloimmune
	Microangiopathic hemolytic anemias
	Hemolytic uremic syndrome
	Thrombotic thrombocytopenic purpura
	Disseminated intravascular coagulation
	Paroxysmal nocturnal hemoglobinuria
Macrocytic anemias	
Megaloblastic	Vitamin B_{12} deficiency
	Folate deficiency
Nonmegaloblastic	Aplastic anemia
	Malignant infiltration of the bone marrow[b]
	Myelosuppressive drug toxicity[b]
	Diamond-Blackfan anemia
	Fanconi anemia
	Hypothyroidism

[a]Anemia of inflammation may be normocytic (75%) or microcytic (25%).
[b]May be normocytic or macrocytic.

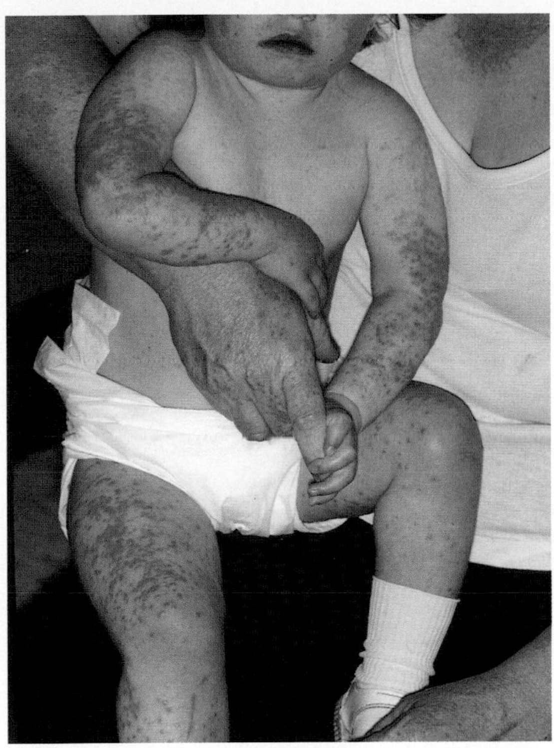

Color Plate 1 • Papular acrodermatitis of childhood. A toddler with erythematous, edematous papules concentrated on the extremities and strikingly sparing the trunk that are typical of this condition. It appears to be a reaction to a viral infection.

(Image courtesy of Anne W. Lucky, MD.)

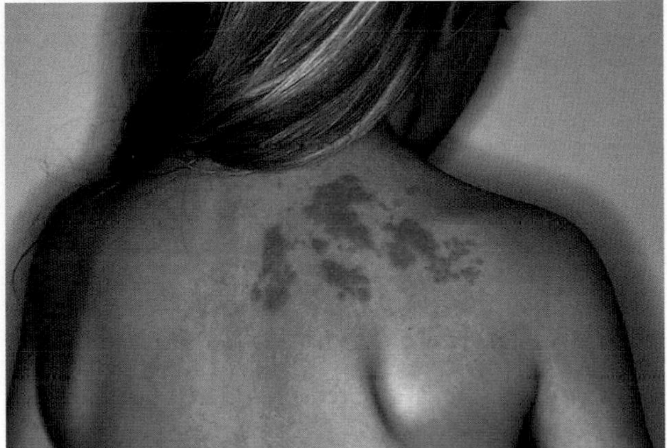

Color Plate 2 • Herpes zoster. Tender grouped papulovesicles on an erythematous base involving the upper right back in a dermatomal distribution.

(Image courtesy of Anne W. Lucky, MD.)

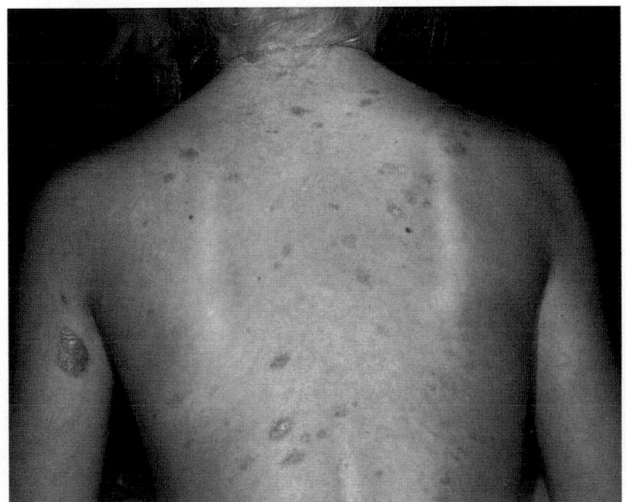

Color Plate 3 • Pityriasis rosea. A salmon-pink annular patch with a collarette of scale developed on the back of the patient's left arm followed several days later by an eruption of smaller salmon-colored lesions in a "Christmas-tree" distribution on the trunk.

(Image courtesy of Anne W. Lucky, MD.)

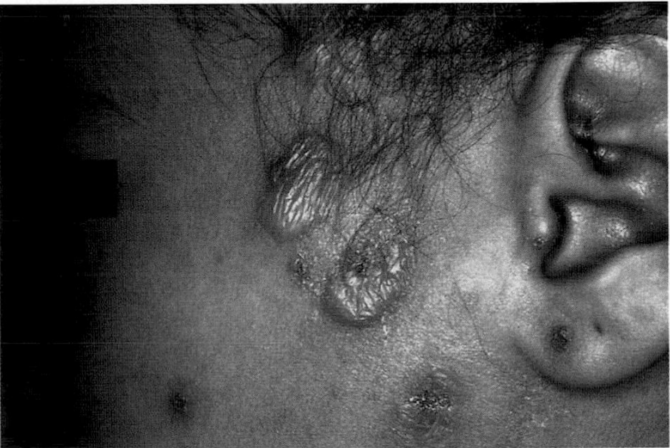

Color Plate 4 • Bullous impetigo. Intact fluid-filled thin bullae with scale peripherally and a hemorrhagic crust centrally that can be mistaken for cigarette burns especially following bullae rupture. Toxin-producing *S. aureus* is causative.

(Image courtesy of Anne W. Lucky, MD.)

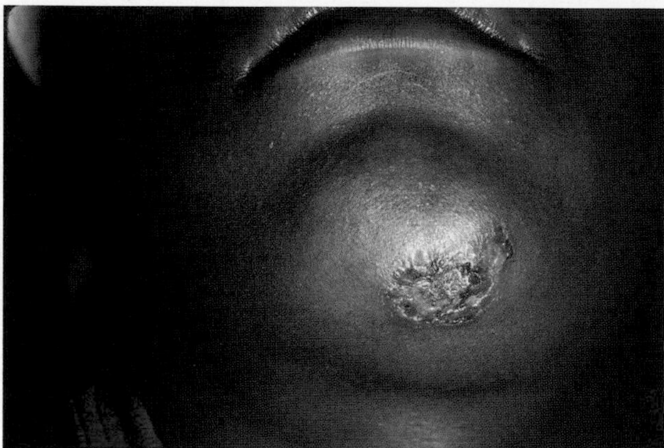

Color Plate 5 • Nonbullous impetigo has a honey-colored crust on an erythematous ulcerated base. *Streptococcus* or *Staphylococcus* species can usually be cultured from the lesion.

(Image courtesy of Anne W. Lucky, MD.)

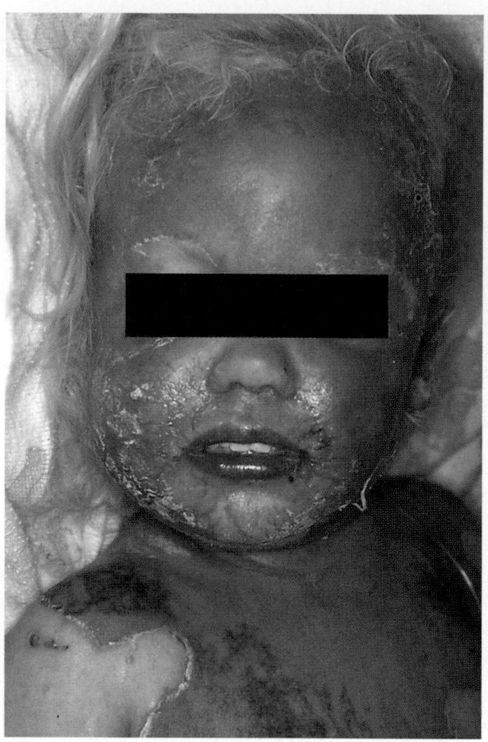

Color Plate 6 • Diffuse areas of erythema with superficial flaccid vesicles and ruptured bullae associated with significant pain and fevers are seen in Staphylococcal Scalded Skin Syndrome due to a toxin-producing strain of *S. aureus*.

(Image courtesy of Anne W. Lucky, MD.)

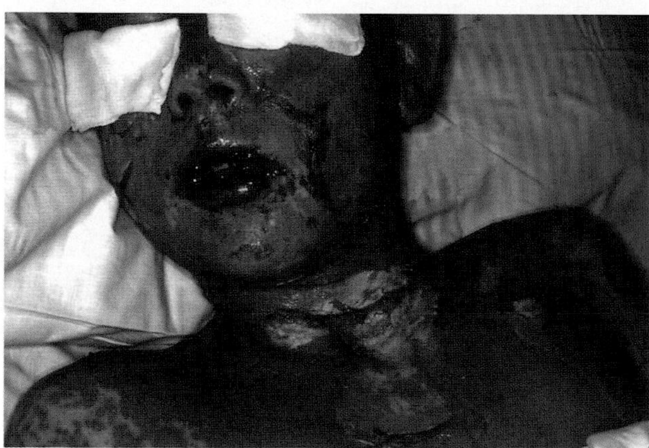

Color Plate 7 • Typical inflammatory hemorrhagic bullae of the oral mucosa noted in Stevens Johnson Syndrome.

(Image courtesy of Anne W. Lucky, MD.)

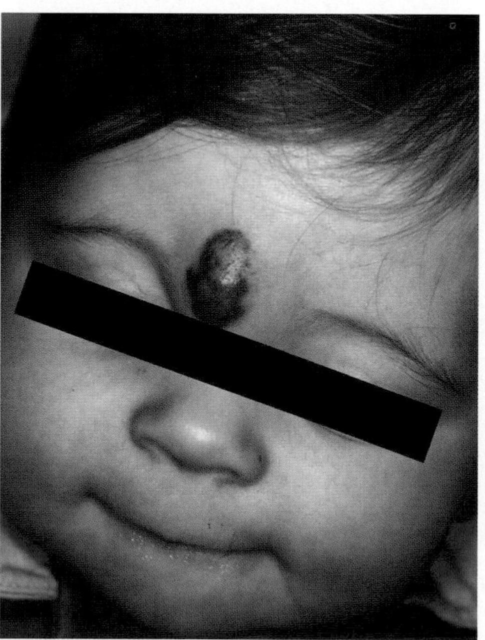

Color Plate 8 • A hemangioma with superficial and deep components involving the glabella.

(Image courtesy of Anne W. Lucky, MD.)

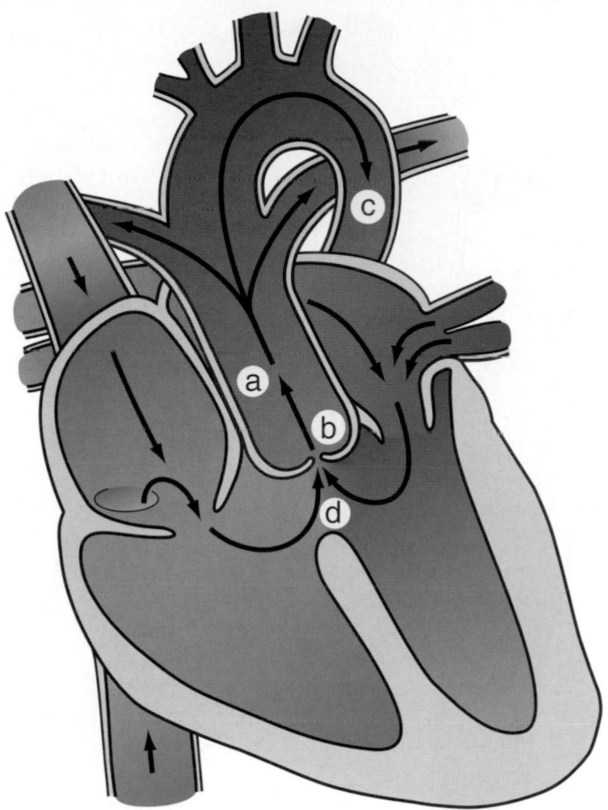

Color Plate 9 • Truncus arteriosus. Typical anatomic findings include (A) a single truncal vessel arising from the heart giving off the coronary arteries, pulmonary arteries, and aortic arch; (B) abnormal truncal valve; (C) left aortic arch shown (right aortic arch occurs in 30% of cases); (D) ventricular septal defect.

(Illustration by Patricia Gast.)

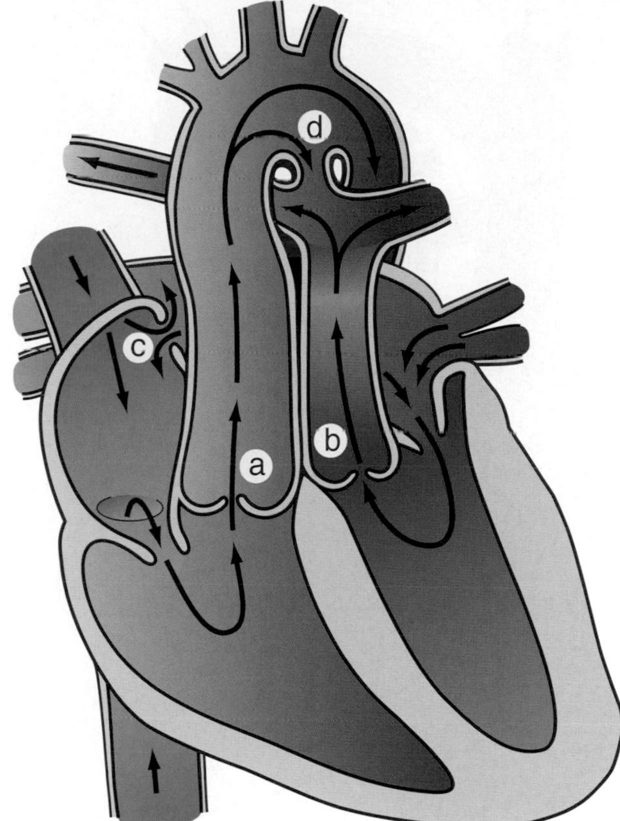

Color Plate 10 • Transposition of the great arteries with an intact ventricular septum, a large patent ductus arteriosus, and an atrial septal defect. Note the following: (A) aorta arises from the morphologic right ventricle; (B) pulmonary artery arises from the morphologic left ventricle; (C) mixing occurs across the atrial septal defect; (D) shunting from the aorta to the pulmonary artery via the ductus arteriosus.

(Illustration by Patricia Gast.)

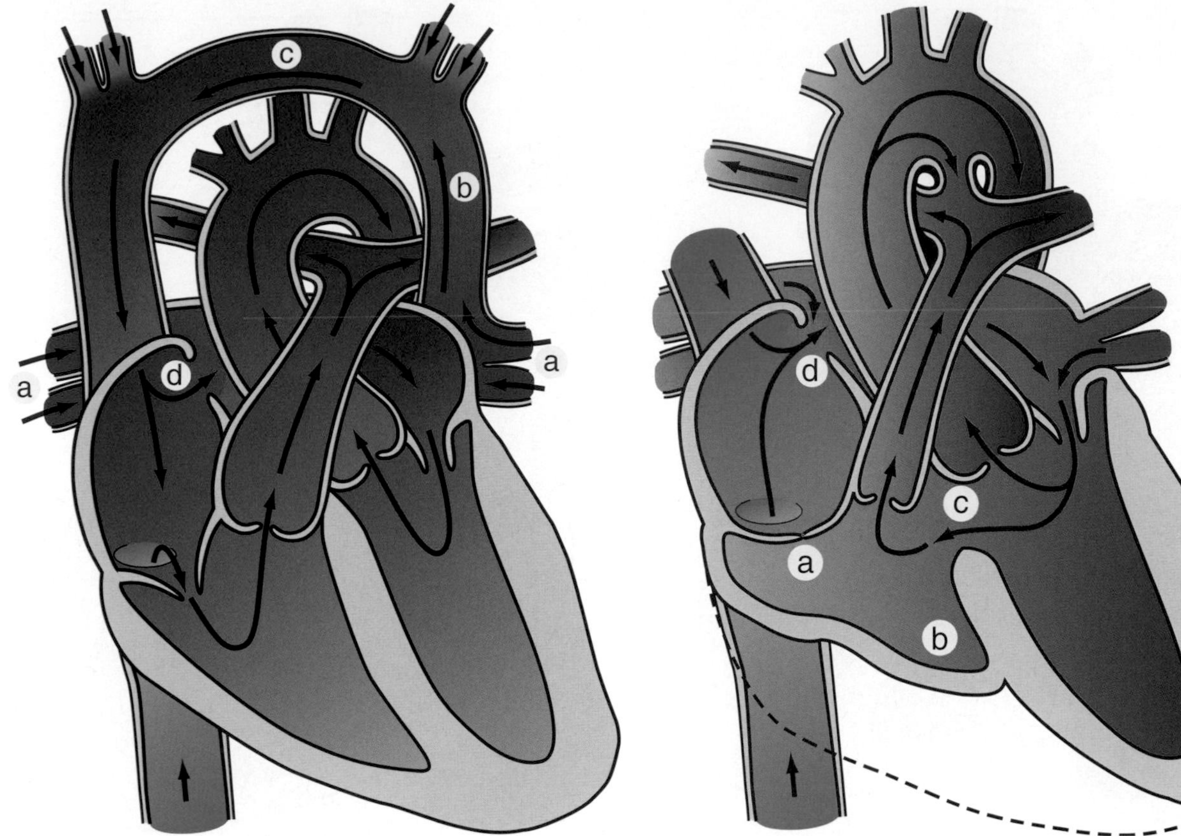

Color Plate 11 • Supradiaphragmatic total anomalous pulmonary venous connection. Note the following: (A) pulmonary veins join into a confluence; (B) the confluence joins a vertical vein which ascends to connect with the (C) innominate vein and then drains via the SVC into the right atrium; (D) venous return must cross the PFO to fill the left atrium.

(Illustration by Patricia Gast.)

Color Plate 12 • Tricuspid atresia with normally related great arteries and a patent ductus arteriosus. Typical anatomic findings include (A) atresia of the tricuspid valve; (B) hypoplasia of the right ventricle; (C) ventricular septal defect; (D) patent foramen ovale (PFO). Note: All systemic venous return must pass through the PFO to reach the left atrium and left ventricle.

(Illustration by Patricia Gast.)

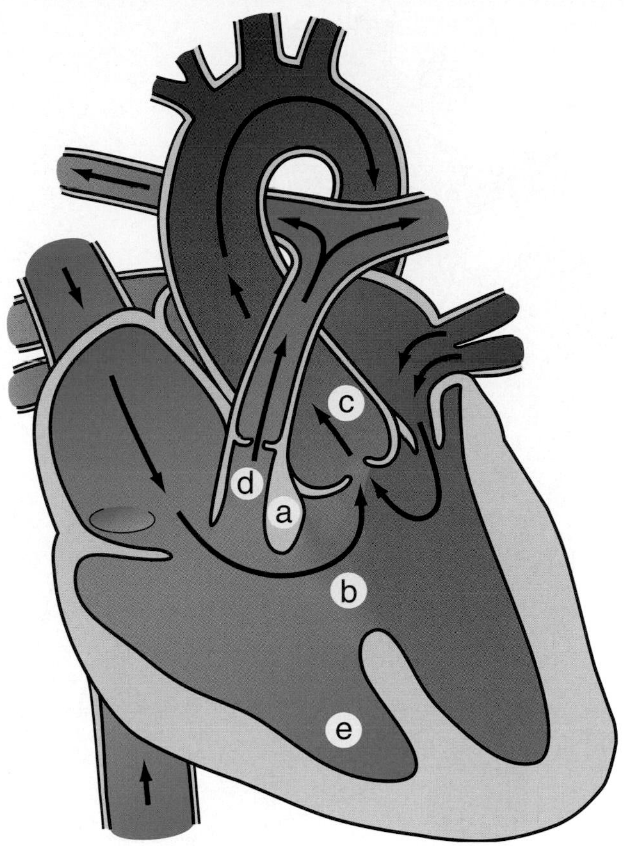

Color Plate 13 • Tetralogy of Fallot. Typical anatomic findings include (A) an anteriorly displaced infundibular septum, resulting in subpulmonary stenosis; (B) large anterior malalignment VSD; (C) overriding of the aorta over the muscular septum; (D) hypoplasia of the pulmonary valve and main pulmonary artery; (E) right ventricular hypertrophy, secondary to right ventricular outflow tract obstruction. (Illustration by Patricia Gast.)

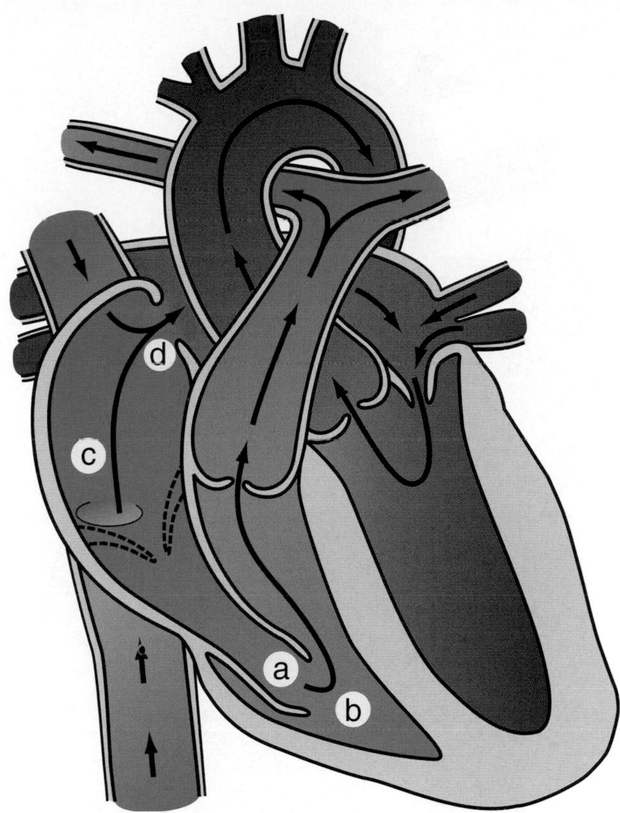

Color Plate 14 • Ebstein anomaly. Typical anatomic findings include (A) inferior displacement of the tricuspid valve into the right ventricle (the normal placement of the tricuspid valve is noted in dashed lines); (B) small right ventricle; (C) marked enlargement of the right atrium because of "atrialized" portion of right ventricle as well as tricuspid regurgitation; (D) right-to-left shunting at the atrial level. (Illustration by Patricia Gast.)

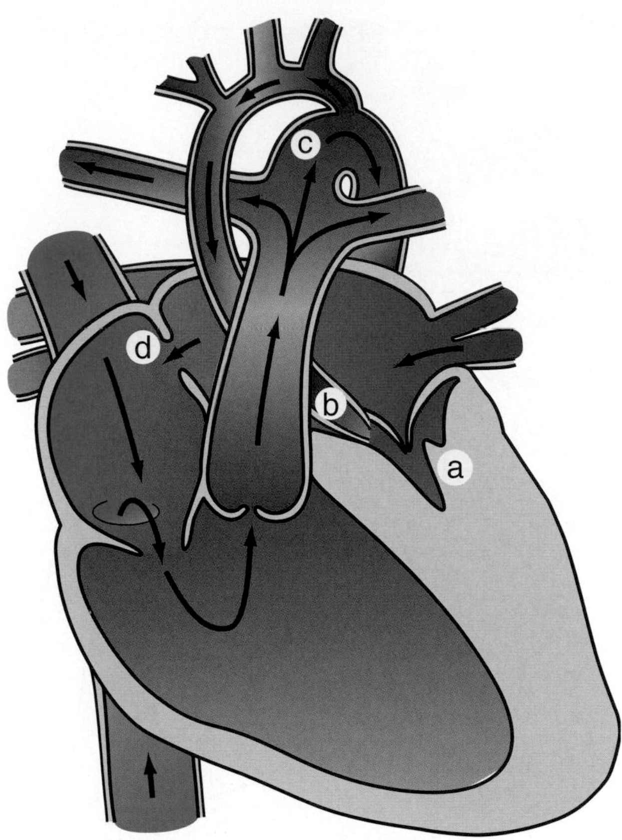

Color Plate 15 • Hypoplastic left heart syndrome. Typical anatomic findings include (A) atresia or hypoplasia of the mitral valve and hypoplasia of the left ventricle; (B) aortic atresia or stenosis and a diminutive ascending aorta and transverse aortic arch; (C) patent ductus arteriosus supplying systemic blood flow; (D) patent foramen ovale, with a left to right shunt.

(Illustration by Patricia Gast.)

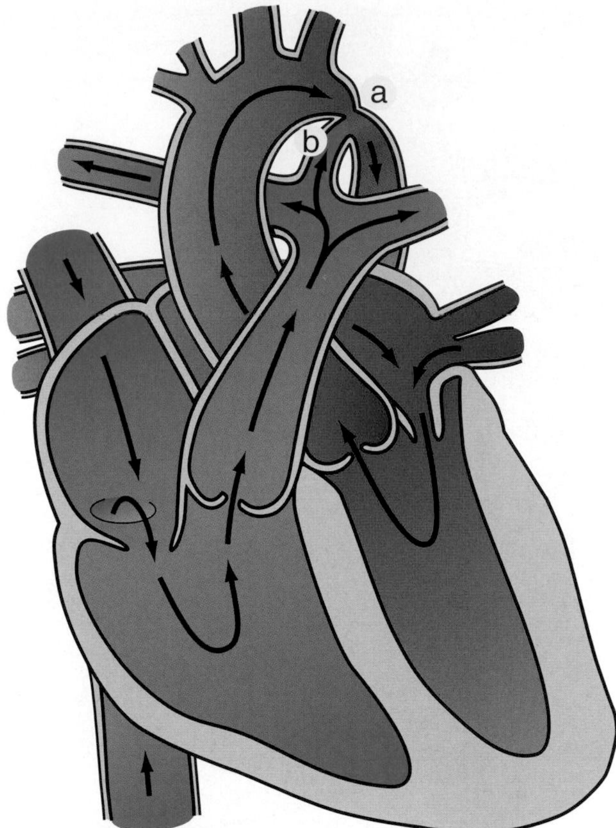

Color Plate 16 • Coarctation of the aorta. Possible anatomic findings include (A) narrowing distal to the left subclavian artery; (B) patent ductus arteriosus supplying systemic flow to descending aorta.

(Illustration by Patricia Gast.)

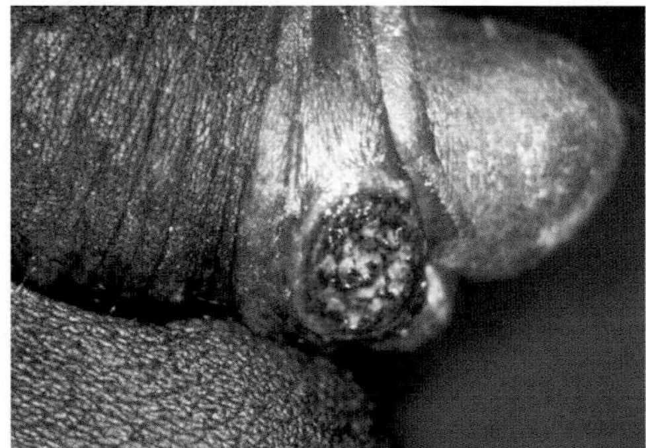

Color Plate 17 • Chancre of primary syphilis.

(From Goodheart HP. *Goodheart's Photoguide of Common Skin Disorders*, 2nd ed. Philadelphia, PA: Lippincott Williams & Wilkins, 2003.)

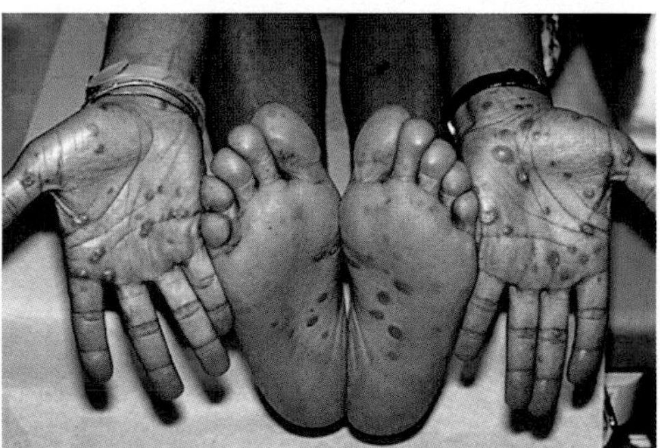

Color Plate 18 • Typical lesions of secondary syphilis (palms, soles).

(From Goodheart HP. *Goodheart's Photoguide of Common Skin Disorders*, 2nd ed. Philadelphia, PA: Lippincott Williams & Wilkins, 2003.)

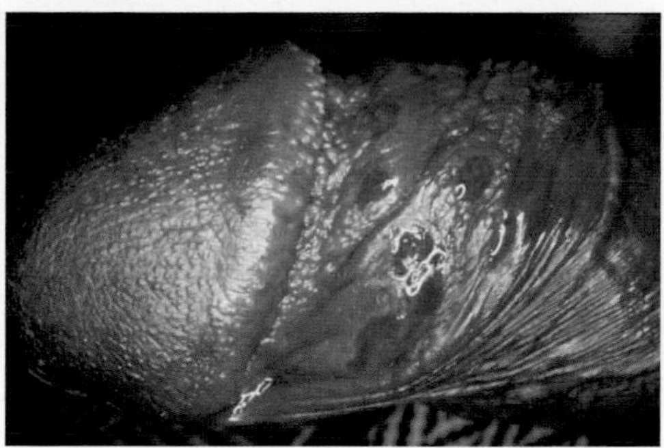

Color Plate 19 • Genital herpes (multiple erythematous ulcerations).
(From Goodheart HP. *Goodheart's Photoguide of Common Skin Disorders*, 2nd ed. Philadelphia, PA: Lippincott Williams & Wilkins, 2003.)

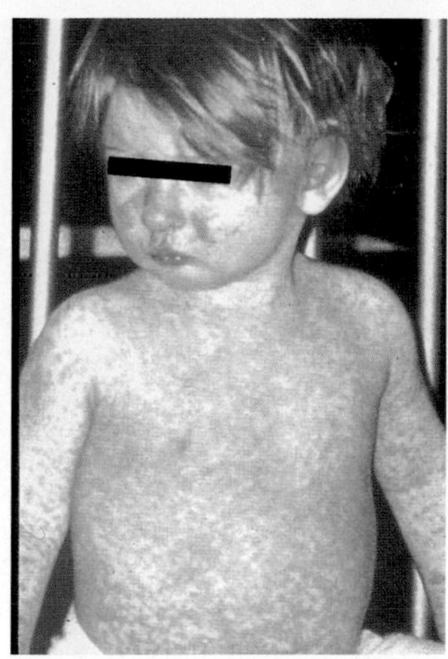

Color Plate 20 • A child with measles.
(Photo courtesy of Centers for Disease Control and Prevention.)

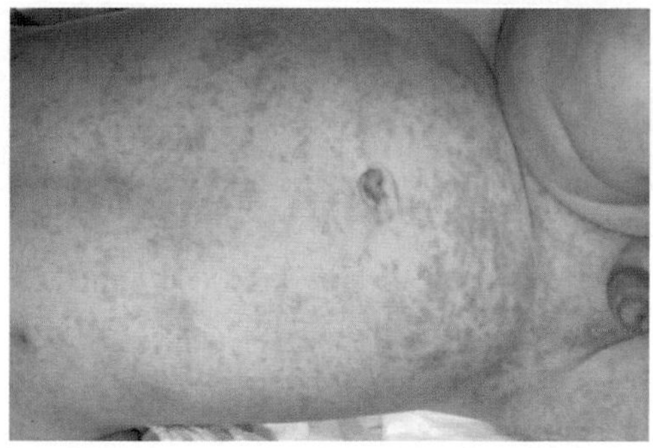

Color Plate 21 • Typical roseola exanthem.
(From Goodheart HP. *Goodheart's Photoguide of Common Skin Disorders*, 2nd ed. Philadelphia, PA: Lippincott Williams & Wilkins, 2003. Image courtesy of Bernard Cohen, MD.)

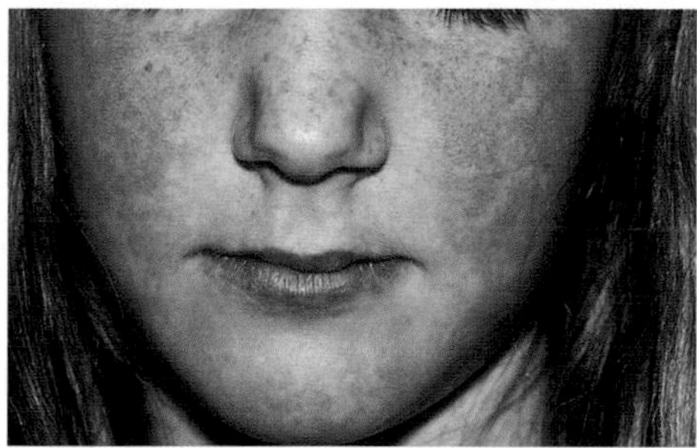

Color Plate 22 • "Slapped cheeks" of erythema infectiosum (fifth disease).
(From Goodheart HP. *Goodheart's Photoguide of Common Skin Disorders*, 2nd ed. Philadelphia, PA: Lippincott Williams & Wilkins, 2003.)

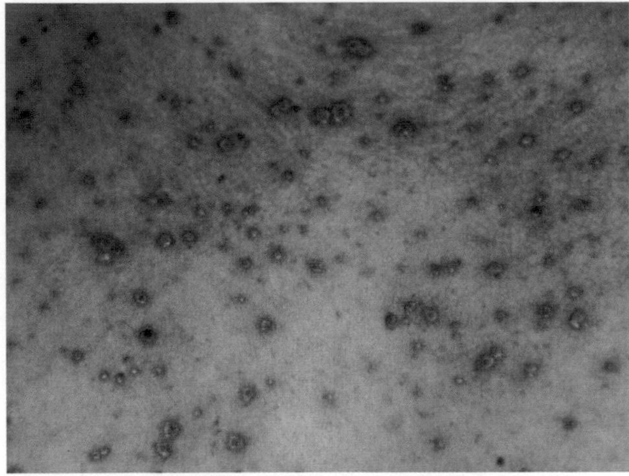

Color Plate 23 • Typical varicella lesions.

(From Sweet RL, Gibbs RS. *Atlas of Infectious Diseases of the Female Genital Tract*. Philadelphia, PA: Lippincott Williams & Wilkins, 2005.)

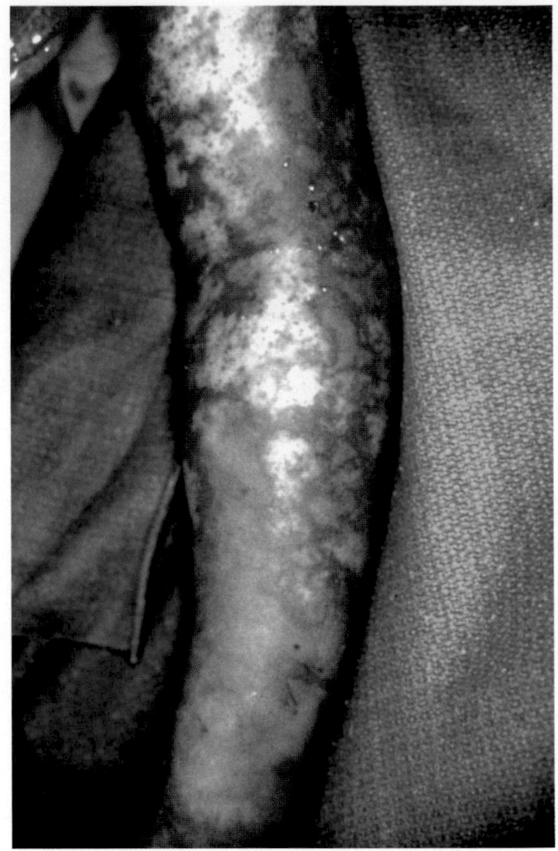

Color Plate 24 • Petechial lesions of Rocky Mountain spotted fever.

(Image from E Rubin, MD, and JL Farber, MD. *Pathology*, 3rd ed. Philadelphia, PA: Lippincott Williams & Wilkins, 1999.)

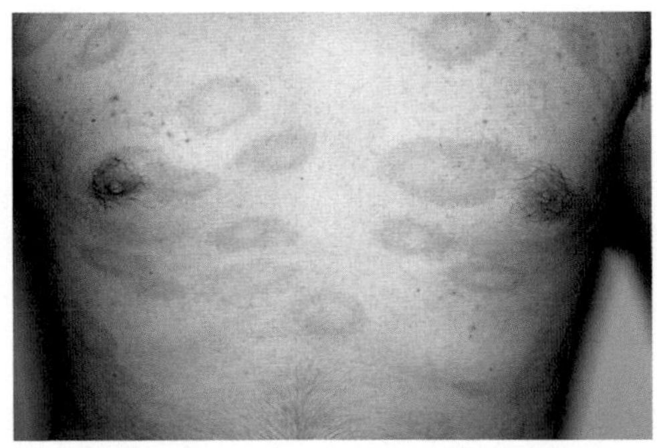

Color Plate 25 • Lyme disease (erythema migrans).

(From Goodheart HP. *Goodheart's Photoguide of Common Skin Disorders*, 2nd ed. Philadelphia, PA: Lippincott Williams & Wilkins, 2003.)

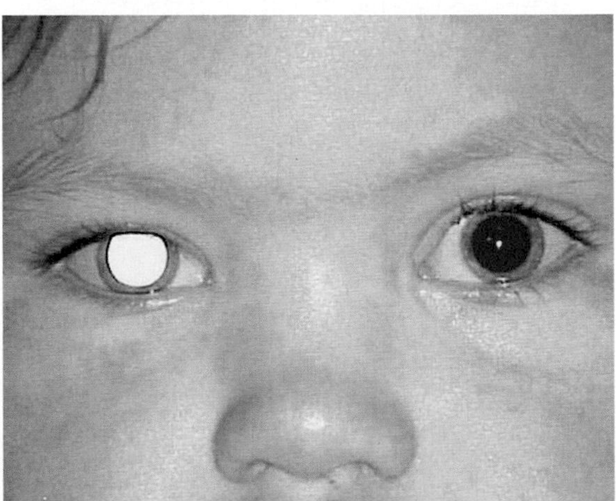

Color Plate 26 • Leukokoria due to advanced intraocular retinoblastoma of right eye.

(From Tasman W, Jaeger E. *The Wills Eye Hospital Atlas of Clinical Ophthalmology*, 2nd ed. Philadelphia, PA: Lippincott Williams & Wilkins, 2001.)

anemic children, especially those with light to medium complexions, may appear yellowish (sallow), and this is important and easy to differentiate from jaundice. Jaundice is a different hue and is also visible in the sclerae (scleral icterus). A flow murmur may be heard in moderate to severe anemia. Tachycardia and postural changes in heart rate and blood pressure are seen with acute blood loss, but compensation to chronic anemia may lessen some of these findings. The examiner should seek clues of specific causes of anemia, such as jaundice (hemolysis); maxillary hyperplasia and frontal bossing (hemolytic anemia and ineffective erythropoiesis); petechiae, purpura, and ecchymosis (bone marrow infiltration or failure); hepatomegaly and/or splenomegaly (leukemia, inherited hemolytic anemias); lymphadenopathy (leukemia or chronic inflammation); and short stature, abnormal facies, café-au-lait macules, and bony abnormalities of the thumb and forearm, which are associated with bone marrow failure syndromes. Table 11-2 lists physical findings that suggest a specific cause of anemia.

DIAGNOSTIC EVALUATION

Initial laboratory tests needed to evaluate anemia include a complete blood count (which includes red cell indices), differential white blood cell count, reticulocyte count, and peripheral blood smear. The most important laboratory clue to the cause of anemia is the reticulocyte count, which provides evidence about the mechanism of anemia. The bone marrow responds to hemolysis by increasing red cell production, releasing into the circulation immature red blood cells called reticulocytes (reticulocytosis). Decreased red blood cell production results in a reticulocyte count that is too low for the degree of anemia (reticulocytopenia). One must take care to interpret the reticulocyte count in the context of the degree of anemia. The second most important laboratory clue to the cause of anemia is red blood cell size, measured as the mean cell volume (MCV). Individual types of anemia may be macrocytic, normocytic, or microcytic. One must take care to interpret the

TABLE 11-2 Significance of Physical Findings Found in the Evaluation of Anemia

Body System	Physical Finding	Potential Significance (Cause of Anemia)
Skin	Hyperpigmentation	Fanconi anemia, dyskeratosis congenita
	Café-au-lait macules	Fanconi anemia
	Jaundice	Hemolysis
	Petechiae, purpura	Bone marrow infiltration, autoimmune hemolysis with autoimmune thrombocytopenia, hemolytic uremic syndrome
Head	Frontal bossing	Thalassemia major, sickle cell anemia
	Maxillary hyperplasia	Thalassemia major, sickle cell anemia
	Microcephaly	Fanconi anemia
Eyes	Microphthalmia	Fanconi anemia
	Retinopathy	Sickle cell disease
Mouth	Glossitis	B_{12} deficiency
	Cleft lip	Diamond-Blackfan anemia
	Hyperpigmentation	Peutz-Jeghers syndrome (GI blood loss)
	Telangiectasia	Osler-Weber-Rendu syndrome (GI blood loss)
	Leukoplakia	Dyskeratosis congenita
Chest	Shield chest (widespread nipples)	Diamond-Blackfan anemia
	Murmur	Prosthetic valve hemolysis
Abdomen	Splenomegaly	Sickle cell disease, thalassemia, immune hemolytic anemia, hereditary spherocytosis, leukemia, lymphoma, Epstein-Barr virus, portal hypertension
	Hepatomegaly	Sickle cell disease, leukemia, lymphoma
Extremities	Absent thumbs	Fanconi anemia
	Absent radii	Thrombocytopenia-absent radius syndrome
	Triphalangeal thumb	Diamond-Blackfan ansmia
	Spoon nails (koilonychia)	Iron deficiency (extremely rare physical finding in children)
	Dystrophic nails	Dyskeratosis congenital

MCV based on age-, sex-, and race-matched normal values. Examination of the peripheral blood smear is also critical for the diagnosis of anemia (Figs. 11-1 and 11-2), as it provides morphologic clues about the red cells, white cells, and platelets that the complete blood count does not. Table 11-1 outlines the most common causes of anemia and classifies them according to mechanism of anemia and red blood cell size.

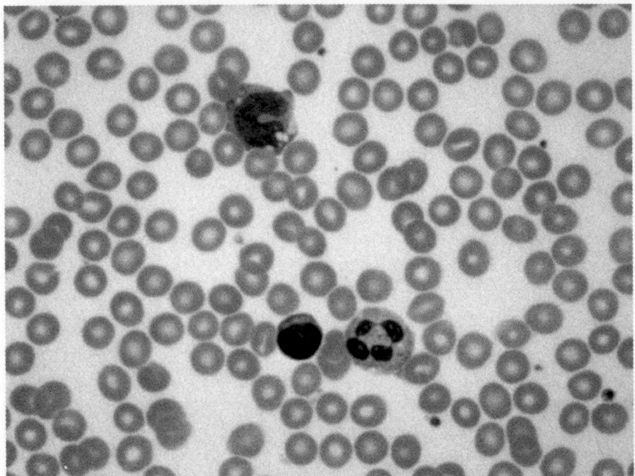

Figure 11-1 • Peripheral blood smear. Generally normal red blood cells are shown with biconcave disc morphology. Also shown are a monocyte (top nucleated cell), lymphocyte (bottom left nucleated cell), and neutrophil (bottom right nucleated cell). The platelets are normal in size and shape, but they appear to be slightly decreased in number in this view.

The combination of a history, physical examination, complete blood count (which includes an MCV), reticulocyte count, and peripheral blood smear is usually sufficient to diagnose accurately the most common forms of anemia without the need for further expensive and unnecessary tests. However, many other tests are available that can clarify or establish the diagnosis when initial testing is insufficient. With hemolysis, serum lactate dehydrogenase and indirect bilirubin can be elevated, whereas haptoglobin may be decreased. Urobilinogen may be detected on urinalysis. A direct antiglobulin test demonstrates the presence of immunoglobulins on the red blood cell surface and is diagnostic of immune hemolytic anemia. A glucose-6-phosphate dehydrogenase (G6PD) assay should be considered in African American and Mediterranean individuals with hemolytic anemia, although it can be falsely negative during acute hemolysis. Hemoglobin separation techniques (isoelectric focusing and high-pressure liquid chromatography) are used to diagnose hemoglobinopathies. Newborn screening procedures to identify infants born with significant hemoglobinopathies, such as sickle cell disease and severe forms of thalassemia, are currently in place in every state in the United States. Serum iron concentration, total iron-binding capacity (TIBC), and serum ferritin levels may confirm a diagnosis of iron deficiency when first-line testing is insufficient. Positive heme tests of stool or gastric contents indicate gastrointestinal bleeding. The erythrocyte sedimentation rate (ESR) is generally elevated in anemia of inflammation. In children, a macrocytic

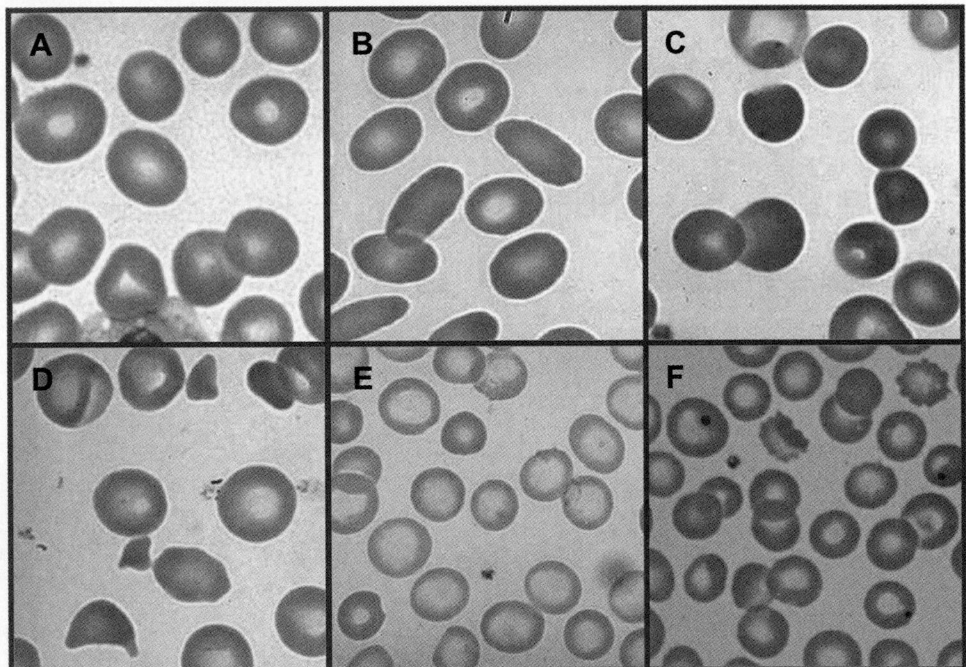

Figure 11-2 • Examples of normal and abnormal red blood cell (RBC) morphology. Panel A: normal RBCs. Panel B: elliptocytes. Panel C: spherocytes. Panel D: schistocytes. Panel E: hypochromic microcytic RBCs. Panel F: Howell-Jolly bodies and acanthocytes. Some images are from Bain B, Diagnosis from the blood smear, *New Engl J Med* 2005; 353:498–507.

anemia is most worrisome for a syndrome of bone marrow failure or infiltration, so a bone marrow examination is often needed. Vitamin B_{12} and red blood cell folate levels may also be measured, although dietary deficiencies of these nutrients are uncommon in children in developed nations.

TREATMENT

Treatment depends on the underlying cause of the anemia. Specific conditions and their treatment are discussed below.

MICROCYTIC ANEMIAS WITH DECREASED RED BLOOD CELL PRODUCTION

Hypochromic microcytic red blood cells result from impaired synthesis of either the heme or globin components of hemoglobin. Inadequate heme synthesis may be the result of iron deficiency, recurrent or chronic inflammation, sideroblastic states, or copper deficiency. Decreased globin synthesis is the hallmark of thalassemia. Iron-deficiency anemia, the thalassemia syndromes, and the anemia of inflammation are the most common causes of hypochromic microcytic anemias. Lead intoxication, whose main hematologic feature is basophilic stippling, not microcytosis, is discussed in detail in Chapter 21. The microcytosis that may be seen with lead intoxication is usually caused by concomitant iron deficiency (iron deficiency causes a microcytic anemia and pica; pica can result in ingestion of lead and the noncausal association between lead and microcytosis).

IRON-DEFICIENCY ANEMIA

Iron deficiency, the most common cause of anemia during childhood, is usually seen between 6 and 24 months of age but is not uncommon during adolescence. Iron deficiency may be caused by inadequate dietary intake of iron, decreased iron endowment at birth, blood loss, or malabsorption of iron. Nutritional iron deficiency develops when rapid growth and an expanding blood volume put excessive demands on iron stores. Dietary risk factors include extended exclusive breastfeeding (more than 6 months) without iron supplementation, consumption of low-iron formula preparations, early institution of low-iron solids, excessive cow milk intake, and the absence of iron supplements in high-risk situations (e.g., prematurity). The iron present in breast milk is much more bioavailable than the iron in cow's milk, but it is still insufficient to provide enough iron beyond 6 months of age.

Iron-deficiency anemia can occur as early as 3 months of age in the premature infant who has inadequate iron stores at birth. It can occur in the infant or toddler who receives a diet exclusively composed of cow's milk, low-iron formula, or breast milk (without iron supplementation after 6 months). Nutritional iron deficiency can also occur during adolescence when rapid growth may coincide with a diet with suboptimal iron content. This is a particular problem in adolescent females because of menstrual iron loss.

Prenatal iron loss can occur from feto-maternal transfusion or from twin-to-twin transfusion. Perinatal bleeding may result from feto-placental transfusion or obstetric complications such as placental abruption or placenta previa. Postnatal blood loss may be overt (bloody stools or traumatic hemorrhage) or occult, as with anomalies of the gastrointestinal tract (e.g., juvenile polyps, Meckel diverticulum), inflammatory bowel disease, parasitic infestations, and idiopathic pulmonary hemosiderosis. Malabsorption of iron is uncommon, but can occur in certain disease states (e.g., celiac disease) or as an inborn error.

Clinical Manifestations

Mild iron deficiency is usually asymptomatic. With moderate iron deficiency (hemoglobin concentration approximately 6–8 g/dL), the child may have decreased appetite, irritability, fatigue, and decreased exercise tolerance. Physical examination shows skin and mucous membrane pallor, tachycardia, and a systolic ejection murmur along the left sternal border. The child with severe anemia (hemoglobin less than 3 g per dL) may show signs of congestive heart failure, which include tachycardia, an S_3 gallop, cardiomegaly, hepatomegaly, distended neck veins, and rales. Children with slowly progressive, chronic anemia may be remarkably hemodynamically compensated. Glossitis, angular stomatitis, and koilonychia (spoon nails) are usually never seen in children with isolated iron-deficiency anemia in developed nations.

Table 11-3 lists the laboratory findings typical for the common causes of microcytic anemia. Bone marrow examination

TABLE 11-3 Classical Laboratory Findings for Common Causes of a Mild Microcytic Anemia

Test	Iron Deficiency	Thalassemia Trait[a]	Anemia of Inflammation
RDW	↑	Normal	Normal
MCV	↓	↓	Normal or ↓
RBC count	↓	↑	↓
Hb A_2	↓	β:↑ α:↓	Normal
Hb F	Normal	β:↑ α: Normal	Normal
Serum iron	↓	Normal	↓
TIBC	↑	Normal	Normal or ↓
Ferritin	↓	Normal	↑

Abbreviations: Hb A_2, hemoglobin A_2; Hb F, hemoglobin F (fetal); MCV, mean cell volume; RBC, red blood cell; RDW, red cell distribution width; TIBC, total iron-binding capacity; ↑, increased; ↓, decreased.
[a]When the result of a test differs between α-thalassemia and β-thalassemia, the result is preceded by an "α:"or "β:"

is not necessary to confirm a diagnosis of iron deficiency, but when performed demonstrates micronormoblastic hyperplasia of the erythroid line and absence of stainable iron. A response to appropriate iron supplementation is the best diagnostic test for iron deficiency.

Treatment

Mild to moderate iron-deficiency anemia without evidence of congestive heart failure is treated with 3 to 6 mg/kg/day of elemental iron by mouth. The reticulocyte count increases within 2 to 3 days of iron therapy, and the hemoglobin increases at a rate of approximately 0.3 g/dL/day after 4 to 5 days. The hemoglobin concentration normalizes within a month. However, iron therapy must continue (at a lower dose: 2 to 3 mg/kg/day of elemental iron) for 2 to 3 months after the hemoglobin normalizes to replenish tissue stores and prevent recurrent iron deficiency. If the hemoglobin does not increase as suspected, considerations include nonadherence to iron, incorrect dose of iron, an incorrect diagnosis of iron deficiency, or malabsorption of iron. Transfusion of packed red blood cells is reserved for those with symptomatic anemia in whom a rapid correction is needed and those with impending or established high-output congestive heart failure. Although infants and young children can tolerate remarkable degrees of anemia, especially if the decline in hemoglobin is gradual, individuals with severe anemia must be transfused very slowly in serial, small (2 to 5 mL per kg) aliquots of packed red blood cells to avoid cardiac decompensation due to volume overload.

ALPHA AND BETA THALASSEMIA

Pathogenesis and Clinical Manifestations

The thalassemias are hereditary anemias characterized by decreased or absent synthesis of one or more globin subunits of the hemoglobin molecule. α thalassemia is classically caused by deletions of one or more of the four α-globin genes, leading to reduced synthesis of α-globin. β thalassemia is classically caused by point mutations of the β-globin gene, leading to reduced (β^+ mutations) or absent (β^0 mutations) synthesis of β- globin. The result of decreased production of either the α- or β-globin is an *imbalance* between the normally matched production of both—the key pathophysiology of thalassemia. This imbalance leads to an excess of one globin type (β in α-thalassemia, α in β-thalassemia) that may pair with itself, is unstable, precipitates, and damages the membrane inside the developing erythroblast, resulting in ineffective erythropoiesis and hemolysis.

Thalassemias are classified by clinical severity. Thalassemia *major* is a transfusion-dependent condition. Thalassemia *minor* is the asymptomatic trait state with only mild anemia. Thalassemia *intermedia* encompasses all the conditions of intermediate severity between the major and minor states. Tables 11-4 and 11-5 classify the common thalassemia syndromes.

The number of deleted globin genes determines the hematologic consequences of α-thalassemia. These deletions can be *cis* or *trans*. *Cis* deletions occur when two α-globin genes are deleted from one chromosome, whereas *trans* deletions signify α-globin gene deletions on each of the two chromosomes. Different races and ethnicities have varying rates of both *cis* and *trans* deletions of α-globin genes in their population.

Homozygous α-thalassemia major occurs when all four α-globin genes are deleted. Failure to produce any α-globin chains results in γ-globin tetramers (hemoglobin Bart's) and small amounts of embryonic hemoglobins. Hemoglobin Bart's has a high affinity for oxygen and does not release it to the tissue. The result is severe anemia, tissue hypoxia, heart failure, hepatosplenomegaly, generalized edema, and death *in utero* because of hydrops fetalis. The *cis* deletion is most prevalent in Southeast Asians, so homozygosity for *cis* deletions also occurs in this population.

TABLE 11-4 Comparison of the Classical α-thalassemia Syndromes

Genotype	Number of Normal α Genes	Description
αα/αα	4	Normal
αα/α-	3	Silent carrier state
--/αα	2	Thalassemia trait (α-thalassemia minor)
α-/α-	2	
--/α-	1	Hb H disease (α-thalassemia intermedia)
--/--	0	Hydrops fetalis (α-thalassemia major)

Abbreviations: α, α-globin gene; -, deleted α-globin gene; /, indicates the distinction between the two chromosomes.

TABLE 11-5 Comparison of the Classical β-Thalassemia Syndromes

Genotype	Description
β / β	Normal
β / β^0	β-thalassemia trait (minor)
β / β^+	
β^+ / β^+	β-thalassemia intermedia
β^+ / β^0	
β^0 / β^0	β-thalassemia major (Cooley's Anemia)

Abbreviations: β^0, null allele (absent globin production); β^+, holomorphic allele (decreased globin production); /, indicates the distinction between the two chromosomes.

Hemoglobin H disease (α-thalassemia intermedia) results from deletion of three of the four α-globin genes. In normal infants, fetal hemoglobin (which consists of two α-globin chains and two γ-globin chains) predominates at birth, but declines thereafter as γ-globin production falls and is replaced by β-globin production. In newborn infants with hemoglobin H disease, the dearth of α-globin leads to the formation of hemoglobin Bart's (γ-globin tetramer), which accounts for 10% to 40% of the total hemoglobin. With the reduction of γ-globin synthesis and the increase in β-globin synthesis at birth, hemoglobin Bart's diminishes and hemoglobin H (β-globin tetramer) predominates after the first few months of life.

Hemoglobin H eventually accounts for 10% to 40% of the total hemoglobin, and normal hemoglobin A accounts for approximately 60% to 90% of the total hemoglobin. This diagnosis is most common in children with Southeast Asian ancestry. Affected individuals have moderate anemia, variable hepatosplenomegaly, and the need for intermittent transfusions.

α thalassemia trait, also known as α-thalassemia minor, results from the deletion of two α globin genes. This defect manifests with mild anemia, hypochromia, and microcytosis. The α-thalassemia trait, present in 3% of U.S. Blacks and 1% to 5% of those of Mediterranean descent, is often confused with mild iron deficiency. The hemoglobin electrophoresis may be normal in these children, or show decreased hemoglobin A_2, and the diagnosis is often one of exclusion. It can be confirmed by parental or genetic studies.

Those with deletion of only one α-globin gene are called "silent carriers" for α-thalassemia because they have a normal or near-normal hemoglobin concentration and normal or near-normal red blood cell indices. The condition can be documented by quantitative measurement of globin chain synthesis or by gene analysis. A carrier can produce offspring, depending on the genotype of the normal parent, who are also silent carriers or have α-thalassemia trait or hemoglobin H disease.

β thalassemia major results either from complete or near-complete absence of β-globin synthesis (classically, the β^0/β^0 genotype). β-Thalassemia intermedia can occur with a variety of genotypes in which there is moderately diminished, but not absent, β-globin production (e.g., β^0/β^+ or β^+/β^+ genotypes). The child with β-thalassemia minor, the heterozygous form, has one normal β-globin gene and one abnormal β-globin gene (e.g., β/β^+ or β/β^0 genotypes).

Newborns with β-thalassemia have normal blood counts, unlike those with α-thalassemia, because the fetus and newborn normally use fetal hemoglobin. In β-thalassemia major, severe anemia, organomegaly, and growth failure progressively develop during the first year of life. If untreated, bone marrow hyperplasia and extramedullary hematopoiesis produce characteristic features such as frontal bossing, maxillary hypertrophy with prominent cheekbones, and an overbite. Failure to thrive is prominent in this population. Untreated, death occurs within the first few years of life because of progressive congestive heart failure. Despite severe anemia, there is a relative reticulocytopenia, reflecting the characteristic ineffective hematopoiesis. Peripheral blood smear reveals marked hypochromia, microcytosis, anisocytosis, and poikilocytosis. Hemoglobin F accounts for 95% of hemoglobin in the β^0/β^0 genotype and lesser amounts in other genotypes (e.g., β^0/β^+).

Children with β-thalassemia intermedia have moderate anemia, variable hepatosplenomegaly, and the need for intermittent transfusions. Children with β-thalassemia minor have only mild microcytic anemia. On blood smear, the hypochromia, microcytosis, and anisocytosis are disproportionately severe given the mild degree of anemia. Hemoglobin separation shows elevation of the hemoglobin A_2 level and sometimes elevation of hemoglobin F.

Epidemiology

Thalassemia is most common in African, Southeast Asian, Mediterranean, and Middle Eastern populations. The most severe forms of α-thalassemia, three- and four-gene deletions, occur frequently in the Southeast Asian population because of the high prevalence of *cis* deletions. Beta thalassemia is most often found in populations originating from the Mediterranean, Middle East, and India, but is found in Southeast Asian populations as well.

Treatment

Therapy for children with thalassemia major includes regular (monthly) packed red blood cell transfusions to ameliorate symptomatic anemia, suppress ineffective and extramedullary erythropoiesis, minimize organomegaly and bone disease, and improve quality and duration of life. The usual goal of transfusion therapy is to maintain the nadir (pretransfusion) hemoglobin concentration ≥10 g per dL. This regimen eliminates an increased erythropoietic drive, allowing normal linear growth and bone development. Suppression of erythropoiesis also decreases the stimulus for increased iron absorption, which helps minimize iron overload.

Splenectomy is considered when transfusion requirements exceed 250 mL/kg/year. Iron overload develops in children with β-thalassemia, whether they are transfused or not, because of hyperabsorption of dietary iron. However, transfusional iron loading is the overriding mechanism. When the bone marrow storage capacity for iron is exceeded, iron accumulates first in the liver and then in the heart, pancreas, and gonads, damaging those organs and producing signs and symptoms of hemochromatosis. As a result, untreated or poorly chelated thalassemia patients develop cardiomyopathy and congestive heart failure as adolescents or young adults. Cardiac disease is the main cause of death in thalassemia major. To minimize the morbidity and mortality associated with iron overload, patients are treated with iron chelating agents such as oral deferasirox or subcutaneous deferoxamine. Bone marrow transplantation can be curative, but because of its associated morbidity and mortality, this procedure is best performed in specialized centers using HLA-matched sibling donors.

Principles of therapy for thalassemia intermedia (α or β) are the same as those for β-thalassemia major, but the need for transfusion and the complications of the disease, therapy depend largely on the severity of the anemia. Because of the constant state of increased erythropoiesis, folic acid supplementation is recommended for patients not maintained on chronic transfusion therapy in order to prevent folate deficiency and megaloblastic anemia.

No treatment is necessary for α- or β-thalassemia minor, although genetic counseling is recommended. Thalassemia trait may be mistaken for iron-deficiency anemia because both may cause a mild, microcytic anemia. Thalassemia trait should be considered in a child with presumed iron-deficiency anemia who is compliant with, but does not respond to, an appropriate dose of iron therapy. The child with α-thalassemia trait has a normal hemoglobin electrophoresis (outside the neonatal period) or a decrease in hemoglobin A_2, whereas the electrophoresis of the child with β-thalassemia minor may show elevations of one or both of hemoglobin A_2 and hemoglobin F.

ANEMIA OF INFLAMMATION

Anemia of inflammation, once called anemia of chronic disease, can result from chronic inflammatory diseases, such as inflammatory bowel disease, juvenile idiopathic arthritis (JIA), chronic infections, and malignancy as well as relatively minor acute or recurrent viral infections. Typically, the anemia of inflammation is normocytic, but it is microcytic in 25% of cases. Inflammation increases the hepatic production of hepcidin, a key regulator of iron metabolism. Hepcidin induces the internalization and degradation of ferroportin, an iron-transport protein, on macrophages and duodenal enterocytes. This impairs the release of iron from macrophages and absorption of iron by the gut, thereby limiting the availability of iron that is necessary for erythropoiesis. Anemia of inflammation can be thought of as a functional state of iron deficiency. This response likely evolved to sequester iron away from invading pathogens, thereby limiting their growth and replication. A modest decrease in the survival time of red blood cells and a relatively limited erythropoietin response also contribute to the anemia of inflammation.

Clinical and Laboratory Features

The anemia is usually mild (hemoglobin concentration approximately 8 to 10 g/dL) and often incidentally discovered. Table 11-3 notes the laboratory findings typical for anemia of inflammation. As in iron-deficiency anemia, the serum iron level is reduced; in contrast to iron-deficiency anemia, the total iron-binding capacity is low, and the serum ferritin level is normal or increased. Bone marrow examination shows micronormoblastic hyperplasia and an increase in storage iron, but a decrease in the number of iron-containing erythroblasts.

Treatment

Treatment should be directed at the cause of the inflammation. The anemia will resolve spontaneously when the underlying inflammatory condition resolves. Therapy with iron supplements is unnecessary and ineffective unless comorbid iron deficiency is clearly documented. Some children with severe anemia of inflammation, such as those with prolonged or critical illness, may need a transfusion of packed red blood cells as a temporizing measure.

NORMOCYTIC ANEMIAS WITH DECREASED RED CELL PRODUCTION

Normocytic anemias with decreased red cell production have many causes. A common theme is impaired or inadequate bone marrow response to anemia, as occurs with replacement of the marrow by fibrosis, infiltration of the marrow by malignant cells, or deficiency of erythropoietin (e.g., chronic renal disease). The bone marrow may also fail because of toxic insults. Transient marrow failure states include transient erythroblastopenia of childhood (TEC), human parvovirus-induced aplastic crisis (in patients with hemolytic anemia), and drug toxicity from myelosuppressive and chemotherapeutic agents. A normocytic anemia also occurs with acute blood loss, in which a compensatory increase in total blood volume results in the anemia before the bone marrow has time to correct the deficit in red cell mass. The anemia of inflammation, discussed above, is often normocytic, especially early in the course of the disease.

TRANSIENT ERYTHROBLASTOPENIA OF CHILDHOOD

TEC is an acquired pure red cell aplasia due to temporary suppression of bone marrow erythropoiesis. The exact cause of TEC is not known, although a number of viruses have been epidemiologically linked to TEC. Human parvovirus is not believed to be the cause of TEC, however. As the name implies, TEC is self-limited and usually associated with normal white blood cell and platelet counts.

Clinical and Laboratory Features

TEC occurs between 6 months and 4 years of age, with a peak incidence at 2 years of age. The history and physical examination are unremarkable except for the gradual onset of pallor over the course of weeks or months. Often this is imperceptible to parents who see the child every day. An outside observer, such as a visiting grandparent, may be the first to recognize the pallor. There is no organomegaly or lymphadenopathy, and the child is otherwise well. The anemia in TEC is normocytic, and the blood counts show reticulocytopenia (unless TEC is identified in the recovery phase characterized by reticulocytosis). Bone marrow examination, if performed, shows few erythroid precursors and normal myeloid and platelet precursors.

The differential diagnosis of TEC includes Diamond-Blackfan anemia (DBA), which is a constitutional bone marrow failure syndrome. DBA usually presents before 6 months of age, produces a macrocytic, and is often associated with physical anomalies, such as characteristic (Cathie) facies, hypoplastic thenar eminence, and triphalangeal thumb.

Treatment

The hemoglobin concentration is usually at its nadir at the time of diagnosis. Spontaneous recovery occurs within 1 to 2 months of diagnosis. Red blood cell transfusions are necessary only if the patient has symptomatic severe anemia or evidence of congestive heart failure.

NORMOCYTIC ANEMIAS WITH INCREASED RED CELL PRODUCTION

HEMOLYTIC ANEMIA

Normocytic anemias with increased red cell production are most commonly caused by hemolysis. Hemolysis is synonymous with increased red blood cell destruction and is defined as a shortened red cell lifespan. The anemia and consequent tissue hypoxemia is sensed by the renal interstitium, which produces erythropoietin in compensation to augment erythropoiesis. The result is a compensatory reticulocytosis. Hemolytic anemias can be caused by defects intrinsic to the red cell (intracorpuscular defects) or factors extrinsic to the red cell (extracorpuscular insults), that is damage from within or damage from without. In general, intrinsic defects are hereditary and extrinsic defects are acquired.

Intrinsic hemolysis can be caused by defects of any of the three components of the red cell: the membrane, cytosol (enzymes), and hemoglobin. Intrinsic membrane defects include hereditary spherocytosis (HS), hereditary elliptocytosis, hereditary stomatocytosis, and paroxysmal nocturnal hemoglobinuria (PNH). PNH is the only intrinsic defect that is not inherited. Hemoglobinopathies (sickle cell disorders, thalassemia) and enzyme disorders (G6PD deficiency, pyruvate kinase deficiency) are also intrinsic defects.

Extrinsic hemolysis can be classified as nonimmune and immune. *Nonimmune hemolytic anemias* can be microangiopathic (disseminated intravascular coagulation, hemolytic uremic syndrome, thrombotic thrombocytopenic purpura), toxin-related (snake venom, copper, and arsenic), due to intraerythrocytic parasites (malaria, babesiosis), or extensive burns. *Immune hemolytic anemia* refers to hemolytic anemia caused by the deposition of antibody, complement, or both on the surface of the red cell that leads to its damage and eventual destruction.

The following is a discussion of four common types of hemolytic anemia in children. Three are examples of intrinsic defects (HS, sickle cell disease, and G6PD deficiency), and one is an example of an extrinsic insult (autoimmune hemolytic anemia).

HEREDITARY SPHEROCYTOSIS

Spherocytes are abnormal red blood cells with a high surface-to-volume ratio (globular or spherical rather than discoid) produced by the loss of membrane without a proportional loss in cell volume. All spherocytosis is not HS. A number of other conditions also produce spherocytes, such as immune hemolytic anemia, sepsis, burns, and toxins.

HS refers to a groups of related diseases caused by a congenital, intrinsic defect in the cytoskeleton of red blood cells, specifically a deficiency or dysfunction of one or more of the membrane-supporting proteins, spectrin, ankyrin, band 3 protein, or protein 4.2, whose role is to maintain the proper deformability and elasticity of the erythrocyte. The defect shortens the red cell lifespan (that is, causes a hemolytic anemia) and produces the characteristic morphology, the spherocyte, after which the condition is named. The hemolysis occurs mainly in the extravascular compartment and in the spleen. The membrane of HS red cells is recognized as abnormal by splenic macrophages, and membrane fragments are removed with each passage of the red cell through the splenic circulation. This progressive loss of membrane produces spherocytes and microspherocytes. The poor deformability and osmotic fragility of spherocytes leads to their early destruction. Inheritance of HS is usually autosomal dominant, but 25% of cases are caused by new mutations or are autosomal recessive.

Clinical Manifestations

HS varies greatly in clinical severity across patients, ranging from incidentally discovered, asymptomatic, mild anemia to severe anemia with growth failure, splenomegaly, and a requirement for chronic transfusions in infancy necessitating early splenectomy. Severe disease is uncommon, however, and HS is often diagnosed incidentally, when anemia is discovered on a blood count obtained for another purpose, or when screening is done for a family history of anemia. HS can also be discovered when investigating the cause of anemia or jaundice.

Newborns may have exaggerated or prolonged neonatal jaundice (unconjugated hyperbilirubinemia) because of the hemolysis superimposed upon physiologic jaundice, and roughly 1/3 may require transfusion for symptomatic anemia during the first few months of life when hemolysis is superimposed upon physiologic anemia of infancy. The need for transfusion during the neonatal period does not indicate that the child will have ongoing severe anemia and need further transfusion therapy later in life. Beyond the newborn period, the typical features of HS include jaundice (especially scleral icterus), which may be intermittent, and variable splenomegaly. Pallor and fatigue occur depending on the degree of anemia. Jaundice may only be noticed during febrile or other inflammatory illnesses when the hemolytic rate may increase. These episodes are called "hyperhemolytic" episodes, marked by increased anemia, pallor, and jaundice. These episodes resolve when the underlying illness abates. Some individuals have recurring hyperhemolytic episodes requiring transfusion. Infection with human parvovirus causes the transient aplastic crisis, a moderate to severe exacerbation of the underlying anemia due to temporary cessation of erythropoiesis. The aplastic crisis resolves when neutralizing antibody is formed 1 to 2 weeks following infection, providing lifelong immunity and protection against further parvovirus infection. Because of chronic hemolysis, and the increased flux of bilirubin through the hepatobiliary system, individuals with HS may develop bilirubinate (pigment) gallstones, even in the first decade of life. These gallstones may be asymptomatic or cause typical signs and symptoms of cholecystitis or choledocholithiasis.

Laboratory Testing

Laboratory studies typically show a mild-to-moderate normocytic anemia, reticulocytosis, elevated MCHC, and indirect hyperbilirubinemia. A conjugated hyperbilirubinemia may indicate cholelithiasis. Failing to obtain a reticulocyte count when evaluating for the cause of anemia, is a common reason that HS and other hemolytic anemias may be missed. During the parvovirus-related transient aplastic crisis the anemia will be more severe, and there will be an inappropriately low reticulocyte count. Upon recovery from the aplastic crisis, nucleated red blood cells will first appear in peripheral blood followed about 1 day later by a burst of reticulocytosis. Aplastic crisis discovered during the recovery phase may be mistaken for a hyper-hemolytic episode, also characterized by increased anemia, in which the reticulocyte count is increased from baseline.

HS can easily be diagnosed with a good history (e.g., intermittent scleral icterus), physical examination (e.g., mild splenomegaly), and family history (e.g., anemia or cholelithiasis), along with a complete blood count, reticulocyte count, and examination of the peripheral smear (showing anemia, reticulocytosis, and spherocytosis). It is wise to exclude immune hemolytic anemia by a direct antiglobulin test (DAT). Further testing is usually not needed to confirm the diagnosis of HS. Osmotic fragility testing is a test for spherocytes, not HS. Any cause of spherocytosis (listed earlier in this chapter) will give a positive osmotic fragility test. Osmotic gradient ektacytometry can also demonstrate defects in red cell water content or volume, but not differentiate the different causes of spherocytes. A newer test, eosin-5-maleimide (EMA) binding, has high sensitivity and specificity for HS and might see increasing use when the diagnosis of HS is unclear.

Treatment

The most important "treatment" for HS is expectant management—awareness of and watchful waiting for possible complications, promptly addressing them if they arise (e.g., cholecystectomy for symptomatic cholelithiasis), and ongoing education of the patient and family about the disease. Folic acid supplementation is needed only for severe hemolytic anemia. Episodic transfusions may be given for symptomatic or life-threatening anemia during the transient aplastic crisis or "hyperhemolytic" episodes. The need for multiple or regularly scheduled transfusions should prompt serious consideration for splenectomy. Splenectomy can often "cure" the hemolytic anemia, although the underlying red cell defect remains. Splenectomy should be reserved for those patients with symptomatic hemolysis affecting quality of life (e.g., fatigue, growth failure, the need for frequent transfusions). The risks of splenectomy include a lifelong, increased risk of overwhelming sepsis with encapsulated organisms (especially, *Streptococcus pneumomiae*) as well as thrombosis and, possibly, pulmonary hypertension. Splenectomy should be delayed, when possible, until after 2 years of age, because the risk of sepsis is higher in the very young. Individuals who have a splenectomy need appropriate immunization before and after surgery (against the pneumococcus and meningococcus) and at least several years of postsplenectomy prophylactic penicillin (if not lifelong). Asplenic individuals also need to seek immediate medical attention for any high fever for the remainder of their lives.

SICKLE CELL DISEASE

Sickle cell disease (SCD) is the name for a group a recessive genetic disorders caused by sickle hemoglobin (Hb S). The most common and severe form of SCD is sickle cell anemia (Hb SS), the homozygous state for the Hb S mutation ($\beta^{6\ glu>val}$). Other forms of SCD result from compound heterozygous states with Hb S and other abnormal hemoglobins, such as Hb C (sickle-hemoglobin C disease). In the United States, approximately 1 in 2,500 newborns and 1 in 400 African American newborns has SCD, and at least 70,000 individuals are affected in the United States. Millions are affected worldwide.

Genetics and Pathophysiology

The common forms of SCD are listed in Table 11-6. Sickle cell trait, which is not a disease, is included in Table 11-6 for comparison.

The two main pathophysiologic consequences of polymerization of Hb SS, or sickling, are hemolysis and vaso-occlusion. The mean RBC lifespan in Hb SS is dramatically shortened to 10 to 20 days from the normal RBC lifespan of 120 days. The rate of hemolysis in SCD usually exceeds the rate at which new RBCs can be produced by the bone marrow. Sickle erythrocytes are also abnormally adhesive and have decreased flexibility. Consequently, they can adhere to and damage the endothelium of blood vessels and block the flow of blood. This microvascular obstruction, called vaso-occlusion, leads to ischemia and infarction of different tissues.

Diagnostic evaluation

In the United States and some other countries, universal newborn screening programs for hemoglobinopathies now identify individuals with SCD shortly after birth. Such early diagnosis is key to preventing early mortality from sepsis and acute splenic sequestration.

Beyond the immediate newborn period, the laboratory evaluation of suspected SCD should include a complete blood count, reticulocyte count, and examination of the peripheral blood smear. Table 11-7 lists the usual hematologic findings in the common forms of SCD. To confirm a diagnosis of SCD, however, some analysis of hemoglobin (Hb) types must be performed. Abnormal Hb must be identified using at least two methods because they can be difficult to differentiate. Contemporary Hb separation methods include isoelectric focusing (IEF) and high-pressure liquid chromatography (HPLC). DNA-based diagnostic methods, which are increasingly available, and family testing may be needed in occasional diagnostic challenges.

It is important to know that a "sickle prep" or the Sickledex™ does not differentiate between SCD and sickle cell trait. These tests only confirm the presence of Hb S, which is found in both SCD and the trait, so it is not helpful for the diagnosis of SCD.

TABLE 11-6 Comparison of the Common Sickle Cell Diseases and Sickle Cell Trait

Condition	Abbreviation	Genes Present	Main Hbs present	Usual Phenotype
Sickle cell anemia	Hb SS	$\beta^S\ \beta^S$	Hb S	Severe
Sickle-β^0-thalassemia	Hb Sβ^0	$\beta^S\ \beta^0$	Hb S	Severe
Sickle-hemoglobin C disease	Hb SC	$\beta^S\ \beta^C$	Hb S, Hb C	Mild–moderate
Sickle-β^+-thalassemia	Hb Sβ^+	$\beta^S\ \beta^+$	Hb S > Hb A	Mild
Sickle cell trait	Hb AS	$\beta\ \beta^S$	Hb A > Hb S	Asymptomatic

TABLE 11-7 Typical Laboratory Findings in the Common Forms of SCD

Disease	Hgb (g/dL)	MCV	Reticulocytes (%)
Sickle cell anemia	6–9	Normal	10–25
Sickle-β^0-thalassemia	6–9	Decreased	10–25
Sickle-hemoglobin C disease	9–12	Normal	5–10
Sickle-β^+-thalassemia	10–12	Decreased	2–10

Because patients with SCD have a chronic hemolytic anemia, they also have unconjugated hyperbilirubinemia and variable elevations of lactate dehydrogenase (LDH) and aspartate transaminase (AST). After the first year of life, the peripheral blood smear in Hb SS and Hb Sβ^0 shows variable numbers of pathognomonic irreversibly sickled cells, as well as polychromasia, Howell-Jolly bodies, poikilocytes, and target cells. Howell-Jolly bodies are indicative of hyposplenism. Patients with Hb SC and Hb Sβ^+ usually do not have significant numbers of irreversibly sickled cells, but they have instead a larger number of target cells. The MCV is normal in Hb SS and Hb SC, unless there is coinheritance of α-thalassemia. The MCV is low in Hb Sβ^0 and Hb Sβ^+. Leukocyte and platelet counts are usually moderately increased in SCD in the absence of infection.

Clinical Course

At birth, newborns with Hb SS have normal birth weight and are not anemic. Anemia and reticulocytosis usually appear between 2 and 6 months of age. Along with the anemia come jaundice and a cardiac flow murmur. Jaundice and flow murmurs are expected findings that should not cause concern. Splenic infarction and hyposplenism may begin to occur by 3 months of age. Therefore, it is necessary to prescribe prophylactic penicillin before this time to prevent pneumococcal sepsis. Before splenic infarction is complete, the spleen may be palpably enlarged. Nevertheless, it is still poorly or nonfunctional. Acute vaso-occlusive events are unusual before 6 months of age. The first painful event is often dactylitis, which is a painful swelling of the hands and feet. Dactylitis is rare beyond 3 years of age.

Infections

Children with SCD have a very high vulnerability to severe pneumococcal sepsis due to their early loss of splenic reticuloendothelial function (functional hyposplenism) because of continuous vaso-occlusive infarction. The damaged, enlarged spleen gradually becomes small and fibrotic, and it is rarely palpable after 6 years of age. Fatal pneumococcal sepsis is now rare in children with SCD in the United States because of universal newborn screening for hemoglobinopathies, prophylactic penicillin, and the protein-conjugated pneumococcal vaccine. Patients with SCD also have a predilection for osteomyelitis. Salmonella species cause about half the cases of osteomyelitis in SCD and staphylococci most of the rest.

Splenic Sequestration

In young children in whom splenic autoinfarction is not yet complete, the spleen may become acutely enlarged and engorged with blood sequestered from the systemic circulation, with consequent severe anemia, hypovolemia, and marked splenic enlargement. The recognition of acute splenic enlargement and the signs and symptoms of acutely severe anemia by both parents and health care professionals is important to prevent a fatal outcome. Transfusion is needed for symptomatic or severe anemia.

Aplastic Crisis

During many viral infections and inflammatory states, erythropoiesis may be modestly reduced, resulting in relative reticulocytopenia and transiently more severe anemia. Human parvovirus, however, temporarily destroys early red cell precursors in the bone marrow and causes a dramatic and potentially life-threatening anemia. This episode of severe anemia without appropriate reticulocytosis is called the aplastic crisis. Transfusion of blood is the most important intervention for symptomatic or severe anemia. Lifelong immunity against parvovirus prevents recurrent episodes.

Acute Painful Episodes

Intermittent episodes of pain are caused by acute vaso-occlusion, primarily in bones and bone marrow, with consequent ischemia and inflammation. Infection, dehydration, and exposure to the cold may precipitate pain. Patients with SCD-related pain, even severe, typically have no accompanying physical signs, such as edema or erythema (an exception to this is dactylitis in infants and very young children). The treatment of the painful episode is symptomatic. Analgesia must be tailored to the degree of pain and the patient. A combination of nonsteroidal anti-inflammatory drugs and opioid analgesics, titrated to effect, will usually achieve adequate pain relief. Overhydration is not helpful, and transfusion is not effective for uncomplicated painful episodes.

Acute Chest Syndrome

Acute chest syndrome is a pneumonia-like illness. Acute chest syndrome often starts as a small infiltrate in one lobe, but it can progress rapidly to involve multiple lobes, resulting in respiratory distress severe enough to require intubation and ventilatory support. Acute chest syndrome is a leading cause of death in adolescents and adults. Management includes oxygen supplementation for hypoxemia, maintenance of hydration without overhydration, adequate but not excessive analgesia, and antibacterials. Transfusions or exchange transfusions may be needed for moderate and especially severe cases.

Stroke

Children and adults with SCD may suffer stroke, causing paralysis and neurocognitive dysfunction. In the past decade, primary stroke prevention strategies using transcranial Doppler ultrasonography and chronic transfusion regimens have been quite effective at preventing stroke in children. Imaging of the brain and cerebral vessels is important for any child presenting with weakness or other signs or symptoms of stroke. Transfusion therapy, oftentimes exchange transfusion, is indicated for acute stroke and prevention of recurrent stroke.

Chronic Organ Dysfunction and Damage

In addition to early splenic dysfunction and involution, other forms of progressive organ dysfunction or damage occur with increasing age in the kidneys, bones, eyes, lungs, heart, and liver.

Treatment

There are three main disease-modifying treatments that can reduce the overall severity of SCD or cure it: hydroxyurea, chronic transfusions, and hematopoietic stem cell transplantation. Hydroxyurea increases the concentration of Hb F, which decreases sickling. Clinically, hydroxyurea reduces the frequency of painful episodes and acute chest syndrome. Chronic, monthly transfusions are effective at preventing most complications of SCD, but the most common indications are primary and secondary stroke prophylaxis. Complications of transfusions include iron overload and alloimmunization. Stem cell (or bone marrow) transplantation is the only potential cure for SCD. Widespread use of transplantation is limited by the lack of donor availability and toxicities of the procedure.

GLUCOSE-6-PHOSPHATE DEHYDROGENASE DEFICIENCY

G6PD deficiency, the most common red blood cell enzyme defect, is an X-linked condition. The deficiency of this enzyme in the hexose monophosphate shunt pathway results in depletion of nicotinamide adenine dinucleotide phosphate (NADPH) and the inability to regenerate reduced glutathione, which is needed to protect the red blood cell from oxidative stress.

The most common forms of G6PD deficiency are the A^- and Mediterranean variants. The mutation that causes the A^- variant, found in approximately 10% of African Americans, produces an enzyme with a shortened half-life of 13 days. The Mediterranean variant occurs predominantly in persons of Greek and Italian descent. This enzyme is extremely unstable and has a half-life of only several hours.

When there the red blood cell experiences oxidative stress, exposed sulfhydryl groups on the hemoglobin are oxidized, leading to dissociation of heme and globin moieties, with the denatured globin precipitating as Heinz bodies, which can be visualized by special stains. Damaged red cells are removed from circulation by the reticuloendothelial system; severely damaged cells may lyse intravascularly. Known chemical oxidants include sulfonamides, nitrofurantoin, primaquine, dimercaprol, and naphthalene. Hemolysis may also be precipitated by infection, inflammation, and, with the Mediterranean variant, ingestion of fava beans.

Laboratory Features and Clinical Manifestations

The typical course of mild G6PD deficiency (as with the A^- variant) is episodic stress- or drug-induced hemolytic anemia. Patients with the A^- variant have a limited degree of hemolysis that is restricted to the older red blood cell population with insufficient G6PD activity (because of the shortened half-life of the enzyme). The younger red blood cells, including the reticulocytes produced in response to hemolysis episode, have sufficient enzyme activity to resist oxidative stress and do not lyse. Hemolysis is most common in males who possess a single abnormal X chromosome. Heterozygous females who have skewed X chromosome inactivation may become symptomatic, as may females homozygous for the A^- variant. One percent of African American females are A^- variant homozygous.

Severe G6PD deficiency, as with the Mediterranean variant, can result in hemolysis that can destroys most of the red cell mass because even the young red cells have insufficient enzyme activity. Hemolysis may be life-threatening, and transfusion may be needed.

During hemolytic episodes, physical examination reveals jaundice and dark urine (caused by hemoglobinuria and high levels of urobilinogen). Laboratory tests reveal elevated indirect bilirubin and lactate dehydrogenase and low haptoglobin. Initially, the hemolysis exceeds the ability of the bone marrow to compensate, so the reticulocyte count may be low for the first 3 to 4 days. On peripheral blood smear, the red cells appear to have "bites" taken out of them (blister cells) or have an asymmetric distribution of hemoglobin (eccentrocytes).

The diagnosis of G6PD deficiency is made by measuring enzyme activity. G6PD levels may be normal in the setting of acute, severe hemolysis because most of the deficient cells have been destroyed (leaving only the younger cells with sufficient enzyme activity). Repeating the test at a later time when the patient is in a steady-state condition is important.

Treatment

Patients with G6PD deficiency associated with acute severe hemolysis need to avoid drugs and chemicals that initiate hemolysis. Treatment is supportive, including packed red blood cell transfusion during significant cardiovascular compromise and vigorous hydration and urine alkalinization to protect the kidneys against damage from precipitated free hemoglobin.

AUTOIMMUNE HEMOLYTIC ANEMIA

Immune hemolytic anemia may be alloimmune or autoimmune. Alloimmune hemolytic anemia results from antibodies produced by one individual against the red blood cells of another individual of the same species, such as hemolytic disease of the newborn caused by maternal–fetal incompatibility for minor RBC antigens (e.g., Kell). Isoimmune hemolytic anemia is a special case of alloimmune hemolytic anemia caused by isohemagglutinins, which are naturally occurring antibodies with specificity against the A or B antigens of the ABO blood group. Isoimmune hemolytic disease of the newborn is caused by maternal–fetal ABO incompatibility (see Chapter 13). In autoimmune hemolytic anemia, the patient produces autoantibodies against autologous (self) antigens on his or her own red blood cells. Autoimmune hemolytic anemias can be idiopathic, postinfectious (*Mycoplasma pneumoniae*, Epstein-Barr virus), drug-induced (penicillin, quinidine, α-methyldopa), or may be a feature of an underlying autoimmune disease (e.g., systemic lupus erythematosus) or malignancy (e.g., lymphoma).

Laboratory Features

The binding of antibodies (with or without complement) to the red blood cell membrane causes immune hemolytic anemia. These antibodies can be identified by the direct antiglobulin test (DAT, previously called the direct Coombs' test), which is the diagnostic test for autoimmune hemolytic anemias.

The antibodies that cause autoimmune hemolytic anemias may be of the IgG or IgM classes. IgG antibodies tend to be warm-reactive (maximal activity at 37°C). They are considered "incomplete" antibodies because they can fix early complement components but cannot agglutinate red blood cells or activate the complement cascade in its entirety. IgG-mediated hemolysis occurs primarily in the extravascular compartment because of the trapping of antibody-coated red blood cells by macrophages in the reticuloendothelial system, especially the spleen. IgG antibodies are associated with idiopathic cases, underlying autoimmune diseases, lymphomas, and viral infections. IgM antibodies are usually cold-reactive (maximal activity at ≈4°C). They are called "complete" antibodies because they can agglutinate red blood cells and activate the complement sequence through C9, causing lysis of red blood cells. Hemolysis occurs primarily in the intravascular compartment. IgM antibodies are associated with *Mycoplasma pneumoniae*, Epstein-Barr virus, and some transfusion reactions.

Clinical Manifestations and Treatment

The typical presentation is a previously healthy young child with the rapid onset of fatigue, pallor, and jaundice. Splenomegaly occurs in a minority, and some have dark urine (hemoglobinuria).

Depending on the degree, there may be tachycardia, a flow murmur, and even impending heart failure. A complete blood count shows anemia, which can be mild to severe, and a compensatory reticulocytosis. The peripheral smear shows anemia and polychromasia and varying degrees of spherocytosis and red cell agglutination. A presentation with mainly jaundice but mild or no hemoglobinuria is most consistent with IgG-mediated extravascular hemolysis, that is, warm autoimmune hemolytic anemia. A presentation with marked hemoglobinuria and mild or no jaundice is consistent with IgM-mediated intravascular hemolysis, that is, cold agglutinin disease.

Therapy for autoimmune hemolytic anemia varies depending on the cause and the clinical condition of the patient. In general, treatment is supportive, with the judicious use of corticosteroids and packed red blood cell transfusions for warm autoimmune hemolytic anemia. Autoantibodies react with virtually all red blood cells, making cross-matching difficult, so close communication with the blood bank is necessary. In some severe chronic cases, other immunosuppressive pharmacotherapy and splenectomy may be indicated. Cold agglutinin disease tends to be steroid nonresponsive, and keeping the patient warm can prevent some of the hemolysis.

MACROCYTIC ANEMIAS WITH DECREASED RED CELL PRODUCTION

Macrocytic anemias can be subclassified based on the presence or absence of megaloblastosis, a marker of ineffective DNA synthesis within a red blood cell precursor. Not all macrocytic anemias are megaloblastic, but all megaloblastic anemias are macrocytic. Causes of megaloblastic anemia include dietary vitamin B_{12} and folate deficiency, drugs that interfere with folate metabolism (methotrexate, trimethoprim), and some metabolic disorders (orotic aciduria, methylmalonic aciduria, Lesch-Nyhan syndrome). Macrocytic anemias without megaloblastosis result from bone marrow injury or failure, including bone marrow failure syndromes (Diamond-Blackfan anemia, Fanconi anemia, idiopathic aplastic anemia, myelodysplasia); drug-induced anemias (azidothymidine, valproic acid, carbamazepine); chronic liver disease; and hypothyroidism.

MEGALOBLASTIC MACROCYTIC ANEMIAS

Vitamin B_{12} Deficiency

Vitamin B_{12}, a coenzyme for 5-methyl-tetrahydrofolate formation, is needed for DNA synthesis. It is found in meat, fish, cheese, and eggs. Dietary vitamin B_{12} deficiency is rare in developed countries except in the breastfed infant whose mother is a vegan with poor attention to dietary sources of vitamin B_{12}. Another cause of vitamin B_{12} deficiency is selective or generalized malabsorption. Vitamin B_{12} combines with intrinsic factor, which is produced by gastric parietal cells, and absorbed in the terminal ileum. Transcobalamin II then transports vitamin B_{12} to the liver for storage. The availability of vitamin B_{12} is reduced by any condition that alters intrinsic factor production, interferes with intestinal absorption, or reduces transcobalamin II levels. Disorders such as congenital pernicious anemia (absent intrinsic factor), juvenile pernicious anemia (autoimmune destruction of intrinsic factor), and transcobalamin II deficiency result in vitamin B_{12} deficiency. Other causes include ileal resection, small bowel bacterial overgrowth, and infection with the fish tapeworm *Diphyllobothrium latum*.

Clinical Manifestations

The effects of vitamin B_{12} deficiency include glossitis, diarrhea, and weight loss. Neurologic sequelae include paresthesias, peripheral neuropathies, and, in the most severe cases, dementia, ataxia, and/or posterior column spinal degeneration. Vitiligo is the main dermatologic manifestation.

Megaloblastic changes on peripheral blood smear include ovalocytosis, neutrophils with hypersegmented nuclei (more than four per cell), nucleated red blood cells, basophilic stippling, and Howell-Jolly bodies. The hallmark of megaloblastic anemia is nuclear-to-cytoplasmic dyssynchrony in RBC precursors (the nucleus matures or develops more slowly than the cytoplasm). The mean corpuscular volume is usually greater than 100 fL. Medullary hemolysis results in elevated levels of serum lactate dehydrogenase, indirect bilirubin, and serum iron. In severe cases, megaloblastic anemia may be accompanied by leukopenia and thrombocytopenia. Diagnosis is confirmed by a subnormal serum level of vitamin B_{12}. The Schilling test is no longer available clinically in the United States. Vitamin B_{12} deficiency also increases the blood concentration of homocysteine and methylmalonic acid, and these are useful markers of deficiency and response to therapy.

Treatment

Treatment for most forms of vitamin B_{12} deficiency, with the exception of bacterial overgrowth and fish tapeworm, is parenteral vitamin B_{12}. The erythropoietic response is rapid, with marrow megaloblastosis improving within hours, reticulocytosis appearing by day 3 of therapy, and anemia resolving within 1 to 2 months.

Folate Deficiency

Dietary folate, found in liver, green vegetables, cereals, and cheese is converted by the body to tetrahydrofolate, which is required for DNA synthesis. Because folate stores are relatively small, deficiency may develop within 1 month and anemia within 4 months of deprivation. Etiologies include inadequate dietary intake, impaired absorption of folate, increased demand for folate, and abnormal folate metabolism. Dietary deficiency of folic acid is unusual in developed countries. Children at risk are infants who were fed goat milk, evaporated milk, or heat-sterilized milk or formula; each has inadequate folate content. Malabsorptive states of the jejunum, such as inflammatory bowel disease and celiac sprue, can cause folate deficiency. Increased demand for folate occurs with an increased rate of red blood cell turnover (hyperthyroidism, pregnancy, chronic hemolysis, malignancy). Relative folate deficiency may develop if the diet does not provide adequate folate to meet these needs. Certain anticonvulsant drugs (phenytoin, phenobarbital) interfere with folate metabolism.

Clinical Manifestations

Specific symptoms are often absent, although pallor, glossitis, malaise, anorexia, poor growth, and recurrent infection may be seen. Unlike vitamin B_{12} deficiency, neurologic disease is not associated with folate deficiency.

Laboratory findings include low red blood cell folate and normal serum vitamin B_{12} levels. Megaloblastic changes on peripheral blood smear and bone marrow aspirate are the same as those noted with vitamin B_{12} deficiency.

Treatment

It is imperative not to misdiagnose B_{12} deficiency as folate deficiency because treatment with folate may result in hematologic improvement and allow for progressive neurologic deterioration. Treatment with 1 mg of folate given orally each day for 1 to 2 months treats the anemia and replenishes body stores. Clinical response is rapid, following a time course similar to that of vitamin B_{12} replacement therapy. Children with chronic hemolytic conditions may require folate supplementation.

NONMEGALOBLASTIC MACROCYTIC ANEMIAS

Dietary vitamin B_{12} and folate deficiency are rare in children in developed nations. So, the evaluation of a child with microcytosis should always include consideration of nonmegaloblastic causes. Bone marrow failure disorders may be congenital or acquired, and it is especially important to consider congenital disorders in children. Prognosis and treatment depend upon the diagnosis. This section briefly discusses two congenital (Diamond-Blackfan anemia, Fanconi anemia) and one acquired bone marrow failure syndrome (severe aplastic anemia).

Diamond-Blackfan Anemia

Diamond-Blackfan anemia (DBA) is a congenital pure red cell aplasia. Both autosomal dominant and recessive patterns are reported. Twenty-five percent of patients have a mutation in the ribosomal protein S19 gene (*RPS19*). Mutations in several other ribosomal protein genes have been described recently.

Clinical Manifestations and Diagnosis

The anemia develops shortly after birth but is not usually detected until later, when symptoms develop; 90% of cases are diagnosed within the first year of life. Infants present with mild macrocytosis and reticulocytopenia. On hemoglobin electrophoresis, there is an elevated hemoglobin F. Red blood cell adenosine deaminase is often elevated. Twenty-five percent of patients have associated congenital anomalies that include short stature, web neck, cleft lip, shield chest, and triphalangeal thumb. TEC is an important consideration in the differential diagnosis of DBA (see above). Generally, DBA tends to present at a younger age than TEC and is usually macrocytic, unlike TEC. Children with DBA are at high risk for multilineage bone marrow failure and leukemia later in life.

Treatment

Two-thirds of patients respond to oral corticosteroids, oftentimes with a very low, "subphysiologic" dose, with an improvement in or resolution of anemia. Steroid responders may maintain their response indefinitely or eventually lose the response. Those who do not respond to steroids, lose their response, or have excessive steroid-related toxicity may be transfusion dependent. Bone marrow transplantation with a matched sibling donor is an option for some patients.

Fanconi Anemia

Fanconi anemia is an autosomal recessive disorder that results in pancytopenia. One form is X-linked. Mutations in over a dozen known genes can cause Fanconi anemia. The disorder results from defective DNA repair mechanisms that lead to excessive chromosomal breaks and recombinations. These chromosomal anomalies are found in all cells of the body, not just the hematopoietic stem cells, although there may be somatic mosaicism. The mean age at onset of pancytopenia is 8 years.

Clinical Manifestations and Diagnosis

Common signs include hyperpigmentation and café au lait spots, microcephaly, microphthalmia, short stature, horseshoe or absent kidney, and absent thumbs. Hematologic manifestations include progressive pancytopenia. Macrocytosis is universal even before the onset of anemia, and elevated hemoglobin F is seen on hemoglobin electrophoresis. Approximately 10% of children with Fanconi anemia develop leukemia during adolescence.

Diagnosis is confirmed by demonstrating increased chromosomal breakage with exposure to diepoxybutane (DEB) or other agents that damage DNA.

Treatment

Patients frequently require red blood cell transfusions for symptomatic anemia. Some patients have hematologic improvement with androgen therapy. Hematopoietic stem cell transplantation is the treatment of choice for progressive bone marrow failure if an HLA-matched donor can be found. Because of Fanconi anemia patients' DNA repair defect, the preparative (pretransplant) doses of radiation and chemotherapy, both of which damage DNA, must be reduced from what is normally used for patients without Fanconi anemia to prevent severe morbidity and death.

Severe Aplastic Anemia

Severe aplastic anemia is an acquired failure of the hematopoietic stem cells that results in pancytopenia. The disorder may result from exposure to chemicals (benzene, phenylbutazone), drugs (chloramphenicol, sulfonamides), infectious agents (hepatitis virus), or ionizing radiation. Most commonly, a specific cause of aplasia is not identified, and it is termed idiopathic severe aplastic anemia. Postinfectious and idiopathic forms of severe aplastic anemia are caused by autoimmune destruction of hematopoietic stem cells and/or the microenvironment of the bone marrow.

Clinical Manifestations and Diagnosis

Patients present with signs and symptoms referable to anemia (fatigue, pallor), thrombocytopenia (easy bruising, bleeding), and/or neutropenia (fevers, infections). The onset of signs and symptoms is usually insidious and slow. Toxic exposures (medications, chemicals, radiation) are very rare causes of aplastic anemia in the United States, but a complete history should elicit any such exposures. The CBC shows cytopenias and almost always microcytosis. Aplastic anemia is diagnosed by the combination of peripheral pancytopenia and a hypocellular bone marrow.

Treatment

Without treatment (historically), 80% of patients die within 3 months of diagnosis from bleeding or infection. The treatment of choice is a bone marrow transplant with an HLA-matched sibling donor. Immunosuppression with antithymocyte globulin (ATG) and cyclosporine is used for patients who do not have a suitable donor. If transplantation is considered, it is important to minimize transfusions to reduce exposure to potentially sensitizing blood products. Neutropenic patients are at risk for serious bacterial infection and usually require antibiotics when they develop fever.

DISORDERS OF WHITE BLOOD CELLS

White blood cells (WBC), or leukocytes, are the primary systemic defense mechanisms against infections. The total white blood cell count and the differential count often provide valuable clues for the diagnosis and treatment of a variety of conditions, hematologic and nonhematologic. Most often, increases or decreases in WBC number are transient or secondary to another condition. The leukocytes are broadly categorized as granulocytes (neutrophils, eosinophils, and basophils), lymphocytes, and mononuclear phagocytes (monocytes). Granulocytes are so named because of the presence of intracytoplasmic granules. Neutrophils are the largest population of granulocytes and are also referred to as segmented neutrophils ("segs")—these are the mature form of neutrophils. "Band" (or stab) is the name for the immature form of the circulating neutrophil (not yet having distinct nuclear segmentation).

An increase in the neutrophil count is often seen in the presence of inflammation and infections, especially bacterial but not exclusively. The terms "left shift" or "bandemia" refers specifically to an absolute increase in the number of bands, whether or not the total WBC count is increased. Neutrophils and monocytes are the phagocytes of the blood. Monocytes also function as antigen presenting cells. An increase in eosinophils is often seen in allergic and atopic conditions as well as parasitic infections. In the presence of neutropenia, there is often a compensatory monocytosis. Basophils are the least numerous of the leukocytes and may also be involved in allergic responses. Lymphocytes are a critical component of the immune system, and are responsible for both humoral and cellular immune responses.

When a child with a suspected WBC dysfunction is encountered, a thorough medical history including the past and family history should be obtained along with a detailed physical examination. In particular, a history of medications, toxins or other environmental exposures, and the frequency and severity of prior infections is absolutely critical. A family history of other similarly affected individuals with a history of early childhood or in utero deaths and any delays in umbilical cord separation should also be obtained. Recurrent fevers and infections of the skin and mucous membranes (especially of the perianal region and mouth) are particularly indicative of WBC dysfunction or deficiency. Gingivitis and oral mucosal ulcerations are common features of chronic neutropenia.

White blood cell disorders can be broadly classified into abnormalities of WBC number (leukopenia or low WBC count; leukocytosis or elevated WBC count) and WBC function (leukocyte function disorders). Leukopenia is generally defined as a total WBC count of less than 4,000 cells/mm^3. Because leukopenia may be due to suppression of one of more types of WBCs, one must pay close attention to the differential count. Neutropenia is arbitrarily defined as an absolute neutrophil count (ANC) less than 1,500/mm^3 for individuals 1 year of age or older and less than 1,000/mm^3 when under 1 year of age. African Americans commonly have lower neutrophil counts than Caucasians, with an ANC *normally* as low as 600 to 800. So, it is very important to consider the patient's race/ancestry when interpreting leukocyte counts. The most common causes of leukopenia and neutropenia are transient responses to infections (bacterial or viral) or drugs. In these cases, the mechanism of leukopenia could be variable, including antibody-mediated destruction, bone marrow suppression, or a shift into the tissue or marginated compartments. Neutropenia resolves when the infection resolves or the offending drug is discontinued. When neutropenia is prolonged, severe, or accompanied by decreases in other cell types, then a bone marrow examination should be considered. Fever or infection in the setting of severe neutropenia (ANC $< 500/mm^3$) often warrants parenteral antibiotic therapy and hospitalization. Decreases in other WBC types is much less common. A marked decrease in lymphocytes, especially in young infants, should prompt further evaluation for an underlying immune disorder, such as severe combined immunodeficiency. Viral infections and corticosteroids can also cause lymphopenia.

An increase in the WBC count above the normal range is called leukocytosis and is most often encountered in response to inflammation, infection, allergy, or as a consequence of some malignancies. Leukocytosis is a normal physiologic finding in the newborn period, during stress, and in pregnancy. Leukocytosis is commonly seen in association with bacterial and viral infections and in chronic inflammatory states. An increase in neutrophils or lymphocytes is the most common cause for leukocytosis. Rarely, an increase in eosinophils (eosinophilia) can also be encountered. Disorders associated with eosinophilia include allergy and drug hypersensitivity, parasitic infestations, skin and connective tissue disorders, gastrointestinal disorders, and the idiopathic hypereosinophilic syndrome.

Disorders of leukocyte function are rare and may involve abnormalities in one or more of their normal physiologic functions which include motility and migration, chemotaxis, and bacterial ingestion and killing. Nonspecific clues to the presence of leukocyte function include chronic leukocytosis (especially in the well state), lack of pus formation, and delayed separation of the umbilical cord. Specialized testing is required for the diagnosis, and if leukocyte dysfunction is suspected, a referral to a pediatric hematologist is warranted.

DISORDERS OF HEMOSTASIS

Normal hemostasis requires the integrity and interaction of blood vessels, platelets, and soluble coagulation ("clotting") factors. Platelets and the vessel wall are the key participants in **primary hemostasis**, which includes vaso-constriction and the formation of a platelet plug at the site of vessel injury. The platelets that are activated at the site of tissue injury, in combination with exposed tissue factor, bring about the **secondary hemostasis**, which involves the formation of a fibrin mesh from the action of soluble coagulation factors on the surface of platelets and other cells. Bleeding can result from abnormalities in any of these systems. Defects in primary hemostasis typically cause bruising and mucocutaneous bleeding. In contrast, defects in secondary hemostasis classically cause hemarthrosis and hematomas.

Disorders of platelets and of coagulation factors are discussed below. Examples of primary vascular anomalies that can cause bruising and bleeding include hereditary (Ehlers-Danlos syndrome) and acquired defects (vitamin C deficiency—scurvy) of collagen synthesis. Vasculitis, such as Henoch-Schönlein purpura (HSP), can mimic a bleeding disorder. HSP produces abdominal pain, arthritis, nephritis, and palpable "purpura" classically distributed over the buttocks and lower extremities. The term "purpura" is a misnomer, because the palpable lesion is vasculitic, and HSP is not a hematologic or bleeding disorder.

DISORDERS OF PLATELETS

Platelets are key participants in primary hemostasis. Platelet disorders can be either quantitative or qualitative. Quantitative abnormalities are identified by the platelet count, whereas qualitative disorders are detected by measures of platelet function. **Thrombocytopenia**, defined as a platelet count below 150,000/mm^3, is a common cause of abnormal bleeding. A low platelet count can result from *decreased production* or *increased destruction* of platelets. The adequacy of platelet production can be estimated, when necessary, by assessing the number of megakaryocytes in the bone marrow.

Decreased platelet production can result from suppression or failure of the bone marrow. Bone marrow failure states causing thrombocytopenia include disorders resulting in pancytopenia (Fanconi anemia, idiopathic aplastic anemia, leukemia); congenital amegakaryocytic thrombocytopenia; thrombocytopenia-absent radius (TAR) syndrome; and Wiskott-Aldrich syndrome. TAR syndrome, also known as congenital megakaryocytic hypoplasia, is an autosomal recessive disorder in which thrombocytopenia develops in the first few months of life and typically resolves spontaneously after 1 year of age. Absence of the radii is pathognomonic (the thumbs are present). Wiskott-Aldrich syndrome is an X-linked disorder characterized by immunodeficiency, eczema, and micothrombocytopenia (the platelets are small and few). Bone marrow transplantation is potentially curative. Examples of thrombocytopenia caused by bone marrow suppression include chemotherapeutic agents; acquired viral infections (human immunodeficiency virus [HIV], Epstein-Barr virus, measles); congenital infections, including toxoplasmosis, syphilis, rubella, cytomegalovirus, and parvovirus B19; and certain drugs (anticonvulsants, sulfonamides, quinidine, quinine, and thiazide diuretics). Acquired postnatal infections (with the exception of HIV) and drug reactions usually cause transient thrombocytopenia, whereas congenital infections may produce prolonged suppression of bone marrow function.

Thrombocytopenia caused by shortened platelet survival is much more common than thrombocytopenia caused by inadequate production. Platelet destruction is most commonly immune-mediated. Thrombocytopenia in the newborn can result from alloimmune or autoimmune antibodies. Alloimmune IgG antibodies are produced against the fetal platelets when the fetal platelet crosses the placenta and presents itself to the maternal immune system. If there is an antigen on the fetal platelet that does not exist on the maternal platelet, it is recognized as foreign and antibodies are created against the antigen. Maternal antiplatelet antibodies then cross the placenta, causing destruction of the fetal platelet. This disorder is known as neonatal alloimmune thrombocytopenia. The maternal antiplatelet antibody does not produce maternal thrombocytopenia. Autoimmune IgG antibodies are transferred to the fetus through the placenta when the mother has immune thrombocytopenia (ITP). These maternal autoantibodies cross the placenta and attack the fetal platelets. In contrast to alloimmune antibodies, autoimmune antibodies also result in maternal thrombocytopenia (unless the mother has had a splenectomy). Depending on the platelet count, the presence of bleeding, and certain risk factors, neonates with alloimmune or autoimmune thrombocytopenia may be treated with corticosteroids and/or intravenous immunoglobulin (IVIG) until the maternal antiplatelet antibodies dissipate in fetal circulation. Washed maternal platelets or antigen-matched platelets are the best platelet product for neonatal alloimmune thrombocytopenia. A discussion of childhood ITP appears later in this chapter. Heparin-induced thrombocytopenia is another form of immune-mediated thrombocytopenia, paradoxically associated with thrombosis.

Microangiopathic hemolytic anemias also cause thrombocytopenia by decreasing platelet survival by entrapment in the small vessels (as with the RBCs) and removal from the circulation. Microangiopathic disorders include disseminated intravascular coagulation (DIC), hemolytic-uremic syndrome (HUS), and thrombotic thrombocytopenic purpura (TTP). DIC is discussed later. HUS, characterized by a microangiopathic hemolytic anemia, renal cortical injury, and thrombocytopenia, is a major cause of acute renal failure in children. Verotoxin-producing Gram-negative organisms (such as *Escherichia coli* O157:H7) that bind to endothelial cells cause HUS. Because of endothelial cell injury, there is localized clotting and platelet activation. Microangiopathic hemolytic anemia results from mechanical injury to red cells as they pass through the injured vascular bed with fibrin deposition across the lumen, and thrombocytopenia results from platelet adhesion to the damaged endothelium with subsequent activation and removal. An estimated 60% to 80% of patients with HUS transiently require dialysis. Most children survive the acute phase and recover normal renal function. In TTP, there is a lack of the von Willebrand factor cleaving protease (ADAMTS 13) with a resultant increase in the large multimeric forms of von Willebrand factor. These large multimers have an increased affinity for platelets which leads to their aggregation, activation, and eventual removal (thrombocytopenia). Other findings in TTP include microangiopathic hemolytic anemia, fever, renal involvement, and neurological findings.

Diminished platelet survival can also result from platelet trapping, as seen with Kaposiform hemangioendotheliomas (Kasabach-Merrit syndrome). Hypersplenism refers to the nonspecific trapping of blood cells in an engorged or enlarged spleen of any cause, which is most commonly seen in sickle cell disease, thalassemia syndromes, Gaucher disease, and portal hypertension. Table 11-8 lists the common causes of thrombocytopenia during the neonatal, infant, and childhood periods. Two causes of thrombocytopenia in children are discussed below: ITP and disseminated intravascular coagulation.

Immune Thrombocytopenia

ITP, previously called idiopathic thrombocytopenic purpura, is condition caused by autoimmune destruction of platelets, primarily by antiplatelet autoantibodies. Antibody-coated platelets are destroyed in the reticuloendothelial system, especially the spleen. ITP may be primary (occurring in isolation) or secondary, as a feature of an underlying disease, such as systemic lupus erythematosus or HIV infection.

Clinical Manifestations

Children typically present 1 to 4 weeks after a febrile or viral illness with the abrupt onset of petechiae and bruising. Sometimes there is no clear antecedent illness. Some children will also have overt bleeding from the mucous membranes, such as epistaxis and oral bleeding. Severe bleeding, including internal and intracranial hemorrhage, is rare in children with ITP and can occur spontaneously or after trauma. There should be no history of fatigue, bone pains, weight loss, or unexplained fevers.

Other than thrombocytopenia, the complete blood count should otherwise be normal, unless there is a clear and satisfactory explanation (e.g., anemia due to overt bleeding). The

TABLE 11-8 Typical Causes of Thrombocytopenia by Age Group at Presentation

Neonate
Maternal immune thrombocytopenia (ITP)[a]
Neonatal alloimmune thrombocytopenia[a]
Sepsis, DIC
Congenital infections
Inherited thrombocytopenia (e.g., Wiskott-Aldrich syndrome)[a]
Thrombocytopenia-absent radius syndrome[a]
Congenital amegakaryocytic thrombocytopenia[a]
Infant
Viral infections
Medications
Sepsis, DIC
ITP[a]
Malignancies (leukemia, neuroblastoma)
Inherited thrombocytopenia (e.g., Wiskott-Aldrich syndrome)[a]
Childhood
ITP[a]
Medications
Hypersplenism (e.g., thalassemia, Gaucher disease, portal hypertension)
Sepsis, DIC
Leukemia
Aplastic anemia
Thrombotic microangiopathies (e.g., hemolytic uremic syndrome)
Hemophagocytic lymphohistiocytosis
HIV infection

[a]Typically characterized by isolated thrombocytopenia (no other abnormalities of the complete blood count).

peripheral smear will show thrombocytopenia with the presence of characteristic large, young platelets (when the platelet count is less than about 20,000/mm^3). Physical examination only shows evidence, if any, of mucocutaneous bleeding (bruising and petechiae), but no splenomegaly, hepatomegaly, or lymphadenopathy. ITP is usually a clinical diagnosis based upon a typical history, physical, and blood count: the abrupt onset of bruising and isolated thrombocytopenia (with large platelets but an otherwise normal blood count) without any other explanation in an otherwise healthy child with no organomegaly or adenopathy. For most cases, the diagnosis of ITP does not require a bone marrow examination, extensive laboratory testing, or the detection of antiplatelet antibodies (which is a poor test for this purpose). However, if there are atypical findings on the history, physical examination, the complete blood count, or the peripheral blood smear, then bone marrow examination is indicated to exclude leukemia and aplastic anemia. If necessary to perform, a bone marrow examination will classically show megakaryocytic hyperplasia but normal myeloid and erythroid elements.

Treatment

Childhood ITP is typically a benign, self-limited disease that does not cause severe bleeding. Seventy-five percent to 80% of the cases of childhood acute ITP resolve spontaneously within 6 months. Treatments to raise the platelet counts are only temporizing measures that do not affect the time to spontaneous remission or cure the underlying disease. A minority of children will have thrombocytopenia that lasts longer than 6 months (persistent ITP) or 12 months (chronic ITP). The progression to chronic ITP does not necessarily mean that a child will have lifelong ITP.

Because childhood ITP is most commonly a benign, self-limited disease that does not cause major bleeding, and all treatments for ITP have side effects, inconveniences, and costs, physicians should take care to ensure that their treatments are not worse than the disease itself. The therapeutic plan should be carefully individualized, with primary attention to the presence of overt bleeding, rather than any arbitrary platelet count. Severe bleeding, although rare, often occurs despite treatment, so treatments do not necessarily prevent severe bleeding. There are two main therapeutic options: (1) watchful waiting with education and reassurance awaiting spontaneous resolution or (2) pharmacotherapy to temporarily increase the platelet count. For the child without troublesome overt bleeding, watchful waiting is most often appropriate. Pharmacotherapy is best reserved for children with troublesome, recurrent, or serious overt bleeding; children engaging in risky physical activities; or excessive parental anxiety despite education and reassurance. Children with oral hemorrhagic bullae ("wet purpura") as well as adolescents and young adults may tend to bleed more than other children, so pharmacotherapy may be indicated in these scenarios. The three most common first-line agents for ITP are corticosteroids, IVIG, and anti-D immunoglobulin. All three temporarily increase the platelet count, lasting for 1 to 3 weeks, so recurrent treatments may be needed. Children with chronic ITP and troublesome bleeding may require other interventions, such as splenectomy or immunosuppressive agents (e.g., rituximab). Newer thrombopoietin mimetics, like romiplostim and eltrombopag, are being studied in children.

Just as important as any pharmacotherapy is education of the patient and family about medications and activities to avoid. Antiplatelet medications, such as aspirin, should be avoided completely. NSAIDs, like ibuprofen, have only weak antiplatelet effects in vivo, but are probably best to avoid as well. Acetaminophen is safe to use in ITP. Children should not engage in contact sports or engage in excessive roughhousing. Prudent protective measures should also be taken, like wearing a helmet when riding a bike, not sleeping on the top bunk of a bunk bed, or climbing to high places with the potential to fall (monkey bars, tree houses). Finally, families should be educated about the signs and symptoms of severe, especially internal, bleeding that require immediate medical attention, such as severe headache, vomiting, lethargy, or loss of consciousness.

Disseminated Intravascular Coagulation (DIC)

Normal homeostasis is a balance between hemorrhage and thrombosis. In DIC, this balance is altered by severe illness so there is activation of both coagulation (thrombin) and fibrinolysis (plasmin). Endothelial injury, release of thromboplastic procoagulant factors into the circulation, and impairment of clearance of activated clotting factors directly activate and amplify the coagulation cascade. Intravascular activation of the coagulation cascade leads to fibrin deposition in the small blood vessels, tissue ischemia, release of tissue thromboplastin, consumption of clotting factors, and activation of the fibrinolytic system. Coagulation elements, especially platelets, fibrinogen, and clotting factors II, V, and VIII, are consumed, as are the anticoagulant proteins, especially antithrombin, protein C, and plasminogen. Platelets are also activated and removed from circulation. Acute and chronic conditions associated with DIC include sepsis, burns, trauma, asphyxia, malignancy, and cirrhosis.

Clinical Manifestations

The bleeding diathesis may be diffuse, with bleeding from venipuncture sites and around indwelling catheters. Gastrointestinal and pulmonary bleeding can be severe, and hematuria is common. Thrombotic lesions affect the extremities, skin, kidneys, and brain. Both ischemic and hemorrhagic strokes can occur.

The diagnosis of DIC is a clinical one bolstered by laboratory evidence. Thrombocytopenia is evident, along with prolonged prothrombin time (PT) and partial thromboplastin time (PTT). Fibrin split products and D-dimers are elevated. Fibrinogen and factor V and VIII levels are low. The peripheral blood smear reveals schistocytes, which are seen with microangiopathic disease.

Treatment

The treatment of DIC is supportive. The disorder that caused DIC must be treated, and hypoxia, acidosis, and perfusion abnormalities need to be corrected. If bleeding persists, the child should be treated with platelets and fresh-frozen plasma, which replaces depleted clotting factors. Heparin may be useful in the presence of significant arterial or venous thrombotic disease unless sites of life-threatening bleeding coexist.

DISORDERS OF COAGULATION

Coagulation disorders can be inherited or acquired. The most common inherited defects are hemophilia A and B and von Willebrand disease, whereas vitamin K deficiency is an important acquired coagulation defect.

Hemophilia A and B

Hemophilia A is caused by deficiency of **factor VIII** and occurs in 1 in 5,000 males, whereas hemophilia B results from **factor IX** deficiency and is found in 1 in 25,000 males. Both are X-linked recessive disorders. All other clotting factors are coded on autosomal chromosomes and are therefore inherited in an autosomal fashion. The lack of factor VIII or IX causes a delay in the production of thrombin, which catalyzes the formation of the primary fibrin clot by the conversion of fibrinogen to fibrin which is then stabilized by the action of factor XIII.

Clinical Manifestations

Hemophilia A and B are indistinguishable clinically (excluding definitive laboratory testing and specific treatment), and the severity of each disorder is determined by the degree of factor deficiency. Children with mild hemophilia (5% to 49% of normal factor levels) require significant trauma to induce bleeding, and spontaneous hemorrhage does not occur. Those with moderate hemophilia (1% to 5% of normal factor levels) require moderate trauma to induce bleeding episodes but may also have infrequent (approximately yearly) spontaneous hemorrhage. Those with severe hemophilia (children with less than 1% of normal factor levels) may have frequent, spontaneous bleeding (approximately monthly) and bleed with very minor trauma. Mild hemophilia may go undiagnosed for many years and is sometimes diagnosed in the setting unexplained postoperative bleeding. Severe hemophilia manifests during infancy. Hemophilia is characterized by spontaneous or traumatic hemorrhages, which can be subcutaneous, intramuscular, or within joints (hemarthrosis). Life-threatening internal hemorrhage may follow trauma or surgery. In newborns with hemophilia, there may be intracranial bleeding from traumatic delivery or after circumcision; otherwise, bleeding complications are uncommon in the first year of life. Circumcision should be avoided in boys with a family history of hemophilia.

In both forms of hemophilia, the PTT is prolonged and the PT is normal. In hemophilia A, factor VIII coagulant activity is low, whereas in hemophilia B, factor IX activity is low. Table 11-9 compares hemophilia A, hemophilia B, and von Willebrand disease.

Treatment

The mainstay of hemophilia treatment is intravenous infusion of the specific (deficient) factor. Factor therapy may be given "on-demand," given when bleeding occurs, or as part of an ongoing prophylactic regimen to prevent bleeding. An important long-term goal of therapy is to prevent crippling joint damage caused by recurrent hemarthrosis (hemophilic arthropathy).

Recombinant factors VIII and IX are now the treatment of first choice. For mild-to-moderate bleeding episodes, such as hemarthroses, a single infusion to increase the factor level to at least 40% is appropriate. Sometimes repeat doses are given, with the frequency depending on the half-life of the factor (VIII: 8–12 hours, IX: 18–24 hours). For life-threatening bleeding, maintaining the factor level at 80% to 100% is necessary.

Desmopressin acetate (DDAVP), a synthetic vasopressin analogue, releases factor VIII from endothelial cells. When administered, it may triple or quadruple the initial factor VIII level of a patient with mild or moderate hemophilia A but has no effect on factor IX levels. If adequate hemostatic levels of factor VIII can be achieved with DDAVP, it can be the initial treatment of bleeding for mild to moderate hemophilia A. Because DDAVP is an antidiuretic hormone analogue, hemophiliacs who frequently use DDAVP should be monitored for hyponatremia caused by water retention.

Mild acute bleeding episodes can be treated in the home once the patient has attained the appropriate age and the parents have learned how to administer recombinant factor VIII or IX or DDAVP. Bleeding associated with surgery, trauma, or dental extraction can be anticipated, and excessive bleeding can be prevented with appropriate replacement therapy. Aminocaproic acid (Amicar), an inhibitor of fibrinolysis, may help treat oral bleeding after a dental procedure. It is generally given before and after the procedure.

Testing of blood products for HIV and hepatitis viruses did not begin until the mid-1980s, and as a result, many hemophiliacs contracted the viruses. Between 1979 and 1984, 90% of hemophiliacs who received plasma-derived factor products

TABLE 11-9 Comparison of the Classical Features of Hemophilia A, hemophilia B, and von Willebrand Disease

Characteristic or Test	Hemophilia A	Hemophilia B	von Willebrand Disease
Inheritance	X-linked	X-linked	Autosomal dominant or recessive
Factor deficiency	Factor VIII	Factor IX	von Willebrand factor (+2° VIII def.)
Bleeding site(s)	Muscle, joint, surgical	Muscle, joint, surgical	Mucous membranes, skin, surgical, menstrual
PT	Normal	Normal	Normal
aPTT	Prolonged	Prolonged	Prolonged or normal
Bleeding time	Normal	Normal	Prolonged or normal
Factor VIII	Low	Normal	Low or normal
Factor IX	Normal	Low	Normal
vWF antigen	Normal	Normal	Low[a]
vWF activity	Normal	Normal	Low[a]
Platelet adhesion	Normal	Normal	Low

[a]Different forms of von Willebrand disease may decrease the antigen alone, activity alone, or both.

became HIV seropositive. Acquired immunodeficiency syndrome (AIDS) is the most common cause of death in older patients with hemophilia. Newer pooled, pathogen-inactivated concentrates are safe, and all recombinant preparations are free of viruses.

The most significant complication of therapy today is the formation of inhibitors, which are neutralizing IgG antibodies directed against factor VIII or IX. These inhibitors prevent infused factor replacement from working. Clinically significant inhibitors occur in 10% of patients with factor VIII deficiency and 1% with factor IX deficiency. The treatment of bleeding patients with an inhibitor is difficult. For low-titer inhibitors, options include continuous factor VIII infusions or administration of porcine factor VIII. For high-titer inhibitors, it usually is necessary to administer a product that bypasses the inhibitor, such as recombinant factor VIIa or an activated prothrombin complex concentrate. Frequent use of high doses of prothrombin complex concentrates, and especially of the activated products, increases the risks of thrombosis, which has resulted in fatal myocardial infarction and stroke in adults. Induction of immune tolerance with continual antigen (factor) exposure can eradicate inhibitors.

von Willebrand Disease

Von Willebrand disease is caused by deficiency of von Willebrand factor (vWF), an adhesive protein that connects subendothelial collagen to activated platelets. vWF also binds circulating factor VIII, protecting it from rapid clearance from the circulation. von Willebrand disease is classified on the basis of whether vWF is quantitatively reduced but not absent (type 1), qualitatively abnormal (type 2), or absent (type 3).

Clinical Manifestations

vWF is necessary to anchor platelets to the injured vessel wall, so the clinical manifestations of von Willebrand disease are similar to thrombocytopenia, including easy bruising, epistaxis, gingival bleeding, menorrhagia, and other mucocutaneous bleeding. In severe von Willebrand disease, there may be a marked, secondary factor VIII deficiency (because there is minimal or no vWF to carry and protect factor VIII from clearance), and the patient will also have manifestations similar to hemophilia (hemarthrosis, hematomas). Approximately 85% of patients with von Willebrand disease have classic type 1 disease, which results in mild to moderate deficiency of vWF. Many individuals with mild reductions in vWF levels have no bleeding at all.

Diagnosis

Laboratory testing includes measurement of the vWF antigen (vWF:Ag), which is the amount of protein whether functional or not, and the vWF activity, which is measured functionally by the ristocetin cofactor assay (vWF:RCoF). Analysis of vWF multimer pattern is required for a specific diagnosis. Other tests may be abnormal. The bleeding time, which is increasingly unavailable, may be prolonged. The PTT may be prolonged if there is a sufficient, secondary deficiency of factor VIII. The PFA-100 (Platelet Function Analyzer) test is a newer test of platelet function which many had hoped would replace the bleeding time. This test measures the time taken for blood, drawn through a fine capillary, to block a membrane coated with collagen and epinephrine or collagen and ADP. This is referred to as the *closure time* and is measured in seconds and is abnormally prolonged in von Willebrand disease and in some platelet function disorders. Anemia, thrombocytopenia, antiplatelet medications, and improper specimen collection, handling, and processing (e.g., "tubing" the sample to the lab) will also prolong the closure time, so a prolonged PFA-100 is not specific for von Willebrand disease. Table 11-9 compares the findings in classic von Willebrand disease with those in hemophilia A and B.

Treatment

The treatment of von Willebrand disease depends on the severity of bleeding, but is usually given to treat active bleeding (e.g., epistaxis) or prevent bleeding in a high-risk situation (e.g., perioperatively). DDAVP, which stimulates the release of vWF from endothelial cells, is the treatment of choice for bleeding episodes in most patients with type I von Willebrand disease. Patients with type 3 disease (who have no vWF to release), or with severe bleeding not responding to DDAVP, can be treated with a virally attenuated vWF-containing concentrate (Humate P). Cryoprecipitate should not be used, because it is not virally attenuated. Hepatitis B vaccine should be given before exposure to plasma-derived products. As in all bleeding disorders, medications that alter platelet function, such as aspirin, should be avoided.

Vitamin K Deficiency

Coagulation factors (factors II, VII, IX, and X) and antithrombotic factors (protein C and protein S) are synthesized in the liver and depend on vitamin K for their activity. The factors must undergo γ-carboxy glutamation to become active, which is catalyzed by a vitamin K-dependent enzyme. When vitamin K is deficient, coagulation is impaired. Vitamin K deficiency often occurs because of malabsorption, especially with cystic fibrosis and with antibiotic-induced suppression of intestinal bacteria that produce vitamin K. Overdose of warfarin, a drug that interferes with vitamin K metabolism, causes severe deficiency of vitamin K-dependent factors. Similarly, maternal use of warfarin or anticonvulsant therapy (phenobarbital, phenytoin) may also result in vitamin K deficiency in the newborn. The most common disorder resulting from vitamin K deficiency is hemorrhagic disease of the newborn, which occurs in neonates who do not receive intramuscular vitamin K at birth.

Clinical Manifestations

Although most newborn infants are born with reduced levels of vitamin K-dependent factors, only a few develop hemorrhagic complications. Because breast milk is a poor source of vitamin K, breastfed infants who do not receive prophylactic vitamin K on the first day of life are at the highest risk for hemorrhagic disease of the newborn. Peak incidence is at 2 to 10 days of life. The recommended preventive dose of vitamin K is 1 mg given intramuscularly. The disorder is marked by generalized ecchymoses, gastrointestinal hemorrhage, and bleeding from the circumcision site and umbilical stump. Affected neonates are at risk for intracranial hemorrhage.

Both the PTT and PT are prolonged in vitamin K deficiency because factors of both the extrinsic (VII), intrinsic (IX), and common pathways (II, X) are affected. Prolongation of the PT is a more sensitive test for vitamin K deficiency because infants normally have a relatively prolonged PTT. The coagulopathy seen with hemorrhagic disease may be confused with liver disease or DIC, both of which have a prolonged PT and decreased factor VII level. Table 11-10 differentiates vitamin K deficiency, liver disease, and DIC by laboratory data.

Treatment

Nutritional disorders and malabsorptive states respond to parenteral administration of vitamin K. Fresh-frozen plasma or prothrombin complex concentrate, which is a mixture of coagulation factors II, VII, IX, and X, is indicated for severe bleeding along with vitamin K.

TABLE 11-10 Differentiation of Vitamin K Deficiency, Liver Disease, and DIC

Laboratory Test	Vitamin K Deficiency	Liver Disease	DIC
PT	↑	↑	↑
Platelets	nl	nl to ↓	↓
Fibrinogen	nl	nl to ↓	↓
Factor VIII	nl	nl to ↑	↓
Factor VII	↓	↓	nl to ↓
Factor V	nl	↓	↓

nl, normal; ↑,••••••; ↓,••••

Deep Vein Thrombosis, Pulmonary Embolism, and Anticoagulation Therapy

Venous thrombosis is rare in children but the incidence is rapidly rising with advances in supportive and intensive care (especially the use of indwelling venous catheters), epidemic obesity, and the increasing use of oral contraceptives. The estimated risk for thrombosis in children in the general population is 0.07/10,000 and about 5.3/10,000 in hospitalized children. The rate of venous thrombosis in children is only one-tenth of that in adults. Thrombosis in infants and teenagers accounts for 70% of the cases seen in children. Venous thrombosis develops under conditions of slow blood flow, an injured vascular endothelium, and in older children, unilateral acute limb swelling, with pain and discoloration, and distended superficial veins should make one suspect a deep vein thrombosis. Childhood thrombosis is usually multifactorial and is precipitated by the concurrence of multiple risk factors. The various risk factors for childhood venous thromboembolism are listed in the Table 11-11.

Indwelling venous catheters (central lines or "ports") are the most common risk factor for thrombosis in children. Several genetic mutations have been identified that are associated with an increased risk of thrombosis. The most common mutations in the Caucasian population are the factor V Leiden and the prothrombin gene G20210A mutations. In addition, hereditary deficiencies in the natural anticoagulant factors, protein C, protein S, and antithrombin are also associated with an increased risk for thrombosis. Diabetes, obesity, and nephrotic syndrome are some examples of concurrent medical illnesses that also increase this risk. Other risk factors

TABLE 11-11 Common Risk Factors for Venous Thromboembolism in Children

- Indwelling venous catheters
- Estrogen-containing oral contraceptives
- Congenital heart disease
- Surgery, trauma, immobility, paresis
- Inherited thrombophilias
- Antiphospholipid antibodies
- Obesity
- Malignancy
- Cancer therapy (asparaginase)
- Inflammatory bowel disease
- Nephrotic syndrome
- Smoking

include estrogen-containing oral contraceptives, smoking, and immobility.

A potentially life-threatening complication of venous thrombosis is pulmonary embolism, which occurs when a thrombus or other substance (i.e., fat, air, bone marrow) enters and obstructs the pulmonary arterial circulation. Pulmonary embolism may lead to significant ventilation-perfusion mismatch and respiratory distress. The lung parenchyma affected by the embolism can undergo necrosis leading to pulmonary infarction. Anticoagulation with various forms of heparin (unfractionated or standard heparin, low molecular weight heparin) or with vitamin K antagonists such as warfarin are used as standard therapy for the treatment of venous thrombosis and pulmonary embolism. In specific cases, thrombolytic therapy with tissue plasminogen activator (tPA) may be indicated to dissolve the thrombus; rarely, surgical embolectomy is performed. A long-term complication of venous thrombosis is the post-thrombotic syndrome, characterized by chronic swelling, pain, skin changes, and prominent veins.

TRANSFUSION OF BLOOD PRODUCTS

Blood products should only be transfused when strict clinical and laboratory criteria are met. Packed red blood cells (PRBCs) and platelets are the most commonly transfused blood products. Transfusion of granulocytes, whole blood, fresh frozen plasma (FFP), and cryoprecipitate may be warranted in special circumstances.

PRBC transfusions are indicated for symptomatic or severe anemia. PRBC transfusions increase the oxygen carrying capacity in anemic patients and help to ensure adequate tissue oxygenation. Sometimes transfusion is used to decrease the proportion of an abnormal hemoglobin, like hemoglobin S. It is more important to base the need for transfusion on an assessment of the patient rather than an arbitrary hemoglobin concentration. Chronicity of anemia, active bleeding, underlying cardiopulmonary disease, and other individual factors influence the decision to transfuse independent of the hemoglobin concentration. The volume of one unit of PRBCs derived from a routine blood donation varies from 250 to 350 mL, so it is important to calculate and consider ordering a specific volume of PRBCs (rather than a specific number of units of PRBCs), especially for younger children. Administration of 10 to 15 mL/kg of PRBCs usually raises the hemoglobin level by 2 to 3 g/dL. This volume can safely be administered over 3 to 4 hours except in severely anemic (hemoglobin <5 g/dL) patients or those at risk for transfusion-associated circulatory overload, where the rate of transfusion has to be much slower (1 mL PRBCs/kg/hour is safe).

Platelet transfusions are normally indicated to prevent or stop bleeding in patients with thrombocytopenia or platelet function disorders. Like PRBC transfusions, there is no "universal" transfusion trigger for platelet transfusions, as bleeding risk and response to transfusion depends on the patient and the disease. Platelet transfusions are usually not indicated in patients with ITP, irrespective of the platelet count, except with life-threatening hemorrhage when given concomitantly with (after) other treatments like steroids and IVIG.

Fresh frozen plasma is indicated for replacement of missing coagulation factors (when the specific factor concentrate is unavailable) or for plasma exchange. *Cryoprecipitate* is a rich source of coagulation factors VIII and XIII, fibrinogen, and von Willebrand factor (vWF) and is commonly used for replacement of fibrinogen in severely ill patients. Cryoprecipitate should not be used for hemophilia von Willebrand disease, or other blood disorders where safe, pathogen-free or pathogen-inactivated products are available. *Granulocyte* infusions can be used for prolonged, severe neutropenia and life-threatening sepsis unresponsive to other therapies. *Whole blood* transfusions are rarely used, except during exchange transfusions in neonates and in autologous blood transfusions.

Blood product transfusion is associated with significant risks and complications, although current monitoring and testing procedures have reduced the incidence of many. These risks must always be considered when making a decision to transfuse a patient. The benefits of transfusion should outweigh these risks. The most common transfusion reactions are summarized below.

1. *Febrile reactions* are common and caused by leukocytes present in PRBC and platelet transfusions and can be prevented by the use of leukocyte filters or leukocyte-depleted blood products. If they occur, the transfusion should be paused, a blood bank transfusion workup should be started, and antipyretics administered.
2. *Allergic reactions* are due to protein antigens in the transfused product and occur in 1% to 2% of PRBC. Pruritus, rash, and urticaria, typically begin minutes after the infusion is started. Sometimes severe allergic or anaphylactic reactions occur. The transfusion should be stopped, and antihistamines should be administered. Corticosteroids may be needed. IgA-deficient individuals who have had anaphylactic reactions to blood products require IgA-reduced products (e.g., washed red blood cells, IgA-deficient plasma).
3. *Acute hemolytic transfusion reactions* are most commonly due to clerical errors resulting in administration of the wrong (incompatible) unit to the wrong patient. These reactions are characterized by a sudden onset of fever, chills, tachycardia, tachypnea, and vomiting with severe hemolysis that may result in multiorgan failure, shock, and DIC unless (or despite) the transfusion is immediately stopped and necessary supportive care given.
4. *Infections*, especially serious viral infections, are now extremely rare due to the intensive screening of donors and testing of products. The current estimated risk of transmission of HIV infection is about 1 in 2 million, that of hepatitis C virus is 1 in 2 million, and that of hepatitis B virus is 1 in 200,000. Other viruses can also be transmitted. Bacterial can also be transmitted by transfusion, especially of platelet products, which are stored at room temperature. Transfusion-transmitted parasitic disease (malaria, babesiosis) should be considered in the appropriate clinical circumstances. A very small number of cases of new variant Creutzfeld-Jakob disease (nvCJD) have been transmitted by blood transfusion.
5. *Transfusion-associated acute lung injury (TRALI)* can be a serious, life-threatening complication of transfusion characterized by noncardiogenic pulmonary edema. The pulmonary injury is thought to be caused by the interaction of neutrophils and transfused antibodies (anti-HLA and antihuman neutrophil antigens), their deposition in, and damage to the pulmonary vascular bed. Pulmonary edema can also occur in another transfusion reaction, *transfusion-associated circulatory overload* (TACO) in which the blood product is transfused at a rate greater than the cardiopulmonary system can handle. TACO may occur, for example, when a severely but chronically anemic individual (who has a normal or high total blood volume in compensation) is given a "normal" transfusion volume (e.g., 11 to 15 mL/kg over 3 to 4 hours).

6. *Transfusion-associated graft versus host disease (TA-GVHD)* occurs when immunocompetent lymphocytes (which are normal passengers in PRBC and platelet products, even following leukofiltration) engraft in a recipient whose immune system cannot reject them. This is a very rare but fatal complication. Irradiation of blood products can prevent this complication, and it is indicated for immunocompromised individuals and neonates.
7. *Alloimmunization and delayed hemolytic transfusion reactions* can occur in multiply transfused individuals who develop antibodies against alloantigens on red blood cells, white blood cells, or platelets. Alloimmunization may hinder the ability to find an appropriate blood product for a person who needs it. Red cell alloantibodies may also cause delayed, posttransfusion hemolysis.
8. *Iron overload* (transfusional hemochromatosis) occurs in chronically transfused patients because the body has no mechanism to increase the elimination of iron. Iron chelation therapy may be needed, depending on the iron burden, to prevent organ injury and death.

KEY POINTS

- Anemia has only three causes: decreased red cell production, increased red cell destruction (hemolysis), and blood loss or sequestration.
- The mean corpuscular volume (MCV) and the reticulocyte count are the most helpful ways to approach and classify the differential diagnosis of anemia.
- The most common hypochromic microcytic anemias are iron-deficiency anemia, the thalassemia syndromes, and anemia of inflammation.
- Transient erythroblastopenia of childhood (TEC) is a normocytic anemia caused by bone marrow suppression and occurs between 6 months and 3 years of age.
- Normocytic anemias with increased red cell production (increased reticulocytes) are most commonly caused by hemolysis.
- Hemolytic anemias are caused by extrinsic factors and intrinsic defects. In general, extrinsic factors are acquired, and intrinsic defects are hereditary. Extrinsic factors may be immune or nonimmune. Intrinsic defects include membrane defects, hemoglobinopathies, and enzymopathies.
- Hereditary spherocytosis (HS) is caused by an intrinsic membrane defect in the major supporting proteins of the red blood cell membrane.
- Sickle cell disease is a group of related disorders resulting from an abnormal β-globin chain in the hemoglobin molecule (i.e., sickle hemoglobin, $\beta^{6\ glu>val}$), which, upon deoxygenation, allows the polymerization of hemoglobin into insoluble rods that distort the red blood cell and damage it. The clinical manifestations of sickle cell disease include chronic hemolytic anemia, pain and other vaso-occlusive events, increased risk of bacterial infection, and chronic, progressive organ damage.
- Glucose-6-phosphate dehydrogenase (G6PD) deficiency is the most common red blood cell enzyme defect. It is X-linked, and the severity depends on the mutation.
- Macrocytic anemias can be subclassified based on the presence or absence of megaloblastosis, a marker of ineffective DNA synthesis within a red blood cell precursor. Not all macrocytic anemias are megaloblastic, but all megaloblastic anemias are macrocytic.
- Megaloblastic, macrocytic anemias reflect ineffective DNA synthesis and can result from vitamin B_{12} or folate deficiency, drugs that interfere with folate metabolism, and some rare metabolic disorders.
- Macrocytic anemias without megaloblastic changes result from bone marrow failure and include bone marrow failure syndromes (Diamond-Blackfan syndrome, Fanconi anemia, idiopathic aplastic anemia, myelodysplasia), drug-induced anemias, chronic liver disease, and hypothyroidism.
- Platelet disorders can be either quantitative or qualitative. Platelets are an important component of primary hemostasis, and either type of defect can cause mucocutaneous bleeding.
- Thrombocytopenia is the most common cause of abnormal bleeding in children. Thrombocytopenia caused by shortened platelet survival, which is much more common than thrombocytopenia caused by inadequate production, is caused by alloantibodies, autoantibodies, and microangiopathic states.
- Idiopathic thrombocytopenic purpura (ITP) results mainly from autoimmune antibody formation against platelets. Childhood ITP is typically a benign, self-limited disease that infrequently causes severe bleeding and often requires no pharmacotherapy at all.
- Disseminated intravascular coagulation (DIC) results from severe illness, causing activation of both coagulation (thrombin) and fibrinolysis (plasmin).
- Deficiencies of coagulation factors (disorders or secondary hemostasis) are characterized by spontaneous or induced internal or external bleeding, such as hemarthrosis and hematomas. In contrast, defects in primary hemostasis (e.g., platelet disorders) cause mucocutaneous bleeding.
- Hemophilia A results from a deficiency of factor VIII, and hemophilia B results from a lack of factor IX. Both types of hemophilia are X-linked and characterized by spontaneous or traumatic hemorrhages, which can be subcutaneous, intramuscular, or within joints (hemarthrosis). Life-threatening internal hemorrhage may follow trauma or surgery. Severity depends upon the level of factor in plasma.
- von Willebrand disease is caused by deficiency of vWF, an adhesive protein that connects subendothelial collagen to activated platelets and also binds to circulating factor VIII, protecting it from rapid clearance. It is characterized by mucocutaneous bleeding, epistaxis, gingival bleeding, cutaneous bruising, and menorrhagia.
- The most common disorder resulting from vitamin K deficiency is hemorrhagic disease of the newborn, which occurs in neonates who do not receive vitamin K at birth.
- The transfusion of blood products should be based on patient-specific indications and not on universal, arbitrary transfusion triggers for hemoglobin concentration or platelet count.
- The many potential complications of transfusion of blood products should be carefully considered before transfusion in consideration of the expected magnitude of the benefits.

C Clinical Vignettes

Vignette 1

An 18-month-old child who was born at term is now brought to you, his pediatrician, by his mother because she is concerned that he has become increasingly irritable and tired over the past few weeks. He is drinking well, mainly milk, and his urine has been light yellow. You notice that the child is markedly pale and that he has no jaundice, adenopathy, or organomegaly. You obtain a blood count in your office that shows the following:

(a) WBC 7,500/mm^3
(b) Hgb 6.5 g/dL
(c) MCV 59 fL
(d) RDW 17.2%
(e) Platelets 525,000/mm^3
(f) Reticulocytes 1.6%

1. What is the mechanism of the anemia?
  a. Increased destruction (hemolysis)
  b. Decreased production
  c. Acute blood loss
  d. Sequestration

2. Given that you now know the child has anemia due to an inadequate bone marrow response (decreased production of RBCs), what is the most likely diagnosis?
  a. Transient erythroblastopenia of childhood (TEC)
  b. Iron-deficiency anemia
  c. Lead intoxication
  d. Severe aplastic anemia
  e. Leukemia

3. What is the most likely cause of this patient's iron-deficiency anemia?
  a. Early introduction of cow's milk
  b. Consumption of goat's milk
  c. Occult gastrointestinal blood loss
  d. Inadequate iron endowment at birth
  e. Hereditary malabsorption of iron

4. You do not transfuse the child; rather you treat him with an oral preparation of ferrous sulfate, dosed at 6 mg elemental iron/kg/d. You have him return in 1 week for a blood count. Assuming the diagnosis is correct, you prescribed the right dose of iron, the parents administered the iron appropriately, and the child does not have malabsorption, which of the following blood counts represents the expected response after 1 week of iron therapy?

	Hgb (g/dL)	MCV (fL)	Reticulocytes (%)
a.	6.5	59	1.6
b.	6.6	60	3
c.	7.6	64	4.5
d.	11.3	70	2.5
e.	11.5	75	1.5

Vignette 2

A 4-month-old baby boy, born at term without complications, is referred to you for an abnormal newborn screening test for hemoglobinopathies. The hemoglobin pattern reported from the first week of life is "F, A" but the newborn screening lab also reports a trace amount of hemoglobin (Hb) Barts.

1. What is the significance of Hb Barts on newborn screening?
  a. The baby has a form of α-thalassemia.
  b. The baby has a form of β-thalassemia.
  c. The baby has a form of γ-thalassemia.
  d. The baby has a form of δ-β-thalassemia.
  e. The baby has a form of HPFH (hereditary persistence of fetal hemoglobin).

2. You choose to obtain an Hgb electrophoresis at 4 months of age. The results show the presence of Hb A (89%) and Hb F (11%), but no Hb Barts. What does the disappearance of Hb Barts indicate?
  a. Laboratory error
  b. This baby had a transient, neonatal form of thalassemia.
  c. The Hb F production has increased since birth.
  d. An expected developmental phenomenon
  e. Nonpaternity

3. Assume that this child is African American and has no Asian ancestry. You determine that he has a two-gene deletion α-thalassemia (α-thalassemia trait). From which parent or parents did he almost certainly inherit his α-gene deletions?
  a. Two deleted genes from the mother
  b. Two deleted genes from the father
  c. One deletion each from the mother and the father
  d. Two deletions each from the mother and the father
  e. One deletion from either parent and one new mutation

Vignette 3

A family presents to you with a newborn baby who was recently identified by newborn screening to have a form of sickle cell disease. The parents are upset because they were told by their obstetrician that they could not have a baby with sickle cell disease because only the mother had sickle cell trait on preconception testing. The father was tested for sickle cell trait preconception, and he did not have it.

1. Assuming that the results of the sickle trait testing were correct and that the father without sickle cell trait is, indeed, the biological father, what type of hematologic abnormality could the father have that could explain the occurrence of sickle cell disease in their child?
   - **a.** G6PD deficiency
   - b. α-thalassemia trait
   - c. β-thalassemia trait
   - **d.** Hereditary elliptocytosis
   - **e.** Hgb G Philadelphia trait

2. By confirmatory testing, you determine that the mother in question indeed has only sickle cell trait and the father has only β^+-thalassemia trait. What is the probability for each of their subsequent pregnancies that the child will have a form of sickle cell disease?
   - **a.** <1%
   - **b.** 25%
   - **c.** 50%
   - **d.** 75%
   - **e.** 100%

3. When this child turns 1 year of age, you obtain a complete blood count. Which of the following blood counts would be most consistent with sickle-β^+-thalassemia ($S\beta^+$)?

	Hgb (g/dL)	MCV (fL)	Reticulocytes (%)
a.	7.5	78	15
b.	7.4	64	18
c.	10.3	79	4
d.	10.1	62	3.5
e.	11.1	75	1.5

Vignette 4

You are caring for a young child undergoing intensive chemotherapy for acute myeloid leukemia (AML). She has expected chemotherapy-related myelosuppression, her Hgb concentration is 6.5 g/dL, and she is symptomatic of the anemia. You decided that she needs a transfusion of packed red blood cells (PRBCs). You choose to irradiate the blood product before transfusing it.

1. What complication of transfusion is prevented by irradiation?
   - **a.** Alloimmunization
   - **b.** Febrile transfusion reaction
   - **c.** Transfusion-associated acute lung injury (TRALI)
   - **d.** Transfusion-associated graft-versus-host disease (TA-GVHD)
   - **e.** Viral transmission

2. You also choose to leukofilter (leuko-deplete or leuko-reduce) the blood to prevent alloimmunization, transmission of CMV, and which of the following complications of transfusion?
   - **a.** Acute hemolytic transfusion reactions
   - **b.** Febrile transfusion reactions
   - **c.** Allergic reactions
   - **d.** Malaria
   - **e.** Transfusion-associated circulatory overload (TACO)

3. You transfuse 10 ml/kg of PRBC over 4 hours. The next day you obtain a CBC. Which posttransfusion Hgb concentration represents a typical response to this volume of PRBCs (assume no hemolysis or ongoing losses of blood)?
   - **a.** 7.0 g/dL
   - **b.** 8.5 g/dL
   - **c.** 10.0 g/dL
   - **d.** 11.5 g/dL
   - **e.** 13.0 g/dL

4. Your patient begins to bleed from her nose and mouth. Her platelet count is 8,000/mm^3, so you decide to give her a transfusion of platelets. Which of the following complications of transfusion is much more common with platelets than PRBCs?
   - **a.** Transmission of bacteria
   - **b.** Transfusion-associated circulatory overload (TACO)
   - **c.** Transfusional hemochromatosis
   - **d.** Transfusion-associated graft-versus-host disease (TA-GVHD)
   - **e.** Delayed hemolytic transfusion reaction

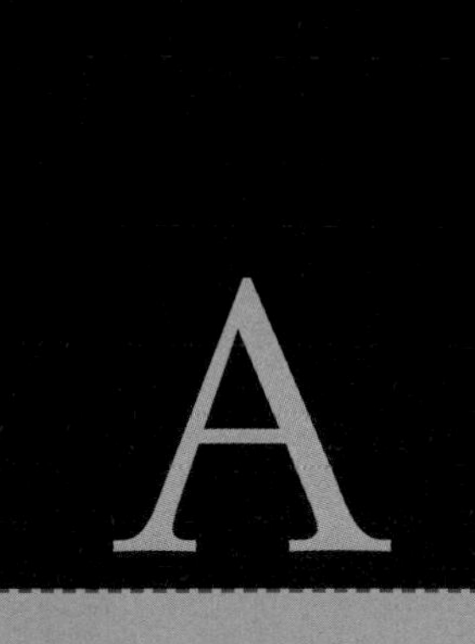

Answers

Vignette 1 Question 1

Answer B: The normal range for the reticulocyte count is 0.5% to 1.5%, but this normal range assumes a normal Hgb concentration. Here, the reticulocyte count is far too low for the degree of anemia. So the mechanism of anemia is decreased production (inadequate bone marrow response). Hemolysis, acute blood loss, and sequestration will cause a compensatory reticulocytosis, which this child does not have. A compensatory reticulocytosis takes 12 to 24 hours to appear, so it may be lacking (temporarily) when a patient presents immediately after the onset of hemolysis, blood loss, or sequestration. The child in this case has been symptomatic for weeks, so this scenario is excluded. Hemolysis would also cause jaundice, dark urine, or both depending on the cause (site) of hemolysis. This child has neither. He also does not have splenomegaly, so splenic sequestration is excluded.

Vignette 1 Question 2

Answer B: Iron-deficiency anemia is consistent with the history, physical examination, all the measurements provided by the CBC (including the microcytosis, increased RDW, and thrombocytosis), and the inadequate reticulocyte response (inadequate iron to make new RBCs). TEC, severe aplastic anemia, and leukemia cause normocytic or macrocytic anemias, not the marked microcytosis seen in this case. Isolated lead intoxication causes marked basophilic stippling but not a marked microcytic anemia. The pica that sometimes accompanies iron-deficiency anemia may lead to secondary lead exposure, but the lead exposure does not cause the anemia.

Vignette 1 Question 3

Answer A: This history gives us a clue that the child is consuming too much milk, but further specific questioning will be needed to determine when cow's milk was introduced and the amount consumed (frequency and volume). This is the most likely diagnosis, however, even though it is a preventable cause of anemia. Occult GI blood loss is a possibility, but dietary iron deficiency would be more common. The child was born at term, so he very likely had a normal endowment of iron at birth (you should also ask about birth weight to be complete). Hereditary malabsorption of iron is rare. Consumption of goat's milk (instead of formula) classically leads to folate deficiency, with or without iron deficiency, which would be macrocytic (isolated folate deficiency) or normocytic (combined iron and folate deficiency), unlike the marked microcytosis in this case.

Vignette 1 Question 4

Answer C: The reticulocyte response occurs first, 3 to 4 days after starting appropriate iron therapy. The Hgb concentration then increases by about 1 g/dL in a week's time. So the correct answer is (C), showing both a reticulocytosis and an increase in the hemoglobin concentration by about 1 g/dL. Answer (A) shows no response, inconsistent with the premises of the question. Answer (B) shows only a reticulocytosis, although the Hgb concentration should be higher after 1 week. Answers (D) and (E) are consistent with several weeks of iron therapy (the Hgb concentration is too high for only 1 week of iron therapy).

Vignette 2 Question 1

Answer A: Newborns make a predominance of fetal Hgb (Hb F) and a lesser amount of adult Hgb (Hb A), giving the normal "F, A" pattern on newborn screening (the predominant hemoglobin is always reported first, so that "F, A" means F $>$ A). Hgb F is composed of 2 α and 2 γ chains ($\alpha_2\gamma_2$). When there is a relative deficiency of α-chains due to α-thalassemia, then the relative excess of unpaired γ-chains self-associate to form Hgb Barts, a tetramer of γ-chains (γ_4). The presence of Hgb Barts indicates the presence of α-thalassemia (the α-globin genes are linked together on chromosome 16). All the other choices are abnormalities of the β-globin locus (the γ-, δ-, and β-globin genes are all linked together on chromosome 11).

Vignette 2 Question 2

Answer D: Fetal Hgb production progressively decreases after birth and approaches the normal adult values of approximately 1.5% to 2.5% by about 6 months of age in hematologically normal infants. Hb F production declines with age because γ-chains synthesis declines. Because γ-chains synthesis declines with age, so will the formation of Hgb Barts, a tetramer of γ-chainss (γ_4). Therefore, the disappearance of Hb Barts as the baby ages is an expected developmental phenomenon. Trace amounts of Hb Barts can be detected by high-sensitivity techniques in older children with one- or two-gene deletion α-thalassemia, but it is not usually detected by Hgb electrophoresis outside of early infancy. Gamma thalassemia, not α-thalassemia, is transient, neonatal form of thalassemia.

Vignette 2 Question 3

Answer C: Two-gene deletion α-thalassemia (α-thalassemia trait) can occur when two α-globin genes are deleted on the same chromosome, in *cis* (--/αα), or when they are deleted on opposite chromosomes, in *trans* (α-/α-). Among individuals of African ancestry, α-thalassemia trait nearly always occurs in *trans* (α-/α-), so this child must have received one α-gene deletion from the mother and the other from the father. In contrast, individuals of Asian ancestry with α-thalassemia trait may carry both deletions in *cis* (--/αα) or in *trans* (α-/α-), so it is possible to inherit two deleted genes from one parent in this scenario.

Vignette 3 Question 1
Answer C: Even when only one parent has sickle cell trait, a couple can still produce children with sickle cell disease. They cannot have a child with sickle cell anemia, which is homozygosity for Hgb S, but they can have children with compound heterozygous forms of sickle cell disease, such as sickle-hemoglobin C disease (Hgb SC), sickle-β^+-thalassemia (Hgb Sβ^+), or sickle-β^0-thalassemia (Hgb Sβ^0). A negative test for the presence of sickle hemoglobin (Hgb S) does not exclude the presence of other abnormal hemoglobins or thalassemia trait. G6PD deficiency and hereditary elliptocytosis, both common among African Americans, do not interact with sickle cell trait to produce a form of sickle cell disease. Alpha thalassemia trait and Hgb G Philadelphia trait are both abnormalities of the α-globin locus; but the coinheritance of Hgb S with certain other β-globin abnormalities is required to produce forms of sickle disease. Among the possible answers, only β-thalassemia trait is an abnormality of the β-globin. So, the child in question has a form of sickle-β-thalassemia.

Vignette 3 Question 2
Answer B: This is straightforward Mendelian inheritance. If one parent has S trait (AS) and the other has β^+-thalassemia trait (Aβ^+), then offspring have a 25% chance of having normal hemoglobin (AA), a 50% chance of having trait (either AS or Aβ^+), and a 25% chance of having sickle-β^+-thalassemia (Sβ^+).

Vignette 3 Question 3
Answer D: Sickle-β^+-thalassemia (Sβ^+) typically produces a mild hemolytic anemia (Hgb 10 to 12 g/dL; reticulocytes 2% to 5%) that is microcytic (MCV ≤70 for a 1-year-old). The anemia is too severe in choices A and B, and there is no microcytosis in choices A, C, and E.

Vignette 4 Question 1
Answer D: Irradiation prevents only one complication: transfusion-associated graft-versus-host disease. TA-GVHD occurs when immunocompetent lymphocytes (which are normal passengers in PRBC and platelet products, even following leukofiltration) engraft in a recipient whose immune system cannot reject them. This is a very rare but fatal complication. Irradiation of blood products can prevent this complication by damaging passenger leukocytes so that they cannot divide, and it is indicated for immunocompromised individuals and neonates.

Vignette 4 Question 2
Answer B: Febrile transfusion reactions are most commonly caused by the recipient's immune response to passenger leukocytes, and leukofiltration is an effective way to reduce the frequency of febrile transfusion reactions. The other complications answers are not mediated be passenger leukocytes (and so are not reduced by leukofiltration). Hemolytic transfusion reactions are caused by host antibody formation against donor RBCs. Allergic reactions are mediated by transfused plasma proteins. Malaria is an intraerythrocyte parasite (and also cell free). TACO is mediated by the volume of the transfused product, given faster than the body can physiologically tolerate.

Vignette 4 Question 3
Answer B: A transfusion of 10 mL/kg of PRBCs will increase the Hgb concentration by about 2 g/dL, so only answer (B) is correct. The posttransfusion increment depends on the volume of the transfusion and the hematocrit of the transfused product. The hematocrit of the transfused product is determined by the hematocrit of the donor (male higher than female) and the anticoagulant/preservative solution that is used. Modern additive solutions produce a PRBC product with an Hct of approximately 55%. Older, but still used, anticoagulant/preservatives such as CPDA-1 (citrate-phosphate-dextrose-adenine) have a higher Hct (approximately 65%), so it is important to know what product your blood bank uses to know how much blood to give your patient.

Vignette 4 Question 4
Answer A: Platelet products are stored at room temperature (in contrast, PRBCs are refrigerated during storage), so bacterial contamination and growth is more common with platelets. TACO can occur from any transfused product, as it is determined by volume. Transfusional hemochromatosis is a complication of PRBC transfusion, specifically. TA-GVHD can occur with either PRBC or platelet products (when the recipient is immunocompromised and the product has not been irradiated). Delayed hemolytic transfusion reactions occur as a consequence of sensitization to transfused RBC antigens and the production of antibodies against the transfused RBC antigens.

Chapter

12 Oncology

Karen C. Burns • Rajaram Nagarajan • Franklin O. Smith • Bradley S. Marino

There are approximately 12,500 new diagnoses of pediatric cancers in patients under the age of 20 years, each year in the United States. Approximately two-thirds occur below the age of 15 years. The most common types of cancers in children under the age of 15 years are leukemia and brain tumors. In the older adolescent group, Hodgkin disease and germ cell tumors predominate (Figs. 12-1 and 12-2).

Common therapeutic modalities for treating childhood cancer include surgery, radiation, chemotherapy, hematopoietic stem cell transplantation, and biologic agents. The most commonly used chemotherapeutic agents are listed in Table 12-1.

Although childhood cancer represents a small number of childhood diseases, it accounts for a substantial number of deaths in children. It is the second most common cause of death below the age of 15 years (11%)—behind only accidents (40%). In older adolescents, cancer-related deaths account for 5% of all deaths—fourth behind accidents, suicide, and homicide. Overall, tremendous progress has been made, with cure rates now exceeding 80%. However, the adolescent and young adult population has not seen this same increase in survival rates. This has led to an emerging field in oncology: Adolescent and Young Adult (AYA) oncology. Research efforts are increasingly focusing on this population.

The number of childhood cancer survivors is growing. Issues relating to survivorship are now being appreciated and need to be acknowledged in pediatric and general practices. Primary care physicians need to be aware that long-term complications of cancer therapies exist and that appropriate lifelong follow-up is needed. It is also important that childhood cancer survivors (and their caregivers) are aware of their history of cancer and the therapies given to them, so that they are empowered to be advocates for their own health as they grow older.

The following sections describe the more common cancers in children and adolescents.

LEUKEMIA

The leukemias account for the greatest percentage of cases of childhood malignancies. There are more than 3,000 new cases of leukemia each year in the United States, and approximately 35 to 40 children per million are affected. Figure 12-1 lists types of childhood cancers (0 to 14 years of age) and the fraction of the total childhood malignancies that each accounts for annually.

PATHOGENESIS

Leukemia results from malignant transformation and clonal expansion of hematopoietic cells at an early stage of differentiation that are then unable to undergo further maturation. Leukemias are classified on the basis of leukemic cell morphology into **lymphoblastic leukemias** (lymphoid lineage cell proliferation) and **myeloid leukemias** (granulocyte, monocyte, erythrocyte, or platelet lineage cell proliferation). **Acute leukemias** constitute 97% of all childhood leukemias and are subdivided into acute lymphoblastic leukemia (ALL) and acute myeloid leukemia, also known as acute myelogenous leukemia (AML). If untreated, they are rapidly fatal within weeks to a few months of diagnosis, but with treatment they are often curable. **Chronic leukemias** make up only 3% of childhood leukemias, the majority of which are chronic myelogenous leukemia (CML) seen in adolescents. Unlike patients with acute leukemias, CML can be indolent and patients may survive without treatment for months to years. If left untreated, the chronic leukemias may undergo an acute transformation that requires immediate therapy to survive. Because CML is so rare in children, a discussion of the chronic leukemias is beyond the scope of this review text. The following discussion focuses on ALL and AML of childhood and adolescence.

CLASSIFICATION

ALL is classified by both morphologic and immunologic methods. **Morphologic classification** is based on the appearance of the lymphoblasts. The L1-type lymphoblast is the most common (85%), followed by the L2 morphology (14%), with L3 lymphoblasts the rarest form. Therapy and outcome are not different for L1 versus L2 lymphoblasts. L3 blasts (or Burkitt or mature B leukemia) are treated more like Burkitt lymphoma with spread to the bone marrow. **Immunologic classification** is based on immunophenotype, which is described by surface antigen expression and flow cytometric analysis. The most

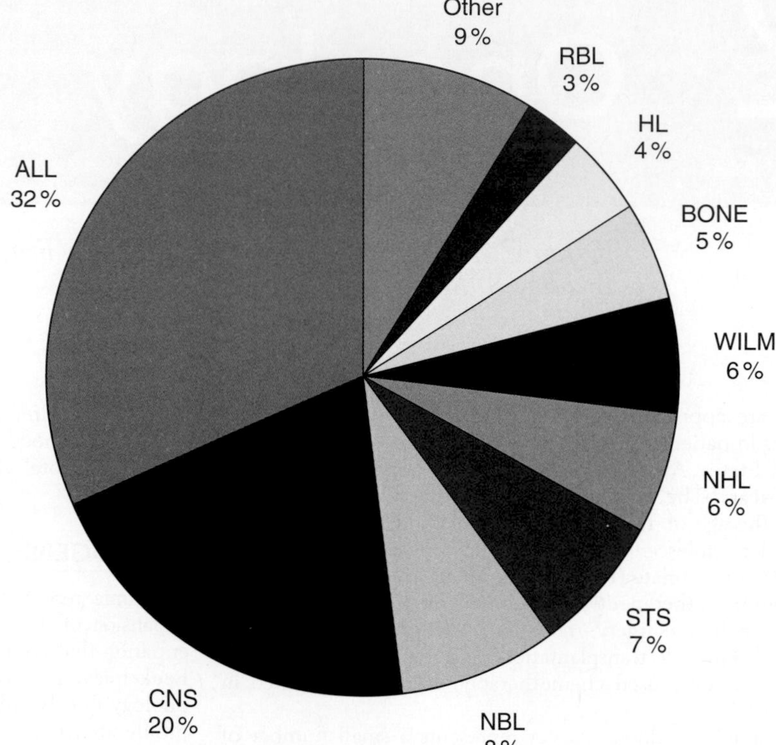

Figure 12-1 • Percent distribution of childhood cancers under the age of 15 years. ALL, acute lymphoblastic leukemia; BONE, osteosarcoma and Ewing sarcoma; CNS, central nervous system tumor; HL, Hodgkin disease; NBL, neuroblastoma; NHL, non-Hodgkin lymphoma; RBL, retinoblastoma; STS, soft tissue sarcoma; WILM, Wilms tumor.
(Compiled from Ries L, Smith MA, Gurney JG, et al., eds. *Cancer Incidence and Survival among Children and Adolescents: United States SEER Program 1975–1995*. Bethesda, MD: National Cancer Institute, SEER program. NIH Pub. No. 99-4649; 1999.)

frequent childhood ALL immunophenotype, precursor B-cell, accounts for 80% of cases and is associated with a good prognosis in the majority of cases. Outcomes for T-cell ALL, which is responsible for 19% of childhood ALL, have improved significantly over the past several years and are now comparable to the outcomes of some precursor B-cell ALL. Mature B-cell ALL or Burkitt leukemia, which accounts for 1% of cases, is treated like Burkitt lymphoma with a good outcome.

AML is classified into eight subtypes based on morphologic and histochemical information using the French–American–British (FAB) classification system: M0 is undifferentiated stem cell leukemia, M1 is myeloblastic leukemia without differentiation, M2 is myeloblastic leukemia with differentiation, M3 is promyelocytic leukemia, M4 is myelomonocytic leukemia, M5 is monoblastic leukemia, M6 is erythroleukemia, and M7 is megakaryoblastic leukemia. The prognosis for AML is dependent on both subtype and risk factors. Patients with M3 AML, and trisomy 21 patients with M7 AML, have a good prognosis, as do patients with favorable risk factors. Patients with poor risk factors have a poor prognosis. Risk factors will be discussed later in this chapter.

EPIDEMIOLOGY AND RISK FACTORS

Table 12-2 compares the epidemiology of ALL and AML. ALL, the most common pediatric cancer, accounts for 75% of all cases of childhood acute leukemia. ALL is 1.3 times more common in boys than in girls and more common in white children than in African American children. The incidence of ALL peaks between 2 and 5 years of age. AML accounts for 20% of all cases of childhood acute leukemia. There is no race or gender predilection in patients with AML. The incidence of AML, in contrast to ALL, is increased in adolescence.

Syndromes with an increased risk for leukemia include trisomy 21, Fanconi anemia, Bloom syndrome, ataxia-telangiectasia, X-linked agammaglobulinemia, and severe combined immunodeficiency. Twins have an increased risk of leukemia if one twin develops ALL or AML during the first 5 years of life. Children who have undergone chemotherapy or radiation therapy for a first malignancy have an increased risk of developing a secondary leukemia 1 to 10 years after treatment. Children with congenital bone marrow failure states, such as Shwachman-Diamond syndrome (exocrine pancreatic insufficiency and neutropenia) and Diamond-Blackfan syndrome (congenital red cell aplasia), have an increased risk of developing AML.

CLINICAL MANIFESTATIONS

History and Physical Examination

Symptoms usually develop days to weeks before diagnosis. Nonspecific constitutional symptoms include lethargy, malaise, and anorexia. Children may complain about bone pain or

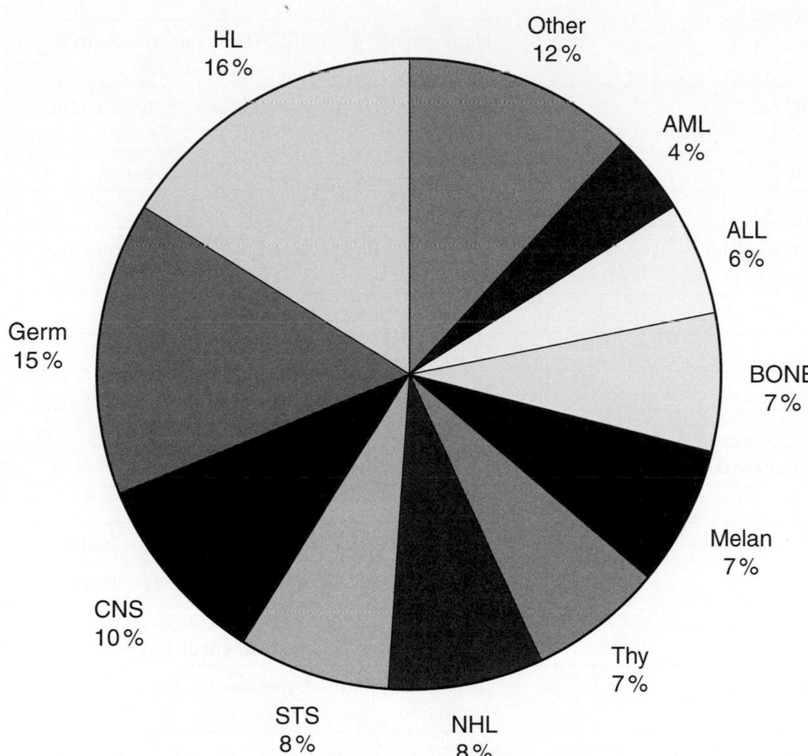

Figure 12-2 • Percent distribution of cancer types for 15- to 19-year-olds. ALL, acute lymphoblastic leukemia; AML, acute myeloid leukemia; BONE, osteosarcoma and Ewing sarcoma; CNS, central nervous system tumor; Germ, germ cell, trophoblastic, and other gonadal tumors; HL, Hodgkin disease; Melan, malignant melanoma; NHL, non-Hodgkin lymphoma; STS, soft tissue sarcoma; Thy, thyroid carcinoma.

(Compiled from Ries L, Smith MA, Gurney JG, et al., eds. *Cancer Incidence and Survival among Children and Adolescents: United States SEER Program 1975–1995*. Bethesda, MD: National Cancer Institute, SEER program. NIH Pub. No. 99-4649; 1999.)

arthralgias caused by leukemic expansion of the marrow cavity. Progressive bone marrow failure may lead to pallor from anemia and ecchymoses or petechiae from thrombocytopenia. The anemia is normochromic and normocytic. Decreased marrow production of RBCs leads to a low reticulocyte count. The WBC count is low (<5,000 per mm^3) in a third of patients, normal (5,000 to 20,000 per mm^3) in a third of patients, and high (>20,000 per mm^3) in a third of patients. Many children have hepatosplenomegaly and cervical lymphadenopathy at diagnosis. Extramedullary involvement is also seen in the CNS, skin, and testicles. CNS infiltration causes neurologic signs and symptoms, such as headache, emesis, papilledema, and sixth cranial nerve palsy. Patients with AML may develop a soft-tissue tumor called a **chloroma** in the spinal cord, brain, or on the skin. Table 12-3 compares the presentations of ALL and AML.

DIFFERENTIAL DIAGNOSIS

The differential diagnosis includes aplastic anemia, idiopathic thrombocytopenic purpura, viral infection (Epstein-Barr virus, parvovirus), metastatic disease secondary to another malignancy, bone marrow suppression secondary to a drug reaction, rheumatologic diseases such as lupus or juvenile rheumatoid arthritis, and viral-induced or familial hemophagocytic syndrome.

DIAGNOSTIC EVALUATION

A complete blood count (CBC) with manual differential and review of the blood smear to look for blast cells should be obtained in any child with suspected leukemia. The peripheral blood can be sent for flow cytometry to determine the type of leukemia. Bone marrow biopsy and aspirate remain the gold standard for diagnosis, even if peripheral blood has been used to type the leukemia. Biopsy and aspirate material are sent for morphology, immunophenotype, and cytogenetics which are critical elements used to risk stratify the leukemia into a treatment group. A comprehensive metabolic panel, LDH, uric acid, calcium, magnesium, and phosphorus are obtained to define baseline values prior to chemotherapy and possible tumor lysis syndrome. Coagulation studies are sent to exclude disseminated intravascular coagulation (DIC). Blood, urine, and viral cultures are obtained if infection is suspected. A chest radiograph is sent to evaluate for mediastinal mass. If mediastinal mass is suspected, an echocardiogram is needed to look for possible cardiac dysfunction or cardiac effusion. A chest CT is frequently obtained to evaluate airway compression. No sedation should be used in the patient with mediastinal mass until these studies are performed and an anesthesia consultation is acquired. A lumbar puncture (LP) is performed to evaluate for central nervous system (CNS) disease. If the patient has thrombocytopenia or coagulation abnormalities, these must be corrected prior to the LP.

TABLE 12-1 Listing of Common Chemotherapeutic Agents and Their Toxicities

Chemotherapy	Mechanism of Action	Acute and Long-Term Toxicity
Alkylating agents		
Cyclophosphamide	Alkylation; cross-linking	Hemorrhagic cystitis; SIADH; cardiactoxicity; fertility
Iphosphamide	Alkylation; cross-linking	Hemorrhagic cystitis; renal toxicity; ototoxicity; fertility
Cisplatinum	Platination; cross-linking	Ototoxicity; renal toxicity; delayed nausea
Antimetabolites		
Methotrexate	Interferes with folate metabolism	Mucositis; Hepatic and renal toxicity; neurotoxicity
Mercaptopurine	Blocks purine synthesis	Mucositis; hepatic toxicity
Thioguanine	Blocks purine synthesis	Mucositis; hepatic toxicity
Cytarabine	Inhibits DNA polymerase	Mucositis; flu-like syndrome; ocular toxicity
Antitumor antibiotic		
Doxorubicin	Intercalation; DNA strand breaks	Mucositis; cardiac toxicity
Plant products		
Vincristine	Mitotic inhibitor; blocks microtubule polymerization	SIADH; neurotoxicity—footdrop, constipation
Etoposide	DNA strand break	Mucositis; infusion reactions; secondary leukemias
Asparaginase	Asparagine depletion	Coagulopathy; pancreatitis; anaphylaxis
Corticosteroids	Receptor-mediated lympholysis	Increased appetite; hypertension; hyperglycemia; myopathy; avascular necrosis; cataracts

Chemotherapy: Brief listing of commonly used chemotherapeutic agents and their toxicities. To a greater or lesser extent the following common toxicities are seen with most chemotherapy: nausea, alopecia, myelosuppression, and immunosuppression. In addition, infertility and second malignancies are a concern following chemotherapy.
Adapted from Pizzo PA, Poplack DG, eds. *Principles and Practice of Pediatric Oncology*, 5th ed. Philadelphia: Lippincott Williams & Wilkins, 2006.

TREATMENT

The treatment strategy for both ALL and AML is to stabilize the patient at diagnosis, put the leukemia in remission, and manage the complications of therapy. Managing leukemic complications at presentation involves blood product transfusions, empirical treatment of potential infection with IV antibiotics, prevention of the sequelae of hyperviscosity, and correcting metabolic abnormalities and renal insufficiency from tumor lysis syndrome. Neutropenia, defined as an absolute neutrophil count less than 500 per mm^3, predisposes children to serious bacterial and fungal infections. The development of fever in a child with neutropenia warrants careful evaluation for bacteremia or sepsis and empiric, broad-spectrum IV antibiotic therapy.

Acute Lymphocytic Leukemia Therapy

Patients with ALL have a high risk of **tumor lysis syndrome**, a triad of metabolic abnormalities (hyperuricemia, hyperphosphatemia, and hyperkalemia) resulting from spontaneous or treatment-induced tumor cell death, with rapid release of intracellular contents into the circulation that exceeds the excretory capacity of the kidneys. Tumor lysis syndrome is generally seen in tumors with high growth rates such as T-cell ALL or Burkitt lymphoma, and patients with mediastinal mass or high white blood cell (WBC) count, but should be anticipated in all cases of acute leukemia. Rapid release of intracellular contents leads to hyperphosphatemia, hyperkalemia, and hyperuricemia. Hyperkalemia can cause cardiac arrhythmias. Initial IV fluids should never contain potassium. Phosphate, especially at high serum levels, binds to calcium, resulting in precipitation of calcium phosphate in renal tubules, hypocalcemia, and tetany. Purines are processed to uric acid. Hyperuricemia can result in precipitation of uric acid in renal tubules and renal failure. Prevention and management of tumor lysis syndrome includes vigorous hydration, urine alkalinization, uric acid reduction with allopurinol or rasburicase, and potassium and phosphate reduction. The risk for tumor lysis is greatest during the first 3 days of chemotherapy.

Hyperleukocytosis (WBC count >200,000 per mm^3) occurs in 9% to 13% of patients with ALL. Hyperleukocytosis can cause significant vascular stasis. This is often seen in the patient with ALL whose WBC count is greater than 300,000 per mm^3. Symptoms include mental status changes, headache, blurry vision, dizziness, seizure, and dyspnea. Without therapy, hyperleukocytosis may cause hypoxemia and secondary acidosis or stroke from sludging in the lungs and CNS, respectively. The WBC count may be lowered using hyperhydration

TABLE 12-2 Epidemiology of Acute Lymphocytic Leukemia and Acute Myelogenous Leukemia

Characteristic	ALL	AML
Incidence	2,500 to 3,000 cases/yr (75%)	350 to 500 cases/yr (15% to 20%)
Peak age	4 yr	Increased in adolescence
Race	White > African American	Equal (APML more common in Hispanic population)
Gender	Male > Female	Equal
Genetics	Trisomy 21, Bloom syndrome, Fanconi anemia, ataxia telangiectasia, Shwachman syndrome, neurofibromatosis, twins, siblings at increased risk	Trisomy 21 (AML much more likely <3 yr), Bloom syndrome, Fanconi anemia, ataxia telangiectasia, Kostmann syndrome, NF-1, Diamond-Blackfan syndrome, Li-Fraumeni syndrome
Noninherited		Aplastic anemia, myelodysplastic syndromes (MDS), PNH
Pathogenesis		
• Environment	Ionizing radiation	Ionizing radiation, benzene, epipodophyllotoxins, alkylating agents (nitrogen mustard, melphalan, cyclophosphamide)
• Viral	Epstein-Barr virus and L3 ALL	None
• Immunodeficiency	Wiskott-Aldrich, congenital hypogammaglobulinemia, ataxia telangiectasia	

APML, acute promyelocytic leukemia; MDS, myelodysplastic syndrome; PNH, paroxysmal nocturnal hemoglobinuria.
From Frank G, Shah SS, Catallozzi M, et al., eds. *The Philadelphia Guide: Inpatient Pediatrics*. Malden, MA: Blackwell; 2005:303.

or leukophoresis. It is recommended that the hemoglobin concentration be kept ≤10 g/dL to minimize viscosity, and that the platelet count be maintained at >20,000/mm^3 to minimize the risk of hemorrhage.

Large collections of malignant cells in the mediastinum (mediastinal mass), common in T-cell leukemia, can compress vital structures and cause tracheal compression or superior vena cava syndrome. Superior vena cava syndrome is characterized by distended neck veins; swelling of the face, neck, and upper limbs; cyanosis; and conjunctival injection. The mass and the compressive symptoms it creates usually resolve with chemotherapy and radiation. Patients with severe symptoms may warrant empiric steroid therapy and/or emergent radiation therapy.

The ALL treatment regimen includes induction, consolidation, interim maintenance, delayed intensification, and maintenance therapies. At diagnosis children with ALL undergo **induction therapy**, during which maximum log kill is achieved. If remission is achieved, leukemic blasts in the bone marrow decrease to less than 5% of marrow cells, and the CBC values return to normal. Induction therapy occurs over 28 days with vincristine, steroids, intrathecal methotrexate, and asparaginase. For high-risk patients, daunomycin is added. The disease response is generally reevaluated every 7 to 14 days. More than 95% of patients with ALL achieve remission after induction therapy. Failure to achieve adequate response by the end of induction requires intensification of therapy. The goals of **consolidation** are to kill additional leukemic cells with further systemic therapy and to prevent leukemic relapse within the CNS by giving intrathecal methotrexate. **Interim maintenance**, which follows induction and consolidation, is less intense and includes vincristine, 6-mercaptopurine, and methotrexate. The delayed intensification course provides another round of intense chemotherapy to induce a deeper remission. **Maintenance therapy** completes the therapeutic course and includes periodic intrathecal methotrexate, vincristine and steroid therapy, as well as weekly oral methotrexate and daily oral 6-mercaptopurine. The objectives of maintenance therapies are to continue the remission achieved in the previous phases and to provide additional cytoreduction to cure the leukemia. Patients with high-risk leukemia receive an additional interim maintenance and delayed intensification course prior to entering maintenance therapy. They also receive CNS directed radiation therapy.

Radiation is used for CNS and testicular disease. It is also used for CNS prophylaxis in those patients who take >14 days to enter remission. Discontinuation of chemotherapy occurs when the patient has remained in remission throughout the prescribed course of maintenance therapy. The total length of therapy is approximately 2.5 years for females and 3.5 years for males. Leukemia can recur during or after the completion of maintenance therapy. The earlier the relapse, the worse the prognosis (<36 months from diagnosis), although isolated extramedullary (CNS, testes) relapses have better outcomes than bone marrow relapses.

Factors associated with poor prognosis in patients with ALL include age greater than 10 years or less than 1 year at diagnosis, WBC count greater than 50,000 per mm^3 at diagnosis, failure to respond to induction therapy, and the presence of the Philadelphia chromosome or hypoploidy in the leukemia

TABLE 12-3 Comparison of the Clinical Presentation of Acute Lymphocytic Leukemia and Acute Myelogenous Leukemia

Characteristic	ALL	AML
Marrow failure		
• Anemia (g/dL)	Hb <7 (43%)	Hb <9 (50%)
• Thrombocytopenia (per mm^3)	Hb 7 to 11 (45%)	Plt <100,000 (75%)
	Hb >11 (12%)	WBC >100,000 (20%)
• Neutropenia (per mm^3)	Plt <20,000 (20%)	
	Plt 21,000 to 99,000 (47%)	
	Plt >100,000 (25%)	
	WBC <10,000 (53%)	
	WBC 10,000 to 49,000 (30%)	
	WBC >50,000 (17%)	
Fever	60%	30% to 40%
Mediastinal mass	10% (mostly in T cell)	
CNS involvement	5%	2%
Chloromas		Common in M4, M5 subtype
		Common in periorbital area
Testicular involvement	2% to 5%	Rare
Disseminated intravascular coagulation		Common (esp. in APML)
Bone pain	20%	20%
Hepatosplenomegaly	60% to 65%	50%
Other		Leukemia cutis (10%)
		• Neonates
		• Blueberry muffin spots
		Gingival hypertrophy (15%)

APML, acute promyelocytic leukemia.
From Frank G, Shah SS, Catallozzi M, et al., eds. *The Philadelphia Guide: Inpatient pediatrics.* Malden, MA: Blackwell; 2005:304.

cells. Factors associated with a particularly good prognosis include trisomy 4, and 10 or a TEL-AML translocation (t[12;22]) in the leukemia cells.

Acute Myeloid Leukemia Therapy

Hyperleukocytosis occurs in 5% to 22% of patients with AML. The most common symptoms for patients with AML-induced hyperleukocytosis include dyspnea and hypoxemia, from pulmonary leukostasis, and mental status change or seizure due to stroke from CNS leukostasis. Patients may require hyperhydration or leukapheresis similar to ALL. In contrast to ALL, patients with AML and hyperleukocytosis are treated at a lower WBC count because AML cells are larger and stickier than the lymphocytes found in ALL. Similar to ALL treatment, a hemoglobin concentration not greater than 10 g/dL is recommended to reduce viscosity, and a platelet count of more than 20,000 is advisable to minimize the risk of CNS hemorrhage.

AML chemotherapy is more intensive than that used for ALL. Induction therapy includes an anthracycline with cytosine arabinoside. Although 70% to 85% of patients with AML achieve remission with induction therapy, many patients relapse within a year. Myelosuppression is severe, and good supportive care is essential. Patients should remain in the hospital for close monitoring for signs of infection until they show signs of bone marrow recovery. If remission can be achieved, patients are assigned a risk group based on chromosome alterations in the leukemic cells. Patients with low-risk disease (including: inv 16, t[16;16], or t[8;21]) are treated with chemotherapy alone. Patients with high-risk disease (including monosomy 5 or 7, or no remission) are treated with bone marrow transplantation from a related or unrelated donor. All other patients are considered intermediate-risk patients. If a matched related donor is available they go on to bone marrow transplant. If no matched related donor is found, they continue with chemotherapy.

Acute promyelocytic leukemia (APML), FAB M3 subtype, has a higher overall survival rate (80%) than the other AML subtypes. Similarly, patients with AML and trisomy 21 also have excellent overall survival. In general, patients who present with a WBC count greater than 100,000/mm^3 at diagnosis have a worse prognosis. Patients with secondary AML/myelodysplastic syndrome have a poor response to therapy.

NON-HODGKIN LYMPHOMA

PATHOGENESIS

Non-Hodgkin lymphomas (NHLs) are a heterogeneous group of diseases characterized by neoplastic proliferation of immature lymphoid cells, which, unlike the malignant lymphoid cells of ALL, accumulate outside the bone marrow. NHLs can be divided into T- and B-cell categories. Histopathologic subtypes in childhood NHL include lymphoblastic (pre-T or pre-B cell), Burkitt lymphoma or large B-cell lymphoma (B-cell), and anaplastic large cell lymphoma (T or null cell). Other peripheral T-cell lymphomas are under the category of NHL but very uncommon in children. Burkitt lymphoma is interesting in that the presentation and pathogenesis in equatorial Africa is different than in developed countries. It almost uniformly presents as a rapidly expanding jaw lesion and 95% of these tumors carry EBV genomes in their cells, whereas only 15% to 20% of North American tumors are associated with EBV and the presentation is more varied.

EPIDEMIOLOGY

Lymphomas are the third most common malignancy in childhood and account for 10% of childhood cancers. There is a distinct geographic frequency of NHL; in equatorial Africa, NHL accounts for 50% of childhood cancer. In the United States, approximately 60% of pediatric lymphomas are NHLs; the remainder is Hodgkin lymphoma. Lymphoblastic lymphoma accounts for 50% of cases, and Burkitt and anaplastic large cell lymphomas account for approximately 35% and 15%, respectively. NHL occurs at least three times more frequently in boys than in girls and has a peak incidence between 7 and 11 years of age.

RISK FACTORS

Children with congenital immunodeficiency (e.g., Wiskott-Aldrich syndrome, X-linked lymphoproliferative disease, severe combined immunodeficiency) and acquired immunodeficiency (e.g., AIDS, iatrogenic immunosuppression in organ and bone marrow transplant recipients) have an increased incidence of NHL. Patients with Bloom syndrome and ataxia-telangiectasia also have a higher incidence of NHL than the general pediatric population.

CLINICAL MANIFESTATIONS

T-cell lymphoblastic lymphoma is most often associated with a mediastinal mass (50% to 70%), whereas B-cell lymphoblastic lymphoma often involves bone, isolated lymph nodes, and skin. Superior vena cava syndrome may be associated with any lymphoma involving a mediastinal mass. Burkitt lymphoma often exhibits extremely rapid growth and can be associated with tumor lysis syndrome even before chemotherapy is started. The sporadic form of Burkitt lymphoma can present as an abdominal tumor associated with nausea, emesis, or intussusception. Other Burkitt locations may include tonsils, bone marrow (20%), and the CNS. The endemic form of Burkitt lymphoma involves the jaw, orbit, and/or maxilla. Anaplastic large cell lymphoma is a slowly progressive disease with fever; weight loss is rare.

DIAGNOSTIC EVALUATION

The evaluation before therapy should include a CBC to look for leukocytosis, thrombocytopenia, and anemia. A comprehensive metabolic panel includes calcium, phosphorus, uric acid, and LDH to evaluate for tumor lysis syndrome. A chest radiograph should be performed to assess for mediastinal mass prior to sedation and biopsy of accessible affected nodes. An echocardiogram and anesthesia consultation is required prior to sedation in the patient with a mediastinal mass. A bone marrow aspiration and biopsy with flow cytometry, cell markers/immunophenotyping, and cytogenetics should be performed to isolate the type of lymphoma. An LP with cytology is performed to evaluate for CNS involvement. A CT scan of the neck, chest, abdomen, and pelvis helps to assess the extent of disease, and a gallium or positron emission tomography (PET) scan is useful for diagnostic purposes and follow-up for residual disease or recurrence.

TREATMENT

Similar to ALL therapy, lymphoblastic non-Hodgkin lymphoma is generally treated with combination chemotherapy. ALL and lymphoblastic non-Hodgkin lymphoma therapy are immunophenotypically similar but with a different distribution of disease (nodal vs. marrow).

Chemotherapy is the mainstay of treatment for Burkitt lymphoma unless the tumor is localized and complete surgical resection is possible. Therapy is quite intense and given over a short period of time (4 to 6 months) using drugs including cyclophosphamide, prednisone, vincristine, methotrexate, cytarabine, doxorubicin, and etoposide. Patients with CNS involvement are known to have a poorer prognosis. Patients with tumor lysis syndrome require extremely careful management with increased fluid intake, alkalinization of the urine, frequent electrolyte observation, and allopurinol. Patients with Burkitt lymphoma are at high risk of developing kidney failure requiring dialysis from their tumor lysis syndrome.

Anaplastic large cell lymphoma is treated with combination chemotherapy. Children are most commonly treated using B-cell lymphoma protocols.

HODGKIN LYMPHOMA

PATHOGENESIS

The cause of **Hodgkin disease** (HD) is unknown, and a number of studies investigating potential etiologies have shown that age, ethnicity, socioeconomic status, and geographic distribution suggest both environmental and genetic components and a multifactorial etiology. Patients who develop HD have an increased incidence of immune dysregulation. There is increased risk in siblings, twins, and an association with EBV, although the EBV genome is not universally found in tumor tissue. In addition, there is an increased risk of HD in patients with ataxia-telangiectasia and Wiskott-Aldrich and Bloom syndromes. Histopathologic subtypes in childhood HD include nodular sclerosing (40% to 55%), lymphocyte predominant (10% to 15%), mixed cellularity (30%), and lymphocyte depleted (5%).

EPIDEMIOLOGY

Hodgkin disease accounts for 5% of all cases of childhood cancer prior to 15 years of age and 9% prior to 20 years of age. Epidemiologic studies have identified three distinct forms of HD: a childhood form (younger than 14 years), a young adult form (15 to 34 years of age), and an older adult form (55 to 74 years of age). Its incidence has a bimodal distribution with peaks occurring at 15 to 30 years of age and after the age of 50. It rarely occurs in children younger than 10 years. There is a 3:1 male predominance in the childhood form of HD.

CLINICAL MANIFESTATIONS

History and Physical Examination

The most common presentation is painless, rubbery, cervical lymphadenopathy in 80% of patients. Two-thirds of patients also have mediastinal lymphadenopathy, and this presentation is more common in adolescent patients. Systemic symptoms ("B" symptoms) are present in 20% to 30% of patients and include unexplained fever, drenching night sweats, and unintentional weight loss of more than 10% over the preceding 6 months. Other common presenting symptoms include anorexia, fatigue, and extreme pruritus.

DIFFERENTIAL DIAGNOSIS

The differential diagnosis for HD includes other diseases that can result in lymphadenopathy with or without systemic symptoms. Reactive or inflammatory nodes as a result of bacterial lymphadenitis, infectious mononucleosis, tuberculosis, atypical mycobacterial infection, cat-scratch disease, HIV infection, histoplasmosis, and toxoplasmosis should be considered. Other primary or metastatic malignant processes resulting in cervical adenopathy or a mediastinal mass include leukemia, NHL, head/neck rhabdomyosarcoma, and germ cell tumors.

DIAGNOSTIC EVALUATION

Evaluation for HD should include a detailed history and physical examination with attention to the signs and symptoms that require a more urgent evaluation including cough, dyspnea, orthopnea, chest pain, bleeding, bruising, jaundice, or pallor. The physical examination should include a careful evaluation of all lymph node groups including the tonsils. Lymphadenopathy in the upper anterior and posterior cervical chains tends to be more commonly associated with childhood infections, whereas nodes in the supraclavicular area are consistent with malignancy. Lymph nodes that are >1 cm, matted, and nontender are of greatest concern. Enlargement of the liver or spleen is consistent with more advanced disease.

Evaluating a child for HD necessitates imaging and should begin with a chest radiograph prior to any biopsy or procedure to determine whether or not there is clinically significant mediastinal involvement, the presence and size of a mediastinal mass, whether there is airway compromise, whether cardiac compression influence the way in which the biopsy is performed, and the type of anesthesia required. Patients with a mediastinal mass should have pulmonary function testing and an echocardiogram before undergoing general anesthesia.

A tissue biopsy is required to make the diagnosis, preferably excisional lymph node biopsy. The hallmark of diagnosis is the identification of Reed-Sternberg cells in tumor tissue.

Recommended basic tests include a CBC, erythrocyte sedimentation rate (ESR), soluble IL-2, C-reactive protein (CRP), chemistry panel including liver function tests (LFTs), direct antibody testing (DAT) if there is evidence of jaundice or anemia, and ferritin. Eosinophilia is seen in 15% to 30% of patients, and anemia is seen either secondary to advanced disease or hemolysis. Global immune defects are common at diagnosis of HD, and anergy is seen in 25% of patients. This immune dysregulation seen at diagnosis predisposes patients to opportunistic infections during their treatment. Imaging studies include a CT scan of the neck, chest, abdomen, and pelvis. PET is quite useful and has a role in diagnosis and in following for residual or recurrent disease. The gallium scan was previously used but has fallen out of favor with the emergence of PET scanning. Although uncommon, evidence of cytopenias should prompt bone marrow aspirate and biopsy, which is routinely performed in patients with extensive disease and "B" symptoms. Bone scan is only recommended for patients with bone pain.

TREATMENT

Treatment depends on the histologic subtype of disease, staging, and response to therapy (Table 12-4).

TABLE 12-4 Staging for Hodgkin Lymphoma

Stage	Definition
I	Involvement of single lymph node region or single extralymphatic site
II	Involvement of two or more lymph node regions on the same side of diaphragm or localized involvement of an extralymphatic site and one or more lymph node regions on the same side of the diaphragm
III	Involvement of lymph node regions on both sides of the diaphragm with involvement of the spleen or localized involvement of an extralymphatic site
IV	Disseminated involvement of one or more extralymphatic organs with or without lymph node involvement
"B" symptoms	Fever higher than 38°C for 3 consecutive days
	Drenching night sweats
	Unexplained weight loss >10% during the prior 6 months
	Those without B symptoms have stage [number] A disease

Most pediatric protocols involve multiagent chemotherapy given in a risk-adapted and response-based manner. Involved field radiation therapy is used for patients with bulky disease or with residual tumor after initial chemotherapy. Vincristine, prednisone, cyclophosphamide, and procarbazine were used commonly in the past, although newer chemotherapy combinations are being used in patients with low- or intermediate-risk disease, given the high risk of infertility for males with the use of cyclophosphamide and procarbazine together. Prognosis varies from 70% to >90% depending on the extent of disease and response to therapy. Recurrent disease is often responsive to therapy but extremely difficult to cure. As in adults, lymphocyte predominance has the most favorable prognosis. There are many late effects secondary to therapy including secondary malignant neoplasms (breast, thyroid, sarcomas); cardiac toxicity (anthracyclines and radiation therapy [XRT]); pulmonary (bleomycin); hypothyroidism (XRT); infertility (alkylating agents as above, pelvic radiation); and musculoskeletal/growth (XRT). Current upfront therapies are now being modified to reduce the occurrence of late effects while maintaining high cure rates.

CENTRAL NERVOUS SYSTEM TUMORS

CNS tumors are the most common solid tumors in children and are second to leukemia in overall incidence of malignant diseases. In contrast to adults, in whom supratentorial brain tumors are more common, brain tumors in children are predominantly infratentorial, involving the cerebellum and brainstem. Table 12-5 denotes the location, clinical manifestations, and prognosis of CNS tumors in children. Childhood brain tumors are differentiated further from those in adults in that they are usually low-grade astrocytomas or malignant neoplasms such as medulloblastomas, whereas most CNS tumors in adults are malignant astrocytomas or metastases from non-CNS cancers.

CLINICAL MANIFESTATIONS

The presenting signs and symptoms of CNS tumors depend on the age of the child and location of the tumor (Table 12-5). Any CNS tumor may cause increased intracranial pressure (ICP) by obstructing CSF flow. Symptoms of

TABLE 12-5 Location and Manifestations of Primary CNS Tumors

Tumor	Age at Onset (yr)	Manifestations[a]	5-Yr Survival (%)	Comments
Infratentorial				
Cerebellar astrocytoma	5 to 8	Ataxia; nystagmus; head tilt; intention tremor	90	20% of all primary CNS tumors
Medulloblastoma	3 to 5	Obstructive hydrocephalus; ataxia; CSF metastasis	50	Acute onset of symptoms; 20% of all primary CNS tumors
Ependymoma	2 to 6	Obstructive hydrocephalus; rarely seeds spinal fluid	50	25% to 40% supratentorial
Brainstem glioma (intrinsic pontine glioma)	5 to 8	Progressive cranial nerve dysfunction; gait disturbance; pyramidal tract and cerebellar signs	<10	Worst prognosis of all childhood CNS tumors
Supratentorial				
Cerebral astrocytoma	5 to 10	Seizures; headache; motor weakness; personality changes	10 to 50	Survival for high-grade glioma is poor
Craniopharyngioma	7 to 12	Bitemporal hemianopsia; endocrine abnormalities; postoperative diabetes insipidus common	70 to 90	Calcification above sella turcica; postoperative diabetes insipidus common
Optic glioma	<2	Poor visual acuity; exophthalmos; nystagmus; optic atrophy; strabismus	50 to 90	Neurofibromatosis in NF-1 in 70% of patients
Germ cell tumor (pineal or pituitary)	—	Paralysis of upward gaze (Parinaud syndrome); lid retraction (Collier sign); precocious puberty; may seed spinal fluid	75	Germ cell line: may secrete BhCG or alpha-feto protein

[a]All CNS tumors may cause increased intracranial pressure.
CNS, central nervous system; CSF, cerebrospinal fluid; hCG, human chorionic gonadotropin.

increased ICP include early morning headaches, vomiting, and lethargy. The headache is usually present upon awakening, improves with standing, and worsens with coughing or straining. It is intermittent but recurs with increasing frequency and intensity. Obstructive hydrocephalus may produce macrocephaly if it occurs before the sutures have fused. Strabismus with diplopia can result from a sixth nerve palsy induced by ICP. Papilledema may be detected on funduscopic examination. The Cushing triad (hypertension, bradycardia, and irregular respirations) is a late finding.

Children with **infratentorial tumors** often present with deficits of balance or brainstem function (truncal ataxia, problems with coordination and gait, cranial nerve dysfunction). Because it can result from increased ICP, a sixth nerve palsy is not considered a localizing focal neurologic deficit, whereas other cranial nerve deficits, by definition, localize the lesion to the brainstem. Head tilt, as a compensation for loss of binocular vision, is noted with focal deficits of cranial nerves III, IV, or VI, which cause extraocular muscle weakness. Nystagmus is usually caused by cerebellovestibular pathway lesions, but it may also be seen with a marked visual deficit (peripheral or cortical blindness).

Children with **supratentorial tumors** commonly present either with signs of increased ICP or seizures. Although most seizures are generalized, less dramatic episodes with incomplete loss of consciousness (complex partial seizures) and transient focal events without loss of consciousness (partial seizures) are also seen. Personality changes, poor school performance, and change in hand preference suggest a cortical lesion. Endocrine abnormalities are noted with pituitary and hypothalamic tumors. Babinski reflex, hyperreflexia, spasticity, and loss of dexterity occur with either brainstem or cortical tumors.

TABLE 12-6 Approach to Treatment of Childhood CNS Tumors

Treatment	Goals
Surgery	Establish diagnosis
	Debulk and/or resect tumor
	Treat increased ICP (ventricular shunt, if required)
Radiation	Control residual disease
	Control tumor dissemination
	Cure
Chemotherapy	Adjuvant therapy for malignant tumors
	Minimize radiation exposure
	Delay and/or obviate need for radiation
Newer approaches	Immunotherapy to scavenge for minimal residual disease
	Antiangiogenic therapy to suppress abnormal tumor blood vessel development
	Molecularly targeted therapy to suppress abnormal growth factor pathways

CNS, central nervous system; ICP, intracranial pressure.
Adapted from Pizzo PA, Poplack DG, eds. *Principles and Practice of Pediatric Oncology*, 3rd ed. Philadelphia: Lippincott-Raven, 1997.

DIFFERENTIAL DIAGNOSIS

The differential diagnosis includes arteriovenous malformation, aneurysm, brain abscess, parasitic infestation, herpes simplex encephalitis, granulomatous disease (tuberculosis, cryptococcal, sarcoid), intracranial hemorrhage, pseudotumor cerebri, primary cerebral lymphoma, vasculitis, and, rarely, metastatic tumors.

DIAGNOSTIC EVALUATION

CT and MRI are the procedures of choice for diagnosing and localizing tumors and other intracranial masses. A head CT can be performed much faster than a head MRI and is safer in an unstable patient. A CT is useful as an initial screen and to assess for hydrocephalus, hemorrhage, or calcification. MRI is the gold standard for localization of brain tumors to assist with surgical planning. Brain MRI is especially helpful in diagnosing tumors of the posterior fossa and spinal cord. Examination of CSF cytology is essential to determine the presence of metastasis in medulloblastoma and germ cell tumors.

TREATMENT

Treatment of CNS tumors is complex and is best managed by a multidisciplinary approach. Table 12-6 outlines the general principles of treatment of primary CNS tumors.

NEUROBLASTOMA

PATHOGENESIS

Neuroblastoma is a childhood embryonal malignancy of the postganglionic sympathetic nervous system. Neuroblastoma can be located in the abdomen, thoracic cavity, or head and neck. Abdominal tumors account for 70% of tumors, a third of which arise from the retroperitoneal sympathetic ganglia and two-thirds from the adrenal medulla itself. Thoracic masses, accounting for 20% of the tumors, tend to arise from paraspinal ganglia in the posterior mediastinum. Neuroblastoma of the neck occurs in 5% of cases and often involves the cervical sympathetic ganglion.

EPIDEMIOLOGY

Neuroblastoma and other sympathetic nervous system tumors account for approximately 8% of all childhood cancers under the age of 15 years. The prevalence is approximately 1 case per 7,000 live births, and there are approximately 800 new cases of neuroblastoma per year. It is also the most common solid tumor outside the CNS under the age of 15 years. The median age at diagnosis is between 17 and 22 months; more than 50% of children are diagnosed before 2 years of age, 90% are diagnosed before 5 years of age, and 97% are diagnosed by 10 years of age. There is a slight male predominance. Neuroblastoma accounts for 15% of the pediatric cancer-related deaths in the United States each year.

RISK FACTORS

The etiology is unknown in most cases, and no causal environmental factor has been isolated. No prenatal or postnatal exposure to drugs, chemicals, viruses, electromagnetic fields, or radiation has been associated strongly or consistently with an increased incidence of neuroblastoma. A family history of the disease can be found in 1% to 2% of cases. Neuroblastoma has been reported in patients with some overgrowth syndromes, Hirschsprung disease, congenital central hypoventilation syndrome (Ondine curse), pheochromocytoma, and/or neurofibromatosis type 1, suggesting the existence of a global disorder of neural crest–derived cells.

CLINICAL MANIFESTATIONS

The clinical manifestations are extremely variable because of the widespread distribution of neural crest tissue and the length of the sympathetic chain. In addition, the biologic behavior is very diverse, from self-resolving asymptomatic disease to widely metastatic disease requiring substantial treatment.

History and Physical Examination

Abdominal tumors are hard, smooth, nontender abdominal masses that are most often palpated in the flank and displace the kidney anterolaterally and inferiorly. Abdominal pain/distension and systemic hypertension occur if the mass compresses the renal vasculature. Respiratory distress can be seen in thoracic neuroblastoma tumors and large abdominal tumors in small children and infants. Sometimes the thoracic variant is asymptomatic, and the tumor is discovered as an incidental finding on chest radiograph obtained for an unrelated reason. Neuroblastoma of the neck presents as a palpable tumor causing Horner syndrome (ipsilateral ptosis, miosis, and anhidrosis) and heterochromia of the iris on the affected side. Sometimes thoracic or abdominal tumors invade the epidural space posteriorly in a dumbbell fashion, compromising the spinal cord and resulting in back pain and symptoms of cord compression.

The signs and symptoms vary according to location of primary disease and degree of dissemination. Metastatic extension occurs in lymphatic and hematogenous patterns. Nonspecific symptoms of metastatic disease include weight loss and fever. Specific metastatic sequelae include bone marrow failure, resulting in pancytopenia; cortical bone pain, causing a limp (Hutchinson syndrome); liver infiltration, resulting in hepatomegaly (Pepper syndrome); periorbital infiltration, resulting in proptosis and periorbital ecchymoses (raccoon eyes); distant lymph node enlargement; and skin infiltration, causing palpable nontender subcutaneous bluish nodules in infants with **International Neuroblastoma Staging System** (INSS) stage IVS tumors (see Table 12-7). Paraneoplastic effects, such as watery diarrhea in patients with differentiated tumors that secrete vasoactive intestinal peptide and opsoclonus-myoclonus (chaotic eye movements, myoclonic jerking, and truncal ataxia), have been noted.

DIFFERENTIAL DIAGNOSIS

The differential diagnosis of abdominal neuroblastoma includes benign lesions such as adrenal hemorrhage, hydronephrosis, polycystic kidney disease, and splenomegaly and malignant tumors such as renal cell carcinoma, Wilms tumor, hepatoblastoma, leukemia, lymphoma, and retroperitoneal rhabdomyosarcoma and others.

DIAGNOSTIC EVALUATION

Once a mass is confirmed by CT of chest, abdomen, and pelvis, the diagnosis of neuroblastoma can be made by pathologic identification of tumor tissue, or by the unequivocal presence of tumor cells on bone marrow aspirate combined with elevated urinary catecholamines (vanillylmandelic acid and homovanillic acid). Tissue biopsy for histology, DNA ploidy, and MYC-related oncogene (MYCN) amplification is important in assessing prognosis and determining treatment. Measurement of urinary catecholamines, which are breakdown products of epinephrine and norepinephrine, is also useful for following response to therapy and for detecting recurrence. Additional imaging required for staging includes bone marrow biopsies, bone scan, metaiodobenzylguanidine (MIBG) scintigraphy, and at times PET scanning.

TREATMENT

Treatment often involves a multimodal and multidisciplinary approach and can involve surgery and chemotherapy and at

TABLE 12-7 Staging for Neuroblastoma: International Neuroblastoma Staging System (INSS)

Stage	Definition
I	Localized tumor with complete gross excision
II	Localized tumor with incomplete gross excision; ipsilateral lymph node sampling (LNS) negative for tumor (IIA), or ipsilateral nodes positive for tumor (IIB)
III	Tumor extends beyond the midline, with or without regional lymph node involvement, or localized unilateral tumor with contralateral regional lymph node involvement
IV	Dissemination of tumor to distant lymph nodes, bone, bone marrow, liver, and/or other organs (except as defined in stage IVS)
IVS	Age younger than 1 year with dissemination of tumor to liver, skin, or bone marrow without bone involvement and with a primary tumor that would otherwise be stage I or II

times radiotherapy and/or biologic therapies. Several biological variables have prognostic values and are used in addition to INSS staging for patients with neuroblastoma. These include age at diagnosis, Shimada histopathology, DNA index of the tumor, and MYCN gene amplification. Loss of heterozygosity is also being explored as a prognostic feature. Depending on stage and biological features, treatment can range from surgery alone to multimodal therapy utilizing surgery and one or more other modalities such as chemotherapy, stem cell transplantation, radiation, and biologic agents (cis-retinoic acid and immunotherapy). Chemotherapy agents used include vincristine, cyclophosphamide, doxorubicin and cisplatin.

Stages I, II, and IVS have a good prognosis, whereas some stage III and IV have a poor prognosis and require aggressive treatment. Stage IVS tumors represent unique biology that has spontaneous regression or only requires very minimal chemotherapy.

WILMS TUMOR

PATHOGENESIS

Wilms tumor is the most common renal tumor in children. It results from neoplastic proliferation of embryonal renal cells of the metanephros. The most often cited genetic anomalies in Wilms tumor involve chromosomal loci 11p13 (WT1) and 11p15 (WT2).

EPIDEMIOLOGY

Renal tumors account for 6% of all childhood cancers under the age of 15 years with Wilms tumor being the most common followed by clear cell sarcoma of the kidney and rhabdoid tumor of the kidney. Renal cell carcinoma is uncommon in the pediatric population, and is more likely seen in the older adolescents. The majority of renal tumors are unilateral with only 7% being bilateral. They are predominantly diagnosed in the first 5 years of life.

RISK FACTORS

Associated anomalies are seen in 10% of Wilms tumor and include sporadic aniridia, hemihypertrophy, cryptorchidism, hypospadias, and other genitourinary anomalies. Associated syndromes include Beckwith-Wiedemann (hemihypertrophy, macroglossia, omphalocele, and genitourinary abnormalities); Denys Drash; Wilms tumor, aniridia, genitourinary abnormalities, and mental retardation (WAGR) and Perlman syndrome (unusual facies, islet cell hypertrophy, macrosomia, hamartomas).

CLINICAL MANIFESTATIONS

History and Physical Examination

Most children (85%) are diagnosed after incidental detection of an asymptomatic abdominal mass by the child's parents while bathing or dressing the child or by the pediatrician during a routine physical examination. Abdominal pain or fever may develop after hemorrhage into the tumor. Other associated findings include microscopic or gross hematuria (33%) and hypertension (25%). Hypertension occurs as a result of either renin secretion by tumor cells or compression of the renal vasculature by the tumor. Additionally, varicocele can be present on physical examination if there is spermatic vein cord compression of the tumor. Von Willebrand disease is present in 8% of patients. It is important to evaluate the patient for associated anomalies and syndromes associated with Wilms tumor.

DIFFERENTIAL DIAGNOSIS

The differential diagnosis of Wilms tumor includes benign lesions such as hydronephrosis, polycystic kidney disease, and splenomegaly, as well as malignant tumors such as renal cell carcinoma, neuroblastoma, lymphoma, retroperitoneal rhabdomyosarcoma, and ovarian tumors.

DIAGNOSTIC EVALUATION

Radiologic studies include abdominal ultrasound to establish the presence of an intrarenal mass, assess the renal vasculature, and examine the contralateral kidney. An abdominal CT scan or MRI assesses the degree of local extension and involvement of the inferior vena cava. A CT scan of the chest and abdomen is routinely performed to detect hematogenous metastases, which are present at diagnosis in 10% to 15% of patients. The most common patterns of spread include the renal capsule, extension through adjacent vessels (inferior vena cava), regional nodes, lung, and liver. The lung is the most common site of metastatic spread. Chest radiograph has been the radiographic standard for evaluation of pulmonary metastases, but the use of chest CT is controversial. Bone scan and MRI of the head are only indicated for clear cell sarcoma or rhabdoid tumor of the kidney, respectively.

TREATMENT

Treatment involves surgical removal of the kidney (unilateral disease) if it can be safely done; otherwise a biopsy can be performed or treatment can be initiated based on radiographic appearance. This decision needs to be made in multidisciplinary setting. Surgery also involves lymph node sampling. Chemotherapy and/or radiation are then prescribed depending on the staging and pathology of the resected kidney. Chemotherapy options range from two drug outpatient treatment to more involved inpatient treatment. Radiation therapy tends to be reserved for those with unfavorable features and can be used to treat metastatic sites. Table 12-8 notes chemotherapeutic and radiation guidelines.

Favorable prognostic factors include small tumor size, younger age at diagnosis, favorable histology, and no lymph node or extrarenal metastases or capsular/vascular invasion. Other potential prognostic factors include loss of heterozygosity at chromosome 1p and 16q but require further evaluation. The 4-year overall survival of patients with favorable Wilms tumor is very good and is approximately 90%.

BONE TUMORS

Primary malignant bone tumors account for 5% of childhood cancers. Two forms predominate: Ewing sarcoma and osteosarcoma.

EWING SARCOMA

Pathogenesis

Ewing sarcoma is an undifferentiated sarcoma that arises primarily in bone. The clonal nature of the disease is revealed by

■ **TABLE 12-8** Chemotherapeutic and Radiation Guidelines

Chemotherapy for favorable histology tumors	
Stage I	Tumor limited to kidney and completely excised.
	Dactinomycin/vincristine × 6 mo.
Stage II	Regional tumor extension, but completely resected.
	Dactinomycin/vincristine × 6 mo.
Stage III	Residual tumor present, but confined to the abdomen.
	Dactinomycin/vincristine × 6 mo. XRT as below.
Stage IV	Metastatic disease. As stage III.
Stage V	Bilateral disease. Special considerations depending on extent of disease in each kidney.
Radiation	
Stage III	XRT to tumor bed and extends across vertebral column to avoid scoliosis.
Stage III as a result of peritoneal spill	Whole abdominal XRT.
Stage IV	XRT to primary disease site (only if stage II) and to lung, liver, or other metastases.

the consistent translocation from chromosome 11 to chromosome 22 in affected cells. Ewing sarcoma is thought to arise from a pluripotent neural crest cell of the parasympathetic nervous system. Other tumors with the same or similar translocations occurring outside of bone are known as peripheral primitive neuroectodermal tumors, and they are also members of the Ewing family of soft-tissue tumors.

Epidemiology

Ewing sarcoma is seen primarily in adolescents and is 1.5 times more common in males than females. It is an extremely rare occurrence in African Americans. Like osteosarcoma, it is more likely to occur in adolescents than in young children.

Clinical Manifestations

Pain and localized swelling at the site of the primary tumor are the most common presenting complaints. Unlike osteosarcoma, in which the long bones are predominantly involved, flat and long bones are equally represented. The most commonly involved sites are the femur (20%), pelvis (20%), fibula (12%), and humerus and tibia (10%). Other sites include ribs, clavicle, and scapulae. In the long bones, Ewing sarcoma often begins midshaft, rather than at the ends as in osteosarcoma. Systemic manifestations are more common in children with metastases and include fever, weight loss, and fatigue.

Differential Diagnosis

The differential diagnosis for Ewing sarcoma includes osteomyelitis, eosinophilic granuloma (Langerhans cell histiocytosis), and osteosarcoma. Metastasis to the bone by neuroblastoma or rhabdomyosarcoma should be considered in younger children with a solitary bone lesion.

Diagnostic Evaluation

Radiographs characteristically reveal a lytic bone lesion with calcified periosteal elevation (onion skin) and/or a soft-tissue mass. An MRI of the bony lesion is needed to assess the extent. Bone scans and chest CTs are needed to assess for other metastatic sites. Bone marrow biopsies are needed to evaluate bone marrow involvement. A biopsy of the lesion confirms the diagnosis, along with genetic studies looking for the t(11;22) which occurs in 85% of patients.

Treatment

Treatment involves both systemic therapy (chemotherapy) and local control therapy (radiation therapy or surgery). Chemotherapy is critical to both reduce the size of the primary tumor and treat metastases, even if overt metastases are not seen, because almost all patients with Ewing sarcoma have microscopic metastatic disease at the time of diagnosis. Specific agents include vincristine, doxorubicin, cyclophosphamide, etoposide, and ifosfamide. Local control generally involves surgical removal of the primary tumor site with a limb-sparing procedure or rarely amputation if it is located in an extremity. Lesions require the use of radiation therapy if appropriate margins cannot be attained.

The approximate 5-year survival rate for patients with distal extremity nonmetastatic tumors is greater than 66% in patients. Children with metastatic disease at diagnosis have less favorable outcomes depending on the extent of metastases.

OSTEOSARCOMA

Pathogenesis

Osteosarcoma, also called osteogenic sarcoma, is a malignant tumor of the bone-producing mesenchymal stem cells. Osteosarcoma arises in either the medullary cavity or the periosteum. The primary tumor is usually located at the metaphyseal portion of bones that are associated with maximum growth velocity, which include the distal femur, proximal tibia, and proximal humerus.

Epidemiology

Osteosarcoma is seen mainly in adolescence, with a male-to-female ratio of 2:1. Peak incidence occurs during the maximum growth velocity period in adolescents and young adults.

Clinical Manifestations

Similar to Ewing sarcoma, pain and localized swelling are the most common presenting complaints, but in contrast to Ewing sarcoma, systemic manifestations are rare. Because these tumors occur most frequently in adolescents, initial complaints may be attributed to trauma. The most common tumor sites are the long bones of the body including the distal femur (40%), proximal tibia (20%), and proximal humerus (10%). Metastases are present at diagnosis in 20% of cases, the majority of which are in the lungs. Gait disturbance and pathologic fractures also may be present.

Differential Diagnosis

The differential diagnoses for osteosarcoma are similar to Ewing sarcoma, and include Ewing sarcoma, benign bone tumors, and chronic osteomyelitis.

Diagnostic Evaluation

A lytic bone lesion with periosteal reaction is characteristic on radiograph. The periosteal inflammation has the appearance of a radial sunburst that results as the tumor breaks through the cortex and new bone spicules are produced. An MRI of the bony lesion is needed to assess the extent. A CT scan of the chest is essential to detect pulmonary metastases, which appear as calcified nodules. In addition, a bone scan is needed to assess for other metastatic bony disease.

Treatment

At diagnosis, 20% of patients have clinically detectable metastatic disease, and most of the remaining patients have microscopic metastatic disease. Management of the primary tumor is surgical, either with amputation or limb-sparing surgery. Unlike Ewing sarcoma, osteosarcoma is relatively resistant to radiation therapy. The addition of both neoadjuvant (before surgery) and adjuvant (after surgery) chemotherapy has raised the survival rate substantially; before chemotherapy, survival from osteosarcoma was 20% with amputation alone. Currently, with aggressive chemotherapy, long-term relapse-free survival is greater than 70%. Specific chemotherapeutic agents include cisplatin, doxorubicin, and methotrexate. Aggressive treatment of metastatic disease is indicated because some patients can be cured with chemotherapy and surgical resection of all metastases.

RETINOBLASTOMA

Pathogenesis

Retinoblastoma (Color Plate 26) is the most common intraocular malignancy in children and is considered a malignant tumor of the embryonic neural retina. The majority of retinoblastoma is sporadic (60%), but the remaining hereditary forms are transmitted as an autosomal trait with high but incomplete penetrance. The genetic mutation associated with retinoblastoma is located at chromosome 13q14 at the RB1 locus.

Epidemiology

Retinoblastoma accounts for approximately 3% of childhood cancers. It occurs in 1 in 18,000 live births in the United States with approximately 300 new cases per year. Two-thirds of cases occur before the age of 2 years, and 95% occur before the age of 5 years. Virtually all bilateral disease (both eyes involved with retinoblastoma) is hereditary and accounts for 25% of cases and presents in the first 2 years of life. Sixty percent of cases are nonhereditary and unilateral (one eye), and the remaining 15% are hereditary and unilateral.

Differential Diagnosis

The differential is rather limited and includes congenital cataract, medulloepithelioma, *Toxocara canis* endophthalmitis, persistent hyperplastic primary vitreous, and Coats disease. It is important that an ophthalmologist with experience in retinoblastoma is involved in the care.

Diagnostic Evaluation

Retinoblastoma is one tumor where routine well-child checks and physical examinations can help detect a cancer and possibly detect it early. The presence of leukocoria (absence of a red reflex) is a finding often seen with retinoblastoma, and its presence can serve as a red flag for further workup. In addition, a parent or guardian may be the first to notice an abnormality in the child's eye (in photographs) and/or vision; such reports should not go unheeded.

The most important aspect of evaluation is the ophthalmologic examination, which should be performed by an experienced ophthalmologist. Both eyes need careful evaluation to determine the extent of the tumor and depending on these findings, further workup is needed. It may include an MRI of the orbits and head to grossly assess involvement of the optic nerve and determine if there is involvement of the pineal or parasellar sites (if involved it is called trilateral retinoblastoma). At times, a bone scan and/or bone marrow biopsies are obtained if there is a high suspicion of systemic retinoblastoma involvement (high-risk features such as optic nerve involvement, choroidal invasion or extraorbital spread, etc.).

Treatment

Treatment for retinoblastoma varies and can include enucleation, chemotherapy, local therapies (laser, cryotherapy), radioplaques, and external beam radiation. Chemotherapy can be used to help shrink the tumors so that local therapies can be more effective. Treatment is dependent on the extent of disease as graded by the Reese-Ellsworth classification. At times, upfront enucleation of the involved eye (if unilateral) is needed if the local therapies (laser or cryotherapy), with or without systemic chemotherapy, are unlikely to cure the eye. Enucleation is also performed in the setting of bilateral disease if one eye is more involved than the other and cannot be salvaged to preserve vision. Subsequent therapy is then based on the pathology of the enucleated eye and whether the remaining eye is involved. It is important that a team approach involving the ophthalmologist, oncologist, and radiation oncologist is used.

Of note, a child born to a parent with bilateral retinoblastoma or to a parent with unilateral retinoblastoma with a known genetic mutation should be screened by an ophthalmologist for retinoblastoma at birth and at regular intervals until the child is at least 4 to 5 years old.

SOFT TISSUE SARCOMAS

PATHOGENESIS

Soft tissue sarcomas (STS) are a very diverse group of tumors. As there are different tumors that develop in different age groups, there are different types of soft tissue sarcomas that tend to develop depending on the age. In general, STS are divided into either rhabdomyosarcomas (slightly less than half) or nonrhabdomyosarcoma sarcomas. Rhabdomyosarcomas have been associated with certain familial syndromes, including neurofibromatosis and Li-Fraumeni syndrome. Nonrhabdomyosarcoma sarcomas are very heterogeneous and their pathogenesis and presentation are dependent on the histology. For example, malignant peripheral nerve sheath tumors are associated with neurofibromatosis type I, while some tumors such as malignant fibrous histiocytoma or leiomyosarcoma are seen in fields of radiation for a prior tumor.

EPIDEMIOLOGY

STS make up 7% to 8% of tumors in children and adolescents, which represent approximately 850 to 900 cases diagnosed each year in the United States. The most common STS in children below the age of 10 years is rhabdomyosarcoma. Rhabdomyosarcoma has two major subtypes, embryonal (53%) and alveolar (21%). As a child gets older nonrhabdomyosarcomas become more common. The nonrhabdomyosarcomas encompass a number of different histologies such as fibrosarcoma, malignant fibrous histiocytoma, synovial sarcoma, and malignant peripheral nerve sheath tumor.

Of note, many of the STS have associated chromosomal abnormalities. Rhabdomyosarcoma has been associated with the t(2;13) and t(1;13) translocations. Synovial sarcoma is associated with t(X;18) translocation.

DIFFERENTIAL DIAGNOSIS

The differential diagnosis is quite variable depending on the site of the primary tumor; therefore, STS may present as a variety of benign and malignant conditions depending on the site. Approximately 35% of rhabdomyosarcoma occurs in the head and neck, 22% in genitourinary sites, and almost 20% in the extremities. The most common sites for nonrhabdomyosarcoma sarcomas are the extremities, trunk/abdomen, and the head and neck.

DIAGNOSTIC EVALUATION

Radiologic evaluation includes appropriate imaging of the primary site of the tumor and may include a CT or MRI scan of the site to assess the extent of disease and involvement of nearby structures. Additional imaging for metastatic disease includes CT of the chest and a bone scan. Further workup involving bone marrow biopsies is dependent on the STS diagnosis and is required for rhabdomyosarcoma. For rhabdomyosarcoma, 25% of newly diagnosed cases have distant metastases with the lung being the most frequent site. Other sites include regional lymph nodes, bone, and bone marrow.

TREATMENT

Treatment is quite variable depending on the diagnosis and the staging of the tumor. For rhabdomyosarcoma, treatment can use all three treatment modalities, surgery, radiation, and chemotherapy. Complete surgical removal, if possible, is key with radiation for residual bulk disease or microscopic tumor. Chemotherapy is used in virtually all cases to help with the reduction of tumor size and eradication of metastasis. The duration and aggressiveness of the chemotherapy are dependent on multiple factors including surgical resection, histology, age at presentation, site of disease, and the presence of metastases.

For nonrhabdomyosarcomas, treatment is dependent on the histology, size of tumor, natural history of the tumor, and the presence of metastatic disease. Again, surgery, radiation, and chemotherapy all play important parts in the treatment.

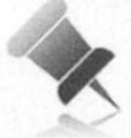

KEY POINTS

- The leukemias account for the greatest percentage of cases of childhood malignancies. Leukemias are classified on the basis of leukemia cell morphology into lymphoblastic leukemias or nonlymphoblastic (myeloblastic) leukemias. ALL is the most common pediatric neoplasm and accounts for about 85% of all childhood acute leukemias.
- NHLs are a heterogeneous group of diseases characterized by neoplastic proliferation of immature lymphoid cells, which, unlike the malignant lymphoid cells of ALL, accumulate outside the bone marrow.
- Hodgkin lymphoma accounts for 40% of the lymphoma cases in the pediatric population.
- The overall prognosis for HD is better than NHL. Late effects of treatment are very common.
- CNS tumors are the most common solid tumors in children and second to leukemia in overall incidence of malignant diseases.
- In contrast to brain tumors in adults, in whom supratentorial tumors are more common, brain tumors in children are predominantly infratentorial (posterior fossa), involving the cerebellum, midbrain, and brainstem.
- Neuroblastoma may occur in the abdomen, thoracic cavity, or head and neck; 70% of children present with abdominal tumors.
- Neuroblastoma has a variable presentation and biological behavior, ranging from spontaneous regression to aggressive dissemination requiring bone marrow transplantation.
- Staging for Wilms tumor is done after exploratory laparotomy, and the therapy involves surgery, chemotherapy, and sometimes radiation.
- Ewing sarcoma is an undifferentiated sarcoma that arises primarily in bone and affects young children and adolescents. Pain and localized swelling are the most common presenting complaints of Ewing sarcoma, and the most common sites for Ewing sarcoma are the femur and the bones of the pelvis.
- Osteogenic sarcoma is a malignant tumor of the bone-producing cells of the mesenchyma and arises most often during maximum growth velocity in the distal femur, proximal tibia, or proximal humerus.
- Similar to Ewing sarcoma, pain and localized swelling are the most common presenting complaints in osteogenic sarcoma, but in contrast to Ewing sarcoma, systemic manifestations are rare.
- Treatment of Ewing sarcoma and osteosarcoma may involve chemotherapy and surgery.
- Well-child checks are important to screen for leukocoria to assess for retinoblastoma.
- The most common soft tissue sarcoma is rhabdomyosarcoma, and the most common site of rhabdomyosarcoma is the head and neck.

C Clinical Vignettes

Vignette 1

A 3-year-old boy is brought to the emergency department (ED) for fever. According to his parents, the fever started about 1 week ago and has been as high as 101.1°F. His fever has been accompanied by increased fatigue. He is less interested in playing with his sister and his favorite toys. His parents report that his appetite also seems to be decreased, but he has not had any nausea or vomiting, nor has he lost any weight. He was seen by his pediatrician 3 days ago, who told he likely has a viral fever. When he awoke from his nap today, he refused to walk on his own and insists on being carried. His pediatrician referred him to the ED for further evaluation. You suspect that this child may have leukemia.

1. Which of the following physical examination findings would support this diagnosis?
   a. Hepatosplenomegaly
   b. Pallor
   c. Bruising and petechiae
   d. B and C
   e. All of the above

2. Both the spleen and liver are reservoir sites for leukemia cells. As a result, both are commonly enlarged at the time of diagnosis. The hepatosplenomegaly will resolve once chemotherapy is started and the patient enters remission. Which of the following laboratory tests is most likely to aid in your diagnosis?
   a. Lactate dehydrogenase
   b. Amylase
   c. Lipase
   d. Complete blood count (CBC) with differential and blood smear
   e. Erythrocyte sedimentation rate

3. The patient's CBC returns with the following values:
   1. White blood cell count: 64,000/mm^3
   2. Hemoglobin: 7.3 g/dL
   3. Platelets: 12,000/μL
   4. Differential:

Neutrophils	10%
Lymphocytes	42%
Monocytes	5%
Eosinophils	1%
Blasts	42%

This child is most likely to have which of the following types of leukemia?
   a. Acute myeloid leukemia
   b. Acute lymphoblastic leukemia
   c. Chronic myeloid leukemia
   d. Chronic lymphoblastic leukemia
   e. Germ cell leukemia

4. Which of the following would be considered a poor prognostic indicator for this patient?
   a. His age
   b. His total white blood cell count
   c. The presence of trisomies 4 and 10 in his leukemia cells
   d. The presence of a TEL/AML rearrangement in his leukemia cells
   e. Good response to induction therapy

Vignette 2

A 14-year-old male has a history of trauma to his knee while playing football. The injury was initially treated conservatively with rest; however, pain persists, with swelling just above the knee 6 weeks later. The review of systems is otherwise negative.

1. Following a thorough history and physical examination, which of the following is the most appropriate next step?
   a. Further observation, with the addition of icing twice a day, compression, and elevation
   b. Magnetic resonance imaging
   c. Radiograph of the knee
   d. Referral to an orthopedic specialist
   e. Referral to an oncology specialist

2. Which of the following represents the most likely oncologic condition in this scenario?
   a. Leukemia
   b. Bone tumor (osteosarcoma or Ewing sarcoma)
   c. Metastasis from another site
   d. Neuroblastoma
   e. Lung cancer

3. Which of the following imaging results is most characteristic of osteosarcoma?
   a. "Radial sunburst" pattern representing periosteal reaction and bone spicules

b. "Onion skin" pattern of calcified periosteal elevation surrounding a lytic bone lesion
c. Pathologic fracture just proximal to the tumor
d. Subluxation of the associated epiphyseal plate
e. Widening of the nearest joint space to >95th percentile of typical findings

Vignette 3

An 18-month-old girl presents to the ED after the mother feels a "lump" in her belly during a bath. The child has been growing well with no acute illnesses. She is eating and drinking with no emesis and there is no history of trauma. Past medical history is negative, as is the review of symptoms. She is on no medications, and immunizations are up-to-date. She has an 18-month health maintenance visit scheduled with her pediatrician in 4 days.

1. Which of the following is the most appropriate next step in the evaluation of this patient?
a. Observation
b. Abdominal plain film
c. Magnetic resonance imaging (MRI) or computed tomography (CT) of the abdomen
d. Abdominal sonography
e. Bone scan

2. An abdominal mass is noted arising from or near the kidney. Which two of the following are the most likely oncologic causes of the mass?
(a) Neuroblastoma
(b) Leukemia
(c) Lymphoma
(d) Wilms tumor
(e) Rhabdomyosarcoma
a. a and b
b. b and c
c. a and e
d. a and d
e. c and e

3. What is the 3rd most common cancer diagnosed under the age of 20?
a. Leukemia
b. Wilms tumor
c. Hodgkin lymphoma
d. Osteosarcoma
e. Neuroblastoma

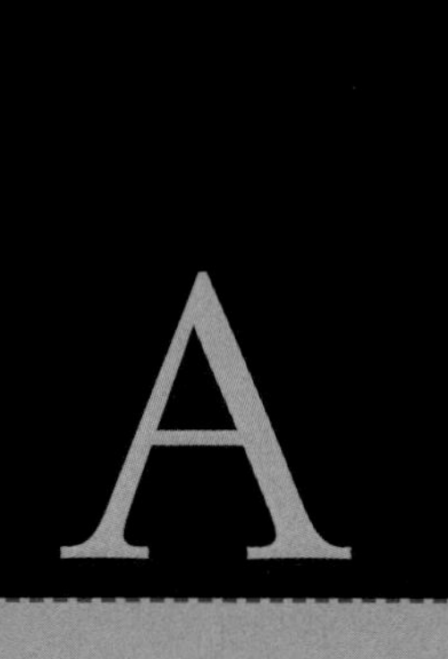

Answers

Vignette 1 Question 1
Answer E: Pallor, bruising, and petechiae are all common symptoms of leukemia because the bone marrow cavity is taken over by the leukemia cells, leaving it unable to produce normal amounts of red blood cells and platelets. As the hemoglobin and platelet counts fall, the symptoms of anemia (pallor) and thrombocytopenia (bruising and petechiae) become obvious.

Vignette 1 Question 2
Answer D: Leukemia typically presents with anemia (low hemoglobin) and thrombocytopenia (low platelets). The white blood cell count may be normal, high, or low. The differential is important because blasts, or circulating leukemia cells, are often seen in the peripheral blood, especially on the blood smear. This profile is very suggestive of the diagnosis of leukemia. The gold standard for confirming the diagnosis would be a bone marrow aspiration and/or biopsy.

Vignette 1 Question 3
Answer B: Acute leukemias account for 97% of all childhood leukemias. Acute lymphoblastic leukemia (ALL) comprises 75% of all acute leukemia diagnoses in children, with acute myeloid leukemia accounting for the remaining 25% of cases. ALL is more common in boys and has a peak incidence between the ages of 2 to 5 years. The incidence of AML does not peak until adolescence. Only 3% of chronic myeloid leukemias occur in pediatric-aged patients. The majority of cases are seen in the adult population. Chronic lymphoblastic leukemia only occurs in adults. Germ cell tumors are found in the pituitary or pineal glands; they do not originate from blood cells.

Vignette 1 Question 4
Answer B: Poor prognostic factors for ALL include a total white blood count greater than 50,000/mm^3 and age less than 1 year or greater than 10 years. This patient's white blood count of 64,000/mm^3 puts him at higher risk for a poor outcome. The presence of trisomies 4 and 10 and/or a TEL/AML rearrangement would be a positive prognostic indicator, as would the patient's age of 3 years. A good response to induction therapy predicts a positive outcome.

Vignette 2 Question 1
Answer C: Plain films (radiographs) are quick and easy to obtain, with instant access to results. Radiographs are the most appropriate initial radiographic modality to assess persistent pain and swelling. If plain films are negative or unrevealing (i.e., demonstrate the observed swelling but no associated abnormality), magnetic resonance imaging should be considered. Although trauma is the most common cause of limb pain in all ambulating ages, the differential diagnosis includes oncologic etiologies.

Vignette 2 Question 2
Answer B: Given the absence of systemic symptoms, including fevers, weight loss, easy bruising and bleeding, and fatigue, an isolated bone tumor is most likely oncologic cause. Although trauma does not cause bone tumors, affected patients often present with a history of trauma at the site, presumably because trauma, especially mild trauma, is so common in children and adolescents. Leukemia tends to have more systemic manifestations. Neuroblastoma is usually diagnosed at a much younger age. Metastasis from another site is rare without other symptoms. Lung cancer is vanishingly rare in this age group.

Vignette 2 Question 3
Answer A: Both osteosarcoma and Ewing sarcoma are more common in adolescents than children, but osteosarcoma is typically not associated with other symptoms such as fever, weight loss, and fatigue. Osteosarcoma arises from the bone-producing mesenchymal stem cells, either in the medullary cavity or the periosteum. The "radial sunburst" pattern is the typical radiographic finding in osteosarcoma. Ewing sarcoma appears to have an "onion skin." Pathologic fractures may occur in the presence of malignancy but typically involve the tumor area. Epiphyseal plate subluxation is not associated with osteosarcoma, nor is widening of the nearest joint space.

Vignette 3 Question 1
Answer D: Given the absence of radiation exposure, the rapidity with which the test can be obtained, the instant interpretation, and the lack of side effects, an abdominal ultrasound is the most appropriate diagnostic study to asses an abdominal mass in a young child. Observation is inappropriate; although constipation can result in small "lumps" in the abdomen, the incidence of serious intra-abdominal pathology is high enough, and the ramifications potentially severe enough, that observation alone is not a viable option. The plain film may show the mass, but the overlay of other tissues limits the detail and will not reveal fluid. If the mass is present on examination, it is unlikely that a plain film would provide any additional information. MRI or CT is indicated if the sonogram

is concerning for a pathologic lesion. Bone tumors do not present as abdominal masses.

Vignette 3 Question 2

Answer D: Neuroblastoma and Wilms occur at this age and present with an abdominal mass. Neuroblastoma is a tumor arising from the postganglionic sympathetic nervous system. Seventy percent are found in the abdomen; of these, the majority initiate in the adrenal medulla. These tumors tend to be firm, smooth, and nontender. Wilms tumor is a tumor of the kidney. Like neuroblastoma, the most common presentation is the presence of an asymptomatic abdominal mass. Often, a parent or caretaker notes the mass. Leukemia does not typically cause a mass. Hodgkin lymphoma is typically diagnosed during an evaluation for persistent, rubbery cervical lymphadenopathy, occasionally associated with fever, weight loss, and fatigue. Non-Hodgkin lymphoma is associated with mediastinal masses. Rhabdomyosarcomas are found primarily in the head, neck, extremities, and genitourinary sites.

Vignette 3 Question 3

Answer E: Neuroblastoma is the 3rd most common pediatric cancer behind leukemias and brain tumors, as a group. This is followed by Wilms tumor, lymphomas, rhabdomyosarcomas, retinoblastoma, and bone cancers.

Chapter 13

Immunology, Allergy, and Rheumatology

Jennifer Huggins • Kimberly A Risma • Katie S. Fine

IMMUNOLOGY

The immune system, composed of specialized cells and molecules, is responsible for recognizing and neutralizing foreign antigens. The **innate immune system** provides the *initial, relatively nonspecific* response to an invading microorganism. Preformed effectors and pathogen-associated molecular patterns (PAMPS) provide the stimulus for inflammation, recruitment and activation of effector cells, and ultimate clearance of the infectious agent. Two to 3 days following foreign antigen exposure, the **adaptive immune system** provides more *specific* pathogen recognition and more complex cellular interactions, resulting in defense against infection and immunological memory. **Immunodeficiency syndromes** increase susceptibility to infection, malignancy, and autoimmune disorders (Table 13-1). Table 13-2 lists clinical criteria that should prompt an evaluation for immunodeficiency.

DISORDERS OF T-CELL IMMUNITY

T-cells modulate most immune responses, providing recruitment of macrophages, assistance to B cells to make immunoglobulins, and direct killing of infected host cells and tumor cells. Therefore, they are the major effectors of cell-mediated immunity, important in the defense against intracellular and opportunistic infections. T-cell-based immunodeficieny is a life-threatening emergency in the neonate, requiring rapid recognition to institute life-saving therapies, Bone marrow transplantation is curative. **Severe combined immunodeficiency (SCID)** and human immunodeficiency virus (HIV) infection represent congenital (SCID) and acquired (HIV) **T-cell immunodeficiencies**.

Clinical Manifestations

History and Physical Examination

T-cell abnormalities predispose patients to infections with intracellular pathogens, including viruses and mycobacteria. Patients with SCID are highly susceptible to opportunistic infections from organisms such as fungi and *Pneumocystis jiroveci*. With the recent recommendation in the United States to vaccinate all children with the live, attenuated rotavirus vaccine at 2 months of age, children with SCID may be at special risk for vaccine-associated diarrhea. Vaccine-associated mortality may be seen in children with SCID in developing countries who still utilize the live poliovirus vaccine and bacille Calmette-Guerin vaccine to prevent tuberculosis. With these children in mind, there is a strong initiative in the United States to develop a newborn screening initiative for SCID, which is already in place in several state screening labs. The incidence of SCID in the United States is predicted to be 1:50,000 to 1:100,000 children. It is significantly higher in populations with consanguineous families.

SCID represents a group of genetically derived disorders of T-cell deficiency. The most commonly identified gene that is defective in boys with SCID is the X-linked gene, *IL2RG*, that encodes the common gamma chain of several interleukin receptors, including Interleukin-2 (IL-2). Boys with X-linked SCID present in the first 6 months of life with severe viral infections, bacterial infections, diarrhea, and failure to thrive. A complete blood count reveals severe lymphopenia (adjusted for age), and enumeration of T cells reveals nearly absent CD4 T cells. Girls may also present with SCID, although the genes responsible include other proteins in the IL-2 receptor signaling pathway.

Children with **DiGeorge syndrome** may also be diagnosed with T-cell immunodeficiency due to a lack of thymus maturation. Occasionally, the defect is so severe that they may present with SCID. It is more common, however, for these children to present in infancy with diseases unrelated to the immune system (e.g., congenital heart disease, hypocalcemic tetany from thymic hypoplasia). Other structures and organs derived from the branchial pouches during embryogenesis may be malformed as well, including the ears and face. The severity of the immunodeficiency is extremely variable. Some children exhibit recurrent and life-threatening infections, while other children have intact thymic (and therefore immune) development.

Diagnostic Evaluation

Absolute lymphocyte counts (calculated by multiplying the percentage of lymphocytes by the total white blood cell count) and T cells are generally decreased. T-cell function, measured by in vitro mitogen stimulation and intradermal delayed hypersensitivity testing, is absent or significantly compromised. Antibody production is generally absent; however, this may not be appreciated during the first 4 to 6 months when maternal antibodies are still present in the blood. No thymic

TABLE 13-1 Causes, Characteristics, and Evaluation of Immune Component Deficiencies

Condition	Mechanism	Sequelae	Laboratory Tests
Disorders of humoral immunity	—Impaired opsonization —Inability to lyse/ agglutinate bacteria —Inability to neutralize bacterial toxins	—Frequent, recurrent pyogenic infections with extracellular encapsulated organisms —Frequent bacterial otitis media, sinusitis, and pneumonia infections	—Quantitative total immunoglobulin levels: IgG, IgA, and IgM —Vaccination antibody titers
Disorders of cell-mediated immunity	—Inability of T cells to direct B-cell antibody synthesis to T-cell-specific antigens	—Frequent, recurrent infections with opportunistic/low-grade organisms and viruses —Increased incidence of autoimmune disorders and malignancies	—Absolute lymphocyte count (ALC) and T-cell enumeration —Abnormal mitogen stimulation response —Delayed hypersensitivity skin testing
Phagocytic disorders: quantitative (neutropenia)	—Insufficient number of neutrophils	—Cellulitis, skin abscesses, furunculosis —Stomatitis, gingivitis, rectal inflammation —Pneumonia, sepsis	—Absolute neutrophil count —Blood smear examination for blasts —Antineutrophil antibodies
Phagocytic disorders: functional (Chronic Granulomatous Disease)	—Inability to kill intracellular bacteria secondary to failure to generate oxygen metabolites such as the superoxide anion	—Increased susceptibility to infections with catalase-positive bacteria and fungi —Chronic lymphadenitis, abscesses, granulomas, osteomyelitis, granulomatous colitis	—Nitroblue tetrazolium test —DHR conversion test
Phagocytic Disorders (Leukocyte Adhesion Deficiency)	Inability of neutrophil to migrate to site of infection	—Increased susceptibility to infections with catalase-positive bacteria and fungi —Severe gingivitis, intestinal fistulas, poor wound healing	Flow cytometry for CD18
Complement disorders	—Impaired opsonization	—Recurrent bacterial infections with encapsulated, extracellular organisms —Increased susceptibility to meningococcal, gonnococcal disease —Increased incidence of autoimmune disease, especially SLE	—Total hemolytic complement (CH_{50}) —Assays of the classical and alternative pathways

TABLE 13-2 Clinical Criteria for Evaluation for Immunodeficiency Syndromes

Severe, persistent, or recurrent sinopulmonary infections
Infection by an unusual[a] or opportunistic pathogen
Family history of immunodeficiency
Infection at an unusual site (e.g., brain or liver abscess)
Failure to thrive, diarrhea, and lymphopenia in an infant
Chronic gingivitis

[a]Including *Aspergillus*, *Serratia marcescens*, *Nocardia* species, *Burkholderia cepacia*, and vaccine-associated pathogens (rotavirus, disseminated BCG).

shadow is seen on chest x-ray in patients with DiGeorge syndrome. Fluorescent in situ hybridization (FISH) testing of chromosome 22 detects the 22q11.2 deletion.

Treatment

SCID is treated initially with immunoglobulin replacement and aggressive identification and treatment of infections. Children are rapidly referred for bone marrow transplantation, which is curative. Future treatments for X-linked SCID will certainly include gene therapy as an alternative to bone marrow transplantation; however, this is available currently only in research trials. SCID due to DiGeorge syndrome has been successfully treated with both thymic and bone marrow transplantation.

Human immunodeficiency virus is discussed in detail in Chapter 10 (Infectious Disease).

DISORDERS OF HUMORAL IMMUNITY

B-cells produce antibodies, the primary effectors of humoral immunity. Antibodies are a vital component of the immune system, particularly in defense against extracellular pathogens such as encapsulated bacteria. A variety of antibodies activate complement, serve as opsonins, inhibit microbial adherence to mucous membranes, and neutralize various toxins and viruses. As a group, **antibody (humoral) deficiency syndromes** are the most common immunodeficiency diseases encountered in pediatric practice.

Clinical Manifestations

History and Physical Examination

A history of recurrent infections with **encapsulated** organisms, such as *Haemophilus influenzae* and *Streptococcus pneumoniae*, and failure to respond to appropriate antibiotic therapy are suggestive of a primary B-cell deficiency. In addition, there is often a history of frequent upper respiratory tract infections beginning after 6 months of age (when maternal antibodies are lost), including otitis media, sinusitis, and pneumonia.

Differential Diagnosis

X-linked agammaglobulinemia (XLA; also termed Bruton tyrosine kinase deficiency or Bruton disease) occurs in affected boys beginning around 6 months of age, which correlates with the waning of maternal antibodies transferred across the placenta. These patients do not produce antibodies and have virtually no mature B cells. In addition to their susceptibility to encapsulated organisms, individuals with this disorder are prone to severe, often life-threatening enterovirus infections.

Common variable immunodeficiency (CVID) is an inherited disorder of hypogammaglobulinemia (particularly IgG and IgA) with equal distribution between the genders. Onset may be in early childhood with recurrent sinopulmonary infections, or later onset (adolescence or even adulthood for unclear reasons). Specific antibody formation to vaccines is defective. In addition to sinopulmonary infections, the incidence of lymphoma and autoimmune disease are increased in these patients.

Selective IgA deficiency is the mildest and most common immunodeficiency syndrome. IgA deficiency is diagnosed when the serum IgA level is less than 5 mg/dL, and serum levels of the other antibody classes are normal. Patients react normally to viral infections but may be susceptible to bacterial infections of the respiratory, gastrointestinal, and urinary tracts. Some patients are asymptomatic.

Diagnostic Evaluation

Quantitative measurement of IgG, IgA, and IgM levels is an important screening test for specific deficiencies and for pan-hypogammaglobulinemia. In order to rule out other causes of hypoproteinemia as etiologies for low immunoglobulins, another serum protein screen such as albumin or transferrin should be ordered at the same time. Antibody titers generated against tetanus and diphtheria (*protein* antigens) and pneumococci and *Haemophilus influenza* (*carbohydrate* antigens) after immunization also assess B-cell function.

A unique scenario arises when considering the etiology for hypogammaglobulinemia in young infants. All serum immunoglobulin classes are present at birth, but most do not reach adult levels until early to middle childhood. Maternal IgG is actively transported across the placenta and is protective throughout the first few months of life. Over the first 6 to 8 weeks of life, maternally derived immunoglobulins decrease and are replaced by the child's growing production. **Transient hypogammaglobulinemia of infancy** is a recognized disorder in which the acquisition of normal infant immunoglobulin levels is delayed. Although some of these patients are subsequently diagnosed with other primary immunodeficiencies, the majority eventually develop normal immunoglobulin levels by 2 to 5 years of age and, in contrast to children with CVID, XLA, or SCID, they have intact responses to vaccination and low (but not absent) immunoglobulin levels. Generally, these children do not require immunoglobulin replacement and receive only supportive care for typical childhood illnesses.

Treatment

The mainstays of therapy for XLA and CVID are appropriate antibiotic use and periodic gammaglobulin administration. **Intravenous immunoglobulin** (IVIG) and/or subcutaneous gammaglobulin provide antibody replacement and have revolutionized the treatment of humoral immunodeficiency syndromes.

COMBINED IMMUNODEFICIENCY SYNDROMES

Combined humoral and cell-mediated immunodeficiencies tend to be inherited and manifest a wide range of clinical severity. Affected patients display increased susceptibility to both traditionally virulent and opportunistic infections or may present with autoimmunity.

Wiskott-Aldrich syndrome is an X-linked recessive disorder of (primarily) B- and (usually) T-cell immunity, atopic dermatitis, and thrombocytopenia. Specifically, the host's antibodies do not respond normally to carbohydrate antigens. Autoimmunity may be present. Survival to adulthood is rare because of bleeding, infections, and associated malignancies. Therefore, bone marrow transplantation is recommended for young infants.

Hyper-IgM syndrome is a group of disorders that have defects in both T-cell and humoral immunity. The most common form is X-linked, due to a mutation in the CD40L gene. The interaction between CD40L on T cells and CD40 on B cells is necessary for immunoglobulin class switching from IgM to IgG, IgA or IgE. Boys present in the first year of life with recurrent sinopulmonary infections and/or *Pneumocystis jiroveci* pneumonia. Diagnosis is made due to the presence of low IgG and IgA, with elevated IgM and absent titers to childhood vaccines. Treatment is bone marrow transplantation.

DISORDERS OF PHAGOCYTIC IMMUNITY

Phagocytes are responsible for removing particulate matter from the blood and tissues by ingesting and destroying microorganisms. These cells must be able to adhere to the endothelium, move through the tissues to their site of action, engulf the harmful matter, and kill it intracellularly. Phagocytic disorders are due to an insufficient number of normal neutrophils (neutropenia); to phagocytic cell dysfunction; or to inability of the phagocytic cell to migrate to the site of action. **Neutropenia** may result from infection (particularly viruses), medication administration (penicillin, sulfonamides, anticonvulsants), circulating antineutrophil antibodies, malignancy in the bone marrow, or aplastic anemia. **Chronic granulomatous disease** (CGD), the most common inherited disorder of phagocytic immunity, occurs when neutrophils and monocytes are unable to kill certain organisms after ingesting them due to a failure to generate superoxide. **Leukocyte adhesion deficiency (LAD)** arises when neutrophils are trapped in the bloodstream and unable to emigrate into the tissues due to a defect in adhesion molecules necessary for binding of the leukocyte to endothelial cells.

Clinical Manifestations

History and Physical Examination

Patients with neutropenia generally do not experience serious or life-threatening infections unless the neutropenia is both *severe* (absolute neutrophil count [ANC] $<0.5 \times 10^3/\mu L$) and *chronic* (lasting longer than 2 to 3 months). Typical complaints include gingivitis, skin infections, rectal inflammation, otitis media, pneumonia, and sepsis. Patients are often infected with *Staphylococcus aureus* and gram-negative organisms. Of note, patients with neutropenia are unable to mount a sufficient inflammatory response, so typical signs of infection such as erythema, warmth, and swelling may be absent even in the presence of significant pathogen load.

CGD is characterized by chronic or recurrent pyogenic infections caused by bacterial and fungal pathogens that produce catalase (*Staphylococcus aureus, Candida albicans, Aspergillus*) and by most gram-negative enteric bacteria. Both X-linked and autosomal inheritance occur. Abscesses and granuloma formation occur in the lymph nodes, liver, spleen, lungs, skin, and gastrointestinal tract. Failure to thrive, chronic diarrhea, and persistent candidiasis of the mouth and diaper area are common. Affected individuals are also at increased risk for opportunistic infections, disseminated viral illnesses, and inflammatory bowel disease.

Children with LAD are susceptible to infections with the same microorganisms as those with CGD. In contrast to CGD, patients with LAD have white blood cell (WBC) counts that are 5 to 10 times normal and are unable to form granulomas. Severe gingivitis, intestinal fistulas, and poor wound healing, such as delayed separation of the umbilical cord, are significant clues for the consideration of LAD.

Diagnostic Evaluation

Severe neutropenia is defined as an ANC $<0.5 \times 10^3/\mu L$. Serial complete blood counts will reveal a leukoerythroblastic response unless the condition is chronic. Bone marrow examination is required if malignancy or aplastic anemia is a consideration.

In CGD, the WBC count typically ranges between 10,000 and 20,000/μL with 60% to 80% polymorphonuclear cells. Leukocyte chemotaxis is normal. The hallmark abnormality is the inability of affected cells to produce an oxidative burst resulting in hydrogen peroxide. The **nitroblue tetrazolium test** (NBT) and the dihydrorhodamine reduction (DHR) test are laboratory studies performed to detect the inability to produce this reduction reaction.

The most common form of LAD results from a genetic defect in CD18, which is the β2 portion of LFA1 and is necessary for tight adhesion between the neutrophil and the endothelial cell. Leukocyte chemotaxis is abnormal. Flow cytometry analysis of CD18 expression on neutrophils will establish the diagnosis.

Treatment

Children with acute neutropenia need no special treatment. Patients with chronic neutropenia and those with infectious complications may respond to recombinant human granulocyte-colony stimulating factor (rhG-CSF) injections. All patients with CGD should receive prophylactic trimethoprim-sulfamethoxazole. Aggressive treatment of deep-seated bacterial and fungal infections is critical. Bone marrow transplantation is frequently recommended, and gene therapy is a promising area of research. Treatment for LAD is adequate treatment of infections and bone marrow transplantation.

DISORDERS OF COMPLEMENT IMMUNITY

Although quantitative deficiencies of virtually all complement components have been described, they are far less common than the immunodeficiencies mentioned earlier. The primary mechanism of disease is impaired opsonization. Patients with **complement disorders** have increased susceptibility to bacterial infections and a higher incidence of rheumatologic disease. In particular, deficiencies of the terminal complement components C5 to C9 increase the likelihood of *Neisseria meningitidis* infections. Deficiencies of the early forms of complement (C1–C4) are seen with increased frequency in patients with systemic lupus erythematosus (SLE).

ALLERGY

An **allergic reaction** is an undesirable immune-mediated response to an environmental stimulus. Allergies have been implicated as a contributing factor in anaphylaxis, asthma, allergic rhinitis, and atopic dermatitis. Allergic reactions range from mild to life-threatening and are *never* considered adaptive.

The **allergic triad** of atopic disease consists of atopic dermatitis (eczema), allergic rhinitis, and asthma. Atopic children will frequently develop *eczema*, followed by *allergic rhinitis* with the eventual development of allergic *asthma*. This is known as the **allergic march**.

ATOPIC DERMATITIS

Atopic dermatitis is a chronic, relapsing and remitting inflammatory skin reaction to specific allergens, including specific foods and environmental allergens. The most common allergens associated with eczema include: milk proteins, egg, fish, wheat, soy, dust mite and animal dander. Eczema usually appears in infancy and affects upwards of 10% of the pediatric population. Genetic predilection is the highest risk factor. About half of patients with atopic dermatitis later develop allergic rhinitis and/or asthma. Early therapeutic intervention may prevent the progression of the allergic march.

Clinical Manifestations

The typical rash consists of a pruritic, erythematous, weeping papulovesicular reaction that progresses to scaling, hypertrophy, and lichenification. In infants younger than 2 years, the eruption involves the extensor surfaces of the arms and legs, the wrists, the face, and the scalp; the diaper area is invariably spared. Flexor areas predominate in older age groups, as well as the neck, wrists, and ankles. The diagnosis of atopic dermatitis is primarily clinical, based on history, physical examination, and response to treatment. The differential diagnosis includes contact dermatitis and psoriasis, a chronic nonallergic skin disorder (see Chapter 6).

Treatment

Eczema is commonly referred to as "the itch that rashes." The goal of treatment is termination of the itch–scratch–itch cycle. Patients should try to keep their 05 dyes skin well-hydrated with lotions that do not contain fragrances. Tight clothing and heat may precipitate exacerbations and should be avoided. Moisturizers are the mainstay of treatment, followed by the use of **topical corticosteroids** for areas of inflammation. Pimecrolimus cream, an inhibitor of T-cell activation, has been approved for patients over 24 months of age who cannot tolerate topical steroids or have resistant disease. Topical tacrolimus is another immunomodulator that may be used in more severe cases. Severe chronic eczema may be complicated by bacterial superinfection.

ALLERGIC RHINITIS

Epidemiology

It is estimated that up to 40% of children are affected by allergic rhinitis by the time they are 6 years of age. Seasonal allergic rhinitis, or **hay fever** , is limited to months of pollination and is uncommon before 4 to 5 years of age. Tree pollens are common during early spring, followed by grass pollens, which are detected until the early summer. Ragweed season starts in the late summer and persists until the first frost. Perennial disease persists year round, usually in response to household allergens (molds, dust mites).

Pathogenesis

Allergic rhinitis is a type 1 hypersensitivity immune response (IgE mediated) to environmental allergens including airborne pollens, animal dander, dust mites, and molds. The offending allergen binds to IgE on mast cells in the upper respiratory tract, with subsequent release of inflammatory mediators. This localized inflammation results in nasal congestion, rhinorrhea and/or postnasal drainage, sneezing, and occasionally itching. Allergic rhinitis is the most frequent cause of chronic or recurrent clear rhinorrhea in the pediatric population.

Risk Factors

Atopy and genetic predisposition are the major risk factors. Smoking in the home in the first year of life also increases the likelihood of subsequent disease. Paradoxically, heavy exposure to animal dander early in life may reduce the risk of subsequent atopic disease.

Clinical Manifestations

History

Patients with allergic rhinitis are plagued with nasal congestion, profuse watery rhinorrhea, and sneezing. Associated allergic conjunctivitis is common. Unrelenting postnasal drip produces frequent coughing and/or throat clearing. Patients may also complain of drowsiness because of recurrent brief awakenings at night. As a group, children with untreated allergic rhinitis have been shown to have decreased school performance when compared with their peers.

Physical Examination

On examination, the nasal mucosa appears boggy and bluish. Two characteristic features of allergic rhinitis are **allergic shiners** (dark circles that develop under the eyes secondary to venous congestion) and the **allergic salute** (a horizontal crease across the middle of the nose due to a constant upward wiping motion with the hand). Because of the severe congestion, patients may become obligate mouth breathers, and a gaping mouth and palatal arching may be seen on physical exam. Children with allergic rhinitis are also prone to recurrent sinusitis and otitis media with effusion.

Differential Diagnosis

Infectious rhinitis is much more common than allergic rhinitis in infants and toddlers and is often mucopurulent. *Sinusitis* causes chronic rhinorrhea and postnasal drip associated with facial tenderness, cough, and/or headache. When a *nasal foreign body* is present, the discharge is usually unilateral, thick, and foul-smelling. Other possible diagnoses include *vasomotor* (idiopathic nonallergic) *rhinitis*, which appears to be due to an exaggerated vascular response to irritants, and *rhinitis medicamentosa*, which results from overuse of topical decongestants.

Diagnostic Evaluation

Usually, a careful history confirms the diagnosis. Patients who do not respond favorably to a trial of second-generation (nonsedating) antihistamines may require further workup. Elevated nasopharyngeal eosinophil levels may support the diagnosis. A serum radioallergosorbant (RAST) test may be used when skin testing cannot be performed, but the sensitivity is 10% to 25% less than the preferred *direct* skin testing for specific allergens.

Treatment

The most effective treatment for any allergic condition is **allergen avoidance**. Switching to air-conditioning in the summer (rather than keeping the windows open) affords some protection to patients with pollen allergies. Limiting the amount of humidity in the home can decrease the presence of dust mites and various fungi. Dust mite mattress and pillow covers as well as frequent washing and/or drying of bedding on high heat help with limiting dust mite exposure. Eliminating animal dander and limiting exposure to cigarette smoke are also helpful.

Pharmacotherapy is an important adjunct if avoidance is not possible. **H_1-histamine blockers** (oral or intranasal) are the mainstay of treatment. They are now available in nonsedating formulations approved for use in children greater than 2 years of age. Intranasal cromolyn is helpful as a preventive medication if taken prior to the onset of symptoms. Nasal topical steroids are very effective treatments with minimal side effects. Oral leukotriene receptor antagonists may be beneficial in some patients. Topical and inhaled sympathomimetics (the most popular being pseudoephedrine) are useful for short-term therapy only and, if taken improperly, may result in severe rebound congestion. Allergy immunotherapy (shots) is indicated and is very effective for the treatment of allergic rhinitis, allergic asthma, and stinging insects. The child must be able to articulate symptoms of a reaction to the immunotherapy before administration. Studies have demonstrated that use of immunotherapy may prevent the developments of both further allergies and subsequent atopic disease.

ASTHMA

Asthma is discussed in detail in Chapter 8. A significant proportion of cases of asthma is allergic in nature. Allergens frequently associated with asthma exacerbations include mold, dust mites, and pet dander. Allergen avoidance is the first step in effective treatment. Other therapies are discussed in Chapter 8.

URTICARIA AND ANGIOEDEMA

Urticaria and angioedema are classic type 1 hypersensitivity reactions. **Urticaria** describes the typical raised edematous hives on the skin or mucous membranes resulting from vascular dilation and increased permeability. The lesions itch, blanch, and generally resolve within a few hours to days. **Angioedema** is a similar process confined to the lower dermis and subcutaneous areas; the depth results in a well-demarcated area of swelling devoid of pruritus, erythema, or warmth. Although acute urticaria and angioedema occur frequently in the pediatric population, chronic forms are rare.

Clinical Manifestations

The diagnosis is based on a detailed history of recent exposures or changes in the patient's environment. The multiple allergens and conditions associated with urticaria and angioedema include foods, medications, insect stings, infections, and some systemic illnesses. Clinical manifestations may be delayed as long as 48 hours after the initial encounter.

Hereditary forms of angioedema exist but are not IgE mediated. Patients with **hereditary angioedema** have an inherited **C1 esterase** inhibitor deficiency. Greater than 50% of the time, the inciting trigger remains a mystery. The angioedema is frequently asymmetric and is not accompanied by urticaria.

Treatment

Treatment depends on severity, which ranges from mild to life-threatening (i.e., swelling around the airway). Subcutaneous epinephrine is the treatment of choice in emergency situations, followed by intravenous diphenhydramine and steroids. Oral antihistamines, sympathomimetics, and occasionally oral steroids are appropriate in milder cases. C1 esterase replacement is a promising therapy that has recently become available for the treatment of hereditary angioedema.

FOOD ALLERGIES

Pathogenesis

Food allergy is an immune-mediated response to a specific food protein. It is important to distinguish between food intolerance (an undesirable nonimmunologic reaction) and true food hypersensitivity, which is an IgE-mediated immune response. Examples of nonimmunologic adverse food reaction include caffeine-induced tachycardia and lactose intolerance.

Epidemiology

Eighty percent of all food allergies present during the first year of life. The overall prevalence of food allergies is also higher in children (5% to 8%) than in adults (1% to 2%). Relatively few foods are represented; **peanuts, eggs, milk proteins, soy, wheat, tree nuts and fish** account for over 90% of reported cases. Exclusive breastfeeding may delay presentation unless the mother is ingesting the offending proteins regularly. One-third of patients with atopic dermatitis and 10% of those with asthma also have a food allergy.

Clinical Manifestations

History and Physical Examination

A detailed history, including daily records of intake and symptoms, is essential for the diagnosis. True food allergies can present with isolated cutaneous reactions, gastrointestinal symptoms, respiratory symptoms, and life-threatening anaphylaxis. Symptoms that develop during weaning are particularly suggestive of food allergies.

Diagnostic Evaluation

Skin testing has a low positive predictive value; it is more helpful for ruling out specific food proteins as causative IgE triggers. A RAST test will identify IgE antibodies to specific foods in the serum. The **double-blind, placebo challenge–food challenge** is the current gold standard. Several foods are eliminated from the patient's diet for a period before testing. Then the foods are disguised and tested, alternating with placebos, over several days. A challenge is considered positive if signs and symptoms recur after ingestion. Such testing must be performed in a hospital setting, as anaphylaxis is a possible complication.

Treatment

Treatment entails eliminating the offending food from the diet. Patients and their caregivers should be educated in the use of an autoinjectable epinephrine pen. For infants with severe, widespread allergies, elemental hypoallergenic formulas are available. Cow milk, soy, egg, and wheat allergies are usually outgrown after avoidance of the offending food. Oral challenges can be conducted safely to reintroduce the food. However, peanut (legume), nut, and fish allergies usually persist. Breastfeeding coupled with delay in the introduction of solid foods until after age 4 to 6 months may prevent the development of certain food allergies.

RHEUMATOLOGY

The modern concept of **rheumatic disease** encompasses a large number of **autoimmune** and **autoinflammatory** conditions. In autoimmune disorders, immune dysregulation of self-tolerance by the adaptive immune system results in production of autoantibodies and self-reactive T cells, leading to inflammation and target organ damage. As a group, autoimmune disorders are not uncommon in pediatrics; examples include most juvenile idiopathic arthritis (JIA), systemic lupus erythematosus (SLE), and juvenile dermatomyositis (JDM). In contrast, autoinflammatory disease develops when the innate immune system is abnormally stimulated, often due to genetic predisposition, leading to overproduction of inflammatory cytokines such as IL-1, TNF-α, and IL-6. Most autoinflammatory diseases are quite rare, with the exceptions of systemic JIA and Crohn disease. The *periodic fever syndromes* are considered to exist within the group of autoinflammatory disorders. The manifestations of rheumatic disease in childhood are protean, and typical presenting signs and symptoms are often seen in nonrheumatic conditions as well. Particularly common are constitutional symptoms such as malaise, fatigue, weight loss or poor weight gain, and/or fever. Clinical manifestations and laboratory abnormalities associated with specific disorders are noted in Table 13-3.

TABLE 13-3 Clinical Manifestations and Laboratory Findings of Rheumatic Disease

Sign/Symptom	Suggested Rheumatic Disease	Sign/Symptom	Suggested Rheumatic Disease
Dry eyes, dry mouth	Sjögren syndrome	***Laboratory findings***	
Oral/nasal ulcers	SLE Granulomatosus with polyangiitis (formerly Wegener granulomatosis) Behçet disease	Leukocytosis	Systemic JIA Kawasaki disease
Chest pain/pleuritis	SLE Systemic JIA Vasculitis	Markedly elevated ESR	Systemic JIA Kawasaki disease Vasculitis
Arthritis (joint swelling, morning stiffness)	JIA SLE Vasculitis	Thrombocytosis	Systemic JIA
Muscle weakness	Juvenile determatomyositis	Proteinuria/hematuria	SLE (lupus nephritis) Small-vessel vasculitis Henoch-Schönlein purpura
Skin tightening/ thickening	Systemic sclerosis Linear scleroderma	Sterile pyuria	Kawasaki disease
Raynaud phenomenon	SLE Systemic sclerosis Vasculitis	Elevated muscle-related enzymes	Juvenile dermatomyositis Juvenile polymyositis SLE
Purpura	Henoch-Schönlein purpura Small- and medium-vessel vasculitis	Antinuclear antibody (ANA)	SLE and related disorders (scleroderma, Sjögren syndrome) JIA (non-systemic)
Malar rash	SLE Juvenile dermatomyositis	Anti-dsDNA, anti-Smith	SLE
Gottron papules (extensor surface rash)	Juvenile dermatomyositis	Antiphospholipid antibodies	SLE
Nailfold capillary changes	SLE Juvenile dermatomyositis Systemic sclerosis Vasculitis	Anti-ssDNA	Linear scleroderma
		Rheumatoid factor	Rheumatoid factor-positive polyarticular JIA
		Low complement C3, C4	SLE

JIA, juvenile idiopathic arthritis; SLE, systemic lupus erythematosus

JUVENILE IDIOPATHIC ARTHRITIS

Epidemiology

Juvenile idiopathic arthritis (JIA) is the most common rheumatic disease in children, with a prevalence of at least 1:1,000 children in the United States. JIA is an umbrella term for the classification of chronic arthritis (>6 weeks) occurring in individuals under 16 years of age. Other causes of arthritis must be excluded before the diagnosis of JIA can be applied. In the past, childhood arthritis was called "juvenile rheumatoid arthritis" (JRA) or "juvenile chronic arthritis" (JCA) and classified according to slightly different criteria. Because the majority of children with juvenile arthritis do not resemble adults with rheumatoid arthritis (RA) and not all children with arthritis have a chronic course, the term JIA was instituted. The most common subtype of JIA is oligoarticular (~45%), followed by polyarticular (~25%), systemic (~10%), psoriatic (~5%), and enthesitis-related arthritis (~15%).

Pathogenesis

The etiology of JIA is unclear, but genetic and environmental factors are likely both involved. Certain human leukocyte antigen (HLA) types are associated with increased risk of disease. The underlying pathophysiology in most forms of chronic inflammatory arthritis is **synovitis** (inflammation and hypertrophy of the synovium), a term that is often used interchangeably with *arthritis*. TNF-α is the major cytokine involved in the development of synovitis/arthritis in JIA; therapeutic blocking of TNF-α has dramatically improved the outcome of many children with JIA.

Clinical Manifestations

History and Physical Examination

Arthritis is a clinical diagnosis defined as swelling within a joint, increased warmth over the joint, painful or limited movement of the joint, and/or joint tenderness. Morning joint stiffness and stiffness after immobility lasting for >30 minutes is a classic symptom of joint inflammation and is particularly common in JIA. Any synovial joint can be affected; often overlooked is the temporomandibular joint. The presence of *severe* joint pain is not characteristic of JIA and suggests an alternate diagnosis (infectious or reactive arthritis, mechanical disorders). JIA subtypes are classified by number and location of joints involved, physical findings, associated diseases or family history, and sometimes extra-articular manifestations (Table 13-4).

Oligoarticular JIA is the most common subtype. The typical patient is a young girl 2 to 4 years of age. Large joints (knee, ankle) are most commonly involved. Long-standing arthritis can result in joint contractures, muscle atrophy, and increased extremity growth in the affected limb (leading to limb length discrepancy). Up to 75% of patients have a positive antinuclear antibody (ANA) test. The majority of patients with oligoarticular JIA experience remission after several years of active arthritis; late recurrences can occur.

Chronic, nongranulomatous anterior uveitis (iridocyclitis) is detected in up to a third of patients with oligoarticular JIA. A positive ANA test is associated with the development of this

TABLE 13-4 Clinical Manifestations of JIA

JIA Subtype	Clinical Features	Onset Age	Sex Ratio
Oligoarthritis	• Arthritis of 4 or fewer joints • Most commonly involves knee, ankle, wrist, elbows	Early childhood; peak at 2 to 4 years	F>>>M
Polyarthritis	Subdivided according to presence of rheumatoid factor (RF)		
Rheumatoid factor-negative	• Arthritis of 5 or more joints	Biphasic distribution; early peak at 2 to 4 years and later peak at 6 to 12 years	F>>M
Rheumatoid factor-positive	• Most commonly distal symmetric arthritis • Rheumatoid nodules	Late childhood or adolescence	F>>M
Systemic arthritis	• Arthritis with or preceded by quotidian (daily) fever for at least 3 days, accompanied by one or more of: 1. Evanescent erythematous rash 2. Lymphadenopathy 3. Hepatomegaly and/or splenomegaly 4. Serositis 5. Mandatory exclusion of infection and malignancy; arthritis may not be present early in course 6. Arthritis can involve large and small joints	Throughout childhood	F = M
Psoriatic arthritis	• Arthritis and psoriasis or arthritis with at least two of the following: 1. Dactylitis 2. Nail pitting or onycholysis 3. Psoriasis in first-degree relative 4. Large and small joint arthritis	Biphasic distribution; early peak at 2 to 4 years and later peak at 9 to 11 years	F>M
Enthesitis-related arthritis	• Arthritis and enthesitis or arthritis or enthesitis with two of the following: 1. Sacro-iliac joint tenderness or infammatory lumbo-sacral pain 2. HLA-B27 antigen 3. Onset after age 6 years in males 4. Acute (symptomatic) anterior uveitis 5. History of HLA-B27 associated disease in a first-degree relative	Late childhood or adolescence	M>>F

condition. Chronic anterior uveitis is typically **asymptomatic** but can be appreciated on slit lamp examination. Due to the risk of visual impairment and blindness, routine screening is indicated in JIA patients at risk for this complication.

Polyarticular JIA , the next most common subtype, can be subdivided into rheumatoid factor (RF)-positive and RF-negative disease. RF-positive JIA resembles adult rheumatoid arthritis, with erosive, predominantly distal, symmetric small joint arthritis (wrist, hand, fingers) and rheumatoid nodules. RF-positive JIA typically has its onset in adolescence and takes a chronic course. RF-negative JIA usually presents in early childhood, may have both large and small joint involvement, and carries a better prognosis than RF-positive disease.

Systemic JIA is quite distinct from the other JIA subtypes, both in the clinical manifestations and the fact that systemic JIA is an **autoinflammatory** disorder. Extra-articular manifestations are prominent and often precede the onset of arthritis. Systemic JIA presents with intermittent high fevers that occur once or twice daily, with normal or below normal temperatures in the interval. The patient appears toxic and suffers from profound malaise during the fever episodes; a faint, evanescent, nonpruritic salmon-colored rash is often present as well. Hepatosplenomegaly, lymphadenopathy, and signs of serositis (pericarditis) may be noted on physical examination. The arthritis can involve both large and small joints and often is destructive. There is a marked acute phase reaction, including leukocytosis, thrombocytosis, anemia, elevated ESR and CRP, and (characteristically) very elevated ferritin. Neither ANA nor rheumatoid factor is present.

A common manifestation of **enthesitis-related arthritis** (ERA) is spondyloarthritis, that is, inflammation of the axial skeleton (sacroiliac joints, small intervertebral joints) and the large weight-bearing joints of the lower extremities. In addition, *enthesitis* (inflammation and tenderness at the site of tendon insertion) is often present in the Achilles tendon, plantar fascia, patellar tendon insertion, and anterior superior iliac spines. ERA is associated with HLA-B27 and occurs predominantly in boys >6 years of age. Extra-articular manifestations include acute anterior uveitis, colitis, and/or aortitis.

Psoriatic arthritis is defined as arthritis in the setting of psoriasis (see Chapter 6) in the patient or a first-degree relative. Findings of psoriasis such as nail pitting or onycholysis may be quite subtle. Dactylitis, when present, is a pathognomonic finding of psoriatic arthritis, and is due to flexor tendon tenosynovitis.

Differential Diagnosis

The differential diagnosis of JIA is extensive. Reactive or postinfectious arthritis (including acute rheumatic fever), other systemic inflammatory conditions (inflammatory bowel disease, connective tissue diseases, Henoch-Schönlein purpura, other forms of vasculitis), and infection (septic arthritis, viral arthritis, Lyme disease) can present with bona fide arthritis. Malignancy (leukemia, neuroblastoma, bone tumors), benign tumors, and musculoskeletal trauma may mimic arthritis.

Diagnostic Evaluation

Laboratory assessment is used primarily to supplement the clinical evaluation. Evidence of a mild acute phase reaction is typically present (excepting the impressive response in systemic JIA), but nonspecific. ANA is often present (except in systemic JIA and ERA) and is associated with an increased frequency of anterior uveitis. Rheumatoid factor, an autoantibody directed against a portion of the IgG molecule, is only present in ~5% of patients with JIA. The presence of the HLA-B27 allele is useful for classification; however, it should not be considered a diagnostic test since it is present in 7% to 8% of the healthy population. Synovial fluid analysis yields a white blood cell count >2,000/mm^3 with predominantly mononuclear cells.

Treatment

Treatment consists of medical management, physical therapy, and rarely surgery. Single large joint arthritis is often best managed with intra-articular corticosteroid injection. When multiple inflamed joints are present, a disease-modifying drug (e.g., methotrexate) is frequently necessary. In recent years, "biologic" therapies designed to neutralize specific cytokines (such as TNF-α,) or provide receptor blockade, as in the case of IL-L, IL-6, or T-cell costimulation have dramatically improved the outcomes for children with JIA that have failed more traditional therapies.

Prognosis and Complications

The prognosis of JIA varies. Generally, the more joints involved in the first 6 months, the more likely the disease course will be chronic. Complications of arthritis include bony erosions, deformities, and growth disturbances (limb overgrowth, growth failure). With the institution of the biologic therapies, crippling arthritis has become very rare.

SYSTEMIC LUPUS ERYTHEMATOSUS

Epidemiology

Systemic lupus erythematosus (SLE) is a chronic autoimmune disease characterized by widespread inflammation that can affect multiple organs. Pediatric SLE is usually diagnosed in late childhood or adolescence, but SLE may be diagnosed well before puberty. When SLE presents before puberty, the male-to-female ratio is equal; after puberty SLE is far more common in females. Asians, African Americans, and Hispanics have higher incidences than Caucasians.

Pathogenesis

The pathophysiology of SLE is complex, but a predominant factor is abnormal handling of cell death leading to an increased exposure to self-nuclear components. The result of abnormal apoptosis is the generation of multiple autoantibodies that cause immune-complex disease and antibody-mediated cellular cytotoxicity, with subsequent target organ injury. Autoantibodies are often directed against components of the cell nucleus (antinuclear antibodies). The etiology of SLE is multifactorial. Individuals with deficiencies of early complement components (C1q, C2, C4) are more prone to develop SLE. The early complement components are needed for normal apoptotic cell clearance.

Differential Diagnosis

Given its ability to affect so many organ systems, SLE is considered a "great masquerader." Adding to diagnostic uncertainty is the fact that overlapping conditions can result in a mixed clinical picture when the patient has features of two or more rheumatic diseases at the same time.

Clinical Manifestations

History and Physical Examination

The diagnosis of SLE is based on the American College of Rheumatology (ACR) classification criteria (Table 13-5). Fever, malaise, fatigue, and weight loss are very common. Mucocutaneous findings include painless oral ulcers, malar rash, discoid lupus, and photosensitivity. The arthritis in SLE is nonerosive but otherwise can mimic JIA. **Lupus nephritis** (LN), glomerulonephritis precipitated by immune-complex deposition, is one of the most severe organ manifestations of SLE and is often present at diagnosis. Renal involvement is described as class I (normal light microscopy), class II (mesangial proliferation), class III (focal proliferative), class IV (diffuse proliferative), or class V (membranous). Renal failure is most common in class IV LN. **CNS lupus** can present with psychosis, depression, confusion, or seizures.

Diagnostic Evaluation

Anemia, leukopenia (most commonly lymphopenia), and thrombocytopenia are characteristic. The ESR is often chronically elevated due to the polyclonal gammopathy of SLE and will increase above baseline during a disease flare, but C-reactive protein is usually normal. A rise in the CRP may indicate infection rather than SLE disease flare. A Coombs test is often positive and may be associated with a hemolytic anemia. Complement levels, including C3, C4, and CH_{50}, may be useful disease-activity markers with a depressed level below baseline indicating active SLE disease. The ANA is virtually always positive, but this finding alone is insufficient for diagnosis, and the ANA is not a disease-activity marker. Antiphospholipid antibodies (including lupus anticoagulant and anticardiolipin antibodies) are associated with an increased risk of arterial and venous thromboses and Libman-Sacks endocarditis. More specific autoantibodies against nuclear components include anti-Smith (Sm), anti-double-stranded DNA (dsDNA), anti-RNP, anti-Ro, and anti-La antibodies. Anti-Sm (present in 30% of SLE patients) and anti-dsDNA (present in 60% of SLE patients) are very specific for lupus. Circulating anti-Ro and anti-La antibodies in an SLE-affected mother may cause congenital heart block and neonatal lupus in her fetus.

TABLE 13-5 Systemic Lupus Erythematosus: Classification Criteria

Four of the following must be present:
Malar rash
Discoid rash
Photosensitivity
Oral ulcers
Arthritis
Serositis
Renal disorder (hematuria, proteinuria)
Neurologic disorder
Hematologic disorder (anemia, leukopenia, thrombocytopenia)
Antinuclear antibody (ANA)
Immunologic disorder (anti-Smith, anti-dsDNA, antiphospholipid antibodies)
From American College of Rheumatology 1982, revised 1997.

Treatment

Although SLE has historically been associated with high morbidity and mortality, prognosis and quality of life are improving. With appropriate therapy, a majority of patients have good long-term survival and normal function. Treatment depends on which organ systems are involved. General considerations include avoidance of sun exposure and use of sunscreen to avoid an increase in cell death; associated photosensitivity can trigger not only skin rashes but also systemic SLE flares. The antimalarial drug hydroxychloroquine is particularly helpful in preventing disease flares and in treating mucocutaneous disease manifestations. Mild cases of SLE with predominantly musculoskeletal involvement are addressed with NSAIDs or disease-modifying drugs if necessary. Renal and CNS involvement require more aggressive treatment. In severe cases, immunosuppressive therapy is necessary. Daily oral or intermittent intravenous pulse corticosteroid administration is often employed. In severe target organ disease, drugs such as cyclophosphamide, mycophenolate mofetil, or azathioprine may be necessary. In the future, biologic therapies (e.g., B-cell depletion) may offer additional benefits to patients with SLE.

DERMATOMYOSITIS

Epidemiology

Juvenile dermatomyositis (JDM) is a multisystem autoimmune disease predominantly involving skin and skeletal muscles. The gastrointestinal tract is less commonly involved. JDM is rare, with an annual incidence ~3:1,000,000. Girls are affected more commonly than boys, with age at presentation typically being between 5 and 10 years.

Pathogenesis

The primary disease process occurs in the small blood vessels (vasculopathy) and is humorally-mediated. Immune complex deposition, complement activation, and infiltration with CD4 lymphocytes in the musculature lead to subsequent capillary and muscle injury. The etiology of JDM is unclear but likely includes genetic and environmental factors. HLA B8/DR3 and HLA DQalpha1*0501 are associated with higher risk for disease. The condition seems to be associated with viral illnesses in some cases.

Differential Diagnosis

Polymyositis, an inflammatory muscular condition without skin findings, has a similar clinical presentation but is less common in children. The pathologic features are distinct from those of JDM; in polymyositis, CD8 lymphocytes infiltrate the muscle fascicles and attack muscle fibers directly.

Clinical Manifestations

History and Physical Examination

Since it predominantly affects the limb girdle musculature, JDM produces characteristic proximal muscle weakness with relative sparing of distal strength. Activities such as climbing stairs, doing sit-ups, and lifting the hands over the head become difficult. Patients often report a history of malaise, fatigue, weight loss, and intermittent fevers. The muscle weakness is accompanied by the pathognomonic **violaceous** dermatitis of the eyelids (heliotrope), hands, elbows, knees, and ankles. **Gottron papules** are characteristic lesions resembling scaly erythematous papules on the extensor surfaces of the metacarpophalangeal and interphalangeal joints of the fingers, the elbows, and the knees. Nailfold capillary changes are common. The weakness may advance to involve bulbar muscle groups used for swallowing and phonation. Longstanding inflammation eventually may result in calcium deposits in the skin and muscle (calcinosis cutis), scarring, and significant muscle atrophy.

Diagnostic Evaluation

The most striking laboratory abnormality is marked elevation of **serum creatine phosphokinase,** an enzyme released during muscle breakdown (as well as other muscle enzymes such as aldolase, aspartate aminotransferase, and lactic dehydrogenase). Von Willebrand factor is typically elevated, presumably secondary to active endothelial inflammation. MRI permits good visualization of muscle inflammation; electromyography is less frequently employed. Definitive diagnosis rests on characteristic muscle biopsy findings, including perivascular inflammatory infiltrate, perifascicular atrophy, loss of capillaries, focal necrosis, and muscle fiber regeneration.

Treatment

Treatment consists of pharmacologic management and physical therapy. The major component of the medical regimen is corticosteroid therapy, either in the form of daily oral prednisone or intermittent pulse (high-dose) methylprednisolone therapy. Corticosteroid-sparing agents such as methotrexate are often given from the onset of treatment. Important second-line agents include intravenous immunoglobulin (IVIG) and cyclosporine. Hydroxychloroquine is thought to be effective in treating the cutaneous manifestations of JDM. Physical therapy is essential and should be tailored to the individual patient based on disease activity and course. Early aggressive therapy with resultant decrease in muscle and skin inflammation within the first 6 months of the start of the disease may prevent subsequent development of calcinosis.

Prognosis

Patients with a limited (monocyclic) disease course generally have a good long-term outcome; those with a more chronic course may suffer from significant disability, especially if calcinosis develops. Spontaneous perforation of the bowel, although rare, is the leading cause of death.

OTHER CONNECTIVE TISSUE DISORDERS

Other connective tissue disorders are quite rare in childhood. Presentations are similar, and clinical differentiation may be difficult.

Systemic sclerosis is characterized by fibrous thickening of the skin (scleroderma), particularly involving the distal extremities and face, and fibrotic disease of internal organs (i.e., esophagus, intestinal tract, heart, lungs, kidneys). Early clinical findings include *Raynaud phenomenon*, the triphasic discoloration of the fingers and toes from white (ischemia) to purple (cyanosis) to red (reactive hyperemia), and *hand and foot edema*, which later progresses to frank sclerodactyly. Mortality risk is related to degree of cardiopulmonary involvement (pulmonary fibrosis), pulmonary arterial hypertension, and renal disease (systemic hypertension, renal failure).

Linear scleroderma and **morphea** are characterized by discrete areas of linear streaks (linear scleroderma) or patchy lesions (morphea). The affected skin initially appears erythematous, later becoming indurated, with thickening and hardening of the skin and underlying soft tissues. Internal organ disease is very rare. Disability can result if the sclerodermatous lesions occur over joints, involve the face, or are large enough to restrict growth.

Sjögren syndrome is characterized by the lymphocytic infiltration of exocrine glands, most commonly the salivary and lacrimal glands, resulting in dry mouth (*xerostomia*) and dry eyes (*xerophthalmia*). Affected individuals may develop chewing and swallowing difficulties and are at risk for severe dental caries. Insufficient tear production may lead to chronic corneal abrasions and resultant corneal scarring. Anti-Ro (SS-A) and anti-La (SS-B) antibodies are often detected. Secondary Sjögren syndrome may be a consequence of other connective tissue diseases.

PRIMARY SYSTEMIC VASCULITIS

Vasculitis is an inflammatory process of the vessel wall with resultant ischemia and necrosis. Apart from **Henoch-Schönlein purpura** and **Kawasaki disease,** *primary systemic vasculitides of the young are relatively rare.* In **Henoch-Schönlein purpura** (HSP), IgA-containing immune complexes are found within vessel walls. The annual incidence of HSP is approximately 1:5,000, but is as high as 1:1,400 in children 4 to 6 years of age. HSP is somewhat more common in boys. **Kawasaki disease** occurs in about 1:10,000 children annually in the United States, is more common in boys, and has a peak age of onset between 2 and 3 years of age.

Clinical Manifestations and Treatment

HSP typically presents with symptoms of skin, joint, gastrointestinal, and kidney disease. Incidence peaks in the winter months, and the condition is often preceded by an upper respiratory infection (most commonly group A *Streptococcus*). The classic rash consists of nonthrombocytopenic purpura localized to dependent areas of the body (lower extremities, buttocks). Distribution of the rash may be atypical (primarily facial) in children less than 2 years of age. Other common findings, particularly early in the disease, consist of scrotal edema and extremity swelling. When present, acute arthritis may be exquisitely painful, even rendering a child immobile. Gastrointestinal involvement is usually significant, including colicky abdominal pain, vomiting, and upper and lower tract bleeding. Bowel wall thickening and intussusception can occur. Glomerulonephritis is present in up to 40% of patients. It is usually mild; however, up to 5% of children with HSP-associated glomerulonephritis will develop end-stage renal disease. Demonstration of IgA deposition in the vessel wall by direct immunofluorescence is pathognomonic. HSP usually requires only supportive treatment. Spontaneous resolution occurs in the majority of patients in less than 4 weeks, although symptoms may persist for up to 12 weeks. Musculoskeletal pain responds to treatment with NSAIDs. Systemic glucocorticoids are reserved for severe gastrointestinal manifestations and significant renal involvement (which may require cyclophosphamide). Fifteen percent of patients experience recurrence of their disease.

The diagnosis of Kawasaki disease rests on the presence of guidelines established by the American Heart Association in 2004 (Table 13-6). The sequential (rather than simultaneous) appearance of disease manifestations may initially result in misdiagnosis. The disease progresses in phases. During the *acute phase* (first 1 to 2 weeks), the typical diagnostic features are accompanied by extreme irritability. Characteristic laboratory findings include leukocytosis, significantly elevated erythrocyte sedimentation rate and C-reactive protein, elevated liver transaminases, and sterile pyuria. Defervescence marks transition to the *subacute phase*, lasting several weeks. Clinical findings subside, but significant thrombocytosis carries a high risk for the development of coronary artery aneurysms; about 25% of untreated patients develop this complication. Aneurysms constitute the most significant cause of morbidity and mortality due to rupture or thrombosis. Current treatment recommendations consist of IVIG (2 g/kg) and high-dose aspirin therapy (80 to 100 mg/kg/day) in four divided doses during the acute stage, followed by low-dose aspirin therapy (3 to 5 mg/kg/day) until the end of the *convalescent phase* (several months later). IVIG typically results in rapid and profound improvement, and administration significantly reduces the risk of formation of coronary artery aneurysms. Repeated IVIG treatment may become necessary if fevers recur or persist. Second-line treatment regimens incorporate high-dose corticosteroids and possibly TNF inhibitors (infliximab). Anticoagulant therapy may be indicated in patients with documented coronary aneurysms.

TABLE 13-6 Clinical Criteria for Diagnosis of Kawasaki Disease

Fever persisting for 5 days or more, together with 4 of the following clinical criteria (by history or physical examination):
1. Changes in extremities • Acute (erythema of palms/soles, swelling of hands/feet) • Chronic (periungual peeling of fingers/toes)
2. Polymorphous exanthem
3. Bilateral bulbar conjunctival injection
4. Changes in lips and/or oral cavity (erythema, cracked lips; diffuse injection of oral mucosa)
5. Cervical lymphadenopathy >1.5 cm (usually unilateral)

PERIODIC FEVER SYNDROMES

The **periodic fever syndromes** (PFS) are frequently included in the rheumatic disease category. Mapping of the human genome in the late 1990s has led to the ability to define the majority of PFS as Mendelian genetic diseases of the innate immune system; thus they are a subset of the hereditary autoinflammatory disorders. The genetically-mutated proteins are linked to pathways of inflammation, apoptosis, and cytokine processing. Common to all PFS is fever that has an abrupt onset and termination and is identical in its presentation with each recurrence. The clinical onset of PFS is typically in childhood or adolescence, and patients are symptom free between attacks but may have subclinical inflammation. The white blood cell count (WBC), C-reactive protein (CRP), and erythrocyte sedimentation rate (ESR) are significantly elevated with fever attack and may remain slightly elevated in between attacks. Amyloidosis may result from chronic, untreated inflammation with any of the PFS. The PFS are distinct in their clinical presentation, ethnicity, inheritance and genetic defects. Thus, clinical history with patient fever diary, family history, ethnicity, and physcial examination are essential to assist in the diagnosis of PFS. A differential diagnosis of recurrent fevers should include the broad categories of infection, neoplasm, and noninfectious inflammatory disorders.

Familial Mediterranean Fever (FMF) is the most common PFS and can be seen worldwide but is concentrated in people of Arabic, Turkish, Armenian, non-Ashkenazi Jews and other Mediterranean populations such as Italians, Greeks and Lebanese. FMF is an autosomal recessive disorder with fevers that occur for 1 to 3 days every 4 to 8 weeks. Other common clinical features include peritonitis, erysipelas-like rash, and oligoarthritis. FMF results from a defect in the *MEFV* gene.

Tumor Necrosis Factor Receptor-associated Periodic Fever Syndrome (TRAPS) is an autosmal dominant disorder seen worldwide with fevers lasting 7 to 21 days and occurring 2 to 3 times per year. Abdominal pain, severe deep muscle aches with overlying erythema, conjunctivitis, periorbital edema and large joint arthritis are hallmarks of TRAPS. Genetic mutations are found in the gene that encodes for the TNF receptor (TNFRSF1A).

Periodic Fever, Apthous Stomatitis, Pharyngitis, Adenitis Syndrome (PFAPA) is a common fever syndrome for which no genetic mutation has been found. Specific diagnostic criteria include (1) three or more episodes of fever lasting no more than 5 days and occurring in regular intervals of 3 to 6 weeks with an early age of onset (typically younger than 5 years); (2) tender cervical lymphadenopathy, pharyngitis, or apthous ulcers; (3) exclusion of cyclic neutropenia or other fever syndromes; (4) normal WBC, CRP and ESR between attacks; and (5) normal growth and development.

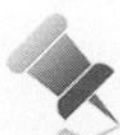

KEY POINTS

- Patients with cell-mediated immune dysfunction are susceptible to autoimmune disorders, intracellular organisms, and opportunistic infections from organisms such as *Pneumocystis jiroveci*.
- Persistent hypocalcemic tetany and/or congenital heart disease coupled with absence of the thymic shadow and cell-mediated immunodeficiency suggest chromosome 22q11 deletion (i.e., DiGeorge) syndrome.

(Continued)

- Humoral immunodeficiency predisposes patients to infection with encapsulated organisms. Common infections include otitis media, pneumonia, and sinusitis. Quantitative immunoglobulin studies and antibody titers against vaccine antigens are abnormal in patients with humoral immune dysfunction. Gammaglobulin therapy (intravenous or intramuscular) provides antibodies to patients with humoral immunodeficiency.
- Severe neutropenia, defined as an ANC $<0.5 \times 10^3/\mu L$, may result from infection, certain medications, circulating antineutrophil antibodies, malignancy, or bone marrow dysfunction. Typical signs of infection (erythema, warmth, swelling) are often absent in the presence of neutropenia.
- Chronic granulomatous disease (CGD) is characterized by chronic or recurrent infections due to catalase-producing bacteria or fungi. In particular, patients develop frequent skin infections and abscesses. The nitroblue tertrazolium test and the dihydrorhodamine reduction (DHR) test are laboratory studies which are useful for detecting CGD. Patients with CGD should receive daily prophylactic trimethoprim-sulfamethaxazole and periodicgamma-interferon.
- Allergic rhinitis may be seasonal or perennial. Nonsedating H_1-histamine blockers and nasal topical steroids are the mainstays of treatment. Peanuts, eggs, milk, soy, wheat, and fish account for the overwhelming majority of food allergies.
- Signs and symptoms of food allergy in infants include rash around the mouth, hives, irritability, diarrhea, and failure to thrive.
- Juvenile idiopathic arthritis is characterized by chronic synovitis and classified by the number and location of joints involved, physical findings, associated diseases or family history, and extra-articular manifestations.
- SLE consists of widespread connective tissue inflammation and vasculitis. The diagnosis of SLE is clinical. Lupus nephritis is the most common clinical manifestation, resulting in significant morbidity. Typical laboratory findings include falling complement levels, a positive antinuclear antibody titer, and a positive double-stranded DNA antibody titer.
- Dermatomyositis is an inflammatory disease of the skin, striated muscle, and occasionally the gastrointestinal tract. Weakness begins in the proximal extremity muscle groups and is accompanied by a characteristic violaceous dermatitis. Serum creatine kinase levels are markedly elevated.
- Henoch-Schönlein purpura is characterized by abdominal pain, vomiting, gastrointestinal bleeding, and palpable, nonthrombocytopenic purpura over dependent regions.
- Kawasaki disease presents with high fever, lymphadenopathy, and mucocutaneous lesions. High-dose IVIG reduces the risk of coronary artery aneurysms in Kawasaki disease.
- PFAPA is a common disorder and seen worldwide. FMF is also seen frequently in multiple but specific ethnic groups. The other PFS are rare, but mapping of the human genome and increased familiarity by the medical community is increasing the frequency of diagnosis. Amyloidosis is a serious long-term complication of chronic inflammation from the PFS.

C Clinical Vignettes

Vignette 1

A 6-year-old girl presents to your pediatric office with a chief complaint of nasal congestion and chronic rhinorrhea. She has had constant nasal congestion for over a year, but her symptoms have worsened now that it is summer and the windows are open. She has an unremitting postnasal drip and continually clears her throat. She is becoming increasingly drowsy because she awakens frequently at night. In addition, her snoring has increased. The physical examination reveals very boggy nasal mucosa and clear rhinorrhea. You are considering a diagnosis of allergic rhinitis.

1. Which of the following examination findings would NOT support a diagnosis of allergic rhinitis?
   a. Eczema
   b. Allergic shiners
   c. Allergic salute
   d. Palatal arching
   e. Urticaria for over 6 weeks

2. You decide to refer your patient to an allergist for direct skin testing for specific allergens. She tests positive to several allergens. You attempt to make a connection between the results of the testing and the fact that your patient has her worst symptoms in the summer. Which of the following associations is **incorrect**?
   a. Tree pollens are common in the early spring.
   b. Dust mites are most common in the fall.
   c. Ragweed season starts in the late summer and persist until the first frost.
   d. Molds are year-round allergens.
   e. Grass pollens are most likely to produce summertime symptoms.

3. You have determined that your patient has allergic rhinitis secondary to cat dander, dust mites, tree pollens, and grass pollens. You are ready to discuss risk factors for allergic rhinitis as well as your treatment recommendations with the parents. Which of the following statements potentially associated with allergic rhinitis education is false?
   a. The fact that both parents suffer from allergic rhinitis does not affect their daughter's risk of having allergic rhinitis.
   b. Nasal topical steroids are a very effective therapy with minimal side effects.
   c. Dust mite exposure can be limited by frequent washing and/or drying of bedding on high heat.
   d. Allergen immunotherapy is an effective therapy for cat dander allergy.
   e. Nonsedating antihistamines are available and are the mainstay of treatment of allergic rhinitis.

Vignette 2

A 15-year-old male is referred to your immunology clinic because he is "always sick" with respiratory and gastrointestinal infections. He did not have any infections during the first 6 months of his life. He attended day care from ages 1 to 5 years with 15 other children, then started kindergarten. During his attendance at day care, he had the usual viral infections but no more than his siblings or other day care attendees. Since the age of 12 years, he has been frequently diagnosed with otitis media, sinusitis, tonsillitis, and intermittent diarrhea. During the past year, he has been hospitalized twice with pneumonia. The first lung infection was caused by *Hemophilus influenza B*; the second was caused by *Streptococcus pneumoniae.* He is up to date on all of his immunizations including vaccination against HiB (*Hemophilus influenza B*). In addition, he received the 7-valent Prevnar vaccination at his 2-year and 5-year health maintenance visits. In the past 6 months, he has lost 5 pounds. Recent studies of his diarrheal stools demonstrated the protozoan parasite *Giardia lamblia*. Physical examination reveals an underweight, pale-appearing teenage male. He has normal tonsils and normal lymph nodes but a mildly enlarged spleen. You are concerned about an immunodeficiency and decide to order some additional studies.

1. Which of the following aspects of this patient's case would NOT support limiting testing to diseases affecting only the humoral system?
   a. No infections during the first 6 months of life
   b. Viral infections while at day care
   c. Pneumonia with encapsulated pyogenic organisms
   d. Infections with organisms against which he has been previously immunized
   e. Frequent gastrointestinal infections including *Giardia lamblia*

2. Which of the following tests is *least* likely to give you information about a patient's humoral immune system?
   a. T and B lymphocyte subpopulations
   b. Quantitative immunoglobulins (IgG, IgA, IgM)

c. Delayed hypersensitivity skin testing
d. Specific antibody testing for *Hemophilus influenza B*
e. Ability to produce antibodies following immunization with *Streptococcus pneumoniae*

3. Your patient's test results confirm a diagnosis of common variable immunodeficiency. You prepare to discuss the results with the patient and his parents. Which of the following statements is FALSE?
   a. This patient is not at increased risk for autoimmune disorders or malignancies.
   b. This patient's B cells are unable to produce antibodies needed to help protect against encapsulated organisms.
   c. This patient's treatment should include replacement therapy with intravenous immunoglobulins (IVIG).
   d. The onset of CVID is most common in late adolescence and early adulthood.
   e. The incidence of CVID is equal in males and females.

Vignette 3

A 3-year-old boy presents to your urgent care center with an 8-day history of high fevers, rash, red eyes, persistent crying, refusal to walk, and decreased oral intake. He goes to day care, so his mother thought that he had "caught a virus" from another child. Upon arrival to urgent care, the nurse informs you that he has a fever of 104.5°F. On physical examination, he is difficult to console and appears uncomfortable. His conjunctivae are injected but without any drainage. He has cracked, red lips, and a red tongue. He has a few enlarged, tender left cervical lymph nodes, with the largest lymph node measuring 2 cm in diameter. His heart examination is normal except for tachycardia, and his lungs are clear to auscultation. His abdomen is nontender, and you do not appreciate any organomegaly or masses. He has diffuse, tender swelling of the hands and feet and an irregular erythematous rash on his trunk and extremities. You are concerned that he may have Kawasaki disease.

1. You recall that Henoch-Schönlein Purpura (HSP) is another systemic vasculitis that occurs in children and consider adding it to your differential diagnosis. Which of the following statements is true?
   a. Kawasaki disease and HSP are equally common in the United States.
   b. The peak ages for Kawasaki disease and HSP are identical.
   c. HSP is characterized by a persistent, high fever.
   d. The rash is similar in both conditions.
   e. Gastrointestinal involvement in HSP is severe and may lead to intussusception.

2. You decide to order some laboratory tests to evaluate your suspicion of Kawasaki disease. Which of the following laboratory results would not support a diagnosis of Kawasaki disease?
   a. Elevated white blood cell count
   b. Normal erythrocyte sedimentation rate (ESR)
   c. Elevated liver transaminases
   d. White blood cells in the urine with a negative urine culture
   e. Elevated platelet count

3. You review this child's clinical findings and determine that he meets the fever requirement (fever for at least 5 days) and has all 5 of the clinical criteria for Kawasaki disease: extremity changes (swelling of the hands and feet), polymorphous exanthem, bilateral bulbar conjunctival injection, lip/oral cavity changes (cracked, red lips and strawberry tongue), and cervical lymphadenopathy > 1.5 cm. All of his laboratory results are also consistent with Kawasaki disease. You decide to initiate treatment for Kawasaki disease with IVIG at 2 gm/kg and aspirin therapy. What major complication of Kawasaki disease are you attempting to avoid with these therapies?
   a. Peeling of the skin of the fingers and toes
   b. Glomerulonephritis
   c. Coronary artery aneurysm
   d. Amyloidosis
   e. None of the above

Vignette 4

A mother brings her 3-year-old daughter to your office for evaluation of left knee swelling. The child's symptoms began approximately 30 days ago with morning stiffness that initially lasted 30 minutes. However, she now limps all day. The review of symptoms is negative for fevers, rash, sore throat, pain, gastrointestinal symptoms, or recent infectious illnesses. The patient's vital signs are within normal limits. Physical examination reveals a well-appearing child with a swollen left knee and ankle. The joints are not erythematous but are warm to the touch, have decreased range of motion, and are tender to palpation. The child has a flexion contracture of the left knee and walks with a limp, but the remainder of the examination is normal. A radiograph of the left knee demonstrates mild soft tissue swelling and effusion without osseous abnormalities. Laboratory testing reveals mild elevation of C-reactive protein (CRP) and the erythrocyte sedimentation rate (ESR). You formulate a differential diagnosis and consider Oligoarticular Juvenile Idiopathic Arthritis (JIA) as a potential diagnosis.

1. Which of the following characteristics of this case would be **least** compatible with a diagnosis of Oligoarticular JIA?
   a. Absence of significant joint pain
   b. Mild elevation of CRP and ESR
   c. Joint swelling for less than 6 weeks' duration
   d. Onset before age 16 years
   e. Arthritis involving 4 or fewer joints

2. Although this patient does not have overt evidence of eye disease, you explain to the patient's mother that an ophthalmologic slit lamp examination is necessary to rule out uveitis. Which of the following laboratory tests would be most helpful in assessing this patient's risk for development of chronic anterior nongranulomatous uveitis?
   a. Rheumatoid factor (RF)
   b. Antinuclear antibody (ANA)
   c. HLA-B27
   d. Serum ferritin
   e. White blood cell count

3. Which of the following statements regarding physical examination findings in juvenile idiopathic arthritis is **FALSE**?
   a. Long-standing arthritis can lead to limb-length discrepancy.
   b. Patients with systemic JIA often have an evanescent salmon-colored rash.
   c. Dactylitis is a common finding across JIA subtypes.
   d. Achilles tendon insertion tenderness is often present in patients with enthesitis-related arthritis.
   e. Rheumatoid factor-positive patients have symmetric polyarthritis of small joints.

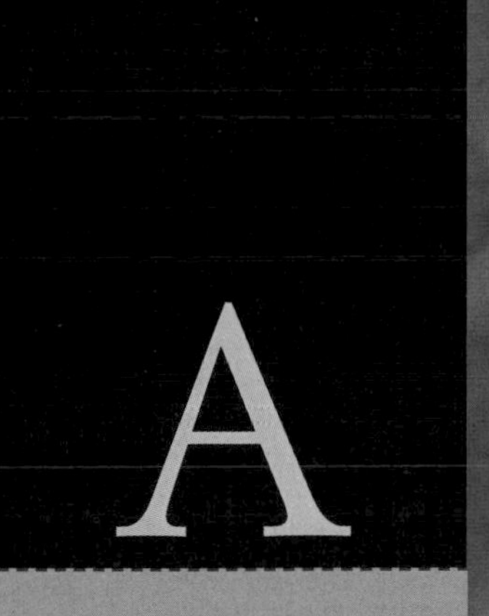

Answers

Vignette 1 Question 1

Answer E: Urticaria that lasts for more than 6 weeks is classified as "chronic urticaria" and is not an IgE-mediated process. Urticaria that develops immediately following exposure to an allergen is most likely IgE-mediated and may accompany allergic rhinitis. Urticaria for 6 weeks is not associated with allergic rhinitis. Eczema may present in infancy or early childhood as the first sign of atopic (allergic) tendencies/illness. The progression of eczema followed by allergic rhinitis which in turn is followed by asthma is known as the **allergic march. Allergic shiners** are dark circles that develop under the eyes secondary to venous congestion and are frequently seen in children with allergic rhinitis. The **allergic salute** is a horizontal crease across the middle of the nose due to the constant upward wiping motion of the nose with the hand. The allergic salute is a hallmark of allergic rhinitis. Severe nasal congestion in patients with allergic rhinitis may lead to obligate mouth breathing; palatal arching may be seen on physical examination as a result.

Vignette 1 Question 2

Answer B: Dust mites, pet dander, and molds are known as **perennial** allergens; all generally produce year-round symptoms. Of note, it is unusual to be allergic to pine trees (i.e., Christmas trees); rather, the mold on the tree produces the allergic symptoms. Rinsing off the tree and letting it dry prior to putting it in the house may prevent allergic symptoms. The other answers contain correct associations. Tree pollens are detected in early spring; followed by grass pollens in late spring and summer; followed by ragweed in late summer until the first frost. The patient's symptoms worsen in the summer, when grass pollens are most prominent. Having air conditioning that would allow the windows to be kept closed would assist in limiting exposure to grass pollens.

Vignette 1 Question 3

Answer A: Parental history of allergic rhinitis is positively associated with the development of allergic rhinitis. Allergen avoidance is the most effective treatment. Dust mites need humans, moisture, and warmth for survival. Hence, high concentrations of dust mites reside in mattresses and bedding. Dust mite covers for mattresses and pillows, and washing or drying bedding on high heat to destroy dust mites, are excellent avoidance measures. It is very difficult for patients and families to give up their pets. In addition, pet owners expose others to animal dander from their clothing on a daily basis. Thus, eliminating the pet from the home will not totally eliminate exposure. Allergen immunotherapy is an effective therapy and reasonable choice for this patient. Topical nasal steroids are safe and effective in the treatment of allergic rhinitis if administered correctly. The nasal steroid inhaler should be directed away from the nasal septum and every effort should be made not to sniff following administration. Even topical steroids may inhibit linear growth. Thus, frequent height measurements should be obtained in patients using inhaled corticosteroids long term. There are a growing number of nonsedating antihistamines for use in the treatment of allergic rhinitis. Many of these agents are now available without prescription.

Vignette 2 Question 1

Answer B: It is common for healthy children to have frequent viral infections when exposed to other children with similar illnesses. Serious viral infections are much more common in children with deficiencies in cellular immunity, as T cells are required to destroy viruses. Prior to 6 months of age, infants are protected by humoral immunity from the mother. IgG crosses the placenta from mother to child and is protective until approximately 6 months of age. Thus, it is not surprising that the patient did not have any infections prior to 6 months of age. A deficiency in cellular or phagocytic immunity would likely lead to infections prior to 6 months of age. Humoral immunity is required for protection against encapsulated organisms such as *Hemophilus influenza B* and *Streptococcus pneumoniae*. Antibodies produced in the humoral immune system serve as opsonins, activating complement to prepare encapsulated organisms for killing. Patients with deficiencies of the humoral immune system lack these protective antibodies even if they have been immunized against these organisms (as seen in this patient). Isolated IgA deficiency is the most common immune deficiency, defined by a serum IgA level of less than 5 mg/dl. IgA deficiency is common to all the humoral immune deficiencies. Frequent gastrointestinal infections, including *Giardia lamblia*, are common in patients with IgA deficiency.

Vignette 2 Question 2

Answer C: Positive results on delayed hypersensitivity skin testing to *Candida* and other infectious agents that humans are commonly exposed to is a measure of cell-mediated immunity. This test would be normal in patients with a disorder affecting exclusively humoral immunity. Lymphocyte sub-populations are a useful test when evaluating deficiencies of the humoral immune system. Patients with X-linked agammaglobulinemia will have very low levels of B cells. Patients with common variable immunodeficiency (CVID) may have normal levels of B cells. Quantitative immunoglobulin testing is required to confirm and help differentiate among humoral immune deficiencies. Levels of immunoglobulins may be only modestly decreased in CVID, but affected patients lack antibodies to infectious agents that they have been immunized against and cannot produce antibodies following a vaccination. Studies for these specific deficiencies are confirmatory tests for the diagnosis of CVID.

Vignette 2 Question 3

Answer A: Patients with CVID are at increased risk of developing autoimmune diseases such as autoimmune thyroiditis, hemolytic anemia, autoimmune thrombocytopenia, and pernicious anemia. In addition, CVID patients have a 300-fold increased risk of lymphoma and a 50-fold increase in risk of gastric carcinoma. Onset of CVID may occur in early childhood but is most common during adolescence or young adulthood. The incidence is equally distributed between males and females. Replacement therapy with IVIG is required to help protect against infections with encapsulated organisms that may be life-threatening in patients with CVID.

Vignette 3 Question 1

Answer E: Henoch-Schönlein Purpura (HSP) is a systemic small vessel vasculitis that affects the skin, joints, kidneys, and gastrointestinal (GI) tract. The GI tract involvement is prominent and may manifest with abdominal pain, vomiting, and GI tract bleeding. Bowel wall thickening occurs, with occasional subsequent intussusception. The annual incidence of HSP in the United States is 1:5,000, which is more common than Kawasaki disease (annual U.S. incidence ~ 1:10,000). The two vasculitides also have slightly different peak ages, with HSP occurring more commonly in children between ages 4 and 6, and Kawasaki disease occurring more commonly in children 2 to 3 years of age. Persistent, high fever is a key disease manifestation of Kawasaki disease, but not HSP. The classic rash associated with HSP is palpable purpura localized to dependent areas of the body, such as the lower extremities and buttocks. In children less than 2 years of age, the rash may be atypical and involve the face. In contrast, the rash in Kawasaki disease is more variable and is often described as a polymorphic exanthem that involves the trunk and extremities.

Vignette 3 Question 2

Answer B: The erythrocyte sedimentation rate (ESR) in Kawasaki disease is significantly elevated, along with an elevated C-reactive protein. Elevated white blood cell count (leukocytosis), elevated platelet count (thrombocytosis), elevated liver transaminases, and white blood cells in the urine with a negative urine culture (sterile pyuria) are all characteristic laboratory findings for Kawasaki disease.

Vignette 3 Question 3

Answer C: Approximately 25% of untreated Kawasaki disease patients develop coronary artery aneurysms. Thrombocytosis related to Kawasaki disease is associated with a high risk of subsequent aneurysms. Aneurysms constitute the most significant cause of morbidity and mortality, due to rupture or thrombosis. In addition to IVIG, high-dose aspirin therapy in the acute stage and low-dose aspirin in the convalescent phase constitute the "standard of care" treatment regimen. Peeling of the skin of the fingers and toes occurs during the course of Kawasaki disease; however, it does not lead to major complications. Glomerulonephritis can be a serious complication of Henoch-Schönlein Purpura (HSP). It is present in up to 40% of HSP patients, and up to 5% of those patients will develop end-stage renal disease. Amyloidosis is a major complication of several of the periodic fever syndromes, and it is related to chronic, untreated inflammation, but not Kawasaki disease.

Vignette 4 Question 1

Answer C: Absence of significant joint pain is typical of JIA. For unknown reasons, children with JIA do not complain of joint pain, even in the setting of obvious joint swelling. Severe joint pain is a red flag that should alert the clinician to consider alternate etiologies such as infection and malignancy. Oligoarthritis patients typically have mild elevation of CRP and ESR; however, these tests can also be normal. A marked acute phase reaction is atypical and should prompt workup for an alternate diagnosis such as infection. Diagnostic criteria for JIA require patients to have objective findings compatible with arthritis for at least 6 weeks' duration. Alternative etiologies in the differential diagnosis that cause arthritis, particularly reactive or postinfectious arthritis, generally resolve within this time frame. The presence of a flexion contracture indicates that this patient has likely had arthritis for longer than the reported 30 days, as this finding is more consistent with long-standing disease. Onset before age 16 years is required to bestow the diagnosis of JIA. The number of affected joints helps differentiate oligoarthritis from polyarthritis. Oligoarticular arthritis affects 4 or fewer joints in the first 6 months of disease, whereas with polyarticular JIA 5 or more joints are affected. Large joints such as the knee and ankle are more commonly affected in oligoarthritis.

Vignette 4 Question 2

Answer B: Rheumatoid factor is an autoantibody directed against a portion of the IgG molecule; it is not associated with an increased risk of anterior uveitis. RF occurs in ~5% of JIA patients and, when present, is more common with polyarticular JIA. RF is considered a poor prognostic indicator regarding overall disease severity and likelihood of persistence into adulthood. Antinuclear antibody is detected in up to 75% of patients with oligoarticular JIA. ANA-positive patients are at increased risk of developing uveitis, which occurs in up to one-third of patients with this type of juvenile arthritis. Because the uveitis is often asymptomatic, patients that are ANA-positive require more frequent slit-lamp examinations to avoid the development of visual impairment and blindness that can occur with untreated disease. HLA-B27 is associated with enthesitis-related arthritis and spondyloarthritis. Affected patients can have anterior uveitis, but it is generally acute rather than chronic, and these patients are often symptomatic, with red painful eyes. Other human leukocyte antigen (HLA) types have been associated with an increased risk of oligoarticular JIA, but not uveitis. Ferritin can be quite elevated in patients with systemic JIA but is not associated with increased risk of iridocyclitis. It is not common for patients with oligoarticular JIA to have a significantly elevated ferritin. The white blood cell count is normal in patients with oligoarticular JIA.

Vignette 4 Question 3

Answer C: Long-standing arthritis can lead to limb-length discrepancy, with the affected limb longer than the unaffected. The presence of joint inflammation leads to increased blood flow to the growth plates of the affected joint, which in turn leads to stimulation of bone growth. This is a common finding in untreated patients with oligoarticular arthritis affecting the knee. Other common physical examination findings in long standing arthritis include joint contractures and muscle atrophy of the affected limb. Patients with systemic JIA often have an evanescent salmon-colored rash, particularly when febrile. Rashes are not commonly found in other subtypes of arthritis. The rash of systemic JIA is generally more prominent during fever episodes and can be missed if not examined in the setting of a fever. Other physical examination findings in these patients can include toxic appearance, arthritis, hepatosplenomegaly, and serositis. Dactylitis is not a common finding across JIA subtypes. Dactylitis, when present, is pathognomonic for psoriatic arthritis. This is commonly referred to as a "sausage digit," and it occurs due to flexor tendon tenosynovitis. Findings of nail pitting or onycholysis may be subtle in patients with psoriatic arthritis. Achilles tendon insertion tenderness is often present in patients with enthesitis-related arthritis. Enthesitis is inflammation and tenderness at the insertion site of tendons to bone. Common sites of tenderness in enthesitis-related arthritis patients include the Achilles tendon, plantar fascia, patellar tendon, and anterior superior iliac spines. Rheumatoid factor-positive patients have symmetric polyarthritis of small joints. RF-positive JIA resembles adult rheumatoid arthritis with a predominantly distal, symmetric arthritis of the small joints including the fingers, wrists, and hands.

Chapter

14 Endocrinology

Deborah Elder • Bradley S. Marino

OVERVIEW

The endocrine system is a system of glands, each of which secretes a type of hormone directly into the bloodstream to regulate the body. Hormones are substances (chemical mediators) released from endocrine tissue into the bloodstream where they travel to target tissue and generate a response. The pituitary gland is considered the master gland and signals other tissue in a specific sequence referred to as an axis. Hormones are often regulated in a feedback loop. The pituitary gland is composed of an anterior and posterior gland. The anterior pituitary gland secretes growth hormone (GH), luteinizing hormone (LH), follicle-stimulating hormone (FSH), prolactin, thyroid-stimulating hormone, and adrenocorticotropic hormone. The posterior pituitary gland consists of axons from neurons with cell bodies in the periventricular nuclei of the hypothalamus. The posterior pituitary gland does not produce hormones. Alternatively, the posterior pituitary hormones arginine vasopressin and oxytocin are synthesized in the hypothalamus and transported along these neurons. Hormones act by binding to specific receptors in the target organ. Hormones regulate various human functions, including growth and development, reproduction, and regulation of metabolism. Hormones are classified based on their chemical composition (amines, proteins, or steroids).

DIABETES MELLITUS

Diabetes mellitus (DM) is a group of metabolic diseases in which a person has high blood sugar most commonly due to either a deficiency of insulin (type 1 diabetes) or a resistance to insulin (type 2 diabetes). The classical symptoms due to the high serum glucose concentration are polyuria (frequent urination), polydipsia (excessive thirst), and polyphagia (increased hunger). Other forms of diabetes include gestational diabetes, congenital diabetes due to genetic defects of insulin secretion, cystic fibrosis–related diabetes, steroid-induced diabetes, and several forms of monogenic diabetes.

TYPE 1 DIABETES MELLITUS

Pathogenesis

Type 1 diabetes mellitus (T1DM) is characterized by autoimmune destruction of pancreatic beta-cells resulting in absent or diminished insulin secretion. T1DM accounts for 10% of all diabetes cases diagnosed.

The overall prevalence of T1DM is 0.25% to 0.5% of the population or 1/400 children and 1/200 adults in the United States. Peak age of onset is 10 to 12 years, but the disease may be diagnosed in children less than 1 year of age. Males and females are equally affected. The presence of anti-islet cell antibodies in 85% of individuals with recent-onset DM and the increased incidence of other autoimmune diseases in children with T1DM suggest an autoimmune etiology. There is a 50% concordance rate among identical twins. Although the precise trigger of T1DM is unknown, genetic, autoimmune, and environmental factors have all been implicated.

The absence of insulin causes a catabolic state due to impaired glucose entry into many cell types and subsequent impairment of cellular actions. The cells are in a starvation state and the body utilizes alternative fuel sources (fat, protein) through the access of gluconeogenesis, lipolysis, and proteolysis. In addition, stress hormones such as epinephrine, cortisol, and GH further up regulate gluconeogenesis. The production of ketoacids is brought about by an increase in lipolysis, fatty acid release, and ketoacid synthesis. When the blood glucose concentration exceeds 180 mg/dL, the resultant glycosuria causes an osmotic diuresis with increased urine output (polyuria). If insulin deficiency is severe, ketones are produced in significant quantities, the blood's native buffering capacity is overwhelmed, and diabetic ketoacidosis (DKA) results with severe dehydration, acidosis, electrolytes abnormalities, and potentially fatal consequences such as coma and death. In addition to DKA, the other major complication seen in T1DM is hypoglycemia from insulin overdose, decreased caloric intake, or increased exercise without a concomitant increase in calories. The only treatment for type 1 diabetes is insulin replacement.

Clinical Manifestations

History and Physical Examination

A history of new-onset weight loss, polydipsia, polyphagia, and polyuria suggests T1DM. The physical examination is generally normal in T1DM unless DKA is present. When DKA is suspected in a child with known T1DM, important historical information includes compliance with insulin therapy, the child's diet over the previous day, and whether the child has been ill and emotionally or physically stressed. The child with DKA appears acutely ill and suffers from moderate to profound dehydration. Symptoms include polyuria, polydipsia, fatigue, headache, nausea, emesis, and abdominal pain. The child's mental status may vary from confused to comatose. On physical examination, tachycardia and hyperpnea (Kussmaul respirations) are generally noted. There may be a fruity odor to the breath because of the ketosis. Intravascular volume depletion may be so marked that hypotension is present. Although cerebral edema is uncommon, it frequently is fatal. Changing mental status, unequal pupils, decorticate or decerebrate posturing, and/or seizures indicate cerebral edema. Early identification and aggressive management of increased intracranial pressure is pivotal to improve outcome. Symptoms of hypoglycemia or insulin toxicity are caused by catecholamine release (trembling, diaphoresis, flushing, and tachycardia) and to cerebral glucopenia (sleepiness, confusion, mood changes, seizures, and coma).

Diagnostic Evaluation

Symptoms suggestive of hyperglycemia, the presence of glucosuria, ketonuria, and a random plasma glucose level greater than 200 mg/dL are consistent with a diagnosis of diabetes mellitus. If early diabetes is suspected, a 2-hour postprandial blood glucose concentration is the first value to become abnormal. A fasting blood glucose concentration greater than 126 mg/dL and a 2-hour postprandial blood glucose concentration after an oral glucose tolerance test greater than 200 mg/dL are suggestive of diabetes. Islet cell antibodies in the serum may be found in 85% of new-onset insulin-dependent diabetics. Poorly controlled diabetics have high levels of glycosylated hemoglobin (HbA1c). Recently, an elevated HbA1c can be used for diagnostic purposes in the adult population. In children with suspected DKA, the serum glucose concentration is grossly elevated, and the venous pH and serum PCO_2 are low. The response to metabolic acidosis is a compensatory respiratory alkalosis and a drop in serum PCO_2. Because of the osmotic diuresis, blood urea nitrogen is elevated, and there is loss of phosphate, calcium, and potassium. Although there is a total body loss of potassium, serum potassium may be low, normal, or even high depending on the level of acidosis. When acidosis is present, protons move from the extracellular space to the intracellular space and potassium moves from the intracellular space to the extracellular space to maintain electroneutrality. Until the catabolic state is reversed with insulin, the urine is positive for ketones; until the serum concentration of glucose falls below 180 mg/dL, the urine is positive for glucose.

Treatment

The immediate goals of treatment of new-onset DM and DKA are reversal of the catabolic state through exogenous insulin therapy and restoration of fluid and electrolyte balances. DKA is a medical emergency. Initial fluid resuscitation consists of administering normal saline or a lactated Ringer solution of 10 mL/kg intravenous bolus. While the fluid bolus is running in, the total fluid deficit is calculated based on the amount of dehydration. The fluid deficit should be replaced over a 48-hour period. The level of hyperglycemia is assessed, and an insulin drip is started at 0.1 unit/kg/hr. The goal is to decrease the serum glucose 50 to 100 mg/dL/hr. A glucose level that falls too quickly could precipitate cerebral edema. When serum glucose approaches 250 to 300 mg/dL, dextrose should be added to normal saline and the electrolyte solution to avoid hypoglycemia. Hyperglycemia, acidosis, and ketone production correct with insulin therapy. Until there is adequate insulin, the body will continue to produce ketoacids. Frequent monitoring of blood glucose level, electrolytes, and acid–base status is crucial.

The child with T1DM is treated through insulin replacement, diet, exercise, psychological support, and regular medical follow-up. Patient education has a vital role. Current therapy requires frequent blood glucose monitoring and carbohydrate counting. The patient learns how to tailor insulin dosing based on the glucose level and the current meal. The newly diagnosed diabetic requires 0.5 to 1.0 units/kg of insulin per day. Most diabetics take insulin four to six times a day. Conventional therapy utilizes doses where two-thirds of the total daily dose is given before breakfast and one-third before dinner and bedtime. The human insulin is divided between short-acting Humalog insulin and intermediate-acting neutral protamine Hagedorn (NPH) insulin. More families are utilizing "Basal-Bolus" methods of insulin administration where a basal insulin is administered (Glargine or levimir) once each day and short-acting insulin (Lispro, Aspart) is given prior to carbohydrate consumption. This allows for a more flexible meal plan and schedule. Insulin pump therapy is available to deliver a basal amount of insulin throughout the day, with bolus doses of short-acting insulin given at mealtimes. At times of medical, surgical, or emotional stress, additional insulin may be needed. Glycosylated hemoglobin levels should be monitored every 3 months to assess average glycemic control. If hypoglycemia occurs, a child may ingest a carbohydrate snack to increase the serum glucose concentration. If the child is vomiting, instant glucose or cake icing may be applied to the buccal mucosa to provide glucose. If the child is having a seizure, intravenous glucose or intramuscular glucagon to release hepatic glucose stores should be given immediately.

Prognosis

The Diabetes Control and Complications Trial demonstrated that intensive management and tight glycemic control reduces the risk of diabetes complications by 50% to 75%. Complications from diabetes include microvascular disease of the eye (retinopathy), kidney (nephropathy), and nerves (neuropathy). Microvascular disease is generally not observed until the child has been insulin dependent for a minimum of 10 years. Accelerated large vessel atherosclerotic disease may lead to myocardial infarction or stroke. Diabetic children should have annual urine collections to screen for microalbuminuria, annual ophthalmologic examinations, and annual screening for hyperlipidemia. Patients with T1DM are at heightened risk to develop other autoimmune diseases, most frequently Hashimoto's thyroiditis and/or celiac disease. These autoimmue diseases are screened for periodically in a patient with T1DM.

TYPE 2 DIABETES MELLITUS

Pathogenesis

Type 2 diabetes mellitus (T2DM) is a polygenic condition that results from relative insulin resistance and beta-cell dysfunction. This insulin resistance initially causes a compensatory increase in insulin secretion; however, with time there is a progressive decline in glucose-stimulated insulin secretion.

Epidemiology

T2DM now accounts for 10% to 40% of newly diagnosed diabetes in adolescents. The increasing incidence parallels the high prevalence of obesity. Most cases occur during early adolescence around the onset of puberty. Prevalence is highest in Native Americans (PIMA Indians), African Americans, and Hispanics but is seen in all ethnic groups. Genetic susceptibility is important; however, environmental factors including obesity, physical inactivity, and diet, play a major role.

History and Physical Examination

Many patients are asymptomatic at presentation. Others may have symptoms similar to those of T1DM. There is usually a positive family history. On physical examination, obesity is noted, with a body mass index (BMI) usually greater than 30 kg/m^2. Often associated with T2DM is acanthosis nigricans, a skin condition involving hyperpigmentation and thickening of the skin folds, found primarily on the back of the neck and flexor areas.

Treatment

Currently, the mainstay of treatment if metabolic derangement is present is insulin therapy. In addition to medical therapy, lifestyle changes in diet and exercise are particularly important. Metformin a biguanide is the only approved oral hypoglycemic agent used for the treatment of T2DM in children older than 10 years. There is not yet any clarity as to the extent and severity of complication of T2DM in children and adolescents. More research is needed in this area.

HYPOGLYCEMIA

The definition of hypoglycemia is a plasma glucose value of less than 50 mg/dL or a whole blood glucose level less than 60 mg/dL.

Etiology

Hypoglycemia may result from (1) hyperinsulinism (congenital, insulinoma, exogenous administration of insulin or insulin-secreting agents); (2) ketotic hypoglycemia (childhood, age 18 months to 5 years, intolerance of fasting states, ketonuria usually present); (3) hormone deficiency (ACTH with or without GH deficiency); (4) glycogen storage disease (glucose 6-phosphatase deficiency); (5) disorders of gluconeogenesis (hereditary fructose intolerance, fructose 1,6-diphosphatase deficiency); and/or (6) defects in fatty acid oxidation.

Clinical Manifestation

Features of hypoglycemia can be classified into two categories. The first is activation of the autonomic nervous system causing a release of epinephrine, which manifests symptoms of sweating, shakiness, tachycardia, and anxiety. The second is of neuroglucopenic origin, resulting in headaches, visual disturbances, lethargy, irritability, mental confusion, loss of consciousness, and/or coma.

Evaluation

During a hypoglycemia event the circulating levels of certain hormones and other biomarkers of fuels can assess the integrity of the metabolic and hormonal systems. It is essential to obtain a "critical sample" when the plasma glucose level is less than 50 mg/dL. The critical sample should assess a chemistry panel with bicarbonate, insulin, c-peptide, cortisol, GH, free fatty acids, beta-hydroxybutyrate, acetoacetate, lactate, and ammonia. A comparison of expected normal values to the critical sample is necessary to determine the etiology of hypoglycemia. In the fasting state of a normal individual, it would be expected for glycogen stores to be depleted and levels of gluconeogenic substrates, free fatty acids, and beta-hydroxybutyrate (the major ketone body) to rise significantly. GH and cortisol will be up-regulated during a fast and certainly elevated during a hypoglycemic event. Insulin levels should then decline to undetectable levels (<2 units/mL). Total and free carnitine, acyl carnitine profile, and serum amino acids should be collected in a nonfasting state.

Infants and children are more susceptible to hypoglycemia than adults and cannot tolerate a prolonged fast. Thirty percent of normal infants who undergo a 6-hour fast will have hypoglycemia. Other risk factors in the newborn period for hypoglycemia include small for gestational age, stress (trauma, asphyxia, sepsis, or cold exposure). Infants of a diabetic mother are at risk for postnatal hypoglycemia. These infants are exposed to intrauterine hyperglycemia and after delivery the glucose source is normalized but resultant endogenous hyper insulin from beta-cell hyperplasia remains hours to a few days after delivery.

Treatment

After the critical sample is obtained, administration of IV glucose is indicated followed by continuous IV infusion of dextrose containing fluids. Long-term management will depend to the etiology of the hypoglycemia.

DISORDERS OF WATER REGULATION

NORMAL VASOPRESSIN REGULATION

Arginine vasopressin is human antidiuretic hormone. It is produced in the periventricular and supra optic nuclei of the hypothalamus. Vasopressin is transported along neurons from these nuclei and terminates in the posterior pituitary gland. An osmotic sensor in located near the supra optic nuclei and detects changes in osmolality as small as 1% to 2%. An increase in osmolality due to dehydration triggers the release of vasopressin signaling the kidney to retain water. Vasopressin has two biological effects: It increases permeability of the collecting duct of the nephron to water and stimulated arterial muscle contraction which increases blood pressure.

DIABETES INSIPIDUS

In central diabetes insipidus, there is loss of arginine vasopressin release (antidiuretic hormone) from the posterior pituitary gland, which results in an inability to concentrate the urine. Diabetes insipidus may occur after head trauma, the presence of any hypothalamic–pituitary tumor or central nervous system (CNS) infection. Histiocytosis X is an infiltrative disease that can cause diabetes insipidus. Most common brain tumors in the pediatric population resulting in DI are craniopharyngiomas or germinomas. Only rarely is diabetes insipidus an isolated idiopathic disorder.

Clinical Manifestations

The child with diabetes insipidus has abrupt-onset polydipsia and polyuria. If water intake is inadequate, severe dehydration and hypernatremia occur. If the cause of the diabetes insipidus is a brain tumor impinging on the pituitary gland, focal neurologic signs and visual abnormalities may be noted. The increased urine output may reach 5 to 10 L/day, with a urine specific gravity and urine osmolality that are quite low. Over time, serum sodium and serum osmolality increase as hemoconcentration occurs from free water loss. In unclear cases, the water deprivation test is used to diagnose diabetes insipidus. To establish a diagnosis of diabetes insipidus, one must have dilute urine (specific gravity < 1.010) and urine osmolality <300 mOsm/kg in the setting of hyper tonicity (hypernatremia and plasma osmolality > 295 mOsm/kg). Demonstration of antidiuretic hormone (ADH) secretion is critical in differentiating ADH-deficient (central) diabetes insipidus from nephrogenic diabetes insipidus, a rare X-linked recessive disease in which the collecting ducts do not respond to ADH.

Treatment

Desmopressin acetate (DDAVP), an ADH analogue, is given intranasally, subcutaneously, or orally to stimulate the kidneys to retain water and reverse the polyuria, polydipsia, and hypernatremia.

SYNDROME OF INAPPROPRIATE SECRETION OF VASOPRESSIN

Syndrome of hyponatremia with inappropriate increased secretion of vasopressin (SIADH) is observed in the presence of vasopressin and excessive water intake resulting in an expansion of intravascular volume with a subsequent dilution effect of Na and serum osmolality. The syndrome is often iatrogenic as a result of excessive IV fluids. SAIDH may be identified in children with encephalitis, brain tumors, head trauma, or psychiatric disease. Many drugs are capable of interfering with free water clearance (lisinopril, carbamazepine, tricyclic antidepressants, and many anticancer drugs). Children with tuberculous meningitis and SIADH have a particularly poor prognosis, as do those with liver failure and SIADH.

Clinical Manifestations

Patients present with normovolemic hyponatremia, relatively concentrated urine, and normal renal, thyroid, and adrenal function. Symptoms are related to the degree of hyponatremia and how rapid the hyponatremia progressed. A patient is unlikely to have symptoms with a sodium of >125 mEq/L. Headache, nausea, lethargy, and other CNS findings may occur when sodium falls <125 mEq/L.

Management

SIADH is a diagnosis of exclusion. Other causes of hyponatremia must be ruled out (hyperglycemia, increased serum lipids or protein, hypothyroidism, and adrenal insufficiency). A serum osmolality <280 mOsm/kg combined with urine osmolality <200 mOsm and urine sodium concentration >20 mEq/L are consistent with SIADH. The patient should appear euvolemic. Most cases of SIADH are self-limited, and the mode of management is fluid restriction. In a child, this involves limiting oral fluid intake to 1,000 mL/m^2/day. In a young child, this may not provide sufficient calories for growth. Demeclocycline, which produces a reversible nephrogenic diabetes insipidus, may also be utilized to treat SIADH, but only in chronic cases. Treatment for the acute symptomatic hyponatremia may be managed by the administration of hypertonic fluids. The goal is to raise the serum sodium level by 0.5 mEq/hr to a maximum of 12 mEq/L in the first 24 hours. Serum sodium should be monitored every 3 to 4 hours.

SHORT STATURE

Short stature or abnormal linear growth is a common concern of parents. Normal causes include familial (genetic) short stature and constitutional delay. Eighty percent of cases of short stature are attributable to these two causes. Pathologic causes may result in either disproportionate or proportionate short stature. Etiologies that result in proportionate short stature are much more prevalent. Disorders that result in disproportionate short stature affects the long bones predominantly and includes rickets, which is caused by activated vitamin D deficiency, and achondroplasia, an autosomal dominant disorder. Diseases that cause proportionate short stature may result from either a prenatal or postnatal insult to the growth process. Prenatal etiologies include intrauterine growth retardation, placental dysfunction, intrauterine infections, teratogens, and chromosomal abnormalities. The most common chromosomal abnormalities that result in short stature are trisomy 21 and Turner syndrome. Postnatal causes include malnutrition, chronic systemic diseases, psychosocial deprivation, drugs, and endocrine disorders. Common endocrine defects that result in short stature include hypothyroidism, GH deficiency, and glucocorticoid excess and precocious puberty. Of note, with precocious puberty there is initial acceleration of growth; however, final adult height is compromised, leaving the individual with subsequent short stature compared to the genetic potential.

DIFFERENTIAL DIAGNOSIS

Children with familial short stature establish growth curves at or below the 5th percentile by 2 years of age. They are otherwise completely healthy, with normal physical examinations. These children have normal bone age values, and puberty occurs at the expected time. Short stature is usually found in at least one parent, but height inheritance is complex, and the diminutive ancestor may be more distant.

Children with constitutional delay of growth develop at or below the 5th percentile at normal growth rate. This results in a curve parallel to the 5th percentile. Puberty is significantly delayed, which results in a delay in the bone age. Because these children fail to enter puberty at the usual age, their short stature and sexual immaturity are accentuated when their peers enter puberty. Family members are usually of average height, but there is often a history of short stature in childhood and delayed puberty. The parents of children with constitutional delay should be counseled that their child's growth is a normal variant and the child will likely mature to the height expected for their family. GH deficiency accounts for approximately 5% of cases of short stature referred to endocrinologists. Children with classic GH deficiency grow at a diminished growth velocity (< 5 cm/yr) and have delayed skeletal maturation. A history of birth asphyxia, neonatal hypoglycemia, or physical findings of microphallus, cleft palate, or other midline defects are suggestive of pituitary dysfunction and increased likelihood of GH deficiency. GH deficiency secondary to hypothalamic or pituitary tumor usually is associated with other neurologic or visual impairments. In an older child with more recent onset of subnormal growth, the index of suspicion for a tumor should be high. Insulin-like growth factor-I (IGF-I) and its binding protein-3 (IGF-BP3) are used to screen for GH deficiency. Formal GH testing with timed sampling for GH is indicated if these screening tests are low for age and pubertal status, or if clinical suspicion is high for GH deficiency. Primary hypothyroidism causes marked growth failure through diminished growth velocity and skeletal maturation. Thyroxine (T4), free T4, triiodothyronine resin uptake (T3RU), thyroid-stimulating hormone (TSH), and thyroid antibodies should be measured (even in the absence of symptoms) to rule out any degree of hypothyroidism when evaluating short stature. Primary hypothyroidism is treated with levothyroxine.

Cushing disease is a rare cause of short stature. Hypercortisolism, from either exogenous steroid therapy or endogenous oversecretion, may have a profound growth-suppression effect. Usually, other stigmata of Cushing syndrome such as moon face, buffalo hump, central obesity, purple striae and hypertension are present if growth suppression has occurred. Chronic systemic diseases may result in short stature from lack of caloric absorption or increased metabolic demands. Cyanotic heart disease, cystic fibrosis, poorly controlled diabetes, chronic renal failure, human immunodeficiency (HIV) infection, and severe rheumatic illness are disorders that increase metabolic demands and diminish growth. Alternatively, inflammatory bowel disease, celiac sprue, and cystic fibrosis may reduce caloric absorption and produce short stature.

Some children who live in emotionally or physically abusive or neglectful environments develop functional GH deficiency. Children with psychosocial deprivation may have bizarre behaviors that include food hoarding, pica, and encopresis, as well as immature speech, disturbed sleep–wake cycles, and an increased pain tolerance. Clinically, they resemble children with primary GH deficiency, with marked retardation of bone age and pubertal delay. If GH testing is done while the child remains in the hostile environment, there is a blunted GH response; when the child is removed from the deprived environment, GH testing reverts to normal and catch-up growth is noted.

A key feature of Turner syndrome is short stature. The clinical manifestations of Turner syndrome may sometimes be subtle. Given that the incidence of Turner syndrome is 1 in 2,500 females, gonadotropins and karyotype testing are indicated in the female adolescent with short stature and delayed puberty. Elevated gonadotropins (indicating primary ovarian failure) and a 45, XO karyotype is diagnostic. Last, chronic administration of certain medications may result in poor growth. Such drugs include steroids, dextroamphetamine (Dexedrine), and methylphenidate (Ritalin).

CLINICAL MANIFESTATIONS

History

Important historical information includes the child's prenatal and birth history, the pattern of growth, presence of chronic disease, long-term medication use, achievement of developmental milestones, and growth and pubertal patterns of the patient's parents and siblings. Evaluating the child's growth charts is vitally important. A thorough feeding history, including what, how, and by whom the child is fed, is also required.

Physical Examination

The majority of physical examinations performed on children with short stature are normal. It is critical to plot the child's height and weight on the appropriate growth curve for age. In addition to height, arm span and upper-to-lower-body segment ratio are measured to check for pathologic disproportionate causes of short stature and suggestive midline defects. In young children, the head circumference should also be evaluated to check for failure to thrive. In children with failure to thrive, weight and height are diminished, and the head circumference is often spared. When examining the child with short stature, the physician may find dysmorphic features in a pattern suggestive of a particular syndrome. The integument should be examined for cyanosis indicating potential congenital heart disease, abnormal pigmentation noted in Cushing syndrome, the stigmata of hypothyroidism, and bruises and poor hygiene indicative of psychosocial deprivation. The thyroid is palpated to determine its size, its consistency, and the presence of thyroid nodules. The lungs and heart are examined to identify chronic cardiopulmonary disease. Abdominal tenderness or bloating may indicate inflammatory bowel or celiac disease. Tanner staging for both boys and girls must be documented to help differentiate among familial short stature, constitutional delay, and precocious puberty. A thorough neurologic and funduscopic examination may reveal underlying CNS disease resulting in GH deficiency.

DIAGNOSTIC EVALUATION

A bone age (anteroposterior radiograph of the left wrist) assessment helps delineate familial short stature from constitutional delay. An advanced bone age likely indicates precocious puberty; a normal bone age, familial short stature, and a delayed bone age, constitutional delay, hormone deficiencies, or chronic illness. Thyroid function tests must be completed to evaluate for hypothyroidism. Urinalysis and renal function tests are needed to rule out chronic renal disease. A complete blood count with differential and an erythrocyte sedimentation rate may reveal evidence of chronic systemic infection. The child's nutritional status may be examined through the serum albumin and total protein counts. A screen for insulin-like growth factor-1 (IGF-1) and insulin-like growth factor binding protein-3 (IGF-BP3) may be ordered to screen for GH deficiency. If a chromosomal anomaly is considered, obtaining a karyotype is necessary. An MRI of the brain should be considered if serum testing documents hormone deficiencies or there are neurological findings to justify the procedure. The MRI may identify a hypothalamic or pituitary process resulting in decreased GH secretion from the pituitary. Other laboratory testing to consider include tissue transglutaminase antibodies (celiac disease) and chemistry profile with Ca, Mg, Phos (renal function), LH, FSH, estrogen or testosterone (to assess puberty status), and prolactin (mild elevation could suggest a disruption of the pituitary stalk).

TREATMENT

For most children with constitutional delay, reassurance that the child's short stature is a normal variant suffices. In some select patients with no signs of puberty by 14 years of age, a 4-to-6-month treatment with the appropriate sex hormone may help to modestly increase stature and pubertal development for psychological support until true pubertal development begins. Children with GH deficiency are managed with biosynthetic human GH by subcutaneous injection. Accelerated growth velocity on GH treatment results in catch-up growth in most children. GH therapy is needed into adulthood because of its effects on bone mass and lipid metabolism. Idiopathic short stature (final adult height prediction below the 3rd percentile) is considered an indication to treat with GH therapy. In addition, children small for gestation age and failure to have catch-up growth by 2 years of age can benefit from increased growth velocity with GH use. Primary hypothyroidism is treated with levothyroxine. After several weeks of therapy, the growth velocity generally returns to normal. Unlike GH therapy, levothyroxine therapy does not promote catch-up growth. To manage the short stature associated with Cushing disease, the physician must identify and treat the etiology. Girls with short stature caused by Turner syndrome may receive GH to increase their final adult height. Short stature caused by psychosocial deprivation is treated by removing the child from the environment. Short stature caused by medications is reversed by discontinuing the offending medication.

THYROID DYSFUNCTION

CONGENITAL HYPOTHYROIDISM

Congenital hypothyroidism (CH) is the most common endocrinopathy affecting newborns. The prevalence of CH in the United States is 1:4000 live births. Mandatory screening for CH is established in the United States and allows the earliest possible treatment. CH is considered a medical emergency as delays in thyroid hormone treatment of weeks or months will result in developmental delays. Classically the TSH is elevated with a normal or low T4. There are two approaches to screening for CH: One is to measure the thyroid hormone level (T4) followed by pituitary TSH if the T4 levels is low, and the second approach is to measure the TSH only. The most common cause of CH is aplasia, hypoplasia, or abnormal migration to its mature location. The second likely etiology is dyshormonogenesis, such as a peroxidase defect responsible for the organification of tyrosine molecules and the creation to thyroid hormone. CH is managed with daily T4 replacement with a goal to normalize the TSH.

HYPOTHYROIDISM

The most common cause of juvenile or acquired hypothyroidism is Hashimoto thyroiditis, a chronic lymphocytic thyroiditis that results in autoimmune destruction of the thyroid gland. Other causes of hypothyroidism include panhypopituitarism, ectopic thyroid dysgenesis, administration of antithyroid medications, and surgical or radioactive iodine ablation for treatment of hyperthyroidism. The incidence of hypothyroidism in girls is four times greater than in boys. There is often a family history autoimmune diseases. Most children present during adolescence; it is unusual to develop thyroiditis before 5 years of age.

Clinical Manifestations

Symptoms include cold intolerance, diminished appetite, lethargy, and constipation. Physical findings include slow linear growth, delayed puberty, immature body proportions, coarse puffy face, dry thin hair, dry skin, and deep tendon reflexes with delayed relaxation.

Diagnostic Evaluation

Thyroid function tests reveal a depressed total T4 serum concentration and a depressed T3RU level. If primary hypothyroidism is present, an elevated serum TSH concentration is noted. If secondary hypothyroidism is present, the TSH level may be normal, or mildly elevated. The detection of thyroid autoantibodies indicates an autoimmune basis for disease, whereas palpation of a thyroid nodule should prompt evaluation with a thyroid scan.

Treatment

Patients with hypothyroidism require thyroid hormone replacement with levothyroxine. Both Free T4 and TSH should be monitored frequently at the outset of therapy and yearly once normal values are achieved. Hypothyroidism which persists untreated for longer than 6 to 9 months results in linear growth attenuation and may have a deleterious effect on final adult height.

HYPERTHYROIDISM

Most cases of hyperthyroidism in children are caused by Graves disease. Other causes include a hyperfunctioning "hot" thyroid nodule or acute suppurative thyroiditis. Graves disease, an autoimmune disorder, is caused by circulating thyroid-stimulating immunoglobulins binding to thyrotropin receptors on thyroid cells, which results in diffuse hyperplasia and increased levels of free T4. Neonatal Graves disease follows transplacental passage of maternal thyroid-stimulating immunoglobulins. In hyperthyroidism, T4 levels are elevated, T3RU is elevated, and TSH is suppressed.

Clinical Manifestations

Symptoms include a voracious appetite (without weight gain or with weight loss), heat intolerance, emotional lability, restlessness, excessive sweating, frequent loose stools, and poor sleep. Exophthalmos is uncommon in children. Older children may complain of palpitations with cardiovascular system being the most sensitive to the effect of excess T4. There is often a change in behavior and deterioration of school performance. Hyperthyroidism should be part of an evaluation for attention deficit disorder as there are many overlapping symptoms. On physical examination, the child may be flushed, fidgety, and warm, with proptosis, a hyperactive precordium, resting tachycardia, and a widened pulse pressure. The thyroid gland is generally enlarged, smooth, firm (but not hard), and nontender, with a bruit on auscultation of the gland. Often a fine tremor is noted, and proximal muscle weakness is present. Acute-onset tachycardia, hyperthermia, diaphoresis, fever, nausea, and vomiting indicate thyroid storm (malignant hyperthyroidism), which may be life threatening but is rare in children. Infants with neonatal Graves disease tend to stare, are jittery and hyperactive, and have an increased appetite and poor weight gain. Tachycardia is usually present, and thyromegaly may be palpable. The cardiovascular system is the most sensitive to elevated thyroxine levels, and these infants may have evidence of congestive heart failure.

Treatment

The use of antithyroid drugs (methimazole) to treat Graves disease requires a prolonged period (usually 2 to 5 years) and close supervision by a physician. Propylthiouracil (PTU) is no longer recommended in the pediatric population due to its safety profile regarding hepatic toxicity. Less than 60% of these patients will achieve permanent remission with drug therapy alone. The antithyroid medication may cause a hypothyroid state necessitating the addition of thyroxin to normalize circulating T4 levels. It may take greater than 1 year for the TSH to recover from suppression and normalize. A small percentage of patients are sensitive to these medications and may experience hives or agranulocytosis. A beta-blocker may be used in early management to slow the heart rate and decrease the drive on the cardiovascular system. Once the T4 is normalized the patient can stop beta-blocker therapy. Most physicians will delay the use of radioiodine (I131) for the treatment of thyrotoxicosis until adolescence so as not to expose a child to radiation. It is preferred in children to ablate the gland and induce a hypothyroid state rather than underdose and create a situation that would require repeat exposure to I131. Total or subtotal thyroidectomy is an alternative therapy. An experienced surgeon should perform this procedure to decrease the complications. Surgical complications from a thyroidectomy include hypocalcemia from permanent or transient hypoparathyroidism and laryngeal nerve paralysis. Neonatal Graves disease generally resolves over the first several months of life as maternal antibodies are cleared. If the infant is hemodynamically compromised by hyperthyroidism, parenteral fluids, digoxin, propranolol, and antithyroid medications may be necessary.

THYROID NODULE

A single firm thyroid nodule is an ominous finding in the pediatric population. Unlike nodules in adults, the thyroid nodule in a child or adolescent is more likely to be malignant. Lack of iodine concentration of a thyroid I123 scan (cold nodule) increases the likelihood of carcinoma. Ultrasound evidence of a cyst is reassuring but the solid component of a cyst should be considered for fine-needle aspiration. The presence of calcification on ultrasound and the palpation of lymph node also suggest cancer. Most recommend that thyroid nodules be surgically removed in the pediatric population.

PAINFUL THYROID GLAND

Subacute thyroiditis (viral infection) or suppurative thyroiditis (bacterial infection can cause tenderness of the thyroid gland. Both of these conditions are associated with an elevation of the sedimentation rate. Subacute thyroiditis may follow a viral illness initially with a course of hyperthyroidism due to release of preformed thyroid hormone from the damaged gland. The TSH may be normal or suppressed. The second phase may include a return to a euthyroid state or followed by hypothyroidism. Suppurative thyroiditis may be accompanied by fever, URI symptoms, and dysphagia. Bacterial infections are treated with antibiotics but the pain experienced in thyroiditis can be managed with anti-inflammatory medications (ibuprofen, steroids).

ADRENAL DYSFUNCTION

The adrenal is made of two parts, the cortex and the medulla originating from different embryonic origins. The cortex is made of three zones, the zona glomerulosa secretes aldosterone, the zona fasciculate and reticularis are involved in the secretion of cortisol and adrenal androgens. Cholesterol is the precursor to all steroid production. The biosynthetic pathway documents sequential action of a series of enzymes in an adrenal cell. The production of cortisol is signaled by pituitary ACTH. Disease states can result in hypoadrenocorticism (congenital adrenal hyperplasia syndromes or Addison disease) or hyperadrenaocortism (Cushing syndrome).

HYPOADRENOCORTICISM

Primary Adrenal Insufficiency

Primary adrenal insufficiency may be congenital or acquired and results in decreased cortisol secretion. Depending on the disease process, there may be a concomitant decrease in aldosterone release. In the newborn, primary adrenal insufficiency may be caused by adrenal hypoplasia, ACTH unresponsiveness, adrenal hemorrhage, or ischemic infarction with sepsis (Waterhouse-Frederickson syndrome). In older children and adolescents, autoimmune adrenal insufficiency is most common. It may occur alone or in association with another autoimmune endocrinopathy such as thyroiditis or type 1 DM. Tuberculosis, hemorrhage, fungal infection, neoplastic infiltration, and HIV infection may also cause destruction of the adrenal gland. Adrenoleukodystrophy is an X-linked recessive disorder of long-chain fatty acid metabolism that results in adrenal insufficiency and progressive neurologic dysfunction. In contrast to primary adrenal insufficiency, secondary adrenal insufficiency is caused by an ACTH deficiency. The most common cause of ACTH deficiency is chronic steroid therapy that results in suppression of pituitary ACTH. Congenital hypopituitarism or pituitary tumors (craniopharyngioma) also result in depressed pituitary ACTH secretion.

Clinical Manifestations

Symptoms of adrenal insufficiency include weakness, nausea, vomiting, weight loss, headache, emotional lability, and salt craving. Postural hypotension is common. Increased pigmentation over joints and on scar tissue, lips, nipples, and the buccal mucosa is observed in primary adrenal insufficiency because of increased ACTH secretion. Melanocyte-stimulating hormone is a byproduct of the ACTH biosynthetic pathway. The postural hypotension and salt craving are caused by a lack of aldosterone. Adrenal crisis is a medical emergency characterized by fever, vomiting, dehydration, and shock. It may be precipitated by intercurrent illness, trauma, or surgery.

Electrolyte abnormalities include hyponatremia due to the inability to excrete free water and hyperkalemia if mineralocorticoid deficiency is involved. In addition, hypoglycemia and mild metabolic acidosis from dehydration can be observed. An elevated baseline ACTH with a concurrent low cortisol level is consistent with primary adrenal insufficiency. Adrenal insufficiency should be suspected if the corticotropin stimulation test is abnormal (cortisol of <20 μg/dL).

Treatment

Adrenal crisis is a life-threatening condition that should be treated without delay. Correction of electrolyte abnormalities and dehydration is required immediately with 5% dextrose in normal saline and stress dose intravenous glucocorticoids.

Long-term management of adrenal insufficiency consists of maintenance doses of oral glucocorticoids and mineralocorticoids. The glucocorticoid dose is increased during times of acute metabolic stress to avoid adrenal insufficiency.

CONGENITAL ADRENAL HYPERPLASIA

The clinical characteristics of congenital adrenal hyperplasia depend on which enzyme in the pathway of steroidogenesis is deficient. Figure 14-1 is a schematic of steroidogenesis in the adrenal cortex. 21-Hydroxylase deficiency accounts for 90% of the cases of congenital adrenal hyperplasia. The disease is inherited as an autosomal recessive trait and tends to occur as either classic salt-wasting 21-hydroxylase deficiency or as virilizing 21-hydroxylase deficiency. 21-Hydroxylase is needed to produce aldosterone and cortisol. 21-Hydroxylase deficiency results in a buildup of the precursors of aldosterone and cortisol. Specifically, 17-hydroxyprogesterone increases, which is then metabolized to dehydroepiandrosterone and androstenedione, which are weak androgens. Androstenedione is then converted to testosterone. Both forms of 21-hydroxylase deficiency result in decreased cortisol and aldosterone secretion, increased adrenocorticotropin hormone (ACTH), and increased 17-hydroxyprogesterone and 17-hydroxypregnenolone. 11-Hydroxylase deficiency accounts for 5% of congenital adrenal hyperplasia and is also inherited as an autosomal recessive trait. Similar to 21-hydroxylase deficiency, 11-hydroxylase deficiency impairs the production of aldosterone and cortisol. 11-Hydroxylase converts 11-deoxycortisol to cortisol and deoxycorticosterone to corticosterone in the aldosterone pathway. With reduction or absence of 11-hydroxylase, cortisol and aldosterone precursors build up and are shunted to androgen synthesis.

Clinical Manifestations

In congenital 21-hydroxylase deficiency, female infants are born with ambiguous genitalia. Clitoromegaly and labioscrotal fusion may result in erroneous male sex assignment. There is normal ovarian development, and internal genital structures are female. Male infants born with the defect have no genital abnormalities. Unless identified by newborn screen, male infants may present with poor feeding, failure to thrive, lethargy, dehydration, hypotension, hyponatremia, and hyperkalemia. Symptoms of emesis, salt wasting, dehydration, and shock develop in the first 2 to 4 weeks of life. Hyponatremia and hyperkalemia result from lack of aldosterone, and hypoglycemia results from decreased levels of cortisol. The diagnosis of 21-hydroxylase deficiency is made by documenting elevated serum levels of 17-hydroxyprogesterone greater than 5,000 ng/dL (usually much higher). In 11-hydroxylase deficiency, there is overproduction of deoxycorticosterone, which has mineralocorticoid activity and results in hypernatremia, hypokalemia, and hypertension. Diagnosis is based on the measurement of increased levels of 11-deoxycortisol and deoxycorticosterone in the serum or their metabolites in the urine. Serum androstenedione and testosterone are also elevated, and renin and aldosterone levels are depressed.

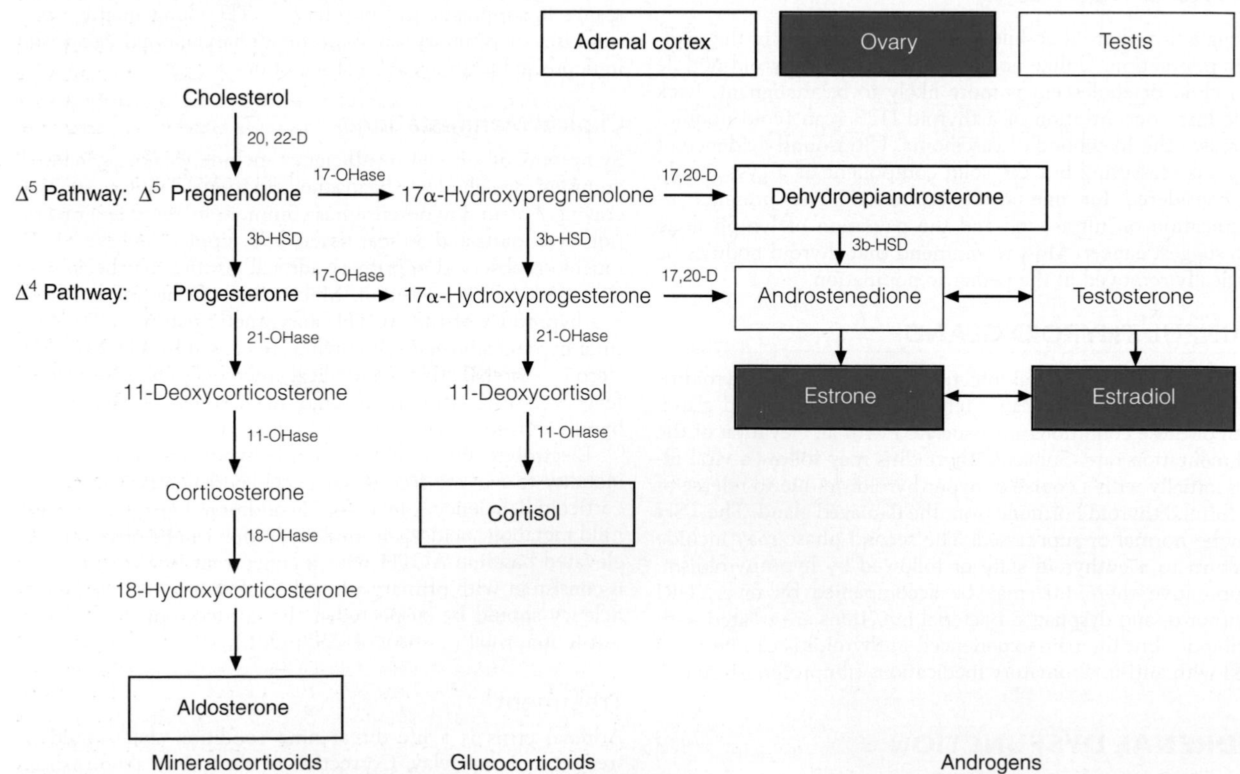

Figure 14-1 • A schematic of steroidogenesis in the adrenal cortex.

Treatment

Cortisol therapy reduces ACTH secretion and overproduction of androgens, and mineralocorticoid administration is adjusted to normalize serum renin levels. Cortisol doses may range from 10 to 20 mg/m^2/day divided 2 to 3 times each day. If salt loss occurs, oral fludrocortisone (florinef) is used for mineralocorticoid replacement (0.05 to 0.1 mg each day). Neonates and infants may require higher florinef dosing and even sodium supplements. Families require education of steroid "stress dosing" of the cortisol. They are asked to give larger doses of the cortisol in times of physiologic stress (fever >101°F, vomiting illness, trauma, surgical procedures). In general, 50 mg/m^2/day as a bolus and then divided every 8 hours for 24 hours until clinically stable is an appropriate stress dose. IM or IV hydrocortisone may be administered in the vomiting child or child with mental status changes.

Surgical correction of female genital abnormalities is accomplished early. The linear growth and sexual development of children with 21-hydroxylase deficiency must be monitored closely. Undertreatment, as indicated by elevated 17-hydroxyprogesterone, androstenedione, and renin levels and by accelerated advancement of skeletal maturity, leads to excessive growth, premature pubarche, and virilization of the child. Ultimately, undertreatment may lead to premature epiphyseal fusion and adult short stature. Over treatment with cortisol suppresses growth and may cause symptoms of hypercortisolism.

HYPERADRENOCORTICISM

Cushing Syndrome

Cushing syndrome is a constellation of symptoms and signs that result from any form of cortisol excess. It is caused by either endogenous overproduction of cortisol or excessive exogenous treatment with pharmacologic doses of glucocorticoids. Endogenous causes include Cushing disease (pituitary overproduction of ACTH) and adrenal tumors. Cushing disease, also known as bilateral adrenal hyperplasia, is the most common etiology of Cushing syndrome in children older than 7 years. In most instances, it is caused by a microadenoma of the pituitary gland resulting in ACTH oversecretion. In infants and children younger than 7 years of age, adrenal tumors predominate. Most adrenal tumors that cause Cushing syndrome are adenomas. Ectopic ACTH secretion may occur with some tumors; however, this is exceedingly rare in children.

Clinical Manifestations

The classic signs and symptoms of Cushing syndrome include slow growth with pubertal arrest, "moon" facies, central obesity, abdominal striae, acne, hirsutism, facial flushing, hyperpigmentation, hypertension, fatigue, muscle weakness, acne, buffalo hump, and emotional and mental changes. Most adrenal tumors are virilizing. Diagnostic testing should include documentation of an increased 24-hour urine free cortisol collection and elevated midnight salivary cortisol test. If hypercortisolism is demonstrated, the low-dose dexamethasone suppression test is performed to document the presence of Cushing syndrome. Dexamethasone is given in the late evening, and a cortisol level is measured the next morning. Failure of the dexamethasone to suppress the morning cortisol level is consistent with Cushing syndrome. A prolonged dexamethasone suppression test is used to differentiate Cushing disease from an adrenal tumor. When evaluating a child with Cushing syndrome, obtaining an MRI scan of the pituitary and CT scan of the adrenal glands is helpful in determining if additional pathology exists.

Treatment

Adrenal tumors require surgical removal. Similarly, bilateral adrenal hyperplasia is treated with surgical excision of the pituitary adenoma. Transsphenoidal microsurgery is the most effective method of microadenoma removal. Perioperative stress dosing of glucocorticoids is needed to avoid adrenal insufficiency. Postoperatively, the patient may develop a mineralocorticoid deficiency in addition to the glucocorticoid deficiency.

DISORDERS OF PUBERTY

PRECOCIOUS PUBERTY

True precocious puberty is defined as secondary sex characteristics presenting in girls before 7 years of age and in boys before 9 years of age and may be either gonadotropin-dependent or gonadotropin independent. True central (gonadotropin-dependent) precocious puberty is more common in girls than in boys. Precocious puberty in girls is usually idiopathic, whereas in boys there is a greater incidence of CNS pathology. Tumors causing gonadotropin-dependent precocious puberty (GDPP) include gliomas, embryonic germ cell tumors, and hamartomas. Other causes of GDPP include hydrocephalus, head injury, and CNS infection or congenital malformation. Gonadotropin-independent precocious puberty (GIPP) is extremely rare but does occur due in McCune-Albright syndrome (polyostotic fibrous dysplasia of bone and café au lait spots), familial precocious puberty in boys (familial testitoxicosis), Leydig cell tumors, and ectopic human chorionic gonadotropin (HCG) production by neoplasms such as hepatic and pineal tumors. Precocious thelarche refers to isolated early breast development. The usual age of onset for precocious thelarche is 12 to 24 months. Premature thelarche is likely caused by small transient bursts of estrogen from the prepubertal ovary or from increased sensitivity to low levels of estrogen in the prepubertal female. This is an isolated finding in a girl with a normal growth rate and bone age. Premature adrenarche refers to the early appearance of sexual hair before 8 years of age in girls and 9 years of age in boys. This benign condition is caused by early maturation of adrenal androgen secretion. This is an isolated finding in children with a normal to slightly advanced growth rate and bone age.

Clinical Manifestations

In precocious thelarche, gonadotropin and serum estrogen levels are in the prepubertal range, and linear growth acceleration and advancing skeletal maturation are not present. This nonprogressive, benign condition is distinguished from true precocious puberty by the normal growth rate and bone age noted with premature thelarche. In premature adrenarche, the levels of adrenal androgens are normal for pubertal stage but elevated for chronologic age. The child's bone age is usually slightly advanced. Children with premature adrenarche must be evaluated for other causes of increased androgen production, such as congenital adrenal hyperplasia, polycystic ovarian syndrome, or adrenal tumor. In children with evidence of significant androgen effect (advanced bone age, growth acceleration, and acne), measurement of adrenal steroids and androgens before and after ACTH administration is used to identify those with congenital adrenal hyperplasia. The clinical manifestations of GDPP include premature development of secondary sexual characteristics and an accompanying growth spurt. If the GDPP is secondary to pathology of the CNS, focal neurologic signs are often present. Diagnosis is based on advanced bone age and pubertal levels of gonadotropins (LH and FSH) and estrogen or testosterone. A pubertal pattern of elevated gonadotropins after infusion of gonadotropin-releasing hormone (GnRH) is indicative of GDPP. In GIPP, gonadotropins are low, and GnRH has no effect on gonadotropin levels.

Treatment

Premature thelarche is a benign condition that does not require any treatment. Premature adrenarche that is not caused by congenital adrenal hyperplasia, tumor, or polycystic ovarian syndrome is also a benign condition. GDPP is treated with injections of long-acting preparations of GnRH (leuprolide). GnRH analogues suppress gonadotropin release and thereby decrease secondary sex characteristics, slow skeletal growth, and prevent the fusion of long bone epiphyseal plates. GIPP is managed by treating the underlying disease process.

PUBERTAL DELAY

Pubertal delay is characterized by a delay in the onset of puberty or in the rate of progression through normal sexual development. In females, this refers to the absence of secondary sex characteristics at 13 years of age or the absence of menarche 3 years from the onset of sexual development. In males, pubertal delay denotes the absence of secondary sex characteristics at 14 years of age or the failure to complete genital growth 5 years from the onset of puberty. Constitutional delay is the cause in 90% to 95% of cases. In these children, the bone age is delayed, growth is slow, and puberty simply appears late. There is usually a positive family history.

Differential Diagnosis

Systemic disease may delay puberty in both sexes. Pubertal delay may be caused by primary gonadal failure (hypergonadotropic hypogonadism). Examples of this include Turner syndrome (45X) or autoimmune ovarian failure (in girls) and Klinefelter syndrome (47XXY) in boys. Hypogonadotropic hypogonadism is caused by hypothalamic/pituitary axis dysfunction. Examples include Kallmann syndrome (mutation in KAL gene), isolated gonadotropic deficiency, hypothalamic and pituitary tumors, hypopituitarism, and anorexia nervosa. Other endocrine disorders (e.g., hypothyroidism) may also delay or advance puberty. All systemic illness can delay puberty.

Clinical Manifestations

The history and physical examination should include an examination of growth trends, the timing of puberty in other family members, and an assessment of the patient's current Tanner staging. Laboratory evaluation is helpful, including bone age, testosterone and estradiol levels, gonadotropins, FSH, LH, prolactin, and thyroid function testing. Screening to look for systemic disease is also indicated.

Treatment

In the case of constitutional delay, a short course of sex steroids may be needed to initiate pubertal development. Psychosocial support is also important. If permanent hypogonadism is determined to be the etiology, sex steroid replacement is initiated at the normal time of puberty and continued for a lifetime.

DISORDERS OF CALCIUM

Disorders of calcium and phosphorus metabolism result from abnormalities in the two major regulators of calcium homeostasis: parathyroid hormone (PTH) and vitamin D. Total serum calcium is tightly regulated within a narrow range normally between 9 and 10.5 mg/dL. Calcium is bound to albumin. As a result, the total calcium may be low while the ionized calcium is normal (1.1 to 1.4 mmol/L). PTH is secreted by the parathyroid glands in response to low levels of calcium. PTH increases serum calcium by releasing stored calcium from bone, increases renal retention of calcium, and increases the production of the active vitamin D metabolite (1-25(OH)2D).

HYPOCALCEMIA

Etiology

Hypocalcemia may be the result of (1) inadequate PTH secretion (hypoparathyroidism) or action (pseudohypoparathyroidism), (2) vitamin D deficiency or resistance, or (3) other disorders such as hypomagnesemia, hyperphosphatemia, hypoproteinemia, and/or drug toxicity. There are congenital and familial forms of hypoparathyroidism. Pseudohypoparathyroidism is due to a PTH receptor mutation and creates a PTH-resistant state. Other causes of hypoparathyroidism include autoimmune disease, surgical removal of the parathyroid glands, and hypomagnesemia (magnesium is required for PTH secretion). Hypoparathyroidism is also seen with DiGeorgesyndrome and Kenny-Caffey syndrome. Of note, many cases of hypoparathyroidism are idiopathic in nature. Vitamin D deficiency may be due to nutritional deprivation. Higher risk individuals include infants who are exclusively breastfed and people who are highly pigmented, take medications that rapidly metabolize vitamin D, and live in areas with limited sunlight exposure. Vitamin D requires enzymes in the liver and kidney to convert the fat soluble form of vitamin D to its most active form (calcitriol 1,25 OH2 vitamin D). In addition, there are vitamin D resistance syndromes. Hypocalcemia may also be seen in Bartter syndrome, renal tubular acidosis, and as a side effect of the administration of particular drugs (furosemide, calcitonin, and antineoplastic agents).

Clinical Manifestations

A patient with hypocalcemia may present with carpo-pedal spasm facial twitching, jitteriness, tetany, or seizures. Laryngospasm may cause shortness of breath or apnea. The electrocardiogram may reveal a prolonged corrected QT interval. Vitamin D deficiency often presents with rachitic bone disease and poor growth parameters in children. The electrolyte pattern may identify and diagnose the defect of hypocalcemia. In hypoparathyroidism, the serum calcium is low and serum phosphorus is elevated due to a lack of renal stimuli by PTH to excrete phosphorus. This pattern is also seen in pseudohypoparathyroidism (ineffective PTH effect). Low serum calcium and low serum phosphorus is consistent with vitamin D deficiency. In vitamin D deficiency, PTH levels are extremely elevated in an attempt to normalize the serum calcium at the expense of bone resorption, resulting in excessive renal phosphorus wasting.

Treatment

The treatment of functional hypoparathyroidism is replacement with oral calcium supplements and an active metabolite of vitamin D (calcitriol 1,25 OH2 vitamin D). Hypocalcemia as a result of vitamin D deficiency may be treated with 25(OH)D. Resistance to vitamin D must be treated with calcitriol 1,25 OH2 vitamin D.

HYPERCALCEMIA

Hypercalcemia is considered when calcium levels are greater than 12 mg/dL. Hypercalcemia may be due to (1) hyperparathyroidism; (2) hypervitaminosis D; (3) immobilization; (4) neoplasia; or (5) familial hypocalciuric hypercalcemia. Hypercalcemia can also be associated with William syndrome or multiple endocrine neoplasia syndrome (hyperparathyroidism).

Clinical Manifestations

Hypercalcemia may be asymptomatic or present with vomiting, lethargy, inability to concentrate, depression, seizures, polyuria, and hypertension. Patients may also present with renal calculi on abdominal ultrasonography, pathological fractures, or a short QT interval on electrocardiograph.

Treatment

Medical management of symptomatic hypercalcemia is hydration with intravenous saline. Furosemide may be given (1 mg/kg) in 6-to-8-hour intervals. Bisphosphonate infusions (pamidronate) has also been found to be useful to inhibit osteoclast function. A sestamibi parathyroid scan may be indicated to identify a surgically removable adenoma of the parathyroid gland. Hypercalcemia caused by vitamin D excess may be treated by glucocorticoids or ketoconazole to suppress the renal activation of 1-25(OH)2D. It is equally important to identify the individual with familial hypocalciuric hypercalcemia, a benign condition, so that unnecessary aggressive management is avoided.

KEY POINTS

- DM is a chronic metabolic disorder characterized by hyperglycemia and abnormal energy metabolism due to absent or diminished insulin secretion or action at the cellular level.
- T1DM results from a lack of insulin production by the ß-cells of the pancreas. Long-term complications from T1DM include microvascular disease (retinopathy, nephropathy, and neuropathy) and accelerated large vessel atherosclerotic disease.
- The percentage of T2DM cases in children is rising.
- The definition of hypoglycemia is a plasma glucose value of less than 50 mg/dL. Hypoglycemia may be the result of hyperinsulinemia, pituitary disease (ACTH deficiency with or without GH deficiency), glycogen storage disease, disorders of gluconeogenesis, or defects in fatty acid oxidation.
- In central diabetes insipidus, there is loss of ADH secretion and an inability to concentrate the urine. This may occur after head trauma, with a brain tumor, or CNS infection.
- A low serum osmolality with inappropriately elevated urine osmolality and urine sodium are consistent with SIADH. SIADH is treated with fluid restriction. Hypertonic fluids may be administered in acute symptomatic hyponatremia as long as the serum sodium is not corrected too rapidly.
- Eighty percent of cases of short stature result from normal growth and development and are caused by either familial (genetic) short stature or constitutional delay of growth and puberty.
- Most cases of hyperthyroidism in children are caused by Graves disease, which is an autoimmune-induced thyroid hyperplasia. Medical therapy for Graves disease consists of antithyroid medication administration. Neonatal Graves disease results from transplacental passage of maternal thyroid-stimulating immunoglobulins.
- The most common cause of juvenile or acquired hypothyroidism is Hashimoto thyroiditis, which is a chronic lymphocytic thyroiditis that results in autoimmune destruction of the thyroid gland. Hypothyroidism is treated with synthetic levothyroxine.
- 21-Hydroxylase deficiency accounts for 90% of the cases of congenital adrenal hyperplasia. In congenital 21-hydroxylase deficiency, female infants are born with ambiguous genitalia, whereas male infants born with the defect have no genital abnormalities. The diagnosis of congenital adrenal hyperplasia is made by documenting elevated levels of 17-hydroxyprogesterone in the serum.
- Primary adrenal insufficiency may be congenital or acquired and results in decreased cortisol and aldosterone secretion, whereas secondary adrenal insufficiency is caused by adrenocorticotropin hormone (ACTH) deficiency.
- Cushing syndrome is a constellation of symptoms and signs that result from high cortisol levels and is caused by either endogenous overproduction of cortisol or excessive exogenous treatment with pharmacologic doses of cortisol.
- True precocious puberty is defined as secondary sex characteristics presenting in girls before 7 years of age and in boys before 9 years of age and may be either gonadotropin-dependent or independent. The most common cause of pubertal delay is constitutional delay.
- Inadequate PTH secretion (hypoparathyroidism) or action (pseudohypoparathyroidism) and vitamin D deficiency are likely causes of hypocalcemia in the pediatric patient. The treatment of functional hypoparathyroidism is replacement with oral calcium supplements and an active metabolite of vitamin D (calcitriol 1,25 OH_2 vitamin D).

C Clinical Vignettes

Vignette 1

A 15-year-old previously healthy male began experiencing fatigue and dizziness upon standing about 2 weeks ago. His appetite is poor. He has had no weight gain over the past 6 months, and pubertal development is delayed. His father completed linear growth by age 17 years, and his mother's age of menarche was 13 years. On physical examination, he appears thin, with weight at the 20th percentile and height at the 75th percentile. Blood pressure is 90/60 mm Hg supine, falling to 60/40 mm Hg upon standing. Supine pulse was 80 beats/min, increasing to 120 beats/min standing. Clinically, he is well hydrated. He appears to have a well-developed sun tan, noticeably different from his parents who are pale in complexion. The thyroid gland is mildly enlarged. Pubic hair and axillary hair are sparse, and testicular volume is 6 milliliters bilaterally. His neurological examination is normal. Radiographs of the skull and chest are normal. Bone age is read as 13 years. Hematocrit is 30%. Serum thyroxine (T_4) is 8.5 μg/dL, TSH was 2.9 μU/ml (normal 0.3–5.0), FSH was 4.6 mU/ml (normal 5–30), prolactin was 4.7 ng/ml (normal 3–24), and IFG-1 level was 252 ng/ml (normal 152–540). Plasma cortisol at 8 a.m. was 2.9 mcg/dL.

1. What is the most likely diagnosis?
   - **a.** Primary adrenal insufficiency
   - **b.** Secondary adrenal insufficiency
   - **c.** Secondary hypothyroidism
   - **d.** Constitutional delay of growth and puberty
   - **e.** Pituitary tumor

2. Which of the results of further laboratory testing would be most likely?
   - **a.** Serum sodium 132 mEq/L, serum potassium 5.8 mEq/L, serum bicarbonate 18 mEq/L, blood urea nitrogen 20 mg/dL, ACTH 230 pmol/L
   - **b.** Serum sodium 130 mEq/L, serum potassium 4.0 mEq/L, serum bicarbonate 27 mEq/L, blood urea nitrogen 12 mg/dL, ACTH 10 pmol/L
   - **c.** Serum sodium 145 mEq/L, serum potassium 4.2 mEq/L, serum bicarbonate 28 mEq/L, blood urea nitrogen 14 mg/dL, ACTH 25 pmol/L

3. What is the most likely pathology involving the adrenal glands in this patient?
   - **a.** Autoimmune destruction
   - **b.** Tuberculosis
   - **c.** Late onset congenital adrenal hyperplasia
   - **d.** Craniopharyngioma

Vignette 2

A 12½-year-old girl presents with short stature (<3rd percentile) and growth failure. She has felt well, but school records indicate that she has not grown in height since age 8 years. She has had mild constipation and cold intolerance. She is an "A" student in school. Her skin is dry, and she has delayed relaxation of her deep tendon reflexes. You note diffuse homogeneous enlargement of the thyroid gland.

1. Which set of thyroid function tests is most likely based on this patient's clinical findings?

	A	B	C	D
Serum T_4 (mcg/dL)	2.0	2.0	8.0	13.0
Free T_4 ng/dL	0.6	0.6	3.2	5.2
TSH mU/ml	75	1.5	2.5	0.1
24-hour radiodine uptake	3%	5%	15%	30%

Normal values T_4 are 5 to 12 mcg/dL, free T_4 are 1.1 to 4.0 ng/dL, and 24h RAIU Scan are 10% to 25%.

2. Which of the following is the most likely underlying cause of this patient's diagnosis?
   - **a.** Iodine deficiency
   - **b.** Autoimmue thyroiditis
   - **c.** Functional nodule
   - **d.** Multinodular goiter

Vignette 3

A 6-year-old female presents with a 6-month history of axillary and pubic hair development. In addition, the family has noticed an occasional acne lesion. There is no history of vaginal discharge or bleeding and no breast tissue on physical examination. The parents deny any known exogenous hormone exposure.

1. Which of the following does not support the diagnosis of premature adrenarche?
   - **a.** Bone age of 7 years
   - **b.** Growth velocity of 10 cm/year
   - **c.** Elevated DHEAS levels
   - **d.** Presence of body odor

2. The patient's bone age is reported to be 10 years. Upon review, the growth chart demonstrates that the height was formerly plotted at the 50th percentile; over the course of 3 years, height is now at the 90th percentile. Which of the following findings would assist in the diagnosis of late-onset 21-OH deficiency?
   a. Hyponatremia
   b. Hyperkalemia
   c. Hypertension
   d. Elevated 17-hydroxyprogesterone

Vignette 4

A 5-year-old girl developed increased thirst and polyuria rather abruptly 2 weeks ago. She is constantly thirsty and becomes angry when fluids are not readily available. She has also begun wetting the bed after being dry for 2 years.

1. Which of the following represents the least likely diagnosis in this child?
   a. Diabetes mellitus
   b. Diabetes insipidus
   c. Hyperthyroidism
   d. Hypocalcemia

2. Initial screening tests include serum Na 150 mEq/L, K 4.5 mEq/L, bicarbonate 28 mmol/L, Cl 110 mEq/L, BUN 10 mg/dL, Ca 9.5 mg/dL, and glucose 80 mg/dL. Serum osmolality is measured at 295 mOsm/L. Osmolality of a first morning void of urine is 100 mOsm/L. What further tests should be completed to confirm the diagnosis and determine possible causes?
   a. Repeat morning testing and renal ultrasound
   b. Water deprivation test and brain MRI if responsive to vasopressin
   c. Oral glucose tolerance test and screening for autoimmune diseases
   d. ACTH stimulation test and measurement of free water excretion

A Answers

Vignette 1 Question 1

Answer B: The symptoms of fatigue, weight loss, and dizziness on standing are relatively nonspecific. However, the delayed puberty and bone age and the finding of postural hypotension suggest adrenal insufficiency. Primary (rather than secondary) insufficiency is suggested by the hyperpigmentation and the effects of ACTH and its melanocyte-stimulating activity. The enlargement of his thyroid gland may be due to risk for primary thyroiditis. The clinical presentations of primary and secondary insufficiency overlap EXCEPT for the finding of hyperpigmentation on physical examination. The presence of high ACTH levels stimulates melanocyte activity; this is seen in primary adrenal insufficiency. The inability to produce ACTH, as seen in hypopituitarism (either congenital or secondary to a brain tumor) would result in ACTH deficiency and symptoms of adrenal insufficiency. Although one may observe delayed puberty and bone age in an adolescent with hypothyroidism, this patient's laboratory values are not suggestive of secondary hypothyroidism. Secondary hypothyroidism infers the pituitary's inability to respond to low thyroxine levels. The TSH may be mildly elevated or normal in the setting of a low T_4. Constitutional delay of growth and puberty is a diagnosis of exclusion. Chronic illnesses that impair linear growth, delay the maturity of the bone, and delay puberty must be excluded. Often there is a family history of delayed puberty in a parent.

Vignette 1 Question 2

Answer A: The most likely laboratory results would be those in (A). Hyperkalemia would be expected because of mineralocorticoid deficiency, which occurs in primary adrenal insufficiency, but not usually in secondary adrenal insufficiency. Lack of mineralocorticoid predisposes to metabolic acidosis due to reduced hydrogen ion excretion. The baseline ACTH level would be high. The results shown in (B) are typical of secondary adrenal insufficiency due to pituitary disease. Here there is no hyperkalemia. The hyponatremia is due to retention of water rather than to renal sodium loss. Baseline ACTH levels are low. The results shown in (C) are compatible with normal pituitary–adrenal function.

Vignette 1 Question 3

Answer A: The majority of cases of spontaneous primary adrenal insufficiency are due to autoimmune destruction of the adrenal glands, also known as Addison disease. This type of insufficiency may occur in association with other autoimmune endocrine deficiencies. Other causes of primary adrenal insufficiency include tuberculosis or other granulomatous diseases, infiltrative diseases, and adrenal hemorrhage. Brian tumors could result in secondary adrenal insufficiency from ACTH deficiency. Late onset congenital adrenal hyperplasia would present with early signs of androgen excess, linear growth acceleration, and bone age advancement, without the salt-wasting as seen in newborns.

Vignette 2 Question 1

Answer A: The patient's history and physical examination findings suggest hypothyroidism. The most likely laboratory findings in uncomplicated primary hypothyroidism are represented in (A). TSH is elevated, and both T_4 and free T_4 are low. The uptake of radioiodine by the thyroid at 24 hours (representing the rate of iodination of thyroglobulin in the thyroid gland) is usually low. (B) is most consistent with *secondary* hypothyroidism (pituitary TSH deficiency). (C) is reflective of a normal subject. (D) represents a set of typical results in a subject with *hyperthyroidism* (suppressed TSH and elevated total and free T_4).

Vignette 2 Question 2

Answer B: The most likely pathologic diagnosis in a spontaneously hypothyroid patient with a goiter is autoimmune thyroiditis. The diagnosis is confirmed in 80% to 90% of cases by demonstrating elevated titers of antithyroid antibodies in the patient's serum. Iodine deficiency can result in a goiter; however, patients who consume diets that are not iodine deficient will not have this as a cause. Hypothyroidism due to iodine deficiency is rare in the United States (due in part to iodized table salt) unless the individual has emigrated from another nation. Functional thyroid nodule would present with thyroid fullness that is unilateral. Laboratory testing of affected patients demonstrates suppressed TSH, either from overproduction of T_4 by the nodule or ongoing recovery from a recent hyperthyroid phase. Multinodular goiters are uncommon in the pediatric population. Upon palpation, multiple discrete nodules can be palpated. Affected patients may have euthyroidism or hypothyroidism.

Vignette 3 Question 1

Answer B: Premature adrenarche is the benign, self-limited appearance of secondary hair growth, body odor, and comedones that usually occurs after age 6 years. Individuals with premature adrenarche grow at a slightly elevated velocity. True pubertal growth rate is typically 9 to 12 cm/year, whereas prepubertal growth rate is 5 to 8 cm/year. Advancement of the bone age is generally considered significant if the reading is 2 years greater than the chronological age. Many typical individuals may have slightly advanced bone age reports not associated with pathology. Elevation of the weak androgen DHEA (measured as serum DHEAS) occurs early in this condition. Gonadal stimulation (ovarian production of estrogen and testicular production of testosterone) will progress normally in patients with premature adrenarche.

Vignette 3 Question 2

Answer D: The characteristic diagnostic finding in children with late-onset congenital adrenal hyperplasia is elevation of 21-OH progesterone, the immediate precursor to the impaired enzyme 21-OHase. Overt salt wasting does not occur in late-onset 21-OH deficiency. Thus, the hyponatremia and hyperkalemia often observed in congenital CAH is not appreciated in the late-onset form. The most common defect leading to all forms of CAH is 21-OH deficiency, resulting in relatively diminished cortisol and aldosterone production and overproduction of androgens. The second most common cause is a diminished effect of the 11-hydroxylase enzyme. Interruption of this pathway leads to overproduction of precursors with mineralocorticoid effects and subsequent hypertension. The 17-OH progesterone levels are usually markedly elevated or will be elevated after stimulation with ACTH.

Vignette 4 Question 1

Answer D: The kidney will begin to diuresis once the blood sugar is greater than 160 to 180 mg/dL. Thus, the combination of polyuria and polydipsia is a common presentation for diabetes at all ages. Diabetes insipidus results when there is inadequate secretion of vasopressin, due to increased serum osmolality or diminished sensitivity to vasopressin at the receptor level. In either setting, the kidney will excrete free water regardless of hydration level (i.e., even when the patient is dehydrated). Other causes of polyuria are hyperthyroidism, hypokalemia and hypercalcemia, and urinary tract infection. Several medications can induce diabetes insipidus (lithium).

Vignette 4 Question 2

Answer B: This patient is very close to meeting the diagnostic criteria for diabetes insipidus, specifically, concentrated serum (NA $>$ 150 mEq/L and or OSM $>$ 300 mOsm/L) in face of dilute urine (urine Osm $<$ 600 mOsm/L and/or urine specific gravity $<$ 1.015). This can at times be diagnosed by random sampling; if not, a water-deprivation test is warranted. Once DI criteria are met, a small dose of Pitressin (vasopressin) is administered to determine if the kidneys are responsive to the hormone. If administration of Pitressin results in concentration of the urine and serum sodium and osmolality improve, this confirms the diagnosis of *central* DI. Because central DI is almost always due to a congenital defect or an acquired lesion of the hypothalamic–pituitary region, a brain MRI is indicated. A repeat sample may not be diagnostic, and there is no role for a renal ultrasound at this stage in the evaluation. Furthermore, restricting fluids in a pediatric patient with possible DI in the home setting (for performance of labs the following morning) may provoke severe hemodynamic instability. There is no indication to perform an OGGT in this patient without elevation of blood glucose or the presence of glucosuria. An ACTH stimulation test will permit evaluation of cortisol secretion after provocation. Cortisol deficiency may result in impaired free water excretion resulting in hyponatremia and concentrated urine.

Chapter

15 Neurology

Amy Harper • Katie S. Fine

NEURODEVELOPMENT

NORMAL DEVELOPMENT

Both intellectual and physical development in infants and children occur in predictable, sequential manners. Table 15-1 presents the typical progression of developmental milestones. Notable skills are subdivided into **gross motor**, **fine motor** (includes visual-motor), **language**, **social/emotional**, and **adaptive** milestones.

The two developmental screens most commonly employed by child psychologists are the **Denver II** developmental screening test and the Clinical Adaptive Test/Clinical Linguistic and Auditory Milestone Scale (**CAT/CLAMS**). The Denver II evaluates children birth to 6 years of age and divides streams of development into gross motor, fine motor–adaptive, language, and personal–social. The CAT rates problem-solving/visual-motor ability and the CLAMS assesses language development between birth and 36 months of age.

DEVELOPMENTAL DELAY

Sometimes development does not progress as expected. **Developmental delay** is diagnosed when performance lags significantly compared with average attainment in a given skill area. The **developmental quotient** (DQ) reflects a child's present developmental achievement: DQ = (developmental age ÷ chronological age) × 100. A DQ below 70 constitutes developmental delay. **Developmental dissociation** refers to a substantial difference in the rates of development between two skill areas. An example of a developmental discrepancy between gross motor and language development is a child with speech delay due to isolated mental retardation whose gross motor development is normal.

Language is the best indicator of future intellectual potential. Language development is divided into two streams, receptive and expressive. Overall, language delay is the most commonly diagnosed form of developmental delay in preschool children.

Age-adjusted parameters are employed when evaluating the developmental achievement of former preterm infants. Until 2 years of age, a child's chronological age should take into account the gestational age at birth. For example, at his or her 9-month checkup, an infant born at 28 weeks' gestation should be able to perform skills typical for a 6-month-old.

SPEECH AND LANGUAGE DELAY

An individual's ability to speak impacts his or her capacity to communicate with others and develop social relationships. Speech delay is the most common developmental concern raised by parents. As many as 15% of young children have some sort of speech/language delay at one time or another during the preschool years. Persistent speech delay which significantly interferes with communication suggests a speech/language disorder. In most cases, there is no underlying biologic abnormality (genetic syndrome, neuromuscular disease) associated with the disorder.

Language disorders result in the inability to understand or acquire the vocabulary, grammatical rules, or conversation patterns of language. **Speech disorders** involve difficulty producing the sounds and rhythms of speech. **Phonetic disorders** are problems with articulation. Speech and phonetic disorders are expressive disorders, whereas language disorders often affect both expressive and receptive language skills.

Dysfluency produces interruptions in the flow of speech. Developmental dysfluency is observed in many preschoolers, resolves by age 4 years, and is not pathologic. True dysfluency (**stuttering**), characterized by signs of tension and struggle when speaking, sound repetition, or complete speech blockage, significantly impedes the ability to communicate.

Parental concern is a good predictor of the need for further workup. Since many young children are uncomfortable speaking freely in front of strangers, a detailed history is often necessary to characterize the quantity and quality of the patient's speech. **Any child with suspected language delay should receive a full audiologic (hearing) assessment**, followed by referral to a speech pathologist for further workup and treatment (if indicated). The most common cause of mild-to-moderate hearing loss in young children is otitis media with effusion. Most children with expressive language delays secondary to middle ear effusions will catch up by preschool age. Early and intensive speech therapy often results in significant and sustained improvement in communication skills over time.

TABLE 15-1 Typical Developmental Milestones

Age	Gross Motor	Fine (Visual) Motor	Language	Social/Adaptive
Birth–1 mo	Raises head slightly in prone position	Follows with eyes to midline only; hands tightly fisted	Alerts/startles to sound	Fixes on face (at birth)
2 mo	Raises chest and head off bed in prone position	Regards object and follows through 180° arc; briefly retains rattle	Coos and vocalizes reciprocally	Social smile; recognizes parent
4 mo	Lifts onto extended elbows in prone position; steady head control with no head lag; rolls over front to back	Reaches for objects with both hands together; bats at objects; grabs and retains objects	Orients to voice; laughs and squeals	Initiates social interaction
6 mo	Sits, but may need support; rolls in both directions	Reaches with one hand; transfers objects hand-to-hand	Babbles	Recognizes object or person as unfamiliar
9 mo	Sits without support; crawls; pulls to stand	Uses pincer grasp; finger-feeds	Imitates speech sounds (nonspecific "mama," "dada"); understands "no"	Plays gesture games ("pat-a-cake"); understands own name; object permanence; stranger anxiety
12 mo	Cruises; stands alone; takes a few independent steps	Can voluntarily release items	Discriminative use of "mama," "dada," plus 1–4 other words; follows command with gesture	Imitates; comes when called; cooperates with dressing
15 mo	Walks well independently	Builds a two-block tower; throws ball underhand	4–6 words in addition to above; uses jargon; responds to one-step verbal command	Begins to use cup; indicates wants or needs
18 mo	Runs; walks up stairs with hand held; stoops and recovers	Builds a three-block tower; uses spoon; spontaneous scribbling	Uses 10–25 words; points to body parts when asked; uses words to communicate needs or wants	Plays near (but not with) other children
24 mo	Walks unassisted up and down stairs; kicks ball; throws ball overhand; jumps with two feet off the floor	Builds four- to six-block tower; uses fork and spoon; copies a straight line	Uses 50+ words, two- and three-word phrases; uses "I" and "me"; 50% of speech intelligible to stranger	Removes simple clothing; parallel play
36 mo	Pedals tricycle; broad jumps	Copies a circle	Uses 5–8 word sentences; 75% of speech intelligible to stranger	Knows age and gender; engages in group play; shares
4 y	Balances on one foot	Copies a cross; catches ball	Tells a story; 100% of speech intelligible to stranger	Dresses self; puts on shoes; washes and dries hands; imaginative play
5 y	Skips with alternating feet	Draws a person with six body parts	Asks what words mean	Names four colors; plays cooperative games; understands "rules" and abides by them
6 y	Rides a bike	Writes name	Identifies written letters and numbers	Knows right from left; knows all color names

GLOBAL DEVELOPMENTAL DELAY

A demonstrable lag in all developmental realms (language, gross motor, fine motor, and adaptive) represents **global developmental delay**. A careful physical examination for unique features and neurological signs, such as small head size or low tone, should be pursued. A significant proportion of these children subsequently will be diagnosed with a genetic disorder, but the etiology remains unclear in as many as 50% of cases.

NEURODEVELOPMENTAL DISABILITIES

INTELLECTUAL DISABILITY

Mental retardation, as defined in the DSM-IV-TR, involves: (1) IQ (intellectual quotient) ≤70; (2) onset prior to 18 years of age; and (3) impaired adaptive functioning (in at least two of the following areas: communication, self-care, home living, social/interpersonal skills, use of community resources, self-direction, academic skills, work, leisure, health, and safety). The most commonly used IQ tests in the pediatric population are the **Wechsler** scales (preschool and school age, WPPSI and WISC) and the **Stanford-Binet** (school age). The Vineland Adaptive Behavior Scale is used by psychologists to measure a child's adaptive functioning based on parent, caregiver and teacher rating forms. An IQ of 50 to 70 denotes **mild** retardation (the great majority of affected individuals), 35 to 55 defines **moderate** retardation, 20 to 40 correlates with **severe** retardation, and below 20 to 25 signifies **profound** retardation.

The cause of mental disability is identified in only about half of cases. Mental retardation may come to the attention of the pediatrician when the child exhibits developmental delay in one or more areas. Obvious dysmorphisms occasionally suggest a specific disorder (e.g., Down, Fragile X, or fetal alcohol syndrome). Laboratory testing may be beneficial when a genetic cause is suspected. Identifying a genetic etiology is important in determining a family's recurrence risk and aiding in prognosis. Comorbid conditions (cerebral palsy, behavioral disorders, seizures) are not uncommon. Treatment is interdisciplinary, supportive, and symptom-specific, with the goal of maximizing adaptive functioning and quality of life.

AUTISM SPECTRUM DISORDERS

Autism spectrum disorders (ASD) encompass a collection of chronic, nonprogressive disabilities characterized by impairments in **social interaction**, **communication**, and **behavior** (Table 15-2). Both autism and **Asperger syndrome** are classified as autism spectrum disorders. The reported prevalence of these conditions has been rising over the past 20 years and is now estimated to be 2 to 7 per 1,000 children in the United States. It is unclear whether this is due to improved reporting, more inclusive criteria, or a higher rate of disease. Autism is more common in males. It is usually diagnosed between 18 months and 3 years of age, although symptoms such as impaired attachment and poor eye contact are often present from infancy. Autism is currently thought to be a multifactorial disorder. Children with genetic conditions such as Fragile X and tuberous sclerosis are known to be at increased risk for ASD. Ongoing research is identifying other genes associated with the development of ASD as well as possible environmental triggers. *Long-term epidemiologic studies have not found any association between the MMR vaccine or thimerosal* (a former vaccine preservative) *and the development of autism.*

TABLE 15-2 Characteristics of Autism Spectrum Disorders

Social interaction
Limited eye contact and facial expression
Difficulty developing peer relationships
Indifference to social overtures
Lack of social reciprocity
Inflexibility
No engagement in pretend play
Communication
Impaired reciprocal communication
Language development deviant, rather than simply delayed
Echolalia, perseverative speech
Behaviors
Restrictive, stereotyped patterns of behavior
Repetitive, self-stimulatory behaviors (e.g., rocking, spinning)
Preoccupation or fascination with a single object or subject

Clinical Manifestations

Children with classic **autism** have significant language and communication abnormalities. They do not engage in meaningful social interactions. They avoid eye contact, exhibit impaired reciprocity, lack understanding of emotions, and do not engage in pretend play. Affected children usually display stereotypic and/or repetitive behavior patterns and may have an attachment to or fascination with unusual objects.

Asperger syndrome is characterized by difficulty forming relationships/relating to others *and* development of intense interest in very specific topics (e.g., dinosaurs, space, electronics). While people with Asperger syndrome may not have disordered language production, they are often hyperverbal and unable to understand abstract forms of language such as metaphors and sarcasm. Children with Asperger syndrome usually want to form friendships, but their inability to pick up on subtle social cues makes this difficult.

Management

Treatment of autism spectrum disorders consists of intensive behavioral intervention (e.g., Applied Behavior Analysis or ABA therapy) and sensory integration therapy, speech and language training, social modeling, and family support. Pharmacologic intervention targets specific symptoms such as anxiety, hyperactivity, and perseverative behaviors. Early recognition and intervention lead to better clinical outcomes. The American Academy of Pediatrics recommends routine screening of all children prior to age 2 years. Common screening tools utilized by pediatricians include the Childhood Autism Rating Scales (CARS) and The Modified Checklist for Autism for Toddlers

(MCHAT). The best prognostic indicators of future success include the extent of language development present during the preschool years and cognitive ability.

ATTENTION-DEFICIT/HYPERACTIVITY DISORDER

Attention-deficit/hyperactivity disorder (ADHD) is a syndrome characterized by **inattention, hyperactivity,** and **impulsivity** which are inconsistent with the developmental stage of the child and manifested through maladaptive behaviors. Classic ADHD is more common in boys and is usually diagnosed in elementary school. School performance and peer relationships often suffer, placing the child at risk for low self-esteem. A variant of ADHD in which inattentiveness is the sole distinguishing feature is more common in girls, who are often diagnosed later than their hyperactive peers. Symptoms persist into adulthood in the majority of patients.

Clinical Manifestations

To be diagnosed with ADHD, a patient must meet specific criteria detailed in the DSM-IV-TR and summarized in Table 15-3. Moreover, the inattention, hyperactivity, and impulsiveness must be present by age 7 years, persist for at least 6 months, and be observed consistently in multiple environments (e.g., school and home). Signs of ADHD may be minimized in settings which are novel, highly supervised, or narrowly focused on the patient. Thus, an affected child may not display any behaviors typical of ADHD in the pediatrician's office.

Assessment

ADHD is a clinical diagnosis. The initial assessment of a child with possible ADHD relies firmly on history obtained from parents and teachers. Age-appropriate rating scales (e.g., Conner's Parent and Teacher Rating Scales, Vanderbilt) are available and standardized. A complete physical examination should be performed. Child psychologists employ more targeted testing to pick up on inattention and lack of sustained focus.

TABLE 15-3 Characteristic Features of Attention-Deficit/Hyperactivity Disorder

Inattention
Has a short attention span, is easily distractible
Fails to attend to details
Demonstrates difficulty organizing activities, completing tasks
Avoids activities that require sustained mental effort
Is forgetful in daily activities
Has difficulty following directions
Hyperactivity
Excessively active for age
Fidgets and squirms; restless
Unable to remain seated
Unable to play quietly or entertain oneself
Talks excessively
Impulsivity
Has difficulty waiting one's turn
Often interrupts others

Management

The goal of therapy is to provide sustained symptom reduction throughout the day with an acceptable minimum of adverse effects. Children with ADHD benefit from a multidisciplinary approach. Emotional supports should be made available for the patient and parents. A behavior management program must be developed to assist both the parents and teachers with positive reinforcement, structure, and discipline. Educational assessment should be considered for children with school underperformance; up to 25% of students with ADHD also have a learning disability. Oppositional defiant disorder is the most common comorbid psychiatric diagnosis; others may include mood, anxiety, and conduct disorders. ADHD may be a comorbid condition with neurologic disorders such as epilepsy or Tourette syndrome.

Pharmacologic intervention *and* behavior modification in combination result in the best outcomes. Psycho-stimulants, including **methylphenidate, dextroamphetamine, mixed amphetamine salts, and lisdexamfetamine** (inactive prodrug metabolized to active form by the body) are available in immediate- and extended-release formulations. All are designated as controlled substances. These drugs work by increasing the availability of dopamine and norepinephrine. Side effects include insomnia, elevated blood pressure, nausea, and anorexia; rarely tics and dyskinesias may develop. Nonstimulant options include **atomoxetine** (a highly-specific norepinephrine reuptake inhibitor), clonidine, and guanfacine. The Food and Drug Administration requires "black box" warning labels on both the stimulants and atomoxetine (risk of sudden cardiac death for the former; suicidal ideation for the latter). Depending on the patient's degree of symptomatology, medication holidays on weekends and vacations may be an option.

CEREBRAL PALSY

Cerebral palsy (CP) is a nonprogressive disorder of movement and posture that results from a static lesion of the developing brain which occurs before, during, or after birth. Approximately one-third of cases develop after full-term birth following an apparently normal gestation. Modern case series have identified a single or mixed etiology for the motor disability in at least 80% of cases of CP. In Shevell's 2003 consecutive case series of children with CP, the top five etiologic entities were periventricular leukomalacia, intrapartum asphyxia, cerebral dysgenesis, intracranial hemorrhage, and vascular infarction. Transient neonatal depression is not predictive of an eventual diagnosis of CP. Excluding extremely premature or low-birth-weight infants, over 90% of infants with Apgar scores of 0 to 3 at 5 minutes do not develop CP. Infants with intrapartum hypoxia-ischemia who have normal neurologic examinations by 1 week of age have a good likelihood of normal outcome. Prenatal factors such as intrauterine infection, prematurity, placental hemorrhage, and multiple gestations raise the risk of CP. Acquired postnatal causes of CP include stroke, trauma, kernicterus from severe hyperbilirubinemia, and infections of the central nervous system.

CLINICAL MANIFESTATIONS

CP is classified by the pattern of motor impairments and by characteristics of muscle tone. The most common form is **spastic** CP, which is the consequence of injury to the pyramidal motor tracts in the brain. Spasticity is velocity-dependent increased muscle resistance in response to passive stretch. Increased tone in CP may have both *spastic* and *dystonic* features. Dystonia is increased muscle tone which is generated by movement. Typically, it is a posturing movement with co-contraction of the extensors and flexors. CP is further classified by which limbs are involved (Table 15-4). Recently, classification systems based on function rather than anatomic location have been introduced. Patients with CP may be initially hypotonic; increased tone develops over time, dependent on the severity of the CNS injury. In infancy, delay in the disappearance of primitive reflexes (such as the Moro or the asymmetric tonic neck reflex) can be early indicators of CP. The diagnosis of cerebral palsy becomes more apparent over time when the child fails to meet gross motor milestones.

Extrapyramidal CP results from damage to the basal ganglia, which is involved in the regulation of muscle tone and coordination. Affected patients exhibit involuntary choreoathetoid movements, dystonia, and postural ataxia, in addition to hypotonic quadriparesis or spastic diplegia. Kernicterus used to be a major cause of extrapyramidal CP; however, improved management of hyperbilirubinemia has decreased the incidence of kernicterus. Now, most patients with extrapyramidal CP have an identifiable risk factor for brain insult (e.g., severe perinatal asphyxia, placental infarction, maternal toxemia, ECMO exposure). Cerebral dysgenesis, including malformations of the cerebellum and brainstem, can cause **ataxic** CP with hypotonia, truncal ataxia, and titubation (bobbing of the head and/or trunk). Hypotonic and ataxic CP often have genetic etiologies.

The American Academy of Neurology and the Practice Committee of the Child Neurology Society published a practice parameter addressing the diagnostic assessment of the child with CP in 2004. The practice parameter suggests that the history and physical examination should be reviewed to exclude a progressive or degenerative brain disorder. The child should be screened for associated conditions including visual or hearing impairments, speech and language delays, problem solving deficits, and feeding and swallowing dysfunction. An electroencephalograph (EEG) should be obtained if there is a history of possible seizures. Neuroimaging with an MRI is recommended to discern an etiology (if possible) for the CP. If cerebral malformation is present, a genetic or metabolic evaluation should be considered. Evaluation for a hypercoagulable state is suggested if a stroke is identified.

TABLE 15-4 Topographic Classification of Spastic (Pyramidal) Cerebral Palsy

Diplegia—bilateral leg spasticity and weakness much greater than arm spasticity and weakness. Often observed in preterm infants with periventricular leukomalacia (PVL).
Quadriplegia—all limbs severely involved. Often related to severe PVL, asphyxia, or cerebral dysgenesis.
Hemiplegia—one side involved. Usually due to a unilateral cortical lesion such as more focal dysgenesis or stroke.

DIFFERENTIAL DIAGNOSIS

Although CP is nonprogressive, periods of rapid growth may transiently make the disorder appear progressive. Metabolic and genetic evaluation should be considered if the child has deterioration or episodic decompensation, no etiology can be determined, or if there is a family history of childhood neurologic disorder. Progressive or degenerative disorders that can be misdiagnosed as CP include metachromatic leukodystrophy, Friedreich ataxia, ataxia-telangiectasia, and certain metabolic and mitochondrial disorders associated with spasticity.

TREATMENT

A multidisciplinary team approach, including a general pediatrician, physical and occupational therapists, nutritionist, speech-language therapist, orthopedist, physiatrist or neurologist, and social support services results in optimal function. Many systemic medicines have been tried to reduce spasticity with variable success. However, significant improvements in motor function have been achieved with botulinum toxin injections along with stretching and/or serial casting to treat joint deformities. Intrathecal baclofen pumps can improve spasticity with fewer central side effects, but the pumps can fail or get infected. Dorsal nerve rhizotomy is used in selected cases to decrease spasticity. Many children ultimately require orthopedic surgery to correct deformities and release contractures.

Comorbidities commonly occur in children with CP. Learning difficulty may be secondary to an intellectual disability, learning disability, or ADHD. These can occur individually or coexist. Up to 50% of patients with CP develop epilepsy. Hearing and visual impairments should be monitored and corrected if possible. If a child with CP is nonverbal or language impaired, it is important to provide for alternate modes of communication including sign language, communication boards, and/or augmentative communication devices. Finally, sleep disorders occur more commonly in children with CP, requiring close monitoring of sleep habits.

NEURODEGENERATIVE DISORDERS

Neural tissue degeneration can occur at any level of the nervous system, from the brain cell bodies to the peripheral nerves. Many degenerative diseases are inherited; most are progressive and debilitating. Neurodegenerative disorders may be divided into **gray matter** disorders, **white matter** disorders, and **systemic** disorders.

Gray matter disorders, which include Tay–Sachs, Gaucher, and Niemann–Pick diseases, result from lipid buildup in neuronal cell bodies. Hypotonia, mental retardation, seizures, retinal degeneration, and ataxia are common. These disorders are further discussed in Chapter 18.

White matter disorders (leukodystrophies) are inherited, progressive degenerative diseases resulting from abnormally formed myelin. The anomalous formation impairs conduction and leads to rapid myelin breakdown. Leukodystrophies present with focal neurological deficits, spasticity, visual disturbances (optic atrophy/blindness), changes in personality, and cognitive decline. **Adrenoleukodystrophy**, so named because of its frequent association with adrenal insufficiency, is an X-linked disorder characterized by areas of periventricular white matter demyelination. Psychomotor retardation progresses to spasticity, extensor posturing, seizures, and early death.

Systemic diseases are categorized according to the particular neural pathway affected. **Rett syndrome** is an X-linked recessive disorder observed almost exclusively in girls; affected males succumb in utero. In the classic form of Rett syndrome, development along all streams is initially normal. Rapid milestone regression begins in the second year of life, with significant slowing of brain growth. **Repetitive hand wringing** is the most characteristic behavioral sign; other manifestations include seizures, ataxia, mental retardation, and autistic behavior. Life expectancy is appreciably shortened.

SEIZURES AND EPILEPSY

A **seizure** is a transient clinical event that results from abnormal and excessive electrical brain activity. The aberrant electrical activity disrupts brain function, leading to **positive signs** (motor, sensory, autonomic changes) and/or **negative signs** (loss of awareness, loss of motor tone), depending on the cortical localization of the seizure. **Epilepsy** is diagnosed when a patient has had two or more unprovoked seizures. In contrast, "provoked" or acute symptomatic seizures occur in the context of an acute brain insult (trauma, intoxication, infection) and are not classified as epilepsy unless they become recurrent following resolution of the acute illness. Some children develop epilepsy due to cortical malformations or have specific age-related epilepsy syndromes. For 60% to 80% of children with epilepsy, no apparent cause can be determined.

FEBRILE SEIZURES

Febrile seizures are typically brief (<10 minutes), generalized seizures associated with fever. They occur in up to 5% of otherwise healthy children ages 6 months to 6 years. Febrile seizures, even when recurrent, are not considered epilepsy. Febrile seizures are divided into simple febrile seizures and complex febrile seizures. **Simple febrile seizures** are generalized, brief, and single (do not recur within 24 hours). **Complex febrile seizures** are focal, prolonged (>10 minutes), or repetitive (recur within 24 hours). One-third of children with febrile seizures present with status epilepticus (>30 minutes). By definition, the diagnosis of febrile seizure *excludes* children with intracranial infection or prior history of nonfebrile seizure. Most febrile seizures occur in the first 24 hours of an illness, in children less than 3 years old and with fevers of 39°C or higher. The rapid rise in the fever often precipitates the seizure.

One-third of children with febrile seizures will have a recurrence. Risk factors for recurrent febrile seizure include: (1) first febrile seizure before age 1 year, (2) family history of febrile seizures, and (3) low-grade fever/short duration of fever at the time of the seizure. Children with all three risk factors or two febrile seizures have a 60% to 70% recurrence rate. A lengthy febrile seizure does not increase the risk of recurrence, but it does increase the risk that a recurrent febrile seizure will be prolonged. Daily anticonvulsant administration is not indicated in children with febrile seizures. Studies show that alternating acetaminophen and ibuprofen during a febrile illness may not prevent the seizure. Education about seizure first aid, seizure precautions, and an emergency plan in case of recurrent seizure is important. Serial seizures and seizures lasting more than 5 minutes can be treated with rectal diazepam. The child should be transported to the emergency department by ambulance if the seizure continues more than 5 minutes or does not resolve following rectal diazepam administration. Febrile status epilepticus should be addressed aggressively to prevent morbidity and mortality.

The American Academy of Pediatrics has practice parameters that address the **evaluation of first simple febrile seizure** in neurologically healthy children between 6 months and 5 years. The diagnosis of febrile seizure is based on a thorough history. It is important to differentiate nonseizure events (such as rigors in a febrile child, breathholding spells, or syncope) from febrile seizure. In the history and physical examination, it is vital to look for evidence that the child may have meningitis or encephalitis causing the seizure and to consider that affected children less than 18 months old may not have meningismus. It is also important to ask about possible ingestions of drugs or toxins and history suggestive of metabolic disorder or derangement from unusual intake or fluid/electrolyte losses. Seizures are the presenting sign in about 15% of children with meningitis, and in about one-third of these children, meningeal signs and symptoms may be absent. The guidelines recommend that lumbar puncture (LP) should be *strongly considered* after first simple febrile seizure in a child less than 12 months and *considered* in the child between 12 and 18 months. In these two age groups signs of meningismus may be subtle. LP should also be considered for children older than 18 months if they have meningeal signs and in children who have recently received antibiotics. Blood glucose, basic serum electrolytes, calcium, phosphorus, magnesium, and CBC are not routinely indicated but can be sent under particular circumstances. EEG and neuroimaging are also not recommended in the evaluation of simple febrile seizures.

Children with febrile seizures have an increased risk of developing epilepsy. Between 2% and 7% of all children with febrile seizures develop epilepsy if followed to age 25 years. Three major risk factors increase the risk of later epilepsy: (1) complex febrile seizures, (2) preexisting neurodevelopmental abnormality, and (3) epilepsy in first-degree relatives. Additional risk factors include history of first febrile seizure under age 1 year, short duration of fever prior to the seizure, and multiple febrile seizures.

It is important to note that over 90% of children who have febrile seizures do not develop epilepsy. Overall, the morbidity and mortality associated with febrile seizures is extremely low. Two large prospective studies showed no differences in cognition between children with a history of febrile seizures and those without.

EPILEPSY

Approximately 5% of all children have a provoked or unprovoked seizure by the age of 20 years. By early adulthood, the cumulative incidence of epilepsy is between 1% and 2%. In children who are observed off of anticonvulsants, the risk for recurrence after a single unprovoked seizure is 30% to 40%. Risk factors for seizure recurrence following a first unprovoked seizure in childhood include: (1) prior history of abnormal brain/development, (2) abnormal EEG, (3) prior febrile seizures, (4) transient focal weakness (Todd paralysis), (5) first degree relative with epilepsy, or (6) seizure arising out of sleep. Healthy, developmentally typical children whose initial seizure occurs while awake have the best prognosis for remaining seizure-free.

After the first unprovoked seizure, generally the child is observed off of daily anticonvulsants, and the parents are provided with an emergency action plan. The recurrence risk is up to 70% to 80% after a second or third unprovoked seizure; at that point most children are started on a daily anticonvulsant.

About 50% of children with epilepsy outgrow their seizures, particularly those with age-related epilepsy syndromes such as benign rolandic epilepsy or childhood absence epilepsy. Some adolescents develop epilepsy due to an age-related epilepsy syndrome (juvenile myoclonic epilepsy) or traumatic brain injury. The probable etiology and prognosis of a seizure vary with the child's age, family history of epilepsy, history of preexisting neurodevelopmental disability, identified epilepsy syndrome, and the acute symptomatic cause for the seizure.

Clinical Manifestations

History and Physical Examination

It is vital to take a thorough history of what occurred before, during, and after an event to determine whether the spell was epileptic or rather a nonepileptic paroxysmal event such as reflux, syncope, or a night terror. The context of the child's age, past medical and family histories, and any prior unusual spells are important in the differentiation of a seizure from a nonseizure event.

The diagnosis of a seizure is based primarily on history. Questions should include what the child was doing and feeling prior to and during the event, how the event evolved over time, how long the event lasted, and how the child behaved following the event. Attempts should be made to differentiate the abnormal movements with regard to whether the movement subsided with gentle restraint, was stereotypic, or *rhythmic* rather than tremulous. Focal features such as head or eye deviation should be noted. It is important to ask if any abnormal spells have occurred previously and whether the child had any recent illness, injury, ingestion, neurological changes/signs, or prior abnormalities of development. The child's past history and family history often provide important supplemental information. At the end of a thorough history, the physician should be able to differentiate an epileptic seizure from a nonseizure paroxysmal event (such as syncope or daydreaming). Occasionally, the available history is not sufficient to make the determination of seizure versus nonseizure. In that case, the family should be educated with regards to the appearance of seizures, as well as seizure first aid and precautions.

The comprehensive physical examination should include vital signs, growth parameters, and presence of neurocutaneous lesions, dysmorphic features, retinal abnormalities, signs of infection, cardiac abnormalities, and/or trauma. A full neurological examination assesses mental status, cranial nerve function (including vision), and evidence of any focal abnormalities of tone or strength, sensation, coordination, reflexes, or gait.

Diagnostic Evaluation

EEG studies can provide supplementary information to support a diagnosis of epilepsy. An abnormal EEG permits classification of the epilepsy as **focal** (localization-related) or **generalized** and may suggest a specific epilepsy syndrome (such as the 3-Hz spike-and-wave pattern typically seen in children with absence epilepsy). The EEG result should be evaluated in light of the child's history. A child with epilepsy can have a normal EEG. Similarly, a child who has had a nonseizure paroxysmal event may have an abnormal EEG. Practice guidelines established by the American Academy of Neurology, the Child Neurology Society, and the American Epilepsy Society recommend a routine EEG as part of the diagnostic evaluation following a first nonfebrile seizure.

If imaging is performed, MRI of the brain is the preferred modality. MRI can demonstrate an abnormality (such as cortical dysgenesis) in about 20% of cases of new-onset seizure. Emergent neuroimaging may be necessary in a child who is not returning to baseline within hours, in the child with a postictal focal deficit, or the patient with signs or symptoms of increased intracranial pressure. Brain MRI may not be necessary if the clinical history and EEG are consistent with certain epilepsy syndromes (such as childhood absence epilepsy). In general, brain MRI should be performed in any child who has a history of a partial-onset seizure, abnormal neurologic examination, or abnormal developmental history. LP should be considered in any child with persistently altered mental status or meningeal signs and in young infants less than 6 months of age. If increased intracranial pressure is suspected or if the child has focal neurologic signs, imaging should precede the LP. Toxicology screening is warranted if there is a question of ingestion of drugs or toxins. Other laboratory tests should be ordered on an individual basis if the child has vomiting, diarrhea, dehydration, or failure to return to baseline alertness.

CLASSIFICATION OF SEIZURES AND EPILEPSY SYNDROMES

Table 15-5 delineates the International Classification of Epileptic Seizures.

Partial seizures are those in which the first clinical and electrographic changes occur in a localized area of the brain. The signs and symptoms of a partial seizure are specific to the focus, and may be motor, sensory, autonomic, or higher cortical psychic symptoms. Partial seizures are further categorized by whether or not consciousness is impaired during the seizure. During **simple partial seizures**, consciousness is fully maintained. In **complex partial seizures**, consciousness is altered, and the individual is not fully aware or responsive.

- **Motor** seizures may manifest as focal rhythmic twitching (the "Jacksonian march" progression of convulsions to involve one side of the body); involuntary movement

TABLE 15-5 International Classification of Epileptic Seizures

Generalized seizures
Tonic–clonic (any combination)
Tonic
Clonic
Atonic
Absence (typical, atypical with special features)
Myoclonic (myoclonic, myoclonic atonic, myoclonic tonic)
Focal seizures
Unknown
Epileptic spasms

Developed by the International League Against Epilepsy (ILAE) in 2009.

(turning of the eyes, head and/or trunk); or vocalization or arrest of speech.

- **Sensory** seizures can include tingling, numbness, an unpleasant odor or taste, vertigo, flashing lights, or auditory symptoms.
- **Autonomic** seizures may include an epigastric "rising" sensation, vomiting, sweating, pupillary changes, or piloerection ("goosebumps").
- Simple partial seizures may generate **higher cortical psychic symptoms** including feelings of familiarity ("déjà-vu"), sudden intense feelings of fear or sadness, dysphasia, and distortions of time. Patients may report vision changes such as formed hallucinations, micropsia (surroundings appear smaller), or macropsia (surroundings appear larger).

During complex partial seizures, the child may have repetitive semipurposeful movements (automatisms) such as picking at the clothes, oral-buccal movements (chewing, swallowing), or more complex motor movements such as kicking or flailing of the arms. When complex partial seizures arise from the frontal lobe, the child may have bilateral motor movements, become combative, or have awakenings from sleep. Both simple and complex partial seizures can evolve into secondarily generalized seizures.

Generalized seizures are those in which the clinical and electrographic changes at seizure onset are bilateral and widespread in both hemispheres. Consciousness is impaired. Seizures may be nonconvulsive (such as absence seizures) or convulsive with bilateral tonic, clonic, or myoclonic movements. In a **generalized tonic–clonic** (GTC) seizure, the tonic phase consists of sustained flexor or extensor contraction followed by the clonic phase (rhythmic, symmetric, generalized contractions of the face and extremities). Often, the patient exhales and remains in exhalation during the tonic phase of a GTC, with breathing commencing in a grunting or irregular fashion during the clonic phase. Convulsive seizures can also manifest as isolated tonic *or* clonic activity. Bowel or bladder incontinence may occur. The child may bite the side of the tongue or buccal mucosa, and can be injured falling to the floor. An **aura** or warning prior to the onset of the GTC implies partial-onset seizure with rapid secondary generalization. Similarly, a postictal transient hemiparesis (Todd paralysis) implies a partial onset to the seizure. The **postictal** phase is characterized by unresponsiveness and flaccid muscle tone. The child should have gradual improvement in level of consciousness over the following 10 to 30 minutes.

Absence seizures begin between ages 4 and 9 years and consist of brief episodes of staring associated with altered consciousness. The typical duration is 5 to 10 seconds. Often, the staring is accompanied by subtle clonic activity in the face or arms or simple automatisms (such as eye blinking, chewing, or perseverative motor activity). Absence seizures start and stop abruptly and have no postictal phase. Although brief, absence seizures can occur in clusters many times a day and interfere with learning and socialization. In a typical absence seizure, the EEG shows abrupt onset and offset of 3-per-second generalized symmetric spike-and-slow wave complexes. In a child with untreated absence epilepsy, 3 to 5 minutes of hyperventilation will often precipitate a typical absence seizure.

Atonic seizures consist of abrupt loss of postural tone in the neck ("head drop") or the entire body ("drop seizure") which can cause injury to the child. **Myoclonic seizures** are quick jerks similar to those experienced by normal subjects while in light sleep.

Every child with epilepsy should be clinically evaluated to determine if he or she has one of the recognized **childhood epilepsy syndromes**. The International League Against Epilepsy syndrome classification is based on age of onset, seizure types involved, and EEG appearance. An epilepsy syndrome diagnosis provides important prognostic, therapeutic, and at times genetic information.

Differential Diagnosis

Neonates can have unusual movements or apneic spells that are not epileptic. Also, encephalopathic neonates may have subclinical seizures that can only be detected with continuous EEG monitoring. Continuous EEG monitoring is often a useful tool for guiding therapy in neonates with encephalopathy or ongoing potential seizures. Apneic spells associated with bradycardia are typically respiratory rather than epileptic in nature.

Young children (particularly toddlers) can have pallid or cyanotic **breathholding spells** precipitated by a sudden pain or upset, followed by a cry, color change, and the child holding his or her breath in exhalation. Some children then lose consciousness briefly and may have stiffening or transient clonic movements. If the history is typical for breathholding spells, potential evaluations beyond thorough history and examination include possibly an EKG to rule out cardiac syncope and assessment for anemia. Breathholding spells are commonly associated with iron deficiency, and resolution may lessen the occurrence of spells.

In pediatric patients, **syncope** is often misdiagnosed as a seizure. Common characteristics of syncope are the proper setting (prolonged standing or kneeling, just stood up, dehydration, sudden pain, or seeing blood); pallor; lightheadedness; visual changes ("vision coning down to black"); and muffled hearing. The loss of consciousness is brief, particularly if the child remains lying down; transient stiffening or clonic movements at the end of syncope (convulsive syncope) reflects transient decreased blood flow in the brain and is not an epileptic seizure. Following common vasovagal syncope, a child should have little if any confusion/mental status change. Findings suggestive of potentially life-threatening cardiac syncope include syncope during exercise, a family history of deafness, or a family history of sudden death in children or young people.

Essential tremor, spasmus nutans, tics, and myoclonus are various movement disorders that may mimic seizures. **Essential tremor** begins in infancy or childhood and may involve the chin, head, neck, and hands; it usually does not interfere with normal functions. **Spasmus nutans** presents in infancy and includes head nodding and tilting and rapid, small-amplitude nystagmus without alteration of consciousness. A child with spasmus nutans should have MRI of the brain to rule out a tumor. **Myoclonic movements** are sudden, involuntary jerk-like motions similar to startle responses.

Tourette complex consists of motor and vocal tics (sudden, involuntary behaviors that are repetitive and stereotyped) that persist for more than a year. Common comorbid conditions include obsessive-compulsive tendencies and attention-deficit/hyperactivity disorder. Children can also have less frequent tics of one type or the other. If tics become disruptive and interfere with social or educational functioning, cognitive behavioral thereapy or medications (such as clonidine) may be beneficial.

Other conditions that are confused with seizures include benign paroxysmal vertigo, temper tantrums, and night terrors.

Pseudoseizures should be suspected in the patient with implausible findings (e.g., alert and responsive during generalized tonic-clonic movements). Continous video EEG monitoring can be helpful to discern epileptic versus nonepileptic spells. The treatment of pseudoseizures is multidisciplinary, involving psyhchiatry, counseling, and social support.

Treatment

Effective treatment of epilepsy combines education and medication management. Both the child and the parents should become knowledgeable about acute seizure care, use of emergency medication (such as rectal valium), and how/when to access local emergency medical services. The choice of antiepileptic treatment is based on multiple factors. When possible, identifying seizure type and epilepsy syndrome helps predict which anticonvulsants may be beneficial (Table 15-6).

With medication, approximately 50% to 70% of patients become seizure free. Another 10% to 30% have significant reductions in seizure frequency and/or intensity. There has been a dramatic increase in the number of medications available for the management of seizures. The newer medications have a better toxicity profile. Conventional anticonvulsants require careful monitoring of serum levels; most newer drugs do not require routine monitoring (Table 15-7).

There is a paucity of classes I and II randomized clinical trials to determine evidence-based recommendations for treatment, particularly for children with generalized seizures. For children with partial-onset epilepsy, oxcarbazepine should be considered for initial monotherapy based on current efficacy evidence. Considering all factors, including cost, carbamazepine, valproic acid, topiramate, and phenytoin are other reasonable choices to treat partial-onset seizures. In terms of generalized epilepsy, valproic acid and ethosuximide have equal efficacy for treatment of childhood absence epilepsy; lamotrigine is more effective than placebo. For other generalized epilepsies, valproic acid, levetiracetam, topiramate, and lamotrigine are reasonable choices.

In most patients, it is reasonable to consider weaning off of anticonvulsant medication after the child has been seizure free for 2 years. In patients with particular epilepsy syndromes such as JME, the seizures are usually life-long, so anticonvulsants are generally not withdrawn. Recommendations to start and stop anticonvulsants must be tailored to the individual patient, with decisions made by the physician together with the patient and family.

For patients with anticonvulsant-refractory seizures (~10%), additional interventions are available. Monitoring a patient's seizures with continuous EEG leads may indicate a focus that can be removed surgically. The risks and benefits of such a procedure need to be explored carefully with the patient and family. Another option is the ketogenic diet. Inducing ketosis through a high-fat, very low-carbohydrate diet may control or reduce symptoms in some children. The vagal nerve stimulator, approved by the Food and Drug Administration in 1997, has proven quite beneficial in some patients.

EMERGENCY MANAGEMENT OF STATUS EPILECTICUS

Status epilepticus is defined as a prolonged episode of seizure activity (>30 minutes) or an extended period of recurrent seizures between which the patient does not return to consciousness. **Status epilepticus is a medical emergency**, leading to hypoxia, brain damage, and death. For treatment purposes, any convulsive seizure lasting more than 5 minutes should be addressed with emergency medication. For out of hospital use, rectal diazepam (Diastat) and midazolam (IV form squirted next to the buccal mucosa or sprayed intranasally) are effective and safe in the setting of prolonged seizures. Airway, breathing, and circulation should be evaluated first and addressed as necessary. Intravenous or rectal short-acting benzodiazepines (lorazepam or diazepam) often stop the seizure. For a prolonged seizure not responsive to initial treatment, fosphenytoin, midazolam, or phenobarbital loading doses are administered to break the seizure as well as to prevent recurrence. Patients with refractory status may require drug-induced comas (pentobarbital or midazolam drips) and continuous EEG monitoring to adjust and evaluate ongoing management. Prognosis after status epilepticus is related to the underlying etiology for the prolonged seizure. If a child has preexisting epilepsy, anticonvulsant levels are drawn. The child who is febrile and toxic-appearing or has new repetitive seizures and altered mental status warrants an evaluation for CNS infection (including LP). A head CT should be obtained prior to LP in a child with focal seizures, postictal focal deficits, or any signs or symptoms of increased intracranial pressure. Targeted or comprehensive toxicology screening is undertaken if there is any concern about ingestion. Historic features consistent with metabolic disorder (unexplained encephalopathy, deterioration during illness, unusual odors) or unexplained acidosis or coma should trigger metabolic evaluation including glucose, lactate, pyruvate, ammonia, carnitine levels, acylcarnitine profile, serum amino acids, and urine organic acids.

ENCEPHALOPATHY

To function normally, the brain needs adequate blood flow, oxygen, energy substrates, removal of metabolic waste, and appropriate electrolyte balance. Disruption of any of these will lead to generalized cerebral dysfunction with alteration in mental status and/or level of consciousness, termed **encephalopathy**.

CLINICAL MANIFESTATIONS

The differential diagnosis of pediatric encephalopathy, or deterioration in mental status due to generalized cerebral dysfunction, is extensive (Table 15-8). Fortunately, the age of the patient, past medical history, history of present illness, and physical examination often suggest the etiology. Encephalopathy secondary to a systemic process such as electrolyte imbalance, infection, or liver failure is characterized by fluctuating mental status and nonlocalizing neurologic manifestations (myoclonus, tremors, temperature instability). In contrast, levels of consciousness are abnormal but fairly stable when encephalopathy results from structural lesions in the brain (tumor, abscess, hemorrhage), and focal neurologic signs are more common. Recent or concurrent febrile illness is consistent with infectious encephalitis. Focal findings (hemiparesis, ataxia, cranial nerve defects) and focal seizures (typically temporal lobe) are more common with **herpes simplex (HSV) encephalitis** than other viral etiologies. **Reye syndrome**, a rare mitochondrial disorder characterized by acute-onset encephalopathy and degenerative liver disease, may follow a

TABLE 15-6 Characteristics of Epilepsy Syndromes and Antiepileptic Drugs

Seizure Type	Epilepsy Syndrome	Clinical Features	First-Line Treatment of Choice (Monotherapy)	Alternative First-Line Treatment	Additional Information
Partial seizures	Simple or complex partial epilepsy	Onset: Any age	Oxcarbazepine Carbamezepine	Levetiracetam Lamotrigine Topiramate	FDA-approved adjunct therapy; Lamotrigine, Tiagabine, Torpiramate, Zonisamide, Felbamate
		Duration: Minutes			
		Aura, staring, automatisms, focal tonic clonic activity, postictal confusion			
		EEG: Localized abnormalities			
	Benign epilepsy with centrotemporal spikes (BECTS), Rolandic epilepsy	Onset: 3–13 y	Majority of children do not require antiepileptic therapy	Oxcarbazepine Carbamazepine	Other: Lamotrigine Levetiracetam
		Duration: 1–2 min			
		Wakes from sleep, paresthesias one side of mouth, ipsilateral facial twitching, drooling.			
		EEG: Unilateral or bilateral centrotemporal spikes			
Generalized seizures	Primary generalized epilepsy	Onset: Any age	Valproic acid (boys only) Lamotrigine or Topiramate (very young, girls, or boys)	Zonisamide (myoclonic seizures present) Levetiracetam	FDA-approved adjunct therapy; Gabapentin, Lamotrigine, Levetiracetam, Topiramate
		Duration: Variable			
		Generalized tonic clonic, myoclonic			

Continued

TABLE 15-6 Characteristics of Epilepsy Syndromes and Antiepileptic Drugs *(contined)*

Seizure Type	Epilepsy Syndrome	Clinical Features	First-Line Treatment of Choice (Monotherapy)	Alternative First-Line Treatment	Additional Information
		EEG: Generalized spike wave, polyspike discharges			
	Childhood and Juvenile Absence Epilepsy	Onset: 4–16 y (varies with syndrome)	Ethosuximide Valproic acid (boys only) Lamotrigine		May worsen seizures: Carbamazepine, Oxcarbazepine, Phenobarbital, Phenytoin, Tiagabine, Vigabatrin
		Duration: 5–30 s up to 100 times a day			
		No aura; abrupt onset, staring, motor arrest, automatisms, no postictal confusion.			
		EEG: 2–3 Hz spike wave complexes			
	Juvenile myoclonic epilepsy	Onset: 7–20 y (varies with seizure type)	Valproic acid (boys only) Lamotrigine Levetiracetam	Valproic acid (girls)	FDA approved adjunct therapy: Levetiracetam.
		Duration: Variable depending on seizure type			May worsen seizures: Carbamazepine, gabapentin, oxcarbazepine, phenytoin, tiagabine, vigabatrin
		Absence, myoclonic (morning), and generalized tonic–clonic			
		EEG: Bilateral spike wave and polyspike and wave discharges 3.5–6 Hz			
	Lennox–Gastaut syndrome	Onset: 3–5 y	Valproic acid	Lamotrigine Topiramate	Typically requires multiple antiepileptic medications.

		Duration: Variable depending on seizure type			Vagal Nerve Stimulator, Ketogenic diet, Rufinamide, Lacosamide, and Felbamate are other considerations for refractory seizures
		Atypical absence, atonic (drop), myoclonic, generalized tonic–clonic, tonic			
		Intellectual disability			
		EEG: Spike wave complexes 1.5–2.5 Hz			
Other seizure types	Infantile Spasms	Onset: <1 y	ACTH Vigabatrin (tuberous sclerosis)	Topiramate ACTH	No evidence exists that any therapy improves long-term outcome.
		Duration: Brief, cluster			Consider Vitamin B6 trial.
		Flexor or extensor movements that generally occur in clusters, head drops			
		High-risk populations include Tuberous Sclerosis and Downs Syndrome			
		EEG: Hypsarrhythmia, burst-suppression, slow spike wave, decrement			
	Neonatal seizures	Onset: <3 mo	Phenobartital	Lorazepam Fosphenytoin	Vitamin B_6 and/or folinic acid trials as well as Levetiracetam are other considerations
		Duration: Variable			
		Apnea, tonic, multifocal clonic, focal clonic, myoclonic			

Note: This table is derived from the treatment guidelines from the International League Against Epilepsy (ILAE), the American Academy of Neurology, and the American Epilepsy Society and Expert Consensus of current practice. Agents listed may or may not have FDA approval for the given indication or age group.
Selection of the initial AED for a child or adolescent with newly diagnosed or untreated seizures requires consideration of other variables, not just efficacy. Other factors which should be considered include: AED-related factors (e.g., adverse effect profile, pharmacokinetics, potential for drug interactions, available formulations, carcinogenic and teratogenic potential), patient-related factors (e.g., age, gender, genetic background, concurrent medications, other disease states, ability to swallow tablets/capsules, capacity to afford, insurance coverage), country-related factors (AED cost, AED availability) (Glauser, 2006).

TABLE 15-7 Side Effects of Anticonvulsants

Medication	Side Effects/Toxicity
Conventional drugs	
Carbamazepine	Diplopia, nausea and vomiting, ataxia, leukopenia, thrombocytopenia
Ethosuximide	Rash, anorexia, leukopenia, aplastic anemia
Phenobarbital	Hyperactivity, sedation, nystagmus, ataxia
Phenytoin	Rash, nystagmus, ataxia, drug-induced lupus, gingival hyperplasia, anemia, leukopenia, polyneuropathy
Valproic acid	Hepatotoxicity, nausea and vomiting, abdominal pain, weight gain, anemia, leukopenia, thrombocytopenia
Felbamate	Decreased appetite, weight loss, nausea, insomnia (sleeplessness), headache
Newer drugs	
Gabapentin	Somnolence, dizziness, ataxia, fatigue
Lamotrigine	Dizziness, ataxia, blurred or double vision, nausea, vomiting, rash (including Stevens–Johnson syndrome)
Oxcarbazepine	Somnolence, hyponatremia, rash
Topiramate	Somnolence, fatigue, confusion, headache, ataxia, weight loss
Zonisamide	Somnolence, ataxia, confusion, irritability, renal stones
Levetiracetam	Somnolence, dizziness, anxiety, mood changes, gastrointestinal upset

viral illness, especially when aspirin has been administered. Signs and symptoms include severe vomiting, delirium, stupor, hypoglycemia, and elevated transaminase and ammonia levels. **Metabolic disorders** typically present with recurrent episodes of mental status changes that clear when the acute process is corrected. A careful history may suggest environmental exposures or drug use. Particular areas of interest on examination include vital signs, liver size, pupil and funduscopic assessment, and neurologic findings (cranial nerves, reflexes, strength, sensation, and cerebellar function).

DIAGNOSTIC EVALUATION

Blood tests evaluate for electrolyte abnormalities, uremia, hypoglycemia, acidemia, and hyperammonemia. The WBC count is elevated in the presence of infection. Urine and blood should be sent for toxicology screening. An emergent head CT scan is indicated in patients with evidence of increased intracranial pressure or focal neurologic signs. A LP is appropriate when meningitis or encephalitis is suspected and increased intracranial pressure has been ruled out. HSV encephalitis is characterized by mediotemporal spikes superimposed on a diffuse slow wave pattern on EEG and temporal lobe abnormalities on CT and MRI.

TREATMENT

Specific identification of the underlying disorder is critical to resolving the encephalopathy and preserving brain function. Treatment depends on the cause and whether increased intracranial pressure is present. Patients with severe disease require intubation and close intracranial pressure monitoring in an ICU. Antibiotics are added in cases of bacterial infection; high-dose IV acyclovir is recommended for patients with HSV. Metabolic disorders are discussed in Chapter 18. Ingestions are discussed in Chapter 21.

HEADACHES

PATHOGENESIS

Headaches are a common complaint in the pediatric population. It is important to determine early in the evaluation whether the headaches are **primary** (benign headaches not associated with underlying neuropathology; includes tension, migraine headaches) or **secondary** (pathologic, with the pain typically generated secondary to increased intracranial pressure).

Benign tension headaches are often associated with psychological stress or fatigue. They are typically described as generalized, constant, and band-like in distribution. Most respond to over-the-counter analgesics, removal of the inciting stressor, and rest. Affected patients who take analgesics more than three to four times a week are at risk for the development of chronic, **analgesic overuse headaches (rebound) headaches**. Frequent tension-type headaches can also be associated with clinical depression.

Migraine headaches are hypothesized to result from sudden progressive depolarization of a hyperexcitable cerebral cortex ("spreading cortical depression"). They are characterized by recurrent attacks of severe, throbbing, typically frontal or frontotemporal pain which lasts for several hours. Photophobia, nausea, and vomiting may also be present. In about one-third of patients, the headaches are preceded by an aura, which is usually visual (e.g., scotomas). Symptoms resolve with sleep. Migraines are classified as **complicated** when they

TABLE 15-8 Causes of Encephalopathy in Children

Infection	**Metabolic disorders**
• Infection of the central nervous system is by far the most common cause of acute encephalopathy in children.	• Aminoacidopathies
• Infections which may present with altered level of consciousness include meningitis, encephalitis, postinfectious encephalomyelitis, brain abscess, and subdural empyema.	• Organic acidopathies
• Sepsis can produce generalized cerebral depression in the absence of central nervous system involvement.	• Disorders of carbohydrate metabolism
• Infection with *Shigella* species occasionally presents with isolated encephalopathy.	• Disorders of fatty acid oxidation
Increased intracranial pressure	**Mitochondrial disorders**
• Trauma/abuse	• Reye syndrome
• Hydrocephalus	**Disorders of the liver**
• Neoplastic infiltration or brain tumor	• Hepatic encephalopathy
• Arteriovenous malformation, embolism, stroke	**Renal disease**
Ingestions (see Chapter 21)	• Hypertensive encephalopathy
Electrolyte imbalances	• Kidney failure/uremia
• Hyponatremia	**Pulmonary disease**
• Hypernatremia	• Acute, chronic hypoxia
• Hypocalcemia	**Cardiovascular disease**
• Hypercalcemia	• Cardiovascular failure/shock/compromised perfusion
• Hypomagnesemia	**Endocrinopathy**
Intracranial shunt infection malfunction	• Hypoglycemia
Seizures postictal phase	• Diabetic ketoacidosis
	• Adrenal insufficiency
	• Hashimoto encephalopathy
	Gastrointestinal disorders
	• Intussusception

are accompanied and/or followed by transient neurologic deficits such as weakness/paralysis, sensory loss, difficulty speaking, or alterations in vision or mental status. Patients who suffer from migraine headaches are asymptomatic and have normal neurologic examinations between episodes of pain. A positive family history of migraine headaches is common.

CLINICAL MANIFESTATIONS

History

Patients should be asked about the history (acute vs. chronic), onset, progression, severity, location, duration, and timing of the headaches. Response to medication and alleviating/exacerbating factors are important factors. Any weakness, visual disturbances, or abnormal sensations should be reported. Questions about stress levels, recent life changes, and precipitating factors (foods, menstruation, exercise) may assist in the diagnosis. Asking the patient or caregiver to keep a headache diary can identify possible triggers, including fatigue, sleep deprivation, fasting, caffeine, menstruation, and stress.

Headaches that wake the patient from sleep or occur primarily in the mornings are suspicious for increased intracranial pressure. These headaches are usually made worse by lying flat or increasing venous pressure by bending, sneezing, or straining. Nausea and vomiting are not uncommon, particularly on wakening, and are concerning in the patient who has no associated complaints of abdominal pain or diarrhea. Pathologic headaches usually increase in both severity and frequency over time. There may be associated personality changes, gait disturbances, and vision abnormalities. Headaches accompanied by worsening focal neurologic deficits warrant emergent evaluation for an intracranial source.

Physical Examination

The physical examination includes assessment of growth parameters, vital signs (including blood pressure), and structures of the head (sinuses, teeth). The funduscopic examination permits detection of **papilledema** (swelling of the optic disc) in cases of increased intracranial pressure; CN VI palsy may also be present. Vision acuity should be documented. Carotid bruits, which may be audible in patients with AVMs, should be ruled out. A full neurologic examination is of paramount importance and includes cranial nerve function, strength, sensation, deep tendon reflexes, gait, balance, and mental status.

DIAGNOSTIC EVALUATION

Neither CT nor MRI of the head is indicated in the patient with nonprogressive recurring headaches and a normal neurologic examination. **Neuroimaging is indicated in the setting**

of any of the following: recent onset of severe, debilitating headaches; headaches which are increasing in severity and/or frequency; headaches in the setting of seizures or a history of neurodevelopmental impairment; and headaches accompanied by neurologic signs (i.e., papilledema, strabismus, unilateral weakness or sensory loss, dysarthria, ataxia, or changes in mental status, cognition [decline in grades], affect, behavior, or arousability). Such signs typically manifest within 6 months of the onset of headaches in patients with underlying neuropathology. Although structural lesions large enough to result in symptomatic increased intracranial pressure are almost always visible on head CT, MRI provides additional detail which may be beneficial in patients with abnormal CT scans or suspected posterior fossa lesions.

DIFFERENTIAL DIAGNOSIS

Pseudotumor cerebri is a benign but important cause of headaches that typically occurs in overweight adolescent females, or in association with thyroid disease or use of certain medications (specific acne medications and antibiotics). It is thought to be caused by impaired CSF resorption. Although the examination is positive for papilledema, the increased intracranial pressure is accompanied by normal neuroimaging. A LP is typically diagnostic (elevated opening pressure) and therapeutic. Acetazolamide, which decreases CSF production, is the standard medication. Refractory cases may require serial LPs or neurosurgical shunting. Pseudotumor cerebri is self-limited and typically resolves without complication. Weight loss for overweight individuals is also recommended.

TREATMENT

Tension headaches respond to nonprescription analgesics and rest. Stress management techniques, massage, and biofeedback training may also be beneficial. Mental health counseling may be beneficial in patients with suspected social or emotional stressors.

Management of the migraine patient begins with reassurance that the headache is not due to underlying neuropathology. Nonpharmacologic interventions (e.g., biofeedback, accupuncture, cognitive therapy, vitamin and herbal supplements) are often very beneficial for controlling migraine headaches. Patients should be instructed to eat regular meals and avoid fatigue, dehydration, and sleep deprivation. Over-the-counter medications (ibuprofen, naprosyn) work well as first choice abortive agents; intranasal or oral **sumatriptan** (as well as other triptan medications) are reserved for older children with headaches which are severe or unresponsive to over-the-counter medications. Subcutaneous sumatriptan is inappropriate for children. Prophylaxis (daily medication) should be considered if headaches occur more than three to six times a month and interfere with daily functions (such as school attendance). Anticonvulsants, antidepressants, and beta-blockers have been prescribed with variable success.

ISCHEMIC/HEMORRHAGIC STROKES

Stroke consists of the sudden onset of focal neurologic impairment caused by an interruption of cerebral blood flow, which may be transient or permanent. In children, stroke is rare and is usually precipitated by one of the following:

- Cardiac disease (congenital heart disease, endocarditis)
- Vascular disease (arteriovenous malformation, aneurysm, dissection, venous thrombosis)
- Hematologic disorders (sickle cell disease and coagulopathy)
- Infection (complications of meningitis or encephalitis)
- Metabolic disease (most commonly homocystinuria)

Most strokes in children occur in the cerebral hemispheres, presenting with hemiparesis, visual field defects, and/or aphasia. Brainstem and cerebellar strokes are less common. The neurologic manifestations correlate with the location of the ischemia. Magnetic resonance angiography (MRA) can evaluate vessels; MRI with diffusion weighted images can detect early strokes (<24 hours). Additional laboratory tests that may prove helpful include coagulation studies, CBC and cultures, connective tissue/vasculitis profiles (ESR, C3, C4, ANA), and workups to rule out lipid and metabolic abnormalities. Depending on the etiology, anticoagulation (low-molecular-weight heparin, warfarin) or antiplatelet therapy (aspirin) is helpful to prevent recurrences. Large clots may require surgical evacuation.

An arteriovenous malformation (AVM) is an abnormal collection of arteries and veins. Occasionally, a cranial bruit is present on physical examination. More commonly, however, AVMs present in a previously asymptomatic individual with the sudden or insidious onset of headache, vomiting, nuchal rigidity, progressive hemiparesis, diplopia, ataxia, and focal or generalized seizures. Arteriography permits determination of the site of the abnormality and feeding vessels. Surgical removal, embolization, or radiotherapy is necessary to prevent recurrent stroke or hemorrhage.

Thrombosis can occur at both arterial and venous sites. Conditions that predispose to thrombosis include sickle cell hemoglobinopathy, coagulation disorders, congenital heart disease, cardiac procedures, arrhythmias, endocarditis, trauma, bacterial meningitis, and infections leading to sinus thrombosis.

WEAKNESS

Abnormalities leading to weakness or paralysis, or both, may occur at any level of the neuromotor axis, from the motor cortex and pyramidal tracts to the anterior horn cell, peripheral nerve, neuromuscular junction, and muscle.

DIFFERENTIAL DIAGNOSIS

Guillain–Barré syndrome (GBS) is an acute-onset, progressive, ascending weakness caused by autoimmune-mediated demyelination of peripheral nerves. More than half of cases develop 7 to 21 days after an acute respiratory or gastrointestinal viral illness. Both sensory and autonomic impairments are often present. Initial symptoms include numbness of the distal extremities followed by progressive (usually) ascending weakness. Deep tendon reflexes wane and disappear. Severity varies from mild weakness to progressive involvement of the trunk and cranial nerves. Respiratory muscle involvement may necessitate mechanical ventilation. A significantly increased CSF protein level supports the diagnosis of GBS. Motor nerve conduction studies demonstrate evidence of demyelination. Symptoms may progress for up to 4 weeks, with resolution typically beginning approximately 4 weeks thereafter. Recovery is usually complete in children, although the rare patient experiences permanent lingering disability. Intravenous immune globulin shortens the duration and severity of the illness.

Tick paralysis resembles GBS, although ocular palsies and pupillary abnormalities are common additional findings. Certain ticks in the Appalachian and Rocky Mountains are capable of producing a neurotoxin that blocks acetylcholine release. The patient recovers completely when the tick is removed from the skin.

Myasthenia gravis (MG) is a chronic autoimmune disorder of the neuromuscular junction. Auto-antibodies bind to the postsynaptic acetylcholine receptor and block transmission. The rate of receptor breakdown also increases, so fewer receptors are present. The principal symptoms are easy fatigability and weakness that are exacerbated by sustained activity and improve with rest. Juvenile MG typically presents in late childhood or adolescence; the onset may be rapid or insidious, and symptoms wax and wane over time. Almost half of patients experience ocular muscle involvement, resulting in ptosis and/or diplopia. Bulbar weakness leads to dysarthria and difficulty swallowing. The classic supportive study is a positive **tensilon test**: intravenous anticholinesterase (edrophonium chloride) results in a transient increase in muscle (particularly ocular) strength by blocking the breakdown of acetylcholine in the synaptic cleft. Repetitive nerve stimulation studies demonstrate a decremental response following repeated stimulation. Acetylcholine receptor antibodies are measurable in the serum. MG may go into complete or partial remission after several years; however, most patients continue to experience periodic exacerbations throughout adulthood. Frequent dosing of an anticholinesterase (pyridostigmine) improves symptoms. Corticosteroids and other immune suppressants are prescribed for maintenance therapy and acute exacerbations. Thymectomy results in significant improvement in many patients with MG, presumably because the thymus is thought to sensitize the lymphocytes producing the offending antibodies.

Duchenne-type muscular dystrophy (DMD), an X-linked recessive disease of muscle tissue, is the most common muscular dystrophy and occurs predominantly in boys. Serum creatinine kinase levels are drastically elevated. The disease presents in early childhood with motor delay. Weakness is greatest in the proximal muscle groups, so the patient has difficulty with standing and climbing. The examiner will note the presence of Gower's sign, in which the boy uses his arms to assist in standing. Hypertrophied calves are also evident on exam. As the disease progresses, ambulation is lost, the muscles atrophy, and contractures develop. Cardiac and cognitive abnormalities often present as well. Treatment is mostly supportive; corticosteroids slow the course. Most children become wheelchair ambulators early in the second decade, with death in adolescence or early adulthood from respiratory failure or cardiomyopathy.

Spinal muscle atrophy (SMA) is an inherited disorder involving degeneration of the anterior horn cells and cranial nerve motor nuclei. The most severe form, SMA type 1 (Werdnig–Hoffmann disease), becomes evident in early infancy with generalized hypotonia and weakness. SMA type 2 presents between 6 and 12 months of age. The child's most advanced motor function is sitting. In SMA type 3, walking is achieved but lost as the disease progresses. Cognitive abilities remain unaffected in SMA. No specific therapy is available; morbidity and mortality are usually respiratory in nature. Diagnostic tests in muscle disease include EMG, muscle biopsy, and specific gene testing.

Tumors that compress the spinal cord result in weakness and paralysis below the lesion and constitute a surgical emergency. Cervical spinal cord injuries produce sudden-onset paresthesias and paralysis. Environmental toxin exposure may induce acquired neuropathies or myopathies. For example, infants in certain endemic areas (or those fed honey) may be exposed to spores of *Clostridium botulinum* and develop progressive paralysis from the elaborated toxin, which irreversibly blocks release of acetylcholine at the motor endplate.

TREATMENT

Diagnostic workup is tailored by findings on history and physical examination. Patients with asymmetric weakness or signs of increased intracranial pressure should undergo neuroimaging to rule out mass effect and hydrocephalus. Findings localized to a particular level of the spinal cord warrant evaluation (including spinal MRI) for cord compression or injury. An LP is helpful when infection is suspected. Supportive treatment may be required at some point; more definitive treatment, if available, is disease-specific.

ATAXIA

Ataxia is the inability to coordinate purposeful movement and control balance. Conditions that affect the cerebellum, connected sensory/motor pathways, and the inner ear are likely to cause ataxia in children. The most common causes in the pediatric population are infectious labyrinthitis, acute cerebellar ataxia, and drug ingestion (e.g., sedatives). Metabolic derangements, hydrocephalus, head trauma, and cerebellar hemorrhages may also cause ataxia. Chronic ataxia may be secondary to a genetic syndrome or brain malformation involving the cerebellum.

DIFFERENTIAL DIAGNOSIS

Viral infection of the labyrinthine structures can cause an acute ataxia which is often associated with horizontal nystagmus. The incoordination resulting from **acute cerebellar ataxia** may be relatively minor; alternatively, the child may be unable to walk or stand. The condition is most common between the ages of 2 and 7 years and often follows a viral illness. The patient appears otherwise well, with no changes in the level of consciousness or mental status. Headache and nuchal rigidity are absent, and the CSF is sterile. The prognosis of acute cerebellar ataxia which involves only the trunk, limbs, and mild nystagmus is quite good, with return of normal coordination within a few weeks. Cases associated with opsoclonus or tremors of the head and neck may require evaluation for a tumor (such as neuroblastoma). In addition, ataxia that is slowly progressive or associated with signs of increased intracranial pressure is more likely to be caused by a brain tumor.

Chronic ataxias typically have a genetic basis such as *ataxia-telangiectasia* or *Friedreich ataxia*. **Ataxia-telangiectasia** is an autosomal recessive neurodegenerative disorder that presents in childhood and progresses to wheelchair dependence. The ataxia is associated with extensive telangiectasias and immunodeficiency. The genetic defect is located on chromosome 11. **Friedreich ataxia** presents later in childhood with progressive ataxia, sensory losses, weakness, and muscle wasting. Skeletal deformities (scoliosis) invariably follow. Most patients die of cardiomyopathy-related heart disease before 30 years of age. Inheritance is autosomal recessive, linked to a defect on chromosome 9.

CLINICAL MANIFESTATIONS

History and Physical Examination

The history should include questions concerning disease onset (acute vs. chronic) and progression (slow vs. rapid). Associated symptoms may include fever, headache, vomiting, vertigo, photophobia, and altered mental status. Recent precipitating events (seizures, infections, head trauma) and exposures (medications, heavy metals, solvents, gases) should be documented. Some ataxias have a genetic basis, so the family history may be positive for neurologic illnesses.

The examination includes evaluation of mental status, truncal balance, gait, deep tendon reflexes, and muscle tone and strength. An abnormal gait may be caused by weakness (reduced reflexes and muscle strength) rather than imbalance. The examiner should note the presence of any nystagmus and/or signs of increased intracranial pressure (bradycardia, hypertension, papilledema, meningismus). If the child is old enough and cooperative, tests such as heel-to-knee, finger-to-nose, and rapid alternating movement help evaluate cerebellar function. The Romberg test evaluates function of the peripheral nerves and posterior columns. With the patient standing balanced with feet together and eyes open, the Romberg sign is present (abnormal) if the child cannot maintain balance when he or she closes the eyes.

DIAGNOSTIC EVALUATION

Toxicology screens should be considered in ambulatory patients or patients with suspected abuse. Neuroimaging permits assessment for cerebellar masses (tumor, abscess, hemorrhage). CT of the head should always precede lumbar puncture in patients with ataxia. A brain MRI is preferred to best evaluate pathology in the posterior fossa. LP permits analysis for abnormalities noted in meningitis, acute disseminated encephalomyelitis (infection-mediated central demyelination), and Guillain–Barré syndrome. Chronic or recurrent ataxia warrants metabolic and genetic workup.

PHAKOMATOSES

Phakomatoses are neurocutaneous diseases characterized by lesions in the nervous system, skin, and eyes. Two autosomal dominant conditions are encountered in children: neurofibromatosis and tuberous sclerosis. Sturge–Weber disease, a sporadic disorder, is traditionally included as well.

NEUROFIBROMATOSIS

Neurofibromatosis types 1 (von Recklinghausen disease) and 2 (bilateral acoustic neuromas) are the most common variants in children. **Neurofibromatosis type 1** is a clinical diagnosis based in part on the presence of six or more café-au-lait spots of a specific size (Table 15-9). A large gene on chromosome 17 coding for neurofibromin has a high spontaneous mutation rate. Patients with neurofibromatosis type 1 are at increased risk for optic pathway gliomas and other low-grade gliomas in the central nervous system. They typically require evaluation and treatment for the associated seizures, learning disorders, renovascular hypertension, and scoliosis. Routine vision screening is critical. Neurofibromas that cause impairment may be surgically removed; however, most will recur.

TABLE 15-9 Diagnosis of Neurofibromatosis Type 1

Two of the following must be present:
1. Six or more café-au-lait spots, >5 mm in size in children and >15 mm in adolescents or adults
2. Axillary or inguinal freckling
3. Two or more Lisch nodules (hamartomas) in the iris
4. Two or more neurofibromas or one plexiform neurofibroma
5. A distinctive osseous lesion, such as sphenoid dysplasia
6. Optic gliomas
7. Affected first-degree relative based on the preceding criteria

Bilateral acoustic neuromas are the hallmark of **neurofibromatosis type 2**. Complications include hearing loss and vestibular disorientation. Brain MRI demonstrates bilateral eighth cranial nerve masses. Neurofibromas, meningiomas, schwannomas, and astrocytomas are also associated with type 2 neurofibromatosis. Cataracts and retinal hamartomas are not uncommon. Surgical debulking is appropriate when hearing impairment becomes pronounced. Cochlear implants have restored hearing in some patients. The genetic abnormality occurs on chromosome 22.

TUBEROUS SCLEROSIS

Tuberous sclerosis, like neurofibromatosis, is a progressive autosomal dominant neurocutaneous disorder, although sporadic cases are more common than inherited ones. Two separate genes have been identified for tuberous sclerosis (chromosome sites 9q34 and 16p13). The normal genetic product is tuberin, a protein thought to suppress the development of tumors.

Disease severity varies greatly. Typical skin lesions include **ash-leaf spots** (flat, hypopigmented macules), **shagreen patches** (areas of abnormal skin thickening), sebaceous adenomas, and ungual fibromas. Ash-leaf spots are the earliest manifestation and are best detected by Wood lamp examination. Neuroimaging demonstrates the distinctive periventricular knob-like areas of localized swelling, or tubers. Subependymal nodules and giant cell astrocytomas may also be present. Mental retardation and seizures (including infantile spasms) are common. Tumors also have a predilection for the kidney, heart (particularly cardiac rhabdomyomas), and retina. Treatment consists of antiepileptic therapy and surgical removal of related tumors when indicated.

STURGE–WEBER SYNDROME

Sturge–Weber syndrome (leptomeningeal angiomatosis) is a disorder of neurologic deterioration associated with a port-wine stain (nevus flammeus) over the area innervated by the first division of the trigeminal nerve. Affected children manifest progressive mental retardation, seizures, hemiparesis, and visual impairment; approximately a third develops glaucoma. *Tunable (pulsed) dye laser therapy* fades the port-wine stain but does not address the underlying neurologic dysfunction. Lesions should be treated early in life to optimize cosmetic outcome. Optimal control of seizures may limit subsequent developmental delay. About 10% of children with a unilateral port wine stain over the dermatome innervated by CNV_1 will be affected with Sturge–Weber syndrome; this percentage is higher if the lesion is bilateral.

NEURAL TUBE DEFECTS

Failure of neural tube closure during the third and fourth weeks of gestation results in a group of related disorders termed **neural tube defects**. Maternal malnutrition, drug exposure (e.g., valproic acid and carbamazepine), maternal hyperthermia, congenital infections, radiation, and genetic factors are all associated with an increased risk of neural tube defects. There is a 3% to 4% risk of a second affected child being born to parents who already have one child with a neural tube defect. Because failure of closure results in persistent leakage of **α-fetoprotein** into the amniotic fluid, the maternal serum α-fetoprotein level at 16 to 18 weeks' gestation is an excellent screening tool for identifying high-risk pregnancies. The incidence of neural tube defects is decreased in infants whose mothers receive at least 400 μg/day of **folic acid** supplementation prior to conception and during the early weeks of pregnancy. The overall incidence of neural tube defects is declining worldwide due to improved maternal nutrition and widespread prenatal diagnosis with subsequent elective termination of the pregnancy.

CLINICAL MANIFESTATIONS

Abnormalities may occur anywhere along the central nervous system (CNS); the higher the lesion, the more severe the sequelae. Neonates with **anencephaly** are born with large skull defects and virtually no cortex. Brainstem function is marginally intact. Many are stillborn; others die within days of birth. **Encephaloceles** are protrusions of cranial contents through a bony skull defect, usually in the occipital region. Affected patients manifest severe mental retardation, seizures, and motor deficits. Hydrocephalus is a frequent complication.

Spina bifida includes a variety of conditions characterized by neural tube defects in the spinal region associated with incomplete fusion of the vertebral arches. **Myelomeningoceles** are protruding sacs of neural and meningeal tissues, whereas **meningoceles** contain meninges only. Both are most common in the lumbosacral region. Bowel and bladder sphincter dysfunction is the rule, and sensorimotor loss exists below the lesion. In **spina bifida occulta**, the bony vertebral lesion occurs without herniation of any spinal contents. Birthmarks, dimples, subcutaneous masses, or hairy tufts at the base of the back suggest an underlying defect. Although the infant may initially appear neurologically intact, the caudal end of the cord is affixed or tethered to the distal spine. As the vertebral column grows throughout childhood, the tethered distal spinal cord develops traction injury, resulting in gait disturbance, sphincter dysfunction, foot deformities, and increasing motor deficits. Spina bifida defects have a high incidence of infectious complications, cortical malformations, and **Chiari type II malformation** (dysgenesis and downward displacement of the lower brainstem and cerebellum that often results in hydrocephalus and stridor, apnea, and dysphagia).

TREATMENT

Cesarean section delivery prior to the onset of labor results in an improved anatomic level of motor function. Early closure of repairable back lesions and prophylactic antibiotics until closure decrease the risk of infection. The majority of infants with myelomeningocele develop hydrocephalus within the first month of life. Early ventriculoperitoneal (VP) shunt placement, even for mild hydrocephalus, appears to improve intellectual outcome. Infants with severe cyanotic episodes, apnea, stridor, and dysphagia from Chiari type II malformations benefit from early cervical decompression. Meticulous attention to urodynamics, anticholinergic medication, and clean intermittent catheterization result in urinary continence for the majority of patients and reduce the risk of urinary tract complications, the major cause of death after the first year of life. Surgical release of tethered spinal cord can prevent deterioration of motor and sphincter dysfunction and may partially reverse acquired deficits. Fetal surgery is associated with measurable preservation of motor and sensory function.

HYDROCEPHALUS

PATHOGENESIS

Hydrocephalus is the pathologic enlargement of the ventricles that occurs when cerebral spinal fluid (CSF) production outpaces absorption, usually secondary to outflow obstruction. In **noncommunicating** hydrocephalus, the block exists somewhere within the ventricular system, and the ventricles proximal to the obstruction are selectively enlarged. Noncommunicating hydrocephalus is most commonly caused by narrowing at the cerebral aqueduct or malformations/enlargements of the posterior fossa. Causes include congenital malformations such as Chiari type II malformations, aqueductal stenosis, arachnoid cyst, and Dandy–Walker malformation; intrauterine infection; and intraventricular hemorrhage. Acquired noncommunicating hydrocephalus in older children is most often due to posterior fossa neoplasms and aqueductal stenosis or gliosis.

In contrast, all ventricles are proportionately enlarged in **communicating** hydrocephalus, which occurs when CSF absorption at the arachnoid villi is impaired secondary to meningitis, subarachnoid hemorrhage, or leukemia. Rarely, communicating hydrocephalus is due to excessive CSF production from a choroid plexus papilloma.

CLINICAL MANIFESTATIONS

History and Physical Examination

The clinical manifestations of hydrocephalus depend on the rate of onset and whether the fontanelles are still open. An inappropriate increase in head circumference or bulging anterior fontanelle may be the only indication in infants; poor feeding, irritability, lethargy, downward deviation of the eyes (the "setting sun" sign), spasticity in the legs, apnea, and bradycardia often provide additional clues that the infant has increased intracranial pressure. In older patients with acute courses, the signs are relatively clear and include morning headache that improves after upright positioning or vomiting, irritability and/or lethargy, and papilledema and diplopia (CN VI palsy). Spasticity, clonus, and hyperreflexia most prominent in the legs are additional neurologic signs of hydrocephalus. The **Cushing triad**, consisting of hypertension, bradycardia, and slow irregular respirations, is a late and ominous sign of increased intracranial pressure implying imminent risk of brain herniation.

DIFFERENTIAL DIAGNOSIS

Conditions that lead to increased intracranial pressure without hydrocephalus include acute intraventricular hemorrhage, diffuse brain edema (secondary to traumatic brain injury, hypoxic-ischemic encephalopathy, large ischemic stroke or encephalitis), cerebral venous sinus thrombosis, abscesses, and many tumors, all of which are easily differentiated by computed tomography (CT) or magnetic resonance imaging (MRI).

DIAGNOSTIC EVALUATION

The CT scan is an important adjunct in the evaluation of hydrocephalus. Anatomic malformations, ventricular size, and source of obstruction are clearly delineated. A head ultrasound (US) may be sufficient in the infant. In children who have a VP shunt, rapid sequence MRI can assess ventricular size without exposing the child to cumulative radiation over time. If a LP is indicated, it **should not** be attempted in the presence of asymmetric or obstructive causes of increased intracranial pressure due to the risk of herniation of the brain across the tentorium or through the foramen magnum.

TREATMENT

Patients with hydrocephalus are at risk for developmental delay, visual impairment, motor disturbances and, in severe cases of obstructive hydrocephalus, death. If the underlying etiology cannot be corrected, surgical diversion with a VP shunt decreases intracranial pressure and relieves the symptoms. An endoscopic **third ventriculostomy** is a surgical alternative to VP shunt when CSF obstruction occurs at or distal to the cerebral aqueduct. This type of ventriculostomy may occasionally close due to gliosis, but this intervention avoids the risks of mechanical failure and infection present with the VP shunt.

Indwelling shunts can be complicated by mechanical failure of the device, problems due to over-shunting or under-shunting, and infection. *Staphylococcus epidermidis* is the most frequently isolated pathogen. Systemic and intraventricular antibiotics are always administered. Shunt removal may also be indicated. The programmable valve is a technological advance in shunts that permits external adjustment to optimize ventricular pressure and helps to avoid over- or undershunting.

ABNORMAL HEAD SHAPES

Microcephaly describes a head circumference that is greater than two standard deviations below mean head size for age. It often results from genetic abnormalities (e.g., trisomy 21, Angelman syndrome) or congenital insults (maternal drug ingestions, congenital infections, or insufficient placental blood flow). Affected children often demonstrate both cognitive and motor delay; associated seizure disorders are not uncommon. "Microcephaly" which mathes weight and length percentiles in an infant without congenital anomalies may be normal.

Macrocephaly, in contrast, refers to a head circumference greater than two standard deviations above the mean. Macrocephaly may be familial; however, cranioskeletal dysplasias, storage diseases, and hydrocephalus should be explored as possible causes, particularly if the growth rate crosses multiple percentile lines over time.

Positional plagiocephaly is the benign flattening of the back of the head often seen in infants placed to sleep exclusively on their backs. A variant results when an infant preferentially lies with the head turned toward one side; flattening of the parieto-occipital area is accompanied by prominence of the forehead on the same side. Most cases require no intervention beyond counseling the parents to encourage the child to lie with the head tilted to the opposite side (by moving a mobile or colorful object to that side). If there is a cosmetic concern, a soft plastic helmet fitted by a plastic surgeon may be successful in gently molding the back of the head into a more acceptable shape when instituted prior to 9 months of age.

Craniosynostosis is the premature fusion of one or more cranial sutures. It may be idiopathic, part of a syndrome, or associated with poor brain growth. Bone growth continues along the open suture lines, resulting in an abnormally shaped head. If early obliteration of the sagittal suture occurs (most common), the child has a long head and a narrow face (scaphocephaly). In contrast, premature closure of the coronal suture results in a very wide face with a short, almost box-like, skull. The need for and timing of surgical intervention, which consists of reopening the sutures and retarding their subsequent fusion, is controversial. Most defects are repaired before 2 years of age for cosmetic reasons.

KEY POINTS

- Until 2 years of age, a child's chronological age should be adjusted for gestational age at birth when assessing developmental achievement.
- The Weschler preschool scale is used to assess IQ in preschoolers.
- Language is the best indicator of intellectual potential.
- Any child with a suspected speech or language disorder should be referred for a full hearing evaluation.
- Dysfluency may be developmental between 3 and 4 years of age. Dysfluency which is accompanied by tension, struggle, and/or total word blockage OR severely limits communication should be considered true dysfluency (stuttering) necessitating referral to a speech therapist.
- Autism spectrum disorder represents a continuum of chronic, nonprogressive developmental disabilities involving

impairments in social interaction, communication, and behavior. Autism and Asperger syndrome are categorized as autism spectrum disorders.

- Any association of autism with administration of the MMR vaccine and/or thimersol has been definitely dispronen.
- The predominant elements of attention-deficit/hyperactivity disorder are inattentiveness, hyperactivity, and impulsivity.
- Pharmacologic interventions for ADHD include stimulant medications, the new prodrug lisdexamfetamine, and the nonstimulant atomoxetine.
- CP is a nonprogressive disorder of movement and posture resulting from a fixed lesion of the brain. If a child with CP exhibits progressive deterioration, an alternate diagnosis should be sought.
- Febrile seizures are typically brief, generalized seizures with fever which occur in up to 5% of otherwise healthy children ages 6 months to 6 years. About a third of children with a history of febrile seizure will have recurrent febrile seizures. Febrile seizures, even when recurrent, are not considered epilepsy. Children with a history of febrile seizure are at slightly greater risk than their peers for the development of epilepsy later in life.
- The context of the child's age, past medical and family histories, and any prior unusual spells are important in the differentiation of a seizure from a nonseizure event. The diagnosis of a seizure is based primarily on the historical account of the episode.
- When evaluating a patient with headaches, it is important to determine whether the headaches are primary (tension or migraine headaches) or secondary (pathologic) in etiology. Clinical manifestations that should prompt consideration of pathologic headaches include symptom focality; frontal or occipital location; debilitating episodes of pain; increasing frequency and/or severity; headaches and vomiting upon awakening; and neurologic signs.
- Abnormalities leading to weakness or paralysis, or both, may occur at any level of the neuromotor axis, from the motor cortex and pyramidal tracts to the anterior horn cell, peripheral nerve, neuromuscular junction, and muscle. Guillain–Barré syndrome is an acute-onset, progressive, ascending weakness caused by autoimmune-mediated demyelination of peripheral nerves. Myasthenia gravis is a chronic autoimmune disorder of the neuromuscular junction. Duchenne-type muscular dystrophy is an X-linked recessive disease involving direct destruction of muscle tissue.
- The most common causes of acute ataxia in the pediatric population are infectious labyrinthitis, acute cerebellar ataxia, and toxic ingestion.
- An elevated maternal serum α-fetoprotein level at 16 to 18 weeks' gestation is an excellent screen for neural tube defects. The incidence of neural tube defects is decreased in infants whose mothers receive folic acid supplementation prior to conception and in the early weeks of pregnancy.
- Clinical manifestations of hydrocephalus include inappropriately large head circumference, bulging fontanelle, and poor feeding (in infants); irritability and/or lethargy; morning headaches and vomiting; papilledema and diplopia; and hyperreflexia of the lower limbs. A LP is contraindicated if herniation of the brain is a concern.
- Positional plagiocephaly is the benign flattening of the back of the head often seen in infants placed to sleep exclusively on their backs. Most cases require no intervention beyond counseling the parents to encourage "tummy time" when the baby is awake and under direct supervisor.

C Clinical Vignettes

Vignette 1

A mother brings her 6-year-old boy to your office with a chief complaint of "staring spells" over the last 6 months. The episodes have been noted by both parents and the patient's teacher. Events last 10 to 20 seconds, during which he stares blankly and is not responsive. There is no clear eye or head deviation. Occasionally, the spells will be associated with lip licking and eye fluttering. The spells have a definite end, after which he quickly returns to baseline and resumes his activity. The boy is unaware of the episodes. He is a good student and there has been no noticeable decline in his schoolwork. There is no family history of seizures. The vital signs and physical examination are normal.

1. Which of the following is the next best step in the evaluation of this patient?
   - **a.** Computed tomography (CT) of the brain
   - **b.** Electroencephalogram (EEG)
   - **c.** Magnetic resonance imaging of the brain
   - **d.** Admission for inpatient video EEG monitoring
   - **e.** Referrel for full psychoeducational testing

2. The EEG reveals 3-Hz symmetric and synchronous spike and wave activity. This result is most consistent with a diagnosis of which of the following conditions?
   - **a.** Complex partial epilepsy
   - **b.** Lennox-Gastaut syndrome
   - **c.** Juvenile myoclonic epilepsy
   - **d.** Absence epilepsy
   - **e.** Transient ischemic events

3. Which of the following represents the most appropriate initial therapy for this patient, given his diagnosis?
   - **a.** Ethosuximide
   - **b.** Carbamazepine
   - **c.** Lorazepam
   - **d.** Phenytoin
   - **e.** Fosphenytoin

Vignette 2

During a routine health maintenance visit, the mother of a 3-year-old male expresses concern regarding his development. The patient spoke his first words at 12 months of age and was speaking in two-word phrases by age 24 months. He was using a pincer grasp at 12 months of age and can currently draw a circle. Review of gross motor milestones reveals that he walked at 18 months of age, but has had difficulty keeping up with his peers when running. He is slow to stand from a seated position. Your examination reveals prominent calves, intact upper and lower extremity reflexes, and normal sensation. The patient demonstrates a toe–toe gait with mild lordosis. He uses his hands to "climb up" his legs when moving from sitting on the floor to standing.

1. This patient's history and physical examination findings are most consistent with which of the following?
   - **a.** Gross motor delay
   - **b.** Global developmental delay
   - **c.** Isolated delays in speech and fine motor skills
   - **d.** Isolated delay in fine motor skills
   - **e.** No developmental delays

2. Which of the following represents the best initial step in the management of this patient?
   - **a.** Serum laboratory testing
   - **b.** MRI of the brain
   - **c.** Referral for pediatric-specific physical therapy
   - **d.** Referral to a specialist in genetics
   - **e.** Electromyography

3. The child's serum CK level is significantly elevated at 20,000 U/L (normal 22 to 198 U/L). A CK level elevated to this degree is virtually diagnostic of which of the following conditions?
   - **a.** Cerebral palsy
   - **b.** Spinal muscular atrophy
   - **c.** Muscular dystrophy
   - **d.** Multiple sclerosis
   - **e.** Adrenoleukodystophy

4. The patient has a 6-month-old brother. Which of the following represents his chance of being similarly affected?
   - **a.** 25%
   - **b.** 50%
   - **c.** 75%
   - **d.** His risk is the same as for the general population.
   - **e.** The brother is affected with the same condition.

Vignette 3

A 2-year-old female is seen in the emergency department for gait changes over the last day or so. Three weeks ago she had a cold with upper respiratory symptoms, which have all resolved. She is otherwise healthy and has shown normal development to date. There is no history of trauma. The parents note that she appears "off balance" and falls easily. These symptoms have been present since she woke up from a nap yesterday. No abnormal eye movements have been observed. On physical examination, all vital signs including temperature are within normal limits. She is alert and shows appropriate social interactions. She has clear tympanic membranes, no skin findings, and a benign abdomen without organomegaly or masses. Pupils are round and reactive, extra-ocular movements are intact, there is no nystagmus, and she has a strong cry. When reaching for a toy, she often misses her target. Upper and lower reflexes are intact. She walks with a wide-based gait and falls after 3 to 4 steps.

1. Your initial diagnostic evaluation would include which of the following?
- **a.** Urine drug screen
- **b.** Computed tomography of the brain
- **c.** Lumbar puncture
- **d.** Urgent EEG
- **e.** (a) and (b)
- **f.** All of the above

2. Computed tomography of the head and laboratory studies are unrevealing. She is admitted to the hospital for further evaluation and monitoring. Which of the following would be the most appropriate next step in the evaluation, given that the above studies are negative?
- **a.** MRI brain
- **b.** Toxicology consult
- **c.** Neurology consult
- **d.** Urine VMA and HVA
- **e.** Skeletal survey

3. MRI of the brain and urine studies are negative. Her gait neither improves nor worsens over the course of hospitalization. Which of the following is the most likely diagnosis?
- **a.** Guillain–Barré syndrome
- **b.** Neuroblastoma
- **c.** Pontine glioma
- **d.** Acute cerebellar ataxia
- **e.** Friedreich's ataxia

Vignette 4

A 14-year-old female is evaluated in your office for a 2-week history of headaches. The headaches are bilateral, frontal, and throbbing in nature. They persist throughout the day without alleviating factors. She denies waking up with a headache and reports no nausea or vomiting. She does report mild photosensitivity and blurred vision. There is no history of photophobia. She reports no recent illnesses or traumas. She recently started a new acne medication and takes an oral contraceptive for dysmenorrhea. On physical examination, her weight is 150 lb (68 kg). Visual acuity is 20/100 in the right eye and 20/40 in the left. Bilateral papilledema is noted. Extraocular movements are intact, with no facial asymmetry or apparent hearing loss. Palatal lift is symmetric and the tongue is midline. The remainder of the neurological examination is normal.

1. Which of the following factors in this patient's history and physical examination is a known risk factor for pseudotumor cerebri?
- **a.** Weight
- **b.** Gender
- **c.** Retinoid-containing acne medication
- **d.** Contraceptive use
- **e.** (a), (b), and (c)
- **f.** All of the above

2. You strongly suspect pseudotumor cerebri. Which of the following tests will further support this diagnosis?
- **a.** Computed tomography of the brain
- **b.** Lumbar puncture with opening pressure
- **c.** Visual evoked responses
- **d.** (a) and (b) only
- **e.** All of the above

3. The head CT is normal, and the lumbar puncture opening pressure is significantly elevated. Which of the following can be effective in the management of pseudotumor cerebri?
- **a.** Amitryptiline
- **b.** Ibuprofen
- **c.** Sumatriptan
- **d.** Acetazolamide
- **e.** Lamotrigine

A Answers

Vignette 1 Question 1

Answer B: Not all paroxysmal events are due to abnormal electrical activity in the brain. Breath holding spells, tics, near-syncope, and daydreaming could be included in the differential diagnosis of this child's behavior. However, when episodes are suspected to be epileptic based on the clinical history and physical examination, the best diagnostic study for possibly confirming and classifying seizures is the electroencephalogram (EEG). Sleep deprivation (sleep-deprived EEG), hyperventilation, and photostimulation often provoke abnormal electrical activity aiding in diagnosing the epileptic syndrome. A normal EEG does not rule out a seizure disorder as the cause of the observable episodes unless they occur while the EEG is recording and the EEG remains unaffected (e.g., pseudoseizures). Inpatient video EEG monitoring is usually not necessary unless the episodes are thought to be consistent with seizure activity and the routine EEG is normal. In that case, continuous video EEG monitoring can be utilized to capture and characterize an event with direct EEG correlation. Video EEG monitoring is also useful in cases of suspected malingering/Munchausen syndrome or when nonepileptic spells represent reflux, tics, or other seizure look-alikes. Computed tomography (CT) of the head is the study of choice following trauma because it is a relatively quick and easy study to obtain under tenuous circumstances. Magnetic resonance imaging (MRI) is preferred when evaluating for underlying structural brain anomalies that may be related to the events. Psychoeducational testing, including IQ and achievement testing, is recommended when a child is experiencing school failure. A psychological and ADHD evaluation, audiology and vision examinations, and measurements of adaptive behavior may help to elucidate source(s) of academic difficulties and formulate a plan to encourage success in learning.

Vignette 1 Question 2

Answer D: The EEG findings above are classic for absence epilepsy, formerly known as petit mal seizures. If the patient is old enough to cooperate, voluntary hyperventilation over several minutes may provoke an episode during testing. Typical absence seizures begin in childhood. Both the onset and ending of the seizure are abrupt, and there is no clinically observable postictal phase. The patient is not responsive to "outside" stimulation during the event but does not lose postural tone. Subtle eye fluttering may be noted during some episodes. Events are brief, lasting less than 30 seconds, and can occur as frequently as 100 times a day. Typical absence seizures are not associated with underlying brain anomalies. Epileptic syndromes differ in clinical presentation and by EEG. Partial seizures present with localized/focal abnormal, involuntary activity which may be motor, somatosensory, or autonomic in manifestation. The patient remains conscious during simple partial seizures. *Complex* partial seizures are accompanied by loss of or impaired consciousness. The epileptic activity originates in the same area of the brain each time but may spread, resulting in generalized tonic/clonic seizure. Lennox–Gastaut syndrome is characterized by multiple seizure types including a combination absence (typical or atypical), generalized tonic–clonic, atonic, or tonic events. The EEG in Lennox–Gastaut syndrome is typically slow with spike-wave and polyspike discharges. Juvenile myoclonic epilepsy (Janz syndrome) is associated with generalized 4 to 6-Hz polyspikes on EEG. The syndrome takes its name from the characteristic involuntary myoclonic "jerks" of the upper limbs. Transient ischemic events are rare in young children, but would be important to rule out if the events were not associated with demonstrable epileptic discharges in EEG.

Vignette 1 Question 3

Answer A: Ethosuximide is the initial drug of choice for patients with childhood absence epilepsy; in fact, this is currently its sole indication. Lamotrigine or valproic acid are second-line agents for patients with excessive side effects or poor control. Intravenous lorazepam is a very important drug for acutely aborting seizures in hospitalized patients; rectal diazepam serves the same purpose for home use. Phenytoin or Fosphenytoin (a prodrug of phenytoin) is utilized in the emergency room in the treatment of status epilepticus. Carbamazepine is contraindicated in this patient as it may potentiate his seizures.

Vignette 2 Question 1

Answer A: Walking is a gross motor skill that is typically acquired by 15 months of age, with population average of about age 12 months. Eighteen months demonstrates a clear delay. This delay would have been picked up at the 15- or 18-month health maintenance visits, either through direct observation by the medical provider or through developmental screening. Attaining the mature pincer grasp by 12 months of age implies that his fine motor skills are progressing appropriately. His language skills, as described, are typical. Since only one stream of development is delayed, this is isolated gross motor rather than global delay.

Vignette 2 Question 2

Answer A: Given the patient's motor delays and weakness on exam, initial serum laboratory testing, in particular serum creatine kinase (CK) levels, will be most sensitive and specific for the suspected diagnosis. An MRI of the brain should be normal in this patient, but would be a consideration in a child with global developmental delays or upper motor neuron signs on examination. Although not the best initial step, a referral to physical therapy is imperative for this patient to optimize his motor function, teach range of motion exercises, and promote stretching to improve his toe–toe gait. A genetics referral may be a consideration in the future if a hereditary muscle disease is apparent on examination and by initial testing. An EMG would be helpful in further discerning the cause of the patient's weakness if he had fatigable weakness, bulbar weakness, or loss of reflexes on exam.

Vignette 2 Question 3

Answer C: The most common muscular dystrophy occurring in boys is Duchenne muscular dystrophy (DMD). In boys with DMD, the CK level can be elevated up to 20-times normal. DMD is an X-linked recessive muscular dystrophy which results from absence of dystrophin. Weakness begins in the proximal muscle groups; the calf muscles appear hypertrophied, and the child rises from a sitting position by leaning on the calves and using the arms to "climb" up the legs (Gower's sign). Becker muscular dystrophy has similar clinical manifestations due to abnormalities in the dystrophin protein, but the onset is later (adolescence), and the disease is generally milder. Cerebral palsy is a nonprogressive disorder of movement and posture resulting from a static brain lesion acquired in the fetal or perinatal period. Spinal muscular atrophy is an inherited disorder that results in the progressive degradation of anterior horn cells. Patients vary in presentation from the infant with profound hypotonia (Wernig-Hoffman) to motor delays. Typically, the examination is significant for tongue fasiculations, proximal greater than distal weakness, and areflexia. Multiple sclerosis is an autoimmune disorder involving demyelination in the brain and spinal cord. Onset is later in life and more common in females, with waxing and waning of symptoms. Adrenoleukodystrophy is X-linked and occurs primarily in boys; this peroxysomal disorder is a neurodegenerative condition involving the white matter of the brain.

Vignette 2 Question 4

Answer B: Genetic diseases that are inherited in an X-linked recessive pattern do not affect females. Females have a 50% chance of being carriers of the gene. As a result, males are at a 50% risk of inheriting the abnormal gene.

Vignette 3 Question 1

Answer E: The initial evaluation in this patient would include a urine drug screen and CT scan. Toddlers in general are at increased risk for ingestions. Reviewing medications available in the home may yield the answer. A stat CT scan would be indicated to rule out any posterior hemorrhage or evidence of cerebellar stroke. A posterior fossa tumor is a consideration, but would be best visualized by an MRI of the brain. An EEG would be considered if the patient had altered mental status in conjunction with her gait changes or if these symptoms were more intermittent. Areflexia or weakness noted on examination would necessitate a lumbar puncture to assess for an elevated protein indicative of Gullian–Barré Syndrome or its ataxic variant, Miller–Fisher.

Vignette 3 Question 2

Answer A: In children, CNS tumors develop predominantly in the posterior fossa. Initial signs and symptoms might include cranial nerve palsies, ataxia, headache (increased intracranial pressure), or seizures. The best imaging modality to visualize the posterior fossa would be an MRI of the brain. Ruling out a tumor would take precedence over consultations. Urine VMA and HVA are metabolites in the urine which are elevated in cases of neuroblastoma. In addition, a paraneoplastic syndrome can be associated with neuroblastoma that includes ataxia as well as dancing eyes (opsoclonus/myoclonus). A skeletal survey would be indicated if there was radiographic evidence of subdural bleeds of varying ages on CT, raising suspicion for nonaccidental trauma.

Vignette 3 Question 3

Answer D: Based on the patient's history of a recent (most likely) viral infection, her age, lack of temperature elevation, normal mental status, negative studies, and lack of deterioration, the most likely diagnosis is acute cerebellar ataxia. In the great majority of cases, coordination returns to baseline (normal) within a few weeks. Guillain–Barré syndrome involves *progressive* ascending weakness with loss of reflexes. Neuroblastomas most commonly produce an abdominal tumor and paraneoplastic syndrome associated with a more subacute onset of ataxia. A pontine glioma is an aggressive tumor arising from the glial cells in the brain or spinal cord. Presentation ranges from signs and symptoms of hydrocephalus to lower extremity weakness/pain/numbness. Adrenoleukodystrophy is a disorder involving the white matter of the brain. Friedreich's Ataxia presents in older children/adolescents with a more insidious onset of incoordination accompanied by nystagmus, weakness, and other neurologic signs.

Vignette 4 Question 1

Answer F: All of the above occur more frequently in patients with pseudotumor cerebri. Other potential associations include medications such as tetracycline; lupus; Addison disease; and hypoparathyroidism.

Vignette 4 Question 2

Answer B: In pseudotumor cerebri, the lumbar puncture is both diagnostic and therapeutic. Obtaining an elevated opening pressure (>20 to 25 cm water) during the lumbar puncture confirms the diagnosis. Removing spinal fluid with a large volume tap reduces the increased intrancranial pressure, and the headache usually improves significantly. However, with papilledema and other signs and symptoms of increased intracranial pressure present, a head CT is indicated prior to the lumbar puncture (to rule out conditions that could potentiate herniation of the brainstem during the procedure). Visual evoked potentials are used to evaluate eye symptoms in patients with multiple sclerosis.

Vignette 4 Question 3

Answer D: Serial lumbar punctures can be employed to alleviate the headaches. Acetazolamide is a pharmacologic agent which decreases CSF production at the choroid plexis. Ibuprofen is often effective as first line in young patients with benign tension or migraine headaches. Sumatriptan often relieves migraine headaches in older children and adolescents. Amitryptiline is a tricyclic antidepressant commonly used as a preventive medication in children with frequent migraines. Lamotrigine is an anticonvulsant that does not affect the symptoms of pseudotumor cerebri.

Chapter

16 Orthopedics

Steven Frick • Katie S. Fine

Pediatricians and family practitioners benefit from a basic knowledge of orthopedics, as musculoskeletal complaints comprise a large percentage of office visits in their patients. The timely diagnosis and management of congenital, developmental, traumatic, and infectious bone and joint conditions in children can minimize potential deformities and loss of function.

DEVELOPMENTAL DISLOCATION OF THE HIP

PATHOGENESIS

Developmental hip dysplasia (DDH) refers to a spectrum of pathological anatomy of the hip joint which occurs in about 1 per 1,000 births. Dysplastic hips at birth may be dislocated and irreducible, dislocated and reducible, reduced and dislocatable, subluxatable (loose but not dislocatable), or stable with abnormal anatomy. DDH may develop in utero, during delivery, or more rarely during childhood. If a dislocation or severe subluxation (i.e., femoral head not centered in the socket) persists, the acetabulum will not develop into a cup-like shape, and the head of the femur can move further out of the socket. Once the ball is repositioned in the socket in an infant, the socket usually regains its cup-like shape.

EPIDEMIOLOGY

DDH is substantially more common in the newborn with breech presentation or a positive family history. Risk is slightly increased in females and first-born children. Association with other anomalies has been described, most commonly metatarsus adductus and congenital muscular torticollis.

CLINICAL MANIFESTATIONS

Early diagnosis of hip dislocation usually results in a better outcome; therefore, careful examination of the newborn is critical. Gluteal fold asymmetry may accompany hip dislocation in the newborn; however up to 71% of normal infants have gluteal fold asymmetry, resulting in very low specificity for this sign. The **Barlow and Ortoloni provocative tests** are most helpful. With the infant's hip and knee each flexed to 90°, the examiner places the fingertips on the greater trochanter, with the thumb webspace over the knee and the thumb on the inner thigh. Gentle pressure is applied to the flexed and adducted hip in a posterior direction during the Barlow maneuver, and a positive result occurs when there is a palpable clunk as the hip dislocates in a posterior–superior direction. This test can be immediately followed by the Ortolani maneuver (hip abduction with a resulting "clunk" as the head relocates into the joint) (Fig. 16-1). DDH can evolve over time, so children should be screened at regular intervals until they are ambulatory. In examining a somewhat older infant (after 3 to 4 months), hip dislocations usually become relatively fixed, and a **Galeazzi** sign should be sought. By holding the ankles with the knees bent and hips flexed 90°, the examiner looks for any foreshortening of the (affected) thigh. Older patients may also present with limited hip abduction, a limp, and apparent shortening of the involved extremity.

Because most of the hip and pelvis are not ossified at birth, radiographs are not helpful until 4 to 6 months of age. Ultrasound is more accurate for the detection of DDH from birth to about 4 months, but screening is best delayed until 4 to 6 weeks of age, when the rate of false positive examinations drops. Routine ultrasound screening of all infants is not recommended but should be considered for babies with a family history of DDH and for those born in the breech position.

TREATMENT

When an abnormal "clunk," limited hip abduction, or limb asymmetry is noted at the newborn examination (or thereafter), the patient should be referred for orthopedic consultation. Most dislocatable hips stabilize without intervention within the first 2 weeks of life. If treatment is indicated in children younger than 6 months, a **Pavlik harness** or another type brace which keeps the hip abducted and flexed is the best initial treatment. Closed reduction (manipulation of the hip ball into the socket) and body casting is used in older patients. Cases that do not respond to conservative measures require surgical reduction or hip reconstruction.

FOOT DEFORMITIES

Flexible foot deformities, such as flexible flatfoot, rarely predispose children to difficulty walking, poor shoe fit, or pain. Almost any deformity of the foot that can be molded by the

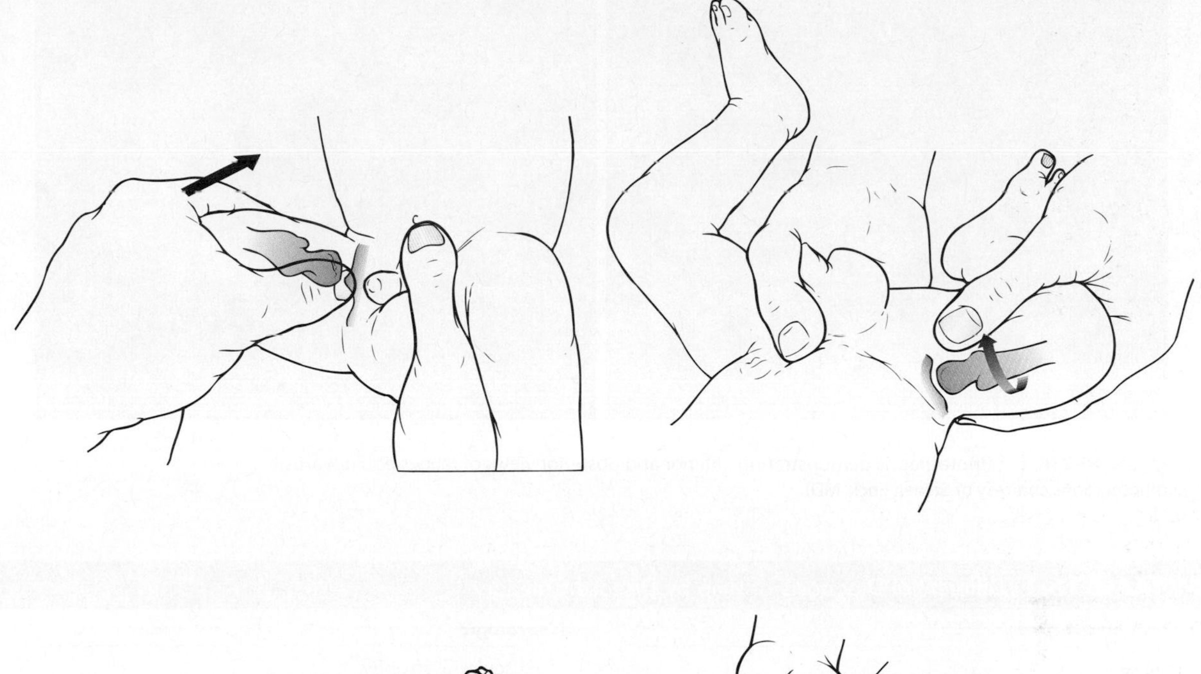

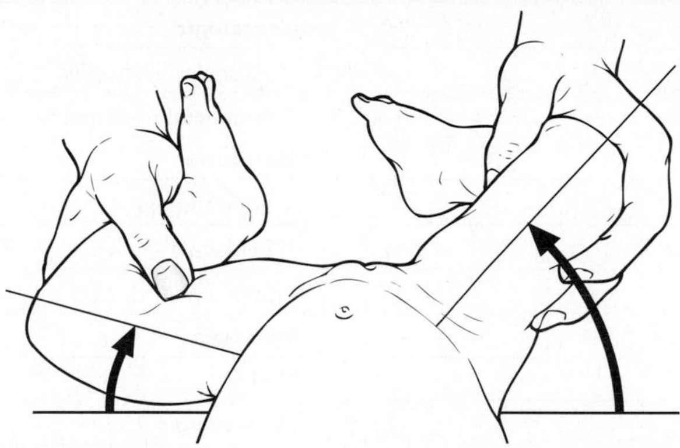

Figure 16-1 • Barlow (*above*) and Ortolani maneuvers.

examiner's hands to an anatomically correct position requires minimal if any intervention.

Metatarsus adductus (in-toeing of the forefoot without hindfoot abnormalities) is a common, benign condition caused by intrauterine positioning. As opposed to clubfoot, ankle motion is unrestricted. Mild metatarsus adductus is flexible, meaning the examiner can straighten out the deformity. In cases of severe metatarsus adductus, the forefoot is inflexible and cannot be corrected into a normal position. Severe cases are treated with serial bracing or casting starting at ages 6 to 12 months. Surgery is rarely indicated.

Talipes equinovarus, or clubfoot, is a rare but potentially debilitating deformity that can be described by the acronym CAVE—Cavus of the forefoot, Adduction of the forefoot, Varus of the hindfoot, and Equinus (plantarflexion) of the ankle (Fig. 16-2). Dorsiflexion at the ankle is impossible in patients with clubfoot. Without treatment, the foot becomes progressively more deformed, and calluses or ulcerations can develop when the child is old enough to ambulate. Early intervention is essential for subsequent normal function and more normal development. Initial treatment usually consists of serial manipulation of the foot with toe-to-groin casting; with appropriate technique over 95% of clubfeet can be corrected. Long-term bracing is then used to avoid relapse. Relapse, however, is common and is addressed with repeat casting and surgery. One in seven children with this condition also has other congenital malformations. **All children with clubfoot should have an examination of active toe movement (especially toe dorsiflexion) to rule out neurological causes of clubfoot.**

LIMP

Limp is probably the most common musculoskeletal complaint prompting medical evaluation in children. Pain, weakness, decreased range of motion, and leg-length discrepancy all disrupt the normal gait.

DIFFERENTIAL DIAGNOSIS

The list of conditions that present with limp is extensive (Table 16-1). Trauma is the most common cause of limp at any age.

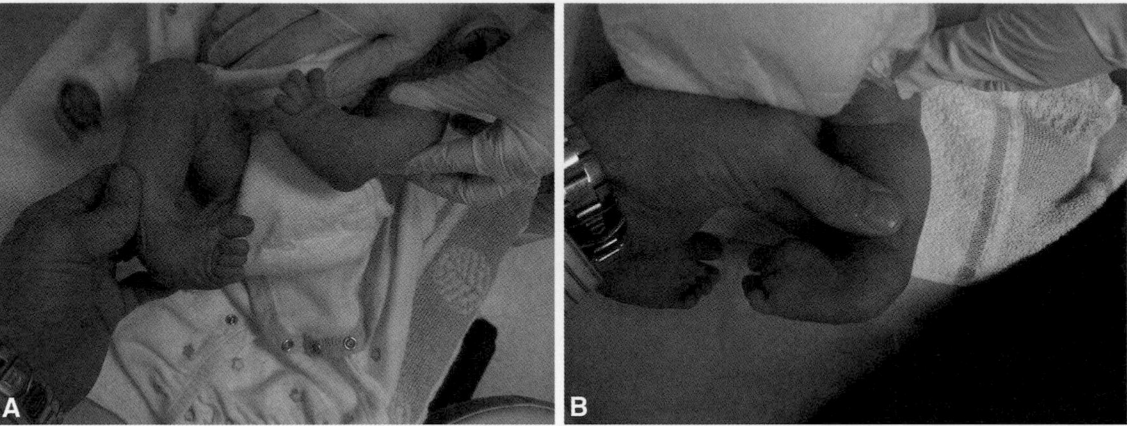

Figure 16-2 (A, B) • Photographs demonstrating anterior and posterior views of talipes equinovarus. (Photographs courtesy of Steven Frick, MD)

TABLE 16-1 Differential Diagnosis of Limp by Disease Category

Trauma or overuse	***Neurologic***
Fracture	Muscular dystrophy
Soft-tissue injury	Peripheral neuropathy
Infectious	***Neoplasia***
Septic arthritis	Bone tumors
Osteomyelitis	Leukemia
Lyme arthritis	Spinal cord tumors
Discitis	***Metabolic***
Inflammatory	Rickets
Transient synovitis	***Hematologic***
Rheumatic disease	Sickle cell disease
Reactive arthritis	Hemophilia
Developmental/acquired	***Other***
Developmental dysplasia of the hip	Appendicitis
Avascular necrosis	Pelvic inflammatory disease
Slipped capital femoral epiphysis	Testicular torsion

The patient's age affects the differential diagnosis. Infection, inflammation, and paralytic syndromes are common etiologies in children from 1 to 3 years of age. From 3 to 10 years of age, Legg-Calvé-Perthes disease, toxic synovitis, and juvenile idiopathic arthritis become more common. Slipped capital femoral epiphysis is a consideration in pubertal patients.

Legg-Calvé-Perthes disease is avascular necrosis (ischemic compromise) of the femoral head. The etiology is unknown. Eventually (over ~ 2 to 5 years), the ischemic bone is resorbed and repaired. Legg-Calvé-Perthes disease occurs more often in males and younger children (4 to 8 years of age). A painless or mildly painful limp that develops insidiously is the most common presenting complaint. The pain is often referred to the knee or thigh, clouding the diagnostic picture. Range of motion is limited, especially internal rotation and abduction. Initial radiographic studies may appear normal; subsequent films demonstrate epiphyseal radiolucency (Fig. 16-3). A bone scan or MRI may be helpful to detect early impairment in the blood supply. Treatment involves containing the softened femoral head within the acetabulum, preserving its spherical contour, and maintaining normal range of motion. Exercises, bracing, casting, or surgery may be prescribed; the best treatment is not currently clear. The amount and area of ischemic damage affects the prognosis. Severe stiffness and subluxation of the femoral head out of the hip socket are the most serious

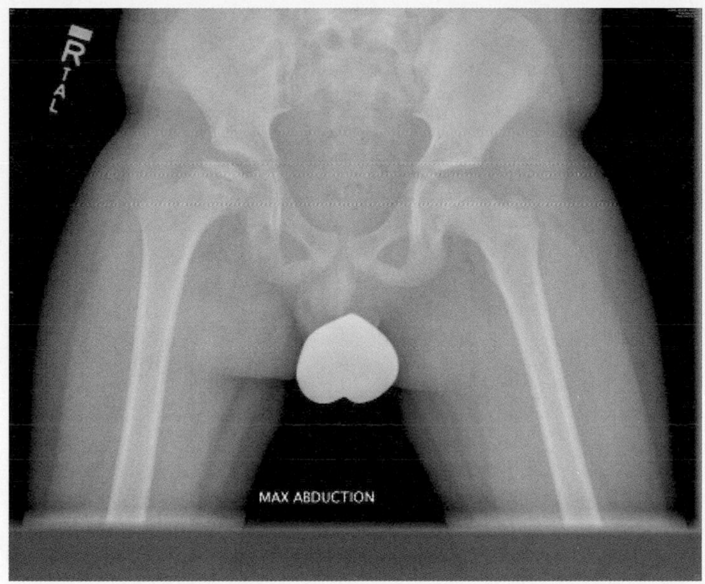

Figure 16-3 • Legg-Calvé-Perthes disease of right hip. Nine-year-old boy with stiffness in right hip who presented with complaint of limp. Radiograph shows 50% collapse with sclerosis of the right femoral head as compared to his normal left hip (*opposite*).
(Courtesy of Cincinnati Children's Hospital Medical Center, Department of Pediatric Orthopaedics.)

acute complications. Long-term disability is related to healing of the femoral head in a misshapen pattern (nonspherical), and the subsequent development of arthritis in the fifth decade of life for 50% of patients.

Slipped capital femoral epiphysis (SCFE) is the gradual or acute separation of the proximal femoral growth plate, with the femur head slipping off the femoral neck and rotating into an inferior/posterior position. The cause is unknown but may be hormonal (the condition is most common during puberty) in origin or related to excessive weight bearing (SCFE is more common in overweight individuals). It occurs slightly more often in males. Antecedent trauma is not a contributing factor. Although usually asymmetric at presentation, 25% to 33% of cases eventually progress to bilateral involvement. The typical patient presents with a limp and pain, which may be centered in the hip or groin but often is referred to the knee. Limited hip internal rotation and outward rotation of the limb with hip flexion are present on examination. Radiographs with the child's hips in the frog-leg lateral position are the study of choice for noting epiphyseal displacement (Fig. 16-4). Radiographs may show physeal plate widening, decreased epiphyseal height and a Klein line (line drawn along the femoral neck) that does not intersect the lateral epiphysis. The primary goal of treatment is prevention of further misalignment. Screw fixation is effective in the acute setting. Chronic cases generally require osteotomy. Long-term complications include avascular necrosis and late degenerative changes similar to those seen with osteoarthritis.

CLINICAL MANIFESTATIONS

History

The history should include questions about the onset, timing, and evolution of the limp. Pain may be severe (fracture, infection), constant, associated with activity (injury), acute, or chronic. The absence of pain suggests weakness or instability. Swelling and stiffness are common in rheumatologic disease. Toxic or transient synovitis often follows a recent viral illness. Any history of bowel or bladder incontinence suggests spinal compression.

Physical Examination

Watching the child walk is particularly important because certain gaits are associated with specific disorders. Each joint should be examined for range of motion, swelling, warmth, erythema, and tenderness. Fractures produce point tenderness and occasionally angulation. Neurologic evaluation includes deep tendon reflexes, strength, and sensation. Extremities are assessed for adequate perfusion and deformities. Muscle atrophy and fasciculation may be present in neuromuscular disease.

DIAGNOSTIC EVALUATION

All patients with significant limp should have a physical examination to localize the area of tenderness or stiffness, followed by plain radiographs of any area(s) with positive findings. A blood test with elevation of the sedimentation rate (ESR), C-reactive protein (CRP) and WBCs can suggest infection, inflammatory arthritis, or occasionally malignancy. MRI has become the preferred screening tool for poorly localized limp or pain, with a screening scan from the lumbar spine to the feet. Bone scan can also occasionally be helpful. Ultrasound and CT scan are most helpful when symptoms localize to a specific bone or joint. Sonography is useful to evaluate for the presence of joint effusion, especially when a septic joint is considered. MRI is also extremely useful for the localized evaluation of joints, bones, cartilage, and soft tissue. It may also be used to evaluate for abscesses or infected bone (gadolinium-enhanced MRI) which may require surgical debridement and drainage. The diagnosis of septic arthritis is made by aspiration of the affected joint for bacterial cultures

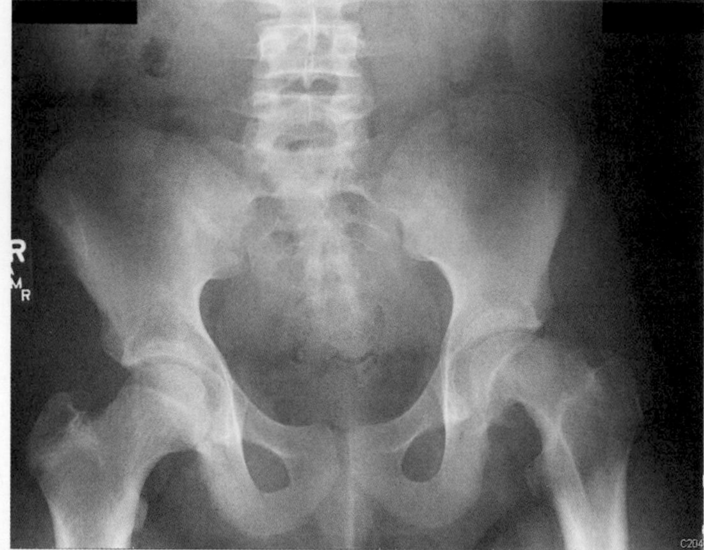

Figure 16-4 • Radiograph of a slipped capital femoral epiphysis. Fourteen-year-old adolescent male with complaint of pain and limp in left thigh. Radiograph shows about 30% slippage of the femoral head off the femoral neck on the left as compared to his normal right hip.
(Courtesy of Cincinnati Children's Hospital Medical Center, Department of Pediatric Orthopaedics.)

and measurement of WBC count. Patients with weakness should have serum creatinine kinase (CPK) checked to evaluate for muscular dystrophy or myopathy; electromyography and nerve conduction studies may also be helpful. If the weakness is progressive and limited to the lower extremities, spinal cord or nerve compression must be ruled out with imaging studies (i.e., MRI).

TREATMENT

Treatment for each condition is specific for that disorder. Fractures and bone/joint infections are discussed below. For traumatic limp with no associated fracture, swelling (sprain or tear), or disability, rest, ice, compression, and pain control are indicated, as well as physical therapy in some cases.

COMMON FRACTURES IN CHILDREN

Children's bones are more flexible than adults' and can bend, bow, or partially break. Incomplete "buckle" and greenstick fractures are more common in children than displaced fractures due to both this flexibility and the presence of a thicker periosteal wrapping around the bones. **Because ligaments and tendons are relatively stronger than bones and growth plates, fractures are much more common than sprains before adolescence**. It is usually safest to assume that any posttraumatic bone or joint pain is a fracture rather than a sprain, even if the initial radiographs are normal.

DIFFERENTIAL DIAGNOSIS

Fractures can disrupt the growth plate, which is the weakest portion of the child's skeletal system. Growth plate fractures are categorized according to the **Salter–Harris classification** (Fig. 16-5). It is important to remember that a small percentage of fractures are not visible on the initial radiograph, only becoming apparent 2 to 3 weeks later on follow-up films. Tenderness over a growth plate is often a nondisplaced fracture even when X-rays are normal. Children's bones may bow or bend without any visible fracture after a trauma ("plastic deformation"). **Stress fractures** due to repetitive stress in athletes are frequently invisible on initial radiographs. **Pathologic fractures** result when underlying disease weakens the bone, as may occur in osteogenesis imperfecta, benign tumors, malignancies, long-term steroid use, infection, endocrine disorders, and some inborn errors of metabolism.

CLINICAL MANIFESTATIONS

History and Physical Examination

The hallmark of a fracture is severe point tenderness over a bone. Localized swelling, bruising, and angulation may also be present. Visual and functional comparison with the opposite (likely uninjured) side is usually very helpful. It is imperative that perfusion and neurologic function (strength, sensation) be evaluated in the area of and distal to the injury.

DIAGNOSTIC EVALUATION

Radiographs should include AP and lateral views of the involved bone as well as the joints immediately adjacent to the injury. Salter–Harris types I and V may not be seen on these views; oblique views or serial radiographs may be needed to confirm the diagnosis. Many childhood fractures are radiographically invisible until 1 to 2 weeks after injury, when the healing bone callus becomes visible.

TREATMENT

Most fractures can be adequately treated with casts or splints. Children with severe limb pain after trauma should be splinted even if X-rays are normal, due to the likelihood of an "occult" fracture. Fractures that are displaced or malaligned often require manipulation in the emergency room. Fractures through the growth plate require particular care because they may result in crooked or shortened limbs. Open fractures that break through the skin usually need antibiotics, operative washout and debridement to minimize the risk of infection. Femur

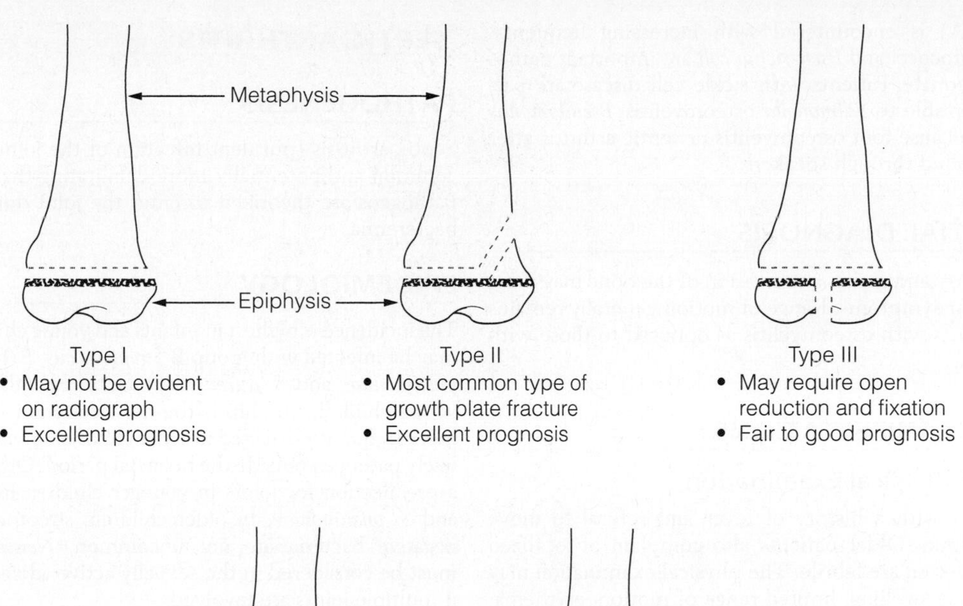

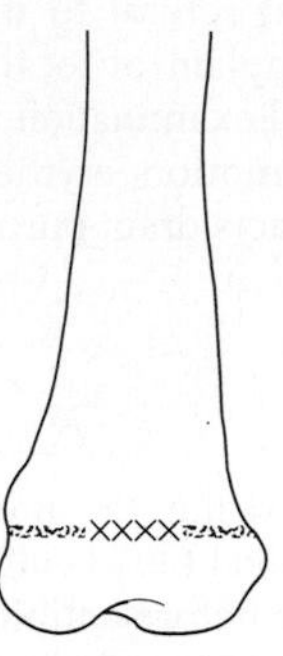

Figure 16-5 • Epiphyseal fractures: Salter–Harris classification.

fractures, elbow fractures and fractures that penetrate the joint often benefit from surgical fixation with pins, plates, or rods.

SUBLUXATION OF THE RADIAL HEAD

"**Nursemaid's elbow**," or radial head subluxation, is a common injury seen in young children. The history is often remarkable for a sudden strong jerking of the child's hand, resulting in rapid extension at the elbow. The child dangles the affected arm close to the body with the elbow slightly flexed and the forearm pronated, often holding the wrist. Motion at the elbow is limited and painful. Treatment consists of extending the elbow and supinating the hand, then fully flexing the elbow, which is often inadvertently performed by the radiology technician when they take an AP radiograph of the elbow. A successful reduction is usually accompanied by a "click" as the entrapped annular ligament pops back into place. "Radial head subluxation" is a misnomer and is never apparent on a radiograph. Usually the child begins to move the arm normally within minutes.

OSTEOMYELITIS

PATHOGENESIS

Bone infections require early recognition and aggressive treatment to bring about a favorable outcome. Hematogenous seeding is the usual source of origin; trauma seems to increase susceptibility. The femur and tibia account for two thirds of cases. Infection usually begins in the metaphysis, an area of relative blood stasis and few phagocytes. Many neonates with bone infection have an associated septic joint.

EPIDEMIOLOGY AND RISK FACTORS

Incidence peaks in the neonatal period and again in older children (9 to 11 years of age), when osteomyelitis becomes more common in males. The predominant organism in all age groups is *Staphylococcus aureus*. Methicillin-resistant *Staphylococcus aureus* (MRSA) is encountered with increasing frequency. Group B streptococci and *Escherichia coli* are important pathogens in the neonate. Patients with sickle cell disease are particularly susceptible to *Salmonella* osteomyelitis. *Pseudomonas aeruginosa* can cause foot osteomyelitis or septic arthritis after a puncture wound through sneakers.

DIFFERENTIAL DIAGNOSIS

Traumatic injury and malignant invasion of the bone may present with similar symptoms. Range of motion generally remains intact in patients with osteomyelitis as opposed to those with septic arthritis.

CLINICAL MANIFESTATIONS

History and Physical Examination

Infants present with a history of fever and refusal to move the involved limb. Older patients also complain of localized bone pain and often are febrile. The physical examination may reveal soft-tissue swelling, limited range of motion, erythema, and point tenderness. Occasionally, sinus tracts drain purulent fluid to the skin surface.

DIAGNOSTIC EVALUATION

The white blood count (WBC) is often within the normal range. Approximately 50% to 60% of peripheral blood cultures are positive. **Aspiration of the involved bone before antibiotics are started is often key to identification of the causative organism**. Identification permits sensitivity testing of the infecting agent, which guides successful antimicrobial management. Radiographs are initially normal but demonstrate periosteal elevation or radiolucent necrotic areas in 2 to 3 weeks. Bone scans are positive within 24 to 72 hours. Gadolinium-enhanced MRI can be obtained to rule out subperiosteal or intraosseous abscess or necrotic bone, especially in patients with severe symptoms or who are refractory to intravenous antibiotics. Serum markers of inflammation are usually elevated. An elevated C-reactive protein value is seen in 98% of cases and returns to normal within 7 days of effective treatment. The ESR is elevated in 90% of cases but requires longer (3 to 4 weeks) to return to normal.

TREATMENT

Treatment consists of intravenous or high-dose oral antibiotics for 4 to 6 weeks. Initially, broad-spectrum antistaphylococcal agents (such as cefazolin, nafcillin, or oxacillin) are appropriate. Vancomycin may be added if suspicion for MRSA is high. Neonates require coverage for group B streptococci and gram-negative bacilli. Patients with sickle cell should initially receive a third-generation cephalosporin for *Salmonella* coverage. When the organism has been recovered and sensitivities are available, therapy may be narrowed. Most patients do not require surgery unless they develop an abscess or necrotic bone (sequestrum). A severe joint infection can destroy cartilage and cause arthritis. Growth arrest can rarely occur if the growth plate is involved.

SEPTIC ARTHRITIS

PATHOGENESIS

Septic arthritis (purulent infection of the joint space) is more common and potentially more debilitating than osteomyelitis. Pathogens are theorized to enter the joint during episodes of bacteremia.

EPIDEMIOLOGY

The incidence is highest in infants and young children. Neonates may be infected with group B *Streptococcus*, *E. coli*, *Streptococcus pneumoniae*, and *S. aureus*. In infants older than 6 weeks and young children, the hip is the most common site. The knee is more frequently affected in older children. *S. aureus* is the most likely pathogen outside the neonatal period. Other bacteria with a predilection for joints in younger children include *K. kingae* and *S. pneumoniae*. In older children, streptococci and gram-negative bacteria are not uncommon. *Neisseria gonorrhoeae* must be considered in the sexually active adolescent, especially if multiple joints are involved.

DIFFERENTIAL DIAGNOSIS

Osteomyelitis and inflammatory arthritis should be considered in the differential diagnosis. In addition, many causes of reactive or postinfectious arthritis may present in a similar manner. **Toxic synovitis** is a frequent cause of hip pain and stiffness in children. It has not been definitively proven to be an infectious condition, although it often follows a viral illness. The hip is most commonly involved. In contrast to septic arthritis, range of motion is minimally limited, the child is generally afebrile and will usually bear weight, the ESR is less than 40 mm/hr, and the WBC count is less than 12,000/mm^3. Toxic synovitis usually resolves without treatment (beyond oral anti-inflammatory medication) over 7 to 14 days.

CLINICAL MANIFESTATIONS

History and Physical Examination

Septic arthritis presents as a painful joint, often accompanied by fever, irritability, and refusal to bear weight. On examination, range of motion is clearly limited. The joint is tender and may be visibly swollen.

DIAGNOSTIC EVALUATION

The standard of care for septic arthritis involves aspiration of the joint. The synovial fluid usually yields a WBC in excess of 25,000/mm^3 and a pathologic organism. The exception is *Neisseria gonorrhoeae*, which is difficult to recover; blood, cervical, rectal, and nasopharyngeal cultures may be additionally helpful.

TREATMENT

Delay in treatment may result in permanent destructive changes and functional impairment. A septic hip is an orthopedic emergency. Intravenous antibiotic therapy remains the treatment of choice; conversion to oral therapy is appropriate when sensitivities are known and symptoms substantially improve. Ceftriaxone is an appropriate initial choice in the young child; a semisynthetic penicillin or (first- or second-generation) cephalosporin are preferred in older children because of the overwhelming presence of *Staphylococcus aureus* arthritis in this age group. Vancomycin is added in cases of suspected MRSA. Cefotaxime is a better choice in the neonate. Antibiotic therapy can be specifically targeted to the pathogen when culture results become available.

OSGOOD–SCHLATTER DISEASE

Osgood–Schlatter disease involves swelling, pain, and tenderness over the *tibial tuberosity*. It is caused by repetitive stress of the distal insertion of the patellar tendon attachment to the proximal tibia. Osgood–Schlatter disease typically occurs between 10 and 15 years of age, during the adolescent growth spurt. Pain is worsened with kneeling, running, jumping, or squatting but is relieved by rest. Radiographs reveal irregularities of the tubercle ossification center and soft tissue swelling. Most cases are mild and treated with activity modification and stretching exercises. Long-term morbidity is quite low; the disorder almost always disappears when skeletal maturity is reached.

IDIOPATHIC SCOLIOSIS

Idiopathic scoliosis is excessive lateral curvature of the spine found in otherwise healthy children with normal bones, muscles, and vertebral discs. The cause is unknown, but heredity definitely plays a role.

EPIDEMIOLOGY

Five percent of children display some degree of spinal deformity. Routine screening is very important. Severe scoliosis requiring bracing or surgery occurs about seven times more often in females than males. Progression of the curve is most rapid during the adolescent growth spurt.

DIFFERENTIAL DIAGNOSIS

Occasionally, scoliosis may be caused by neuromuscular abnormalities or congenital deformities. Kyphosis is an abnormally large roundback of the spine. Kyphosis is usually postural and responds well to observation or physical therapy; inflexible kyphosis may be associated with wedge-shaped vertebral bodies (Scheuermann disease) and may require bracing or corrective surgery.

CLINICAL MANIFESTATIONS

Idiopathic scoliosis is usually not associated with back pain or fatigue; such symptoms warrant further investigation. The physical examination consists of two parts. First, the child is examined from the rear while standing up. Shoulder girdle and iliac crest areas are noted for asymmetry and unequal height. Then, the Adams forward bending test is performed. The child bends forward from the waist with the arms hanging freely. The examiner should examine the patient's back for a rib cage or low back prominence on one side of the spine versus the other. Patients with evidence of curvature on exam should receive standing posteroanterior (PA) and lateral spine radiographs to allow angular measurement of the deformity.

TREATMENT

Treatment depends on the degree of curvature, skeletal maturation, body habitus, and gender of the child. Premenarchal females are the most likely to experience progression of their curvature and should be treated more aggressively. Curvatures less than 25° need only be followed. More pronounced deformity (25° to 40°) in a child who is still growing may benefit from external bracing until the growth spurt is completed. Bracing does not reduce the curve, but it can halt progression and is 50% to 85% effective if used correctly. Unfortunately, compliance tends to be low. Curvature greater than 50° after the growth spurt may continue to progress; such patients often have spinal fusion to reduce the curve and stabilize the spine. Curves of >90° are associated with clinically significant decreased vital capacity and low functional pulmonary reserve.

ACHONDROPLASIA

Achondroplasia is a disorder of physeal cartilage calcification and remodeling. Inheritance is autosomal dominant. The physical appearance is strikingly characteristic: these patients are very short, with large heads. Long bones tend to be wide, short, and curved, and digits are short and stubby. Kyphoscoliosis and lumbar lordosis may be quite pronounced. Heterozygotes have fairly normal intelligence, sexual function, and life expectancy. Homozygotes fare less well, given their increased susceptibility to pulmonary complications, an abnormally small foramen magnum that predisposes to brainstem compression early in life, and lower spinal stenosis that results in pain, numbness, and possibly disordered lower extremity neurologic function in young adulthood.

OSTEOGENESIS IMPERFECTA

Osteogenesis imperfecta (OI) describes a group of closely related genetic disorders resulting in fragile, brittle bones. The common denominator in all variants is the abnormal synthesis of type I collagen, which normally constitutes approximately 90% of the bone matrix but is also dispersed in the teeth, ligaments, skin, ears, and sclerae. The most severe form is type II, or fetal OI, which results in multiple intrauterine and birth fractures and is uniformly fatal in the perinatal period. Clinical severity depends on the subclass of OI (Table 16-2). Some variants cause death early in life; others present with only moderately increased susceptibility to fractures. Blue sclerae are a characteristic feature in some forms of the disease. Short stature is not uncommon as a result of recurrent fractures. Fractures associated with OI occasionally raise the suspicion of child abuse. Patients with severe disease may benefit from pamidronate therapy, which inhibits osteoclastic resorption.

TABLE 16-2 Classification of Osteogenesis Imperfecta

Syndrome	Mode of Inheritance	Orthopedic Manifestations	Nonorthopedic Manifestations	Life Expectancy
Type I	Autosomal dominant	Frequent fractures from the neonatal period through adolescence;[a] severe bone fragility; bow legs; joint laxity; short stature	Blue/gray sclerae; adult-onset sensorineural hearing loss (deafness); abnormal dentition	Generally shortened
Type II	Autosomal recessive	Short, deformed limbs; multiple in utero and neonatal fractures; severe bone fragility	Intrauterine growth retardation; stillbirth; blue/gray sclerae	Days
Type III	Autosomal recessive	Frequent fractures which heal with deformation; severe bone fragility; lower limb deformities; short stature	Normal or mildly blue/gray sclerae	Generally shortened
Type IV	Autosomal dominant	Increased susceptibility to fractures[a]	Normal sclerae; increased risk for aortic dilation	Near normal

[a]Susceptibility to fractures progressively decreases during adolescence; pathologic fractures in adulthood are rare.

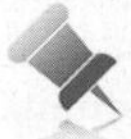

KEY POINTS

- Developmental dysplasia of the hip (DDH) may be demonstrated on physical examination by performing the Barlow and Ortolani maneuvers (in newborns) and evaluating limb length and hip adduction in infants older than 3 months. DDH must be diagnosed and treated early in life to obtain a favorable outcome.
- Plantar and dorsiflexion are intact in metatarsus adductus, whereas in talipes equinovarus, the ankle and hindfoot are fixed in plantar flexion.
- Trauma is the most common cause of limp in all age groups. Plain radiographs are helpful screening tools.
- When evaluating a complaint of limp, any evidence of neurologic involvement (weakness, bowel and/or bladder incontinence) necessitates aggressive workup to rule out spinal cord compression.
- The typical patient with Legg-Calvé-Perthes disease is a young male child who presents with a painless or moderately painful limp and knee pain.
- The typical SCFE patient is an obese adolescent male who presents with hip or knee pain and no history of trauma.
- Fractures through the growth plate may result in deformity or limb-length discrepancy. Epiphyseal fractures categorized as Salter–Harris type III or IV have the greatest risk of disruption of growth.
- The peak incidence of osteomyelitis is bimodal (neonatal period and 9 to 11 years of age). Only approximately half of blood cultures are positive, so aspiration of the bone yields invaluable information.
- *Staphylococcus aureus* is the most common pathogen implicated in osteomyelitis in all age groups. It is also the most common pathogen in sickle cell patients, who are also particularly susceptible to *Salmonella*.
- In cases of osteomyelitis, the MRI or bone scan is more sensitive than plain films early in the disease process.
- The most common cause of septic arthritis in infants and children is *Staphylococcus aureus*. *Neisseria gonorrhoeae* must be considered in the sexually active adolescent.
- Children with toxic synovitis have lower sedimentation rates and WBC counts than those with septic arthritis. Generally, although the joint is tender, children with toxic synovitis will bear weight.
- Scoliosis is more common in adolescent females than in males. Idiopathic scoliosis does not result in back pain or fatigue.
- Bracing is recommended for scoliotic curves from 25° to 40° until the growth spurt is complete. Bracing halts curve progression; it does not correct the curvature already there.
- Patients with osteogenesis imperfecta types I and II often have bluish sclera. Type II OI is the most severe form, resulting in intrauterine or perinatal death.

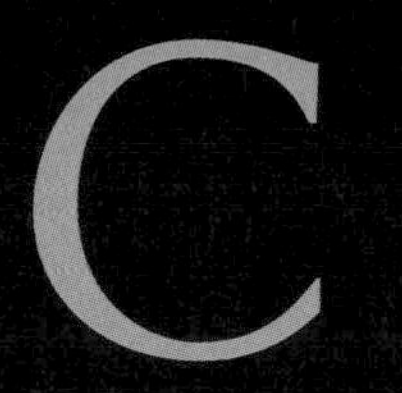

C Clinical Vignettes

Vignette 1

A male infant is born after full-term gestation to a primigravida mother and noted at birth to have bilateral foot deformities. He does not have any other deformities in the extremities and is able to move his feet and toes up and down. His feet are both in a position of adduction and equinus (pointing inward and downward).

1. What are the deformities that describe a congenital clubfoot?
   a. Abduction, eversion, planus, and neutral hindfoot
   b. Adduction, inversion, neutral hindfoot with normal dorsiflexion
   c. Abduction, inversion, neutral hindfoot with normal dorsiflextion
   d. Cavus, adduction, varus, and equinus
   e. Planus, abduction, valgus, and calcaneus

2. What other deformities or systemic problems are commonly associated with clubfoot?
   a. None
   b. Congenital heart defects
   c. Spinal dysraphism
   d. Developmental hip dysplasia
   e. Congenital constriction bands

3. What is the best initial treatment for this patient?
   a. Special orthopedic shoes
   b. Physical therapy
   c. Serial manipulations and casting
   d. Early surgical correction
   e. Surgery at 1 year of age

Vignette 2

A healthy 22-year-old primigravida women delivers a healthy, full-term female infant via Cesarean section after it was discovered during labor that the infant was in breech position. On the first day of life, examination in the newborn nursery reveals no apparent facial or musculoskeletal malformations, but her presentation makes you suspicious she may have developmental dysplasia of the hip (DDH). A careful hip examination demonstrates the left hip is Ortolani positive.

1. The risk factors that should raise your index of suspicion for DDH include all of the following except:
   a. Female gender
   b. Breech presentation
   c. Family history of DDH
   d. Polydacytyly of feet
   e. First-born child

2. The newborn hip examination is critical to identify unstable, abnormal hips and permit early treatment. The description of a hip examination as Ortolani positive means which of the following?
   a. The hip is loose (subluxatable) but is normally located.
   b. The hip is dislocated and irreducible.
   c. The hip is normally located and dislocatable.
   d. The hip is dislocated and reducible.
   e. The hip clicks during examination.

3. Which of the following is the best treatment for a dislocated, reducible hip recognized in infancy?
   a. Observation
   b. Abduction bracing (Pavlik harness or hip abduction brace)
   c. Denis-Browne foot abduction splint
   d. Closed reduction and spica cast
   e. Open reduction and spica cast

4. What is the most significant long-term sequelae of properly treated DDH?
   a. Limb length inequality
   b. Weakness
   c. Early osteoarthritis
   d. Stiffness
   e. Scoliosis

Vignette 3

A 3-year-old male presents with a 24-hour history of irritability, limping on his left leg, and fever at home to 102°F by oral thermometer. He is now refusing to bear weight on his left side. He has no chronic medical problems, was the product of a normal gestation and delivery, and has had normal developmental milestones. One week ago, he had a mild viral upper respiratory illness, and he also had some bruising on his left leg after falling off some playground equipment. On examination, he is supine on the table and is irritable with any movement. His pulse and blood pressure are normal, and he does not appear in distress when he is at rest. Any movement of his left lower extremity causes him to cry out, and he holds his left hip in a position of flexion, external rotation, and slight abduction. Some laboratory studies were ordered by the emergency room physician and show an elevated WBC count with a normal hemoglobin. The three leading possible diagnoses for this patient are believed to be toxic synovitis, septic arthritis, and acute hematogenous osteomyelitis.

1. What additional bloodwork will help narrow the diagnostic possibilities?
   a. Creatinine phosphokinase
   b. Erythrocyte sedimentation rate
   c. Alkaline phosphatase
   d. Serum calcium
   e. Albumin

2. In addition to a WBC count of 18,000/mm^3, the patient's ESR was 90 mm/hr. Manipulation of the left hip made the child very irritable, and any attempt at passive internal rotation of the hip resulted in extreme guarding by the patient and complaints of pain. What laboratory study is definitive for the diagnosis of septic arthritis (SA) of the left hip?
   a. C-reactive protein
   b. Ultrasound evaluation of the hip
   c. MRI imaging
   d. Aspiration of the hip
   e. AP pelvis radiograph

3. The patient had blood cultures obtained in the emergency department, then went to the radiology suite where a left hip aspirate was performed. Three milliliters of thick yellow fluid were aspirated. The initial gram stain was negative, cultures were started, and the WBC count of the fluid was 90,000 cells/mm^3. What antibiotics should be started?
   a. Penicillin
   b. First-generation cephalosporin
   c. Gentamicin
   d. Vancomycin
   e. Second-generation cephalosporin

4. The patient was taken to the operating room and underwent incision, arthrotomy, and drainage of the hip. What is the major concern if diagnosis and treatment of SA of the hip is not carried out promptly?
   a. Chronic osteomyelitis
   b. Destruction of the hip joint (osteonecrosis)
   c. Dissemination of infection to knee and ankle
   d. Development of bacterial pneumonia
   e. Development of infection in opposite hip

Vignette 4

A 13-year-old female presents complaining of right knee pain for 6 weeks. She is obese, with a body mass index of 34 kg/m^2. She denies any injury or recent illness/infection. She does not have pain at rest or at night. Her mom notes she has been limping. Her knee examination is benign. She has no knee effusion and no tenderness, and both knee and patellofemoral joints are normally mobile. She walks with an antalgic gait on the right, with limited time in stance phase on the affected side.

1. The next focused examination should carefully assess which of the following?
   a. Spine
   b. Hips
   c. Ankle
   d. Foot
   e. Contralateral knee

2. The patient has very limited internal rotation of the right hip when supine and has pain at the end of range of motion testing. She also has limited internal rotation of the left hip in the supine position, but does not complain of pain. Flexion of the right hip is possible only to 90° and is accompanied by obligatory external rotation of the hip as the thigh flexes. Which of the following represents the best next step in the evaluation?
   a. Bloodwork to assess for an inflammatory problem (CBC, ESR, CRP)
   b. AP radiograph of the right hip
   c. AP radiograph of the pelvis
   d. AP pelvis and frog lateral pelvis radiographs
   e. MRI of the right hip

3. The patient was found to have bilateral SCFE on the radiographs, with the right side being slightly more displaced. Which of the following is the best initial treatment for this patient?
   a. Referral to an orthopedic surgeon within the next week
   b. Elective referral to orthopedic surgeon
   c. Crutches and physical therapy
   d. Referral today to an orthopedic surgeon for surgical stabilization
   e. MRI of the hips

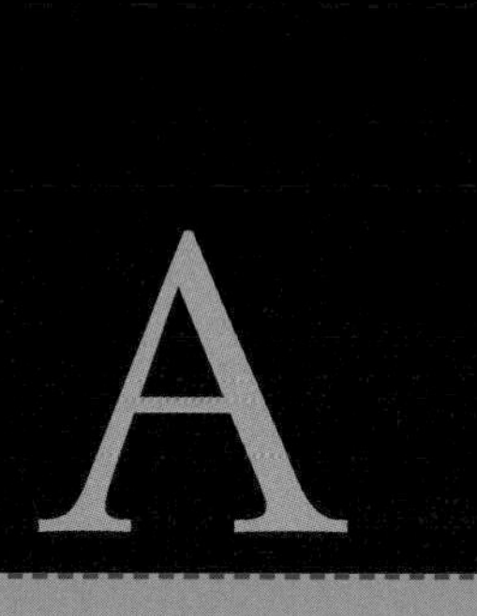

Answers

Vignette 1 Question 1

Answer D: The four components of foot deformity in a congenital clubfoot can be described by the acronym CAVE. **Cavus** is a high arch of the foot with the first ray/great toe metatarsal in plantarflexion. **Adduction** is medial deviation of the forefoot, with the forefoot pointing inward. **Varus** describes the position of the heel, with the inferior part of the heel pointing inward. **Equinus** describes the plantarflexion of the foot, with the toes and foot pointing downward. The key physical examination finding in the newborn to diagnose clubfoot is that all of these deformities are present and the deformities are rigid. In particular, the foot cannot be dorsiflexed to a neutral plantigrade position. In addition, the feet will typically have deep creases in the middle of the foot medially and often a single deep crease in the posterior heel. The small, fine multiple transverse creases that are seen in normal infant feet are usually missing in clubfeet. Clubfeet will not improve without treatment. Feet that are flexible and can be dorsiflexed above neutral (such as most cases of metatarsus adductus) are positional deformities that may improve without treatment.

Vignette 1 Question 2

Answer A: Congenital clubfoot is usually an isolated deformity found in otherwise healthy children. It is more common in boys and is bilateral in 50% of cases. Examination of the infant with clubfoot should include a careful neurological examination to rule out a neurological cause of the foot deformities (make sure the infant can actively dorsiflex and plantarflex the toes), and as in all infants a careful hip examination should be performed to assess for hip instability/developmental hip dysplasia. Some authors have suggested that hip dysplasia is more common in children with clubfeet, but larger and more recent studies have refuted this. Up to one-third of children with congenital constriction bands have a clubfoot, but these patients make up an extremely small percentage of children who have clubfoot. The infant physical examination should include a careful search for constriction bands when a clubfoot deformity is noted, although these will be found rarely.

Vignette 1 Question 3

Answer C: Serial manipulations and casting to hold the foot in the stretched position is the standard treatment for congenital clubfoot, and in the past decade a specific method of manipulation and casting has been shown to be superior to all other methods. This method was developed by Ignacio Ponseti from the University of Iowa over five decades of studying clubfoot patients. The patients are treated with toe-to-groin casts that are changed weekly, and when correctly applied the deformity can be successfully corrected in over 95% of patients. Seventy percent to 90% of patients will have an Achilles tendon tenotomy at the completion of casting to assist in treating the equinus component of the deformity. Ponseti method casting should begin soon after the diagnosis of clubfoot is confirmed by physical examination, but it does not have to begin immediately. Many studies and the experience of multiple practitioners have shown that clubfoot deformities can be successfully corrected when treatment is begun weeks and even months after birth.

Vignette 2 Question 1

Answer D: The major risk factors for DDH are female gender and breech position. Other risk factors are family history of DDH and primigravida mother. DDH is believed to be multifactorial in etiology, with genetic predisposition and intrauterine positional factors playing a role. Musculoskeletal abnormalities in newborns can be thought of as either production defects (abnormal development of a part or parts leading to deformity) or packaging problems (intrauterine pressure or constraints imposed on a developing part result in deformity). In general, production abnormalities lead to progressive deformities if not treated after birth, and are commonly treated with manipulations and casting or bracing, or surgery. Packaging problems may improve with growth and time once outside the constraints of the uterus. DDH is believed to be part production, part packaging as reflected by the risk factors. Female gender and family history relate to the possible production defect, and first born child and breech presentation contribute to packaging abnormalities.

Vignette 2 Question 2

Answer D: The newborn hip physical examination is an essential skill to identify DDH in its earliest stages, when it can be treated most successfully. The hip examination to detect DDH is classically described as the Barlow and Ortolani maneuvers. The Barlow maneuver involves first flexing the hip being tested to 90°; then the hip is adducted (knee across midline) and a gentle force directed posteriorly is applied to see if the hip dislocates. The Ortolani maneuver involves taking the tested hip from a position of 90° flexion and maximum abduction (knee away from midline) and lifting up on the thigh/greater trochanter to see if the hip can be felt to reduce. Thus, the Barlow test detects a hip that is located and unstable/dislocatable, and the Ortolani test detects a hip that is dislocated and reducible. Because of confusion that can be created by describing the physical examination tests by the Barlow or Ortolani monickers, it may be better to describe the hip by the findings of the examination, with five options: normal, stable examination; loose/subluxatable but not dislocatable hip (difficult to determine without extensive experience); reduced/dislocatable hip; dislocated/reducible hip; and dislocated/irreducible hip (also can be difficult to detect). The sensation of the femoral head sliding over the edge of the acetabulum has been described as a "clunk" of dislocation and a "clunk" of relocation—unfortunately this has been mischaracterized by some as a hip "click." Hip "clicks" are palpable brief sensations caused by either soft tissues impinging between the femoral head and socket, or tendons snapping around the hip, and do not signify DDH. DDH in infancy is diagnosed by the examiner sensing instability of the femoral head, feeling the head exit and reenter the socket.

Vignette 2 Question 3

Answer B: The safest and most effective way to reduce and stabilize a dislocated hip in an infant with DDH is with abduction bracing, with the Pavlik harness being a commonly employed device. Although some dislocated hips in infants may spontaneously reduce, the reliability of the hip stabilizing is unknown. Many orthopedic surgeons may monitor a reduced, dislocatable hip (Barlow positive) because many of these will stabilize as the hip matures and the influence of maternal hormones recedes. Closed- and open-reduction techniques are reserved for hips that fail to reduce with abduction splinting.

Vignette 2 Question 4

Answer C: A hip that develops in an abnormal position with the femoral head not centered in the acetabulum (socket) is at high risk for developing early osteoarthritis and hip pain in adulthood.

Vignette 3 Question 1

Answer B: In patients presenting with possible musculoskeletal sepsis, one of the most helpful laboratory tests is the erythrocyte sedimentation rate (ESR). The ESR is nonspecific, but is usually very helpful to rule out significant infection. It is an acute phase reactant, will be abnormally elevated in conditions associated with inflammation, and is usually greater than 40 mm/hr in children with septic arthritis (SA) and/or acute hematogenous osteomyelitis (AHO). A normal ESR is reassuring, as it is unusual to have SA or AHO and have a normal ESR. The following criteria have been studied to differentiate SA from transient synovitis of the hip: (1) inability to bear weight on affected lower extremity, (2) history of fever, (3) WBC above 12,000/mm^3, and (4) ESR greater than 40 mm/hr. Patients with none of these criteria have almost zero chance of having SA; those with one of four have approximately a 5% chance; two of four a 40% chance; three of four a 75% chance; and four of four a 95% chance. The C-reactive protein (CRP) is another test of inflammation and is also frequently used to assess the risk of SA or AHO. It is more time sensitive than the ESR, as it will become abnormal earlier in musculoskeletal sepsis, and will also return to normal earlier if the infection is being successfully treated. It is thus more helpful for monitoring the response to therapy for infections of the musculoskeletal system. The complete blood count is helpful to assess for the risk of SA, but it is also useful to look at the hemoglobin. It is important to remember that many young patients with leukemia will present with complaints of musculoskeletal pain, and a leukemic hip effusion can mimic SA in its presentation. Typically these patients will be anemic, so a normal hemoglobin is reassuring. The other blood laboratory study that should be ordered in patients suspected of musculoskeletal sepsis is a blood culture. Patients do not have to be febrile at the time the blood culture is drawn, and in up to 50% of patients with SA or AHO, the only culture that returns positive is the blood culture.

Vignette 3 Question 2

Answer D: The definitive test for septic arthritis is aspiration of the affected joint. The aspirate is sent for gram stain and bacterial cultures as well as cell count analysis. Bacterial growth from cultures or a WBC count of greater than 25,000/mm^3 with negative cultures is considered diagnostic of septic arthritis. Aspiration of superficial joints can be accomplished without fluoroscopic/radiographic control, but for the hip joint the aspiration should be performed under fluoroscopic control with an arthogram (inject radio-opaque dye into the joint) to confirm that the hip joint has been entered/aspirated. The other tests are nonspecific.

Vignette 3 Question 3

Answer B: The most likely organism in septic arthritis of the hip in a 3-year-old healthy child is *Staphylococcus aureus*. The other likely organism is *Streptococcus*, with other organisms less likely. Before widespread HiB immunizations were instituted, *Haemophilus influenza* type B was commonly seen in this age group. It is now rare and has been replaced by *Kingella kingae* as another common organism causing musculoskeletal sepsis in children. All of these organisms are typically susceptible to first generation cephalosporins, which are usually administered at much higher doses for serious musculoskeletal infections. The controversy over the initial choice of antibiotics now involves coverage for community acquired methicillin-resistant *S. aureus* (MRSA). The best plan for empirical coverage likely involves discussion with local pediatric infectious disease experts and assessment of the bacteriological sensitivities of MRSA infections. In many communities, MRSA infections are commonly susceptible to clindamycin and trimethoprim-sulfa combinations, and many experts recommend adding one of these to the initial antibiotic treatment with a first-generation cephalosporin until culture results return. In this case the child is ill but not toxic or septic; use of vancomycin in these settings may contribute to the development of vancomycin resistance. In the setting of systemic sepsis vancomycin is preferred to make sure that MRSA is covered.

Vignette 3 Question 4

Answer B: Failure to diagnose and treat SA of the hip can result in complete destruction of the hip, as bacterial enzymes may cause lysis of the articular cartilage cells, and pressure from pus in the hip joint can limit blood flow to the proximal femur and cause osteonecrosis/avascular necrosis. *S. aureus* infections are known to occasionally be very aggressive and to cause permanent damage to the hip joint. The major issues with destruction of the hip in a young child are development of substantial limb-length difference over time as the proximal femoral growth plate is lost and with it 30% of the growth potential of the femur. With loss of the femoral head, the hip will lose significant biomechanical function, resulting in a permanent limp and abnormal gait. While the other options mentioned are possible, they are not likely.

Vignette 4 Question 1

Answer B: Skeletally immature patients who present with complaints of knee pain frequently have hip pathology. Hip pain is commonly referred to the knee in children and adolescents; this referral can result in no complaints of hip pain in patients with serious hip pathology where timely diagnosis is necessary to prevent significant complications. Thus, the examiner should carefully examine the hips in every skeletally immature patient who presents complaining of knee pain, especially when the knee examination is unremarkable. Patients with hip pathology will most frequently have pain with hip provocation by internal rotation, and will have increased hip/groin pain or weakness with active straight leg raising. Radiographs of the hip are indicated if the physical examination is abnormal.

Vignette 4 Question 2

Answer D: The presentation of an obese adolescent with knee pain, limp, and painful, limited internal rotation of the ipsilateral hip strongly suggests the diagnosis of slipped capital femoral epiphysis (SCFE). This is supported by the finding of obligatory external rotation of the hip with thigh flexion (Drennan sign), which usually signifies impingement of the femoral neck on the anterior acetabulum. The diagnosis of SCFE is radiographic and can be made at times on an anteroposterior view alone, but the frog lateral radiograph of the hip is the most sensitive test. Thus, if SCFE is suspected, a both lateral and frog-leg views should be ordered. As up to one third of patients with SCFE have a silent slip on the contralateral hip, it is recommended that both hips be imaged.

Vignette 4 Question 3

Answer D: Patients with SCFE who are able to weight bear are described as having stable slips. The standard treatment for stable SCFE is surgical stabilization of the slip with a single screw. The patient should be referred to an orthopedic surgeon on the day of diagnosis for evaluation and scheduling of surgery. There are many documented cases of stable SCFE patients progressing to unstable SCFE (inability to bear weight, increase in deformity of the proximal femur) while awaiting referral or surgery. Progression from stable to unstable SCFE carries a substantial risk of complication, primarily osteonecrosis of the femoral epiphysis/head. The risk of osteonecrosis for stable SCFE treated with screw stabilization is essentially zero, and increases to 20% to 50% if the SCFE progresses to unstable. Osteonecrosis can result in complete destruction of the proximal femur and hip, causing a permanent limp and early painful arthritis. Thus, patients diagnosed with SCFE should be referred for orthopedic evaluation when the diagnosis is made.

Chapter 17

Nephrology and Urology

René VanDeVoorde • Shumyle Alam • Katie S. Fine

The kidneys are the primary regulator of fluid and electrolyte status in the body. They preserve equilibrium by conserving or excreting electrolytes and water. They also excrete waste products of metabolism, such as urea, creatinine, and organic acids. These dual functions are the primary means of maintaining the ionic, osmolar, and pH status of the body. In addition, the kidneys contribute to other bodily functions through the synthesis of erythropoietin, the production of vitamin D, and the regulation of blood pressure. Thus, the kidneys play a central role in the growth and development of children, placing them at risk when faced with anatomic or physiologic stressors to their function. Infants are particularly susceptible as their kidneys are less effective in filtering plasma, regulating electrolytes, and concentrating urine.

Although the kidneys and urinary tract are separate systems, they are interrelated; irregularities in one system may affect the other. These abnormalities may be congenital (anatomic, cellular, or genetic) or acquired (infectious, inflammatory, or traumatic).

RENAL DYSPLASTIC AND CYSTIC DISEASES

Renal dysplasia is a condition in which the renal parenchymal tissue does not form correctly throughout. Typically, both kidneys are affected. There may be areas of normal parenchyma interspersed with areas of fibrosis, immature development, or even other tissue (such as cartilage). Severity ranges from minimal to severe renal impairment, sometimes with the development of isolated cysts or hypoplasia of the kidney. The presence of renal dysplasia is associated with an increased risk of abnormal development elsewhere, particularly in the urinary collecting system, but also in conjunction with other syndromes.

DIFFERENTIAL DIAGNOSIS

In **renal agenesis**, one or both kidneys fail to form. Bilateral renal agenesis is typically noted prenatally with marked oligohydramnios on ultrasound. This results in **Potter sequence** (clubbed feet, cranial anomalies); affected infants are stillborn or die shortly after birth due to associated pulmonary hypoplasia. Unilateral agenesis is usually an isolated defect but may be associated with other abnormalities.

In **multicystic dysplastic kidney (MDK)**, the most common renal cystic disease of childhood, the kidney consists of numerous noncommunicating, fluid-filled cysts. Affected organs are nonfunctional, but the condition is virtually always unilateral. MDK is a common cause of abdominal mass in the newborn (exceeded only by hydronephrosis from ureteropelvic junction obstruction). Diagnosis is confirmed by postnatal ultrasound (noncommunicating cysts) and renogram (demonstrates lack of function). Most cases undergo spontaneous involution. Follow-up imaging with renal ultrasound is necessary until involution or surgical removal. Nephrectomy is only recommended when the kidney changes in size or appearance (increased risk of Wilms tumor), when the patient is persistently hypertensive, experiences pain, or has recurrent infections of the involved side.

Polycystic kidney disease is an inherited disorder that occurs in two forms: the autosomal recessive (ARPKD) and the autosomal dominant types (ADPKD). In the former, both kidneys appear enlarged but maintain their symmetric, reniform shape. The renal collecting tubules are dilated, producing small cysts which are visible only as increased echogenicity on ultrasound. The condition is usually discovered prenatally (with the advances in obstetric ultrasound) or during evaluation of a palpable renal mass in an infant. Similar dilation is found in the hepatic bile ducts, with varying degrees of periportal fibrosis. In general, the kidneys function poorly, and life expectancy is appreciably shortened. Severely affected infants may die within weeks without dialysis; less affected infants suffer from hypertension and an eventual decline in renal function during childhood. The autosomal dominant form of polycystic kidney disease is usually not detected until adulthood, but may be diagnosed earlier on ultrasound for a positive family history, hypertension, or hematuria. The cysts can be quite large and distort the normal shape of the kidney. Hypertension and renal insufficiency develop over time, but do not always follow typical courses even within family cohorts. Early intervention to treat hypertension or proteinuria is currently indicated, with transplant as a viable option when renal function diminishes.

CLINICAL MANIFESTATIONS

The most prominent defect with renal dysplasia is inability to concentrate the urine. Dysplasia of the renal tubules affects their ability to reabsorb fluids; affected patients have an obligate amount of urine output which is unable to change based on fluid status. They may have frequent urination, difficulty in attaining urinary continence, and be particularly susceptible to dehydration if they are unable to maintain volume status through impaired intake (vomiting) or increased losses (diarrhea) of fluid. Additionally, these children are at risk for poor growth if they have increased losses of electrolytes, especially sodium, in their urine.

DIAGNOSTIC EVALUATION

The diagnosis is typically made by renal ultrasound, with the kidneys appearing more hyperechoic than normal. These patients often do not present with hypertension, but the diagnosis is sometimes stumbled upon during an evaluation for elevated blood pressure if the serum creatinine is elevated. Urine specific gravity is often low, but the urine sodium may be elevated in some patients.

TREATMENT

Treatment for the specific disorders is discussed under "Differential Diagnosis" above.

URETEROPELVIC JUNCTION OBSTRUCTION

Ureteropelvic junction obstruction (UPJO) is the most common cause of **hydronephrosis** in childhood. Etiologies of *primary* UPJO include intrinsic narrowing at the junction of the renal pelvis and ureter or angulation of the ureter from a crossing renal vessel. *Secondary* UPJO can result from scarring at the ureteropelvic junction, angulation secondary to massive ureteral dilation (as seen with high-grade vesicoureteral reflux [VUR]), or stones. The obstruction leads to elevated intrapelvic pressure, dilation of the renal pelvis and calyces, urinary stasis, and possible loss of the renal parenchyma. Between 10% and 40% of UPJO cases are bilateral.

CLINICAL MANIFESTATIONS

Hydronephrosis due to UPJO is often detected on prenatal ultrasound, but a palpable abdominal mass is the most common presentation in newborns. Older children may present with abdominal or flank pain, cyclic vomiting, and hematuria in addition to a mass.

DIAGNOSIS

Renal ultrasound confirms the presence of a hydronephrotic kidney. A subsequent diuretic nuclear renogram can further characterize the severity of the obstruction and the relative function of the kidneys.

TREATMENT

Surgical correction is indicated when a proven obstruction progresses, results in deterioration of function, or causes symptoms. The most common approach to correction of UPJO in children is minimally invasive surgery or open pyeloplasty to correct the narrowing between the renal pelvis and the ureter.

VESICOURETERAL REFLUX

VUR results when the length of the tunel of the ureter through the bladder submucosa is insufficient to prevent retrograde flow of urine. The condition may be bilateral or unilateral.

CLINICAL MANIFESTATIONS

The most frequent presentation is recurrent urinary tract infections (UTIs), though it is important to realize the VUR in itself does not cause infection. Retrograde flow of infected urine can result in pyelonephritis. Like UPJO, VUR can cause fetal hydronephrosis, but it is a much less frequent etiology.

DIAGNOSIS

A radiographic voiding cystourethrogram (VCUG) detects abnormalities at ureteral insertion sites and permits classification of the grade of reflux based on the extent of retrograde flow and associated dilation of the ureter and pelvis (Fig. 17-1). It is the initial study of choice when VUR is suspected due to the ability to obtain superior anatomic detail. Higher grades are associated with large, tortuous ureters and marked distortion of the renal pelvis and calyces. Radionuclide cystography exposes patients to a lower radiation dose and is useful for following reflux.

TREATMENT

Antibiotic prophylaxis is the first-line treatment for VUR, as the associated recurrent UTIs and pyelonephritis can lead to progressive renal injury and scarring. Amoxicillin is preferred in infants ≤3 months of age; older patients can be treated with trimethoprim-sulfamethoxazole or nitrofurantoin. There is current controversy in the literature regarding the need for antibiotic prophylaxis in patients with low-grade VUR; however, antibiotic prophylaxis is still recommended for all children with Grade 2 or greater VUR, especially infants and small children.

Low grades of reflux may resolve spontaneously and preclude the need for further antibiotics. However, surgical correction is indicated when the grade of reflux worsens, multiple antibiotic sensitivities or allergies develop, there is evidence of diminishment of renal function, the patient has recurrent UTIs or pyelonephritis, or noncompliance is an issue. Surgery involves lengthening the intravesicular segment of the tunnel through which the ureter enters the bladder (ureteral reimplantation). An alternative to surgery is injection with bulking agents such as Deflux to recreate the tunnel mechanism.

POSTERIOR URETHRAL VALVES

Occurring only in males, posterior urethral valves (PUV) consist of obstructing leaflets within the posterior urethra which result in partial-to-complete bladder outlet obstruction. The increased pressure causes urethral dilation, bladder neck hypertrophy, and bladder trabeculation. VUR occurs with increased frequency and may lead to renal dysplasia. Posterior urethral valves is one of the most common causes of **end-stage renal disease** in the male child.

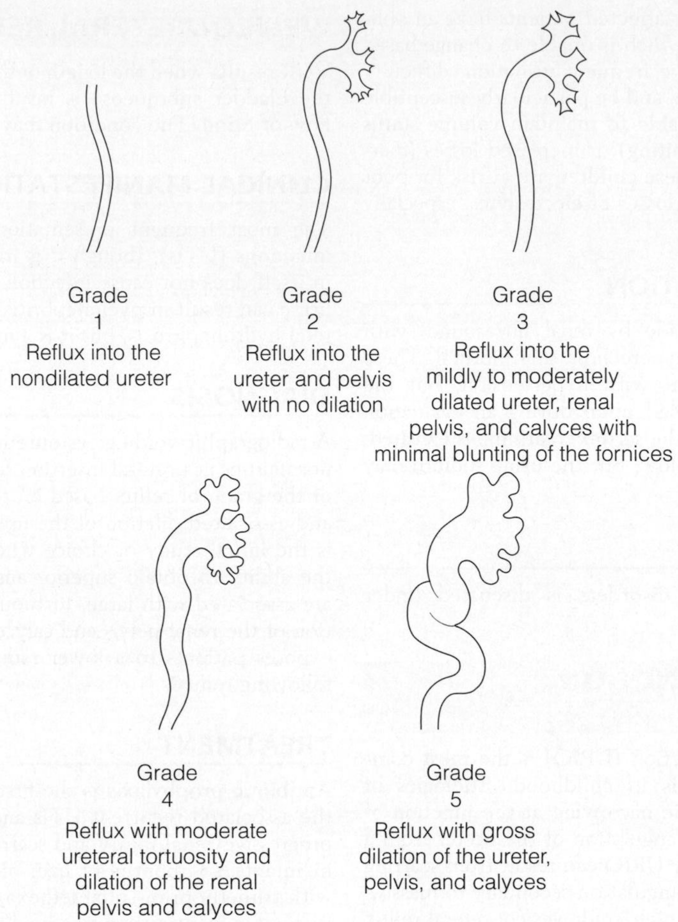
Grade
1
Reflux into the nondilated ureter
Grade
2
Reflux into the ureter and pelvis with no dilation
Grade
3
Reflux into the mildly to moderately dilated ureter, renal pelvis, and calyces with minimal blunting of the fornices
Grade
4
Reflux with moderate ureteral tortuosity and dilation of the renal pelvis and calyces
Grade
5
Reflux with gross dilation of the ureter, pelvis, and calyces

Figure 17-1 • International classification of vesicoureteral reflux.

CLINICAL MANIFESTATIONS

This disorder may be suspected by detecting hydronephrosis and bladder distention on prenatal ultrasound or by palpating a distended bladder or renal mass during the newborn examination. In older infants, parents may note a weak or dribbling urinary stream or unexplained daytime wetting. Occasionally, the condition is diagnosed in boys during radiologic evaluation following a UTI.

DIAGNOSTIC EVALUATION

Renal ultrasound demonstrates evidence of chronic obstruction of the bladder neck. The bladder will be distended, with thickened walls and possible trabeculation. Bilateral hydronephrosis may be present. Posterior urethral valves are clearly visualized on a radiographic VCUG. Reflux is often present and high grade. The bladder is dilated with possible trabeculations or diverticulae. The bladder neck is hypertrophied and may be visualized separate from the body of the bladder. The posterior urethra is also very dilated and may be described as shield-shaped or having a **spinnaker-sail appearance**.

TREATMENT

First-line treatment involves ablation of the obstructing valve leaflets and, if VUR is present, antibiotic prophylaxis. Sometimes intermittent catheterization or temporary diversion of urine with a vesicostomy is necessary. When VUR is secondary to PUV, resolution of reflux is roughly equal for all grades with adequate bladder management. Early surgical correction of the reflux is discouraged, as the bladder pathophysiology can change over time and early surgery has a high failure rate. Prognosis is related to the degree of renal and bladder impairment at the time of PUV ablation; however, nearly all males will need to be followed long-term due to increased risk of development of chronic kidney disease.

HYPOSPADIAS

Hypospadias is the most common congenital anomaly of the penis, occurring in 1 in 250 male newborns. Incomplete development of the distal urethra leads to malposition of the urethral meatus along the ventral side of the penis toward the perineum. The ventral foreskin is usually deficient, and there may be an associated curvature of the penis known as chordee.

Circumcision is contraindicated because surgical repair may require the preputial tissue. The aims of therapy are to extend the urethral meatus to the tip of the glans penis, create a straight erection, and produce the appearance of a normal circumcised phallus. Prognosis is excellent for distal hypospadias; proximal hypospadias may require a staged surgical approach in order to achieve an acceptable cosmetic and functional result. The association of hypospadias with any degree of testicular cryptorchidism should prompt an ambiguous genitalia workup, including genetic karyotyping.

CRYPTORCHIDISM

Cryptorchidism is defined as testes that have not fully descended into the scrotum and, unlike retractile testes, cannot be manipulated into the scrotum with gentle pressure. Isolated cryptorchidism is common at birth, occurring in roughly 3% of term male newborns. Preterm infants have a higher incidence of undescended testes, although this may be related more to low birth weight than gestational age. Testes that remain outside the scrotum may develop impaired sperm and hormone production, with both the undescended and the contralateral descended testes at increased risk for malignancy. Bilateral cryptorchidism can result in oligospermia and infertility.

CLINICAL MANIFESTATIONS

One or both testes may be positioned in the abdomen or anywhere along the inguinal canal. Most are palpable on examination. Ninety percent of patients also have inguinal hernias.

TREATMENT

By 12 months of age, 99% of males have bilateral descended testicles, but spontaneous descent after age 3 months is unlikely. Surgical repair (orchiopexy) takes place at 6 to 12 months of age and has a high success rate (99%). Orchiopexy does not appear to alter the incidence of malignant degeneration (2% to 3%), but it does render the testis accessible for regular self-examination.

TESTICULAR TORSION

Testicular torsion is a **surgical emergency**, requiring prompt recognition and correction to prevent loss of the testicle. Most patients with testicular torsion lack the posterior attachment to the tunica vaginalis that keeps the testis from rotating around the spermatic cord. This creates a mobile testis and results in a **bell-clapper deformity** (the ability of the untethered testis to twist on its stalk).

CLINICAL MANIFESTATIONS

Testicular torsion is a clinical diagnosis with a hallmark presentation of acute onset of unilateral scrotal pain typically sufficient to wake the child from sleep. Nausea and vomiting are common. Right-sided torsion sometimes is confused with appendicitis, necessitating examination of the external genitalia in males with abdominal pain. In torsion, the scrotum often appears swollen and erythematous, while the testis is exquisitely tender. **Epididymitis**, which is more common during adolescence, presents with a similar clinical picture. Epididymitis may be infectious or secondary to torsion of a testicular or epididymal **appendix**.

DIAGNOSIS

The cremasteric reflex is typically absent in testicular torsion. The presence of the "blue dot" sign (on the upper aspect of the scrotum) and a normal cremasteric reflex suggest torsion of the appendix testes rather than the entire testicle. Doppler ultrasound of the scrotum is helpful in differentiating between epididymitis and testicular torsion but may delay appropriate treatment. The diagnosis of torsion is a clinical diagnosis; ultrasound is a helpful tool but should not delay prompt surgical exploration and correction if the index of suspicion for torsion is high.

TREATMENT

Early surgical detorsion is critical and should ideally take place within 6 hours of the onset of pain. If the testis is manually detorsed in the emergency room, ultrasound confirmation of detorsion and surgical exploration should be performed during the admission. Necrotic testes must be removed, and the contralateral testis is fixed to the fibrous layer of the posterior scrotal envelope during surgery to prevent asynchronous torsion. Torsion of a testicular or epididymal appendix resolves spontaneously; epididymitis is often treated with antibiotics.

HYDROCELES AND VARICOCELES

Hydroceles are fluid-filled sacs in the scrotal cavity consisting of remnants of the processus vaginalis. They are often diagnosed in the newborn period or early childhood. Hydroceles communicate with the peritoneal cavity through a patent processus and are at risk for incarceration. These **communicating** hydroceles and hernias should be repaired as soon as possible to prevent the development of an incarcerated hernia. Most noncommunicating or simple hydroceles involute by 12 months of age.

A **varicocele** is defined as dilation of the testicular veins and enlargement of the pampiniform plexus. Varicoceles become detectable in boys during adolescence, occur more commonly on the left, and are usually nontender. They are generally not visible when the patient is supine, but become evident upon standing when the veins distend and produce the characteristic "bag of worms" within the scrotum. Indications for surgical repair include pain, progressive enlargement, and discordant testicular growth. Unrepaired varicoceles may place the patient at an increased risk for infertility.

URINARY TRACT INFECTION (UTI)

Bacterial UTIs may be limited to the bladder (**cystitis**) or may also involve the kidney (**pyelonephritis**). Children with pyelonephritis can sustain damage to the infected area of the renal parenchyma, resulting in localized scarring, decreased function, and hypertension. Common pathogens include *Escherichia coli* (80%), *Proteus*, and *Klebsiella* species.

RISK FACTORS

The most significant risk factor is the presence of an anatomic or physiologic urinary tract abnormality that predisposes to stasis of urine, such as bladder outlet obstruction, vesicoureteral reflux, and dysfunctional voiding. These risk factors may be known from prenatal evaluations or may first become evident with a UTI. Thus, a history of previous UTI is also a significant risk factor.

After the first year of life (equal incidence), girls have almost a 10-fold increased incidence over boys. Although uncircumcised male infants are more prone to UTIs, this risk diminishes after the first year of life and is not a sufficient indication for universal routine circumcision.

DIFFERENTIAL DIAGNOSIS

The differential diagnosis for cystitis includes external genital irritation, meatal stenosis in the circumcised male, vulvovaginitis, vaginal foreign body, sexual abuse, and pinworm infestation. Adenovirus can cause a self-limited hemorrhagic cystitis that does not respond to antibiotics but may be mistaken for a UTI. In the adolescent, the possibility of a sexually transmitted disease must be entertained. Posterior urethralgia is a benign, self-limiting inflammation of the posterior urethra in boys which may mimic a UTI. For the febrile child, lower lobe pneumonia often presents with fever, chills, and flank pain, a reminder that other sources of infection must also be contemplated. Urolithiasis should be considered in the patient presenting with dysuria, hematuria, and flank pain.

CLINICAL MANIFESTATIONS

In febrile infants, the urinary tract is the most common site of bacterial infection. Fever may be the only manifestation of illness. However, infants may also present with other signs of systemic illness, such as lethargy, vital sign instability, poor oral intake, mottled appearance, and even jaundice. The source of infection is almost always hematogenous seeding of the kidneys, which explains the high rate of renal scarring observed in this group of patients. Also, a UTI can be the first clinical suggestion of an obstructive anomaly or vesicoureteral reflux in this age group. Ideally, the urine should be examined in all febrile patients younger than 1 to 2 years.

In older children, UTIs more often result from ascent of exterior fecal flora into the urinary tract. The signs and symptoms of cystitis are similar to those in adults and include low-grade fever, frequency, urgency, dysuria, incontinence, abdominal pain, and hematuria. In contrast, pyelonephritis presents with high fever, chills, nausea, vomiting, and flank pain. Older children are more likely to have an isolated infection of the bladder; upper tract involvement is suggested by elevation of the peripheral white blood count, erythrocyte sedimentation rate, and C-reactive protein.

DIAGNOSTIC EVALUATION

A positive urine culture is the gold standard for diagnosis, although urine microscopy or dipstick findings may suggest a UTI. The presence of nitrites on urine dipstick findings has a high specificity but a relatively low sensitivity for bacterial infection, as not all bacteria produce nitrites. The absence of leukocyte esterase has a fairly high sensitivity. Additionally, urine microscopy findings of both pyuria and bacteriuria are fairly specific for infection. However, the absence of these findings in the urine of a high-risk patient, such as a febrile or ill-appearing infant, does not rule out UTI; for instance, pyuria is often absent in infants with pyelonephritis. Urine may be obtained by suprapubic tap (in neonates), sterile catheterization of the bladder, or clean catch in continent children; these are listed in their order of increasing likelihood of contamination. Bagged specimens are inadequate for evaluation of UTIs.

A urine culture (results in 24 to 48 hours) and dipstick urinalysis should be obtained in all febrile infants without a definitive source of infection (and older patients with suspected UTIs). Patients with positive dipstick results for leukocyte esterase (with or without positive nitrites) should be treated for a presumed UTI until culture results are available. Susceptibility testing is performed on any singular bacteria isolated to ensure appropriate antibiotic treatment.

The workup of initial confirmed UTIs in children is controversial and depends on the patient's age, severity of infection, and response to treatment. Figure 17-2 provides a suggested diagnostic algorithm for children with UTIs. Current American Academy of Pediatrics guidelines recommend that all children younger than 24 months undergo renal ultrasound to rule out hydronephrosis or structural lesions that predispose to infection. Those with hydronephrosis and those with normal ultrasound who do not respond to appropriate antibiotic therapy within 48 hours should also receive a VCUG. In prompt responders with normal ultrasounds, the VCUG is not mandaton. Other experts argue that all infected children younger than a certain age (6 to 12 months) receive a VCUG regardless of response to treatment. It is likely that further studies will result in more evidence-based recommendations. In cases of suspected pyelonephritis, a nuclear imaging study such as a DMSA is helpful to document areas of injury and possible scar formation.

TREATMENT

Children with suspected cystitis should be treated with an appropriate oral antibiotic such as amoxicillin, ampicillin, nitrofurantoin, or trimethoprim-sulfamethoxazole. If the culture is negative, antibiotics may be discontinued. A positive urine culture should prompt a 5- to 7-day course with an appropriate oral antibiotic (based on sensitivity results).

Nontoxic-appearing children with suspected pyelonephritis should be treated with an oral cephalosporin or intravenous ampicillin plus gentamicin or a cephalosporin until culture results are available. Patients who are toxic-appearing, unable to tolerate oral medications, or younger than 6 months must be admitted to the hospital for intravenous antibiotics and observation. Patients older than 6 months may be discharged on a culture-specific oral antibiotic to finish the course of therapy provided their clinical picture improves. Large defects on DMSA scan suggestive of severe pyelonephritis may benefit from a full course of intravenous antibiotics.

The prognosis for patients with isolated cystitis is excellent; morbidity increases with recurrent infection. Most UTI-related complications are the result of pyelonephritis, including perinephric abscesses, renal scarring, and renal failure.

NEPHROTIC SYNDROME

Nephrotic syndrome is a glomerular disorder characterized by marked proteinuria, hypoalbuminemia, hyperlipidemia, and edema. Its etiology may be idiopathic (primary) or secondary (Table 17-1), with most cases (>90%) in children from industrialized nations being idiopathic. **Minimal change disease** (MCD) is by far the most common cause of primary nephrotic

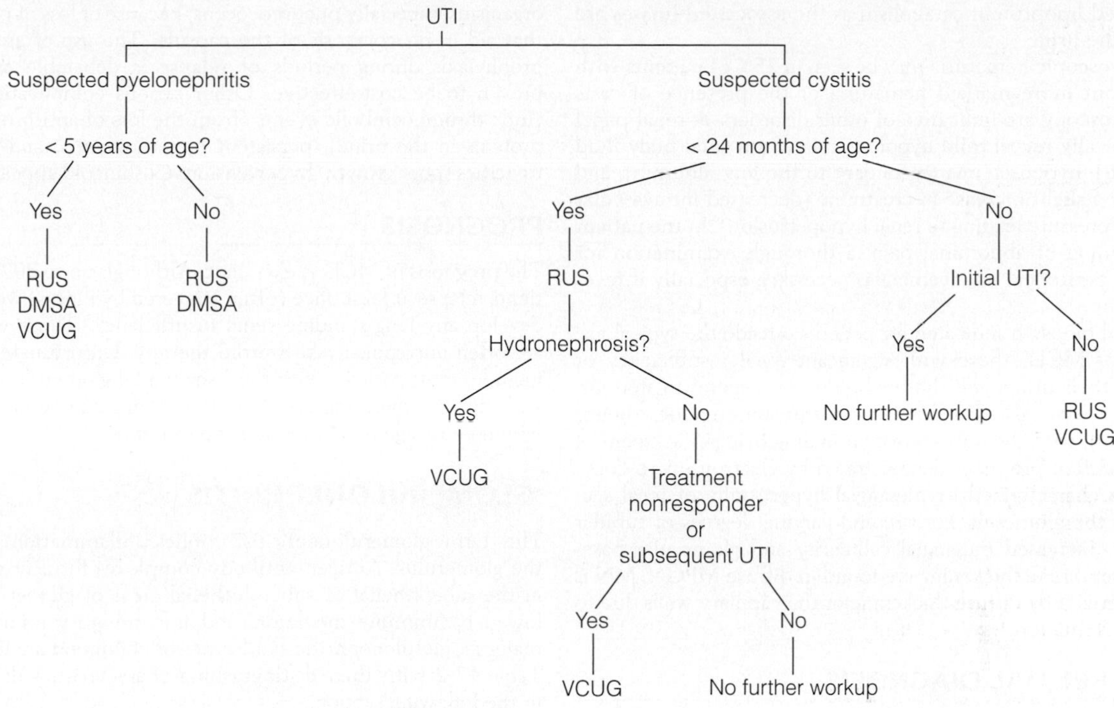

RUS, renal ultrasound; DMSA, technetium-99 dimercaptosuccinic acid renal scan; VCUG, voiding cystourethrogram

Figure 17-2 • Suggested diagnostic algorithm for pediatric urinary tract infection.

TABLE 17-1 Causes of Childhood Nephrotic Syndrome

Primary
• Minimal change disease (MCD)
• Focal segmental glomerulosclerosis (FSGS)
• Membranoproliferative glomerulonephritis(MPGN)
• Membranous nephropathy (MN)
Secondary
• Infections (hepatitis B, hepatitis C, HIV, malaria, syphilis)
• Systemic diseases (SLE, Henoch-Schönlein purpura, IgA nephropathy)
• Drugs (nonsteroidal anti-inflammatory drugs, heroin)
• Malignancies (lymphoma, leukemia)
• Genetic (Finnish-type congenital nephrotic syndrome, Denys-Drash syndrome)

syndrome in children, accounting for more than 80% of all cases. Typical patients present between 2 and 6 years of age, with boys outnumbering girls 2:1. **Focal segmental glomerulosclerosis** (FSGS), **membranoproliferative glomerulonephritis** (MPGN), and **membranous nephropathy** (MN) account for the remainder of idiopathic cases of pediatric nephrotic syndrome; these are typically encountered in older age groups.

CLINICAL MANIFESTATIONS

Patients with early nephrotic syndrome appear quite well, with a fairly insidious onset of symptoms. There may be a history of nonspecific illness a few weeks prior to the associated findings. Periorbital edema is commonly the first abnormality noted; occasionally patients are treated for allergies because of their mild initial presentations. This is followed by dependent (lower-extremity) edema, weight gain, and generalized edema (ascites, perinealedema). Anorexia and diarrhea are variably present, often from intestinal edema. Gross hematuria and hypertension are typically absent; these should raise suspicion of FSGS, secondary etiologies, or glomerulonephritis.

DIAGNOSTIC EVALUATION

The hallmark of nephrotic syndrome is **marked proteinuria**. Nephrotic-range proteinuria is usually defined as proteinuria exceeding 1,000 mg/m^2/day or a spot (random) urinary protein-creatinine ratio exceeding 2.0 (mg/mg). The proteinuria in childhood nephrotic syndrome is relatively selective, consisting primarily of albumin, with resultant hypoalbuminemia (<2.5 g/dL). Hyperlipidemia, with elevated serum cholesterol and triglyceride concentrations, is a consistent feature of nephrotic syndrome but does not always need to be confirmed. Hyperlipidemia is usually transient, resulting from decreased lipoprotein catabolism as the associated lipases are lost in the urine.

Microscopic hematuria may be seen in 25% of patients with MCD, but more marked hematuria or the presence of casts on microscopy are indicative of other disorders. A renal panel will typically reveal mild hyponatremia (from total body fluid overload), hypocalcemia (secondary to the low albumin), and possibly a slight increase in creatinine (decreased intravascular oncotic pressure leading to renal hypoperfusion). In the patient complaining of abdominal pain, a thorough examination for signs of peritoneal involvement is necessary, especially if fever is present.

Renal biopsy is indicated for patients outside the typical age range for MCD, those with significant renal insufficiency or casts in their urine, and those who do not respond to steroids. Gross sections in MCD show few if any abnormalities (hence the name), with the only consistent finding being effacement of epithelial foot processes demonstrated by electron microscopy. **FSGS** is characterized by mesangial hypertrophy of focal sections of the glomeruli, fibrosis, and varying degrees of tubular atrophy. Increased mesangial cellularity and glomerular basement membrane thickening are found in **diffuse MPGN. MN** is characterized by diffuse thickening of the capillary walls due to deposit formation.

DIFFERENTIAL DIAGNOSIS

Generalized edema may be present in hepatic, nutritional, cardiac, and other renal disorders. If the patient is edematous without low serum albumin, then conditions with fluid and salt overload (heart failure, renal failure, cirrhosis) should be considered. If hypoalbuminemia is present without proteinuria, then intestinal losses of protein or hepatic failure may be more likely. Other conditions associated with proteinuria include exercise, trauma, UTI, dehydration, and acute tubular necrosis; however, none of these causes the degree of protein loss seen in nephrotic syndrome.

TREATMENT

If the clinical presentation is consistent with uncomplicated primary nephrotic syndrome, strict dietary salt restriction and oral steroid therapy are appropriate. Steroids result in prompt remission in most cases of MCD, often within 4 weeks. Nephrotic syndrome that does not respond to oral steroids may require treatment with stronger immunosuppressants, such as cyclophosphamide or calcineurin inhibitors. If symptoms do not resolve within 8 to 12 weeks, or if the patient experiences frequent or severe relapses while on steroids, renal biopsy is indicated to confirm the diagnosis and identify the histologic subtype.

Intravenous albumin (followed by a diuretic) assists in inducing temporary diuresis in the presence of incapacitating anasarca or edema-related respiratory compromise. Albumin without diuretics would be indicated in patients presenting with hypotensive shock; rapid expansion with colloid is needed in these patients because of their low intravascular oncotic pressures.

COMPLICATIONS

Bacterial infections, particularly **spontaneous bacterial peritonitis**, are frequent complications of nephrotic syndrome. Patients in relapse are at particular risk of infection from encapsulated organisms, especially pneumococcus, because of loss of proteins that aid in phagocytosis of the capsule. The use of antibiotic prophylaxis during periods of relapse is debatable and not proven to be cost-effective. Other serious complications include thromboembolic events (from the loss of antithrombotic proteins in the urine), persistent hyperlipidemia, and steroid toxicities (poor growth, hypertension, Cushingoid appearance).

PROGNOSIS

The prognosis of MCD is excellent. Although up to 80% of patients relapse at least once (often triggered by illness), very few develop any long-standing renal insufficiency. Those who do are often unresponsive to steroid therapy. Unfortunately, this includes most patients with focal segmental glomerulosclerosis and diffuse membranoproliferative glomerulonephritis, in whom end-stage renal disease is common.

GLOMERULONEPHRITIS

The term **glomerulonephritis** implies inflammation within the glomerulus. Antigen-antibody complexes form or deposit in the subepithelial or subendothelial areas of glomeruli, followed by immune mediators and inflammatory injury. The major glomerulonephritic syndromes of childhood are listed in Table 17-2 with their distinguishing characteristics discussed in the following section.

CLINICAL MANIFESTATIONS

The initial presentation of glomerulonephritis typically includes hematuria (overt or microscopic), proteinuria, azotemia, oliguria, edema, and **hypertension,** findings also referred to as **nephritic syndrome**. Red cell casts are invariably present; in fact, the urine is often described as "tea-colored" by parents. Proteinuria is present, but is usually much less prominent than in nephrotic syndrome. Glomerular filtration is compromised by the inflammation, leading to salt and water retention and circulatory overload, manifested by edema and hypertension. Decreased filtration leads to increasing serum BUN and creatinine levels along with temporary sodium and potassium

TABLE 17-2 Diseases that Present with Nephritic Syndrome
Acute poststreptococcal glomerulonephritis (AGN or PSGN)
Henoch-Schönlein purpura (HSP)
IgA nephropathy
Hemolytic-uremic syndrome (HUS)
Systemic lupus erythematosus (SLE)
Alport syndrome
Membranoproliferative glomerulonephritis (MPGN)
Pauci-immune glomerulonephritides (Wegener's granulomatosis, microscopic polyangiitis, Goodpasture disease)
Shunt nephritis

dysregulation. Patients may complain of malaise (likely from decreased clearance of acid and uremic waste products) and fatigue (from fluid retention). Also, acute inflammation of the kidneys may cause them to swell, resulting in flank pain from the stretching of the renal capsule in some patients.

DIAGNOSTIC EVALUATION

As there are several different glomerulonephritides, each with its own distinctive features, the initial evaluation should first focus on determining whether nephritis is present or not. The differential diagnosis of hematuria, the most prominent manifestation of glomerulonephritis, includes other conditions (infection, trauma, stones, cystic disease) and hematologic disorders. Important laboratory studies include urinalysis (possibly with urine culture), urine microscopy, serum electrolytes with BUN and creatinine, complete blood count (CBC), and coagulation studies.

The first step of the evaluation is confirmation of blood in the urine by microscopy. Both hemoglobin and myoglobin test positive for blood on urine dipstick; however, there are no red blood cells on microscopic urine examination in the presence of myoglobinuria. The presence of red blood cell casts on urine microscopy confirms the diagnosis of a glomerulonephritis.

If glomerulonephritis is confirmed, the first test should be evaluation of serum complement levels. A low level of complement C3 is typical of acute poststreptococcal glomerulonephritis, whereas a persistently decreased level of C3 (and possibly C4) is highly suggestive of lupus or MPGN. Other tests that may assist if the patient is hypocomplementemic include an anti-streptolysin O (ASO) titer, anti-DNAse B titer, antinuclear antibody (ANA), and anti–double stranded DNA antibody. If the patient is normocomplementemic, an antinuclear cytoplasmic antibody (ANCA) may assist in detecting certain pauci-immune glomerulonephritides. However, many of the nephritides are best diagnosed through a thorough history and physical examination along with a diagnostic renal biopsy. As each of these nephritides are diagnosed and treated differently, they are hereafter discussed separately.

Acute poststreptococcal glomerulonephritis (APGN), the most common glomerulonephritis in childhood, occurs sporadically in early school-age children and is twice as common in males. Streptococcal infections involving either the throat (pharyngitis) or skin (impetigo) precede the clinical syndrome by 1 to 4 weeks. Although treating the streptococcal illness does not prevent APGN, obtaining a recent history of infection is important. Elevated antistreptolysin-O or anti-DNAse B titers suggest recent infection. The C3 component of the complement pathway is low and typically recovers in 6 to 8 weeks following the onset of nephritis. Biopsies are not usually performed, as the renal involvement is typically transient, with complete recovery in a majority of patients. Hypertension and edema are often the most significant sequelae and may be controlled through salt and fluid restriction, diuretics, and vasodilators.

Membranoproliferative glomerulonephritis (MPGN) is an uncommon disorder that has no typical features outside of nephritis. It is diagnosed by renal biopsy and should be suspected in older patients with persistently low C3 levels after 6 to 8 weeks. It is treated by high-dose steroids or other immunosuppressants with variable success, often progressing to end stage renal disease. Glomerulonephritis associated with systemic lupus erythematosus is associated with decreased C3 and C4 levels; SLE is further discussed in Chapter 13.

Henoch-Schönlein purpura (HSP) can present acutely with glomerulonephritis, often following symptoms of infection which are thought to be a trigger of the disorder. It is a systemic vasculitis characterized by a purpuric rash often involving the lower extremities and buttocks, crampy abdominal pain, and arthritis. The C3 levels remain normal. About 50% of patients may have an elevated IgA level, though this is not diagnostic of the disorder. Patients may be treated with steroids for severe arthritic or abdominal pain, though this does not necessarily alter the course of the nephritis. Most children with HSP nephritis recover without intervention, but those with greater renal involvement (characterized by significant proteinuria, hypertension, or elevation of creatinine) may require prolonged courses of immunosuppressants such as steroids, calcineurin inhibitors, and antimetabolites. Two percent of children with HSP develop long-term renal impairment.

IgA nephropathy is the most common glomerulonephritis worldwide, with an increased prevalence in pan-Pacific Asian countries. Once thought to be a benign condition, it is now known to slowly progress to renal failure in 25% of cases. Most patients present with either asymptomatic gross hematuria occurring a few days after an upper respiratory or gastrointestinal infection or with persistent microscopic hematuria. However, some patients may present with fulminant nephritis. C3 levels are normal. The only method of confirmation is renal biopsy, which demonstrates mesangial deposits of IgA in the glomeruli. Treatment varies from potent immunosuppression (in those with rapid progression of disease or severe proteinuria), antiproteinuric agents and antioxidants (in moderate disease), to no therapy in the majority of mild cases.

Rapidly progressive glomerulonephritis is the description given to a number of acute glomerulopathies that, for unknown reasons, deteriorate over a few weeks or months to renal failure and even death. Many of these disorders are also systemic vasculitides and may have pulmonary involvement as well. Some of the pauci-immune glomerulonephritides have positive anti-nuclear cytoplasmic antibodies (ANCA) or antibodies against the glomerular basement membrane. All forms demonstrate generalized crescent formation in the glomeruli, thought to represent cellular destruction by macrophages with subsequent necrosis and fibrin deposition. Fortunately, rapidly progressive glomerulonephritis is rare in children. When present, it must be treated immediately with strong immunosuppressants or pheresis.

Alport syndrome, or hereditary nephritis, is caused by mutations in the gene encoding type IV collagen that result in an abnormal glomerular basement membrane. Inheritance is X-linked in the classic form of the disorder, although defective genes encoding other glomerular basement membrane components can cause similar disease. Because type IV collagen is an important component of the cochlea, Alport syndrome is associated with sensorineural hearing loss. A family history of renal failure or hearing loss, especially in males, should raise suspicion for the disease. The diagnosis is usually confirmed through renal biopsy, which reveals a characteristic splitting of the basement membranes, although early high-frequency hearing loss and ophthalmologic features of the disease can also assist in diagnosis. Patients inevitably progress to end-stage renal disease over time, as there is little to be done to prevent progression. Significant progression of renal disease typically occurs toward the end of the second decade in most men and is often mirrored by the degree of hearing loss.

Benign familial hematuria, or thin membrane disease, is a common cause of asymptomatic microscopic and occasionally gross hematuria. Renal function is normal, and biopsy, although unnecessary, reveals diffuse thinning of the glomerular basement membrane on electron microscopy. Because transmission is autosomal dominant, asymptomatic microscopic hematuria is usually found in other family members.

HEMOLYTIC UREMIC SYNDROME

Hemolytic uremic syndrome (HUS) is technically not a glomerulonephritis, but presents with a similar nephritic picture. It is caused by endothelial injury of the renal vasculature with subsequent cascade of microthrombi formation and shearing of erythrocytes passing over the thrombi. A majority of cases are caused by a Shiga-like toxin produced by an enterohemorrhagic strain of *E. coli* (O157:H7), though atypical cases not associated with diarrhea also occur.

CLINICAL MANIFESTATIONS

Children with diarrhea-associated HUS often have an exposure to *E. coli*, either through undercooked meat or an exposure to farm animal feces (via water runoff or foods exposed to manure). Patients present with a prodromal diarrheal illness for 4 to 7 days before the other manifestations of the disorder. Diarrhea is often bloody and associated with significant abdominal pain. This is followed by pallor, jaundice, petechiae, and/or oliguria. Some patients are noted to be edematous from continued fluid intake with declining urine output, such that they may be hypertensive as well.

DIAGNOSTIC EVALUATION

HUS is characterized by the classic trio of microangiopathic hemolytic anemia, thrombocytopenia, and azotemia. The anemia and thrombocytopenia of the disease can be significant, with hemoglobin levels dropping to <8 g/dL and platelet counts often <100,000/mcL. As red cells are hemolyzed, LDH levels are often very elevated. The blood smear demonstrates the hallmark schistocytes of microangiopathic hemolysis. Coagulation studies should be normal.

In patients with diarrhea, a stool culture for *E. coli* O157:H7 should be obtained to confirm typical HUS as well as for epidemiologic investigation, as this is a reportable disease to local and state health units. If the patient does not have associated diarrhea, an evaluation for atypical HUS should be carried out, as its treatment and prevention is altogether different.

TREATMENT

Most therapies for HUS are supportive, as there are no current treatments for the cascade of events following endothelial injury. Transfusion with packed red cells is needed in half of all patients, generally provided if the serum hemoglobin is <7 gm/dL or the patient is symptomatic. Platelet transfusions are usually unnecessary except in the face of active bleeding or for planned surgical intervention if the platelet count is <20,000/mcL. Fluid and electrolyte restriction is often required when oliguria is present. Dialysis (either peritoneal or hemodialysis) may be needed in up to 25% of all patients. A majority of patients recover after the acute period, but there can be long-term sequelae to the kidneys. However, a percentage of patients never recover function and progress to end-stage renal disease. Those with atypical presentations often have more significant disease sequelae which may recur, particularly if they have a genetic form of the disease.

RENAL TUBULAR ACIDOSIS

All forms of renal tubular acidosis (RTA) are characterized by normal anion gap **hyperchloremic metabolic acidosis**, resulting from insufficient renal transport of bicarbonate or acids. The tubules are the site of reabsorption and secretion. Most bicarbonate filtered from the plasma is reabsorbed in the proximal tubule, along with amino acids, glucose, sodium, potassium, calcium, phosphate, and water. In the distal tubule, the remainder of the bicarbonate is reabsorbed and hydrogen ions are secreted into the tubular lumen. Defects in either transport site compromise the kidney's ability to maintain pH homeostasis.

CLINICAL MANIFESTATIONS

Patients with RTA typically present with failure to thrive during their infant or toddler years, though they may be older if the disorder was acquired later in life. This stems from their chronic acidotic state, which may also be associated with vomiting and anorexia. Polydipsia and polyuria with volume contraction may also be seen, especially in proximal RTA. Other presenting signs and symptoms may include findings of rickets or kidney stones.

DIAGNOSTIC EVALUATION

Any patient with nongap metabolic acidosis of unclear etiology warrants further workup to rule out RTA (Fig. 17-3). Patients with bicarbonate losses in the stool, primarily from diarrhea but also with other fistula drainage, may also present with hyperchloremic acidosis. Hypokalemia is seen in both distal (type 1) and proximal (type 2) RTA, while the hyperkalemia of type 4 RTA is secondary to a lack of aldosterone responsiveness in the collecting tubule. Urine pH is typically elevated in distal and proximal RTA; however, it may drop below 6 with proximal RTA if the patient is acidotic enough. Another way to discern between these two is by calculating a urine anion gap (urine Na + K–Cl). If the urine anion gap is positive, then ammonia production is likely impaired (as seen with a distal RTA).

Renal ultrasound may reveal nephrocalcinosis with distal RTA. Most patients with proximal (type 2) RTA have it in conjunction with **Fanconi syndrome**, a generalized disorder of proximal tubule transport. Urinalysis may reveal mild glucosuria and proteinuria, while urine concentrations of potassium and phosphorus are elevated. Additionally, Fanconi syndrome has been associated with other disorders, including cystinosis, Wilson disease, and Lowe syndrome.

TREATMENT

Treatment consists of providing children with sufficient amounts of an **alkalinizing agent** (bicarbonate or citrate) to correct the acidosis completely and restore normal growth. Thiazide diuretics may be administered in proximal RTA to increase proximal tubular reabsorption of bicarbonate. Hypokalemia is treated concurrently when the alkali is coupled with

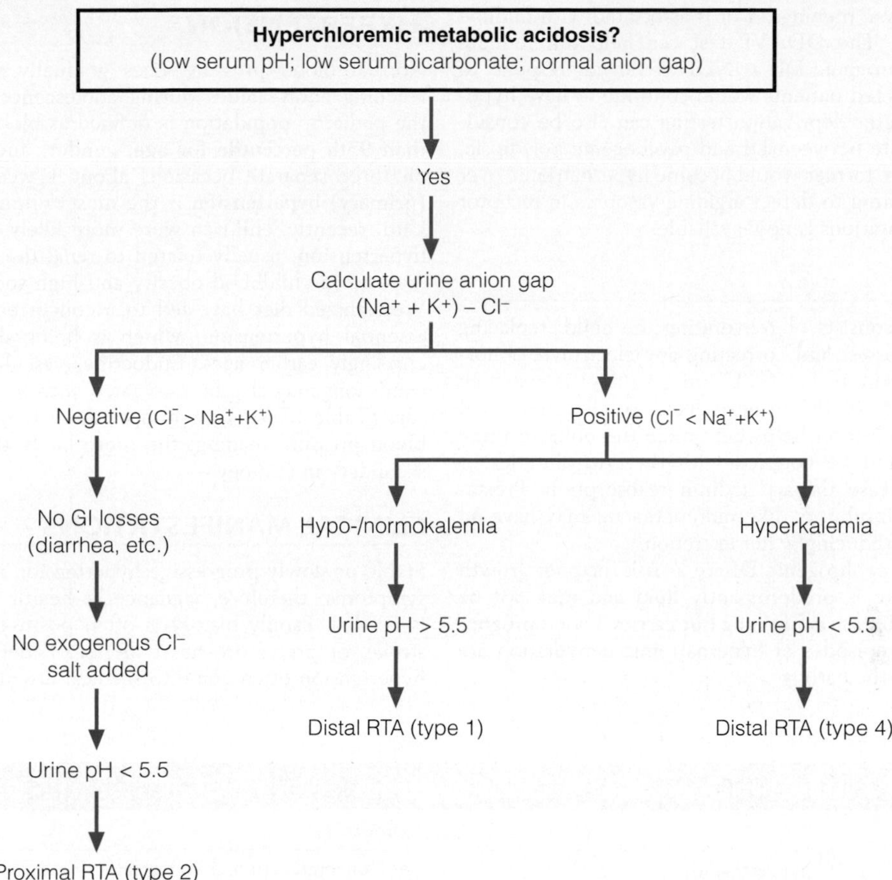

Figure 17-3 • Suggested diagnostic algorithm for hyperchloremic metabolic acidosis of unknown etiology.

potassium as a salt. If RTA is associated with an underlying condition, the primary disorder must be addressed.

NEPHROGENIC DIABETES INSIPIDUS

Diabetes insipidus (DI) is a disorder in renal concentrating ability, secondary to a lack of efficacy of arginine vasopressin (antidiuretic hormone) on aquaporin-mediated transport of water in the renal collecting duct. It may be central or nephrogenic in origin. In central DI, the production or release of hormone is insufficient (see Chapter 14). Nephrogenic DI (NDI) arises from end-organ resistance to the hormone, either from a receptor defect or from other processes that interfere with receptor action. Nephrogenic DI may be congenital, with 90% of cases being X-linked, or acquired. Acquired NDI has been associated with polycystic kidney disease, pyelonephritis, lithium toxicity, and sickle cell disease.

CLINICAL MANIFESTATIONS

Patients with NDI produce large amounts of very dilute urine regardless of their hydration status. This polyuria necessitates excessive water intake (polydipsia) to compensate for these losses. Congenital NDI typically manifests in the first weeks of life with hypernatremic dehydration, as such infants are unable to maintain sufficient fluid intake. Other features may include intermittent fever, irritability, vomiting, and poor growth. Interestingly, associated pregnancies are not associated with polyhydramnios, as the mechanisms affecting urine concentration do not develop until after delivery. Developmental delay may occur as a result of frequent hypernatremic seizures.

Some patients may not manifest symptoms until they are stressed with illness. Older children may present with polyuria, nocturnal enuresis (or significant nocturia), and constipation.

DIAGNOSTIC EVALUATION

Patients with DI are unable to concentrate their urine, even with significant dehydration. Urine specific gravity and osmolarity remain inappropriately low, while serum osmolarity is elevated. A urine osmolality below 500 mOsm/kg in a dehydrated child should suggest DI; in fact, the urine osmolality often is below 200 mOsm/kg. Other causes of polyuria, such as diabetes mellitus and renal salt wasting, can be ruled out by urine dipstick results for glucose, urine electrolytes, and decreased serum sodium levels.

Differentiating central DI from NDI is not possible based on symptomatology alone, although the former more commonly follows head trauma, meningitis, or is associated with midline cranial anomalies. The DDAVP test can help differentiate central from nephrogenic DI, as NDI would not respond to the hormone; affected patients would continue to have hypo-osmolar urine. Water deprivation testing can also be considered to differentiate between DI and psychogenic polydipsia, as patients with the former would become hypernatremic over time. Perinatal testing to detect arginine vasopressin receptor gene (*AVPR2*) mutations is now available.

TREATMENT

Acute treatment consists of rehydrating the child, replacing ongoing urinary losses, and correcting any electrolyte abnormalities. A low-sodium diet (<0.7 mEq/kg/day) is essential; maximal osmolality of the urine is fixed, so the amount of sodium urinary excretion helps determine the obligate urine output. This should be coupled with thiazide diuretics or amiloride to decrease urinary sodium reabsorption. Prostaglandin synthesis inhibitors, like indomethacin, may have an additive effect on reducing water excretion.

Children with nephrogenic DI are at risk for poor growth as their oral intake is predominantly fluid and may not be calorie-rich. The disease is life-long but carries a good prognosis, provided that episodes of hypernatremic dehydration are minimized during the early years.

HYPERTENSION

Normal blood pressure rises gradually as a child grows, reaching adult values during adolescence. Hypertension in the pediatric population is defined as blood pressure **greater than 95th percentile for age, gender, and height** measured on three separate occasions about 1 week apart. **Essential (primary) hypertension** is the most common form in adults. Until recently, children were more likely to have **secondary hypertension**, usually related to renal disease. However, the increase in childhood obesity and high sodium intake of the Westernized diet have led to a concurrent rise in pediatric essential hypertension, which is being documented at increasingly earlier ages. Endocrine, vascular, and neurologic conditions may also be associated with increased blood pressure (Table 17-3). The younger the patient or the higher the blood pressure reading, the more likely the hypertension is secondary in etiology.

CLINICAL MANIFESTATIONS

Stable or slowly progressive hypertension is unlikely to cause symptoms; therefore, vigilance at health maintenance visits is needed. Family history is often positive for hypertension, stroke, or premature heart disease. Patients with secondary hypertension often come to medical attention for complaints

TABLE 17-3 Differential Diagnosis of Pediatric Hypertension

Factitious	***Endocrine***
• Anxiety ("white coat" hypertension)	• Congenital adrenal hyperplasia
• Inappropriate cuff size	• Cushing syndrome
Primary (essential) hypertension	• Hyper- or hypothyroidism
Renal	• Pheochromocytoma
• Glomerulonephritis	• Hyperaldosteronism
• Renal scarring from pyelonephritis	• Hypercalcemia
• Cystic diseases	***Vascular***
• Obstructive uropathy	• Renal artery stenosis
• Renal trauma	• Coarctation of the aorta
• Renal tumor	• Renal artery or vein thrombosis (including from umbilical catheters in newborns)
• Renal failure (acute or chronic)	• Arteriovenous fistula
Neurologic	• Vasculitis
• Pain	***Other***
• Increased intracranial pressure	• Chronic lung disease (infants)
• Traumatic brain injury	• Acute intermittent porphyria
• Malignant hyperthermia	
Drugs and toxins	
• Oral contraceptives	
• Corticosteroids	
• Calcineurin inhibitors	
• Cocaine and other street drugs	

related to their underlying disease (e.g., growth failure, edema). Past medical history (including neonatal history of vascular catheters), recent medication use, and review of systems for urinary tract symptoms provide pertinent information.

Severe hypertension or hypertension that has developed over a short period of time can cause headache, dizziness, and vision changes. **Hypertensive encephalopathy** is characterized by vomiting, ataxia, mental status changes, and seizures. Other symptoms of hypertension may include epistaxis, chest pain, palpitations, and flushing.

DIAGNOSTIC EVALUATION

Obtaining an accurate blood pressure reading is essential in the diagnosis of hypertension. The air bladder portion of the cuff should encircle the patient's arm and be wide enough to cover 75% of the upper limb. A cuff that is too small will give a falsely elevated reading; likewise a cuff that is too large may yield lower pressure readings. Also, the patient should be calmly seated for at least 1 to 2 minutes prior to measurement, with the arm kept still and at heart level during the measurement.

If this measurement is elevated, then the remainder of the physical examination should focus on evaluating for secondary causes of hypertension. At least once, the blood pressure should be taken in all four extremities to exclude aortic coarctation. Particular attention should be given to the presence of tachycardia (sympathetic stimulation), heart murmur (as seen in coarctation) or gallop (heard with significant fluid overload). Retinal examination should be performed to make sure there is no papilledema to rule out intracranial causes of hypertension, especially in patients complaining of headache. Poor growth, flank pain, a retroperitoneal mass, large bladder, or abdominal bruit suggests a renal or renovascular etiology. Obesity contributes to hypertension in a genetically predisposed patient. Other secondary findings to consider include the appearance of Cushingoid features and the presence of thyromegaly or nodules.

The initial laboratory evaluation should include a CBC, serum electrolytes, BUN, creatinine, and urinalysis. This is mainly to screen for any evidence of renal disease, such as anemia, elevated creatinine, or proteinuria. The presence of hypernatremia with hypokalemia may be associated with hyperaldosteronism, while hypercalcemia may also cause elevated blood pressure. Ultrasound of the kidneys permits assessment of anatomy, while a Doppler ultrasound may show the renal vasculature but is rarely diagnostic of renal artery stenosis alone. Chest radiograph, electrocardiogram, and echocardiogram to evaluate heart size and function are often indicated, but more to evaluate for the presence of end organ injury than the etiology of the hypertension. Other secondary tests to consider include thyroid function tests, serum renin and aldosterone, serum metanephrines, and urine catecholamines.

TREATMENT

The best treatment for essential hypertension is **preventive health care**. High-salt diet, sedentary lifestyle, cigarette use, alcohol or drug abuse, high serum cholesterol levels, and obesity compound the disorder and increase the morbidity and mortality. First-line treatment recommendations include decreasing daily dietary sodium intake, decreased total caloric intake, and increased cardiovascular activities. When these measures fail after 3 to 6 months, either from patient nonadherence or nonefficacy, then pharmacologic therapy may be indicated. However, if patients present with symptoms from their hypertension or blood pressure readings >99th percentile, initial use of antihypertensives is warranted. Secondary hypertension responds to treatment of the underlying disorder when possible. Antihypertensives may be necessary in the short term to address the blood pressure elevation associated with the secondary cause.

The choice of pharmacologic therapy is varied, with several different classes of agents available in pediatric patients. Diuretics are often effective in patients with salt or fluid overload and may be used with few minor side effects (increased risk of dehydration). Calcium channel blockers are used in all age groups with very little side effects, but may not directly address the etiology of the hypertension. β-Blockers may be used for catecholamine-induced hypertension, but are contraindicated in athletes or patients with asthma. Angiotensin-converting enzyme (ACE) inhibitors are effective first-line agents in children with renal disease (especially for unilateral renal artery stenosis) *and* in adolescents and athletes because of relatively few side effects and potential long-term benefits, but do require monitoring of renal function. α-Blockers may also be effective for intracranial causes of hypertension. Additional vasodilators are available for pediatric use, but often not as first-line agents.

In patients with severe hypertension, rapid decreases in blood pressure compromise organ perfusion. Hypertensive crisis is an emergency and may be treated with sublingual nifedipine, intravenous labetalol, or intravenous drips of nicardipine or nitroprusside. Hydralazine is also effective, especially in neonates. Close monitoring in the intensive care setting is essential to prevent a rapid drop in blood pressure.

ACUTE KIDNEY INJURY

Renal failure is a potentially life-threatening condition. The incidence in children is increasing. **Acute renal failure** (ARF) consists of an abrupt reduction in renal function, occurring over hours to days, with retention of nitrogenous waste products such as BUN and creatinine (azotemia). Recently, the term **acute kidney injury** (AKI) has been proposed to reflect a complex disorder that occurs in a wide variety of settings with clinical manifestations ranging from a minimal elevation in serum creatinine to anuric failure.

The mechanisms of AKI include prerenal, intrinsic, or postrenal injury (Table 17-4). **Prerenal** injury is the functional response of a structurally normal kidney to hypoperfusion. This is the most common form, accounting for about 55% of AKI, with hypovolemia as the most common underlying mechanism. The decreasing GFR produces oliguria (urine output <400 mL/m^2/day) or anuria. Most patients recover completely from prerenal injury unless it is unrecognized or inappropriately treated.

By contrast, **intrinsic** renal injury results from a structural or functional abnormality in the kidney itself, accounting for about 40% of AKI cases. The most common underlying mechanism is acute tubular necrosis (ATN), and the terms *intrinsic ARF* and *ATN* are frequently used interchangeably. ATN is a poorly understood condition in which damaged tubules become obstructed with cellular debris. It may result

TABLE 17-4 Causes of Acute Kidney Injury

Prerenal
• Hypovolemia (dehydration, shock, hemorrhage, nephrotic syndrome)
• Hypotension (decreased cardiac output, shock, sepsis, anaphylaxis)
• Renal vasoconstriction (NSAIDs, ACE inhibitors, hepatorenal syndrome, renal artery stenosis, abdominal compartment syndrome)
Intrinsic
• Acute tubular necrosis (prolonged prerenal failure, nephrotoxins)
• Acute glomerulonephritis (poststreptococcal, membranoproliferative, crescentic)
• Acute interstitial nephritis (idiopathic, antibiotics)
• Renal vascular disease (hemolytic-uremic syndrome, vasculitis)
Postrenal
• Congenital (posterior urethral valves, ureteropelvic junction obstruction)
• Acquired (stones, clots, neurogenic bladder, tumor)

ACE, angiotensin converting enzyme; NSAID, nonsteroidal anti-inflammatory drugs.

from prolonged prerenal injury, sepsis, the use of nephrotoxic medications (such as aminoglycosides, vancomycin, and radio-contrast media), or infection. Intrinsic renal injury can also occur in patients with glomerulonephritis, interstitial nephritis, and renal vasculitis. While hemolytic-uremic syndrome was the most common cause of intrinsic AKI a decade ago, the epidemiology has shifted in recent years, with sepsis accounting for the majority of cases today. Intrarenal conditions can present with oliguria or anuria, although the urine output may also be normal when nephrotoxins are the cause (nonoliguric renal failure). While many patients can recover from intrinsic renal injury, a significant number progress to chronic kidney disease.

In **postrenal** injury, obstructive lesions at or below the collecting ducts produce increased intrarenal pressure and result in a rapidly declining GFR and hydronephrosis. The lesions may be congenital (a majority of cases in pediatrics) or acquired. Patients with complete obstruction are anuric, while partial obstructions may present with normal or increased urine output.

CLINICAL MANIFESTATIONS

Oliguria is one of the more frequently noted findings with AKI, though this may not be a feature of interstitial nephritis or nephrotoxin-induced injury. Edema is usually evident but often insidious in onset, first presenting with poorly fitting clothing or decreased energy levels. Findings of congestive heart failure (respiratory difficulty, diffuse crackles on lung examination, hepatomegaly) are very late findings but require immediate intervention. Other generalized symptoms may be nonspecific and include malaise, fatigue, anorexia, and vomiting. Flank or abdominal pain may be seen with swelling of the kidneys or urinary tract, such as from obstruction.

Most cases of AKI are diagnosed in hospitalized patients, so their recent medical histories are known. A history of recent dehydration, shock, cardiac surgery, or previous renal conditions may help clarify the etiology. A complete list of recent medications (including radiocontrast) is also very helpful in diagnosing nephrotoxic medication injury, especially as most injury occurs with cumulative administrations of nephrotoxic drugs. Depending on the etiology, the physical examination may reveal dehydration, cardiovascular instability, and abdominal or suprapubic masses. Other historical and examination findings include those seen in the different glomerulonephrhitides.

DIAGNOSTIC EVALUATION

AKI is defined by an acute rise in creatinine, but is also characterized by hyperkalemia, azotemia, and metabolic acidosis. Anemia is variably present. Urinalysis for hematuria, proteinuria, leukocytes, and presence of casts also provides useful information. Red cell casts are typical of acute glomerulonephritis, white cell casts are seen in interstitial nephritis or pyelonephritis, and pigmented coarsely granular casts indicate ATN. Urine and plasma urea nitrogen, creatinine, osmolarity, and sodium can be used to differentiate between prerenal and intrinsic injury (Table 17-5). Urine culture is indicated if pyelonephritis is suspected.

TABLE 17-5 Typical Findings in Prerenal and Intrinsic AKI

Diagnostic Index	Prerenal	Intrinsic Renal
Urinalysis	***Few if any abnormalities***	***Hematuria, proteinuria, casts***
Urine specific gravity	>1.020	<1.020
Urine osmolality (mOsm/kg H_2O)	>500	<350
Urine/plasma creatinine	>40	<20
Serum BUN/creatinine	>20	<15
Fractional excretion of sodium (FENa)	<1	>2

FENa (%) = ([U/P]Na)/([U/P]Cr) × 100

Renal US is the single best noninvasive radiographic test for determining the site of obstruction in postrenal injury, as well as kidney size and shape and renal blood flow. It may also be useful to differentiate between acute and chronic kidney injury, since kidneys are normal or enlarged in AKI and potentially shrunken in chronic kidney disease. Renal nuclear scans can delineate renal perfusion and functional differences. Voiding cystourethrogram and CTs may also be indicated in certain cases as directed by initial imaging studies.

Renal biopsy is indicated when the diagnosis remains unclear or the extent of involvement is unknown. Other laboratory tests for the different glomerulonephritides may also be considered.

TREATMENT

Major complications of AKI may be metabolic (hyperkalemia, hyponatremia, hypocalcemia, metabolic acidosis with high anion gap), cardiovascular (hypertension, pulmonary edema, arrythmias), gastrointestinal (gastritis, bleeding), neurologic (somnolence, seizures, coma), hematologic (anemia, bleeding), and/or infectious (increased susceptibility to infections). These sequelae often need to be treated directly while also addressing the cause of the AKI.

Specific treatments for AKI depend on the etiology. Prerenal injury usually responds to prompt and vigorous correction of the renal hypoperfusion, with either intravenous fluid resuscitation or vasopressor use. Postrenal injury often responds to correction of the obstruction, either through placement of a bypassing catheter or surgical correction.

Once intrinsic AKI is established, treatment is largely supportive, consisting of appropriate fluid management (careful replacement of insensible water loss and ongoing losses), correction of electrolyte abnormalities, and dialysis (for fluid overload, hyperkalemia, or acidosis that is unresponsive to medical therapies). Medications that undergo renal clearance require dosing adjustments in AKI to avoid toxicity or further worsening of the renal injury. The underlying abnormality must be corrected to achieve optimal resolution and to prevent recurrence; these treatments vary greatly depending on the primary etiology. Examples include immunosuppression (immune-mediated disorders), antibiotics (pyelonephritis), removal of the offending agent (nephrotoxins or interstitial nephritis), and occasionally watchful observation. The prognosis of AKI depends on the underlying etiology, length of impairment, and severity of functional disturbance.

CHRONIC KIDNEY DISEASE

Chronic kidney disease (CKD) implies that renal function has dropped below 30% of normal over a longer period of time, typically greater than three months. Function at 10% or less than normal is defined as **end-stage renal disease** (ESRD). The most common causes of CKD in the pediatric population are congenital, most often due to obstructive uropathy, followed by renal dysplasia and other hereditary renal conditions. Some acquired glomerulopathic disorders, such as focal segmental glomerulosclerosis, are also common causes in older children.

CLINICAL MANIFESTATIONS

Unlike acute kidney injury, the different etiologies of CKD typically do not produce oliguria except when it results from an acquired disorder or obstruction. Often there may be an issue with renal concentrating ability, as described in renal dysplasia, resulting in polyuria, episodic unexplained dehydration, or salt craving. Other subjective complaints may include anorexia, nausea, malaise, lethargy, and decreased exercise tolerance—all from the gradual accumulation of unfiltered toxins. Growth failure frequently prompts evaluation for renal disease in the outpatient setting. Rickets may also be present. Other initial presentations include "isolated" hypertension or anemia. With improvements in prenatal imaging, many abnormalities are noted before delivery.

DIAGNOSTIC EVALUATION

Patients with CKD demonstrate many of the same laboratory abnormalities seen in AKI, including azotemia, acidosis, sodium imbalance, and hyperkalemia. The diagnostic evaluations (urinalysis, CBC, renal panel, BUN, creatinine, calcium, and phosphorus) are also very similar. Urinalysis may show a low specific gravity if renal concentrating ability has been lost, while proteinuria may also be present. Anemia is usually more pronounced in CKD than AKI, as there is prolonged cessation of erythropoietin production by the kidney combined with iron deficiency from impaired nutritional intake. Chronic hypocalcemia leads to secondary hyperparathyroidism (elevated intact PTH levels), which may present with renal osteodystrophy on skeletal radiographs. Hyperphosphatemia may also be found in earlier stages of CKD. Renal ultrasound may demonstrate changes in renal size (often small), density (often hyperechoic), and loss of corticomedullary differentiation.

TREATMENT

Treatment for CKD includes nutritional, pharmacologic, and additional interventions to address the clinical manifestations of the disorder and hopefully prevent rapid progression. Close monitoring of clinical and laboratory status is required. Progression of CKD is best avoided by controlling any associated hypertension while minimizing proteinuria through use of ACE inhibitors and angiotensin receptor blockers (ARBs). Protein restriction is controversial, since it lessens azotemia but can also adversely affect growth and development. Sodium and fluid intake may need to be restricted to control hypertension; antihypertensive medication is often needed with advancing disease.

Hyperkalemia is best avoided through dietary potassium restriction or use of potassium binding resins, like Kayexalate. Acidosis may require bicarbonate supplementation. Calcium supplementation and activated vitamin D are used to treat renal osteodystrophy, while phosphate binders and dietary restriction address hyperphosphatemia. Iron supplementation and recombinant erythropoietin address the anemia. Complete catch-up growth is unlikely, even when optimal caloric intake and normalization of metabolic parameters occur; growth hormone may also be needed.

Children with less than 10% of normal renal function (creatinine >3 to 10 mg/dL depending on size) require either dialysis or renal transplant. **Peritoneal dialysis**, which can be performed at home, is the standard for children requiring long-term dialysis. Infectious complications, like exit site infections or peritonitis, are the most commonly reported problems, but can usually be treated in the outpatient setting. Hemodialysis, performed at specialized pediatric dialysis centers, provides close to 10% of normal renal function but is time consuming. Hemodialysis-associated mortality is low, but complications of hemodialysis are not uncommon. They include bleeding (from the anticoagulation of the procedure), thrombosis or infection of vascular access, and too rapid or little fluid or electrolyte removal. Acute dehydration may occur with any treatment. **Dysequilibrium syndrome**, which occurs when the serum urea nitrogen level drops too rapidly (resulting in cerebral edema), may be seen, more commonly with initial hemodialysis treatments. Signs and symptoms of dysequilibrium syndrome include headache, nausea, vomiting, mental statues changes, seizures, and coma.

Renal transplantation is the ultimate therapy for all children with end-stage renal disease, with few absolute contraindications. The donated kidney may come from a related living or deceased donor. Living related donor transplants historically have better host and graft survival rates, though the differences are narrowing.

Children with CKD require complex and time-consuming treatment and, as a consequence, often experience a decrease in quality of life and are predisposed to developmental and social delays.

ENURESIS

Successful bladder control is typically achieved between 24 and 36 months of age, although many developmentally normal children take significantly longer. Enuresis is the involuntary loss of urine in a child older than 5 years. It may be nocturnal and/or daytime, primary or secondary. **Primary** enuretics are patients who have never successfully maintained a dry period, whereas **secondary** enuretics are usually dry for several months before regular wetting recurs.

CLINICAL MANIFESTATIONS

The most important goal is determining whether there is inherent impairment of renal or bladder function causing the enuresis. The ability to maintain continence for some period of time, whether during the day or night or for several weeks to months (such as in secondary enuresis) is somewhat reassuring of functional normalcy.

A careful history of urinary habits is essential and may pinpoint the problem in and of itself. Frequency of urination, urgency, and small volume of voids may assist in determining if the patient has some instability of the bladder. Inquiry about urine withholding symptoms is also essential, as many enuretics know when they need to void but simply ignore these signals and instead will nervously "dance" ("pee-pee dance") or hold themselves (grab the crotch, sit cross-legged, or perform Vincent's curtsy). Parents sometimes witness the patient urinating and may be able to describe the urinary stream, whether strong, weak, deflected, or interrupted. Bowel habits are also essential to know as constipation may contribute to bladder sensitivity, while bowel incontinence may suggest a tendency for fecal and urinary retention, possibly from a neurologic cause.

Physical examination should also focus on findings of secondary causes of enuresis including developmental delay, obstruction, or neurologic impairment. Thorough examination should include the abdomen (masses, palpable bladder), genitalia (urethral abnormalities), anus (tone, signs of constipation), and spine (hair tufts, dimples).

DIAGNOSTIC EVALUATION

Urinalysis, electrolytes, and osmolarity can be considered to rule out renal concentrating defects or cystitis. An abdominal radiograph to look for constipation may be considered. Sonography of the kidneys and bladder will evaluate for potential obstruction.

TREATMENT

For most patients with enuresis, improvement occurs with behavioral modification and elimination of factors that increase bladder sensitivity. Regular timed voiding may help avoid prolonged bladder holding, especially in young children. Treatment of constipation, if present, decreases any extrinsic pressure on the bladder. Avoidance of carbonated, caffeinated, chocolate, and citrus food items may also help to desensitize the bladder. Occasionally, patients require anticholinergic medication to help decrease their bladder detrusor instability.

Primary nocturnal enuresis is thought to be caused by delayed maturational control or inadequate levels of antidiuretic hormone secretion during sleep. Behavior modification programs are moderately effective. The most popular method of treatment is a nighttime audio alarm that sounds as soon as the child starts to urinate, eventually conditioning controlled bladder emptying before enuresis. Intranasal desmopressin acetate (generic name for DDAVP; analogous to endogenous vasopressin) acts to concentrate the urine. If given in the evening, less urine is produced overnight, decreasing the likelihood of wetting. Given the potential for central nervous system side effects, DDAVP is limited to situational use in this population (e.g., in conjunction with a sleepover or during overnight camp). With any of the above therapies, the cure rate is 15% per year after 5 years of age; children who remain enuretic past 8 years of age have a 10% risk of never resolving their condition.

KEY POINTS

- Infants with bilateral renal agenesis develop Potter sequence (clubbed feet, cranial anomalies) and typically are stillborn or die shortly after birth due to associated pulmonary hypoplasia.
- Ureteropelvic junction obstruction (UPJO) is the most common cause of hydronephrosis in childhood.
- The most common presentation of VUR is recurrent UTIs.
- Posterior urethral valves is one of the most common causes of end-stage renal disease in the male child. PUV may be suspected by detecting hydronephrosis and bladder distention on prenatal ultrasound or by palpating a distended bladder or renal mass during the newborn examination.
- Circumcision is contraindicated in infant males with hypospadias because surgical repair may require the preputial tissue.
- Orchiopexy (surgical repair of cryptorchidism) does not appear to alter the incidence of malignant degeneration, but it does render the testis accessible for regular self-examination.
- Testicular torsion is a surgical emergency, requiring prompt recognition and correction to prevent loss of the testicle. The diagnosis of torsion is a clinical diagnosis; ultrasound is a helpful tool but should not delay prompt surgical exploration and correction if the index of suspicion for torsion is high.
- Hydroceles are fluid-filled sacs in the scrotal cavity consisting of remnants of the processus vaginalis, often diagnosed in the newborn period or early childhood. Communicating hydroceles and hernias should be repaired as soon as possible to prevent the development of an incarcerated hernia. Most noncommunicating or simple hydroceles involute by 12 months of age.
- Varicoceles, defined as dilation of the testicular veins and enlargement of the pampiniform plexus, become detectable in boys during adolescence, occur more commonly on the left, are usually nontender, and become evident upon standing when the veins distend and produce the characteristic "bag of worms" within the scrotum.
- Urinary tract infections (UTIs) are the most common bacterial infections in febrile infants. The most significant risk factor for recurrent UTIs is the presence of a urinary tract abnormality that causes urinary stasis, obstruction, reflux, or dysfunctional voiding.
- Nephrotic syndrome is characterized by severe proteinuria, hypoalbuminemia, hyperlipidemia, and edema. Minimal change disease is the most common type of pediatric idiopathic nephrotic syndrome; it typically responds to high-dose steroids within 4 weeks.
- Glomerulonephritides are characterized by hematuria, azotemia, oliguria, edema, and hypertension. The presence of red cell casts on urine microscopy is pathognomonic for glomerulonephritis.
- Acute poststreptococcal glomerulonephritis is the most common glomerulonephritis in children. Its prognosis is excellent, with normalization of C3 levels in 6 to 8 weeks and resolution of clinical manifestations in 90% of cases.
- Henoch-Schönlein purpura (HSP) is a systemic vasculitis characterized by a purpuric rash often involving the lower extremities and buttocks, crampy abdominal pain, and arthritis. About 50% of patients may have an elevated IgA level, though this is not diagnostic of the disorder. C3 levels remain normal.
- Alport syndrome is a form of hereditary nephritis associated with sensorineural hearing loss.
- Hemolytic uremic syndrome (HUS) is characterized by the classic trio of microangiopathic hemolytic anemia, thrombocytopenia, and azotemia. A majority of cases are caused by a Shiga-like toxin produced by an enterohemorrhagic strain of *E. coli* (O157:H7).
- Renal tubular acidosis (RTA) is characterized by hyperchloremic metabolic acidosis with a normal plasma anion gap. The most common type in children is distal RTA type 4 with hyperkalemia (from hypoaldosteronism or pseudohypoaldosteronism), often seen with obstruction of the urinary tract.
- Diabetes insipidus (DI) is a disorder of urine concentration and can be central or nephrogenic. Clinical manifestations include polyuria, polydipsia, and growth retardation. Therapy for nephrogenic DI includes a low-sodium diet, thiazide diuretics, and indomethacin.
- Blood pressure norms for children are related to age, gender, and height. Three blood pressure readings on separate occasions that are greater than the 95th percentile for age, height, and gender constitute hypertension. The younger the hypertensive child and the higher the blood pressure, the more likely that the etiology of the hypertension is secondary.
- The causes of acute kidney injury include prerenal (55%), intrarenal (40%), or postrenal (5%). Laboratory findings include increasing levels of BUN and creatinine, hyperkalemia, and metabolic acidosis.
- The most common causes of chronic kidney disease in the pediatric population are congenital, most often due to obstructive uropathy, followed by renal dysplasia and other hereditary renal conditions. Function at 10% or less than normal is defined as end-stage renal disease (ESRD).
- Patients with primary enuresis are patients who have never successfully maintained a dry period, whereas those with secondary enuresis are usually dry for several months before regular wetting recurs. Regardless of the therapy employed, the cure rate is 15% per year after 5 years of age; children who remain enuretic past 8 years of age have a 10% risk of never resolving their condition.
- Children with growth failure should be screened for renal disease.

C Clinical Vignettes

Vignette 1

A 7-year-old boy presents to the emergency room for gross hematuria of 1 day's duration. He also has had decreased appetite and energy levels for the past 2 days. He has not had any fevers or vomiting, but had been ill about 3 weeks ago with 1 day of fever and abdominal pain. On vital signs, he is afebrile with a heart rate of 82 bpm and blood pressure 120/78 mm Hg. He has some eyelid swelling and pretibial edema but an otherwise negative physical examination. His urine dipstick results show 4+ blood and 2+ protein, but are negative for nitrite and leukocyte esterase. Microscopic examination confirms the presence of red cells in the urine, along with some red cell casts. Serum electrolytes are within normal limits, but creatinine is slightly elevated at 0.7 mg/dL.

1. Which of the following represents the most appropriate next laboratory test?
   a. Serum cholesterol level
   b. Antinuclear antibody (ANA)
   c. Serum IgA level
   d. Complement level (C3)
   e. Serum and urine osmolarity

2. The C3 level is low at 22 mg/dL (normal >75), while a C4 level is normal at 25 mg/dL. Complete blood count is notable for a slightly increased WBC count at 12,000/μL and normal hemoglobin of 12.5 gm/dL. Which of the following is the most likely etiology of his symptoms?
   a. Systemic lupus erythematosis (SLE)
   b. Poststreptococcal glomerulonephritis (PSGN)
   c. Henoch schonlein purpura (HSP) nephritis
   d. IgA nephropathy
   e. Hemolytic uremic syndrome (HUS)

3. ASO titer is also found to be elevated in this patient. Which of the following presents the best therapy for this patient?
   a. Prednisone use (2 mg/kg/day) for 4 to 6 weeks
   b. Prompt antibiotic therapy to prevent disease progression
   c. Diuretic use for hypertension
   d. High-protein diet for proteinuria
   e. Prophylactic antibiotic use to prevent nephritis recurrence

Vignette 2

A 5-year-old boy is being evaluated in the clinic for several days of swelling. His mother first noted some upper respiratory symptoms (rhinorrhea, nonproductive cough) about 2 weeks ago with no fevers. He initially seemed to get better, but the swelling of his eyelids started 2 days ago, prompting her to give him an antihistamine the past two evenings. The swelling has persisted and spread to his face, abdomen, and hands. The child has a decreased appetite and fatigue, but primarily complains of some abdominal discomfort with no vomiting or diarrhea. His weight is 20.2 kg, heart rate is 122 beats per minute, and blood pressure is 85/52 mm Hg. He has notable swelling of his face, eyelids, and distal extremities. His lungs are clear. The abdomen is fairly distended. The remainder of his physical examination is negative. Urinalysis reveals trace blood with 4+ protein and pH 5, but is otherwise negative.

1. Which of the following laboratory results would be MOST unexpected?
   a. Serum sodium of 129 mEq/L
   b. Serum bicarbonate of 12 mEq/L
   c. Serum albumin of 1.8 g/dL
   d. Serum calcium of 7.0 mg/dL
   e. Serum creatinine of 0.6 mg/dL

2. Laboratory results return and indeed show a low serum albumin at 1.7 gm/dL and calcium of 7.9 mg/dL, but otherwise normal electrolytes and creatinine. Complete blood count results and C3 level are normal. Which of the following is the most likely diagnosis?
   a. Minimal change disease (MCD)
   b. Henoch Schönlein Purpura (HSP) nephritis
   c. Systemic Lupus Erythematosis (SLE)
   d. Interstitial nephritis
   e. Focal segmental glomerulosclerosis (FSGS)

3. The patient is started on prednisone 2 mg/kg daily along with an H2 blocker and mild diuretic. A week later, he presents in the office with fever and abdominal pain. He has not been eating as he has felt nauseous, but has kept most of his medication down the past 2 days. He appears ill with a temperature of 102.3° F, pulse of 142 beats per minute, and BP 80/45 mm Hg. His weight is 22.2 kg. His abdomen is distended and he flinches in pain with light palpation to each quadrant. You direct the family to the local emergency department as you call to make certain treatment recommendations. Which of the following recommendations is most appropriate?
   a. Type and screen patient for expectant blood transfusion.
   b. Fluid restrict the patient to <400 mL/m^2/day to prevent acute kidney injury.

c. Place an IV for intravenous steroids.
d. Perform a right upper quadrant US for probable cholecystitis.
e. Place an IV for antibiotics, including vancomycin and a third-generation cephalosporin.

Vignette 3

A 14-month-old female presents to the office with concerns about poor growth. She had been seen in another provider's office for all of her routine childhood visits and was told that she was likely just "petite." The family's concern is that she drinks all day and just cannot seem to gain weight. She was born full-term and was discharged to home on day-of-life 2. She has not had any emergency room visits or hospital admissions since then and has received all of her recommended immunizations to date. She has no reported problems with recurrent fevers or diarrhea, but often has nonbloody, nonbilious vomiting. She was formula fed and would often require feedings every 2 to 3 hours including through the night, only being spaced out in frequency by her parents' necessity at 8 months of age. Even then she had occasional vomiting. She is now eating solid foods, but has a limited appetite. She continues to have very good urine output, soaking through her disposable diapers at times. In the office, she is a small toddler who is cruising about the examination room. Her height and weight are both less than third percentile for age; vital signs are stable. The rest of her examination is normal.

1. All of the following screening laboratory and radiologic evaluations are potentially indicated, EXCEPT:
   a. Renal ultrasound
   b. Voiding cystourethrogram (VCUG)
   c. Urinalysis
   d. Serum electrolytes, BUN, and creatinine
   e. Urine and serum osmolarity

2. The following results were obtained from this patient's samples:
   1. Urinalysis: specific gravity 1.007, pH 7
   2. Trace glucose and protein; negative for blood, LE, or nitrite
   3. Serum electrolytes: sodium 133 mEq/L, potassium 3.0 mEq/L, chloride 116 mEq/L, bicarbonate 14 mEq/L, BUN 8 mg/dL, creatinine 0.2 mg/dL, glucose 106 mg/dL
   4. Serum osmolarity: 275 mOsm/L
   5. Urine osmolarity: 800 mOsm/L
   6. Renal ultrasound: Both kidneys are normal in length, shape, and position.
   7. There is normal corticomedullary differentiation without evidence of calcification. No hydronephrosis is noted and the bladder appears to have normal wall thickness.

Which of the following is the most likely diagnosis in this patient?
   a. Nephrogenic diabetes insipidus
   b. Central diabetes insipidus
   c. Renal dysplasia
   d. Diabetes mellitus
   e. Renal tubular acidosis

3. Which of the following is the best next step in the evaluation of this patient?
   a. Urine electrolytes
   b. DDAVP stimulation test
   c. Sterile urine catheterization
   d. Hemoglobin A1C level
   e. Serum lithium level

Vignette 4

An 8-day-old male infant presents to your office with a 3-day history of decreased number of wet diapers and an abdominal mass noted by the parents. His mother states that he is not feeding well. He continues to breastfeed, as he has since discharge from the nursery. He is having regular, typical bowel movements. Findings on physical examination include a temperature of 38.5°C, respiratory rate of 30 breaths per minute, pulse of 180 beats per minute, and blood pressure of 70/40 mm Hg. He has an oxygen saturation of 100% on room air. He has sunken eyelids and diminished capillary refill. His heart and lung examinations are normal save for his tachycardia. You feel a fullness in his lower abdomen.

1. Which of the following is the most likely diagnosis?
   a. Ureteropelvic junction (UPJ) obstruction
   b. Pyloric stenosis
   c. Posterior urethral valves
   d. Primary vesicoureteral reflux
   e. Duodenal atresia

2. The patient is referred to the emergency department. A urine culture is obtained and he is placed on intravenous fluids and appropriate antibiotics. What is the most appropriate next step in this patient's evaluation and management?
   a. Renal ultrasound
   b. Voiding cystourethrogram (VCUG)
   c. Karyotype
   d. Lasix renogram
   e. Cystoscopy

3. The child is admitted to the hospital. An ultrasound shows bilateral hydronephrosis with a distended trabeculated bladder. Initial laboratory results are now returning. All of the following results would be expected in this patient, EXCEPT:
   a. Urine pH 7.5
   b. Positive urine nitrite and leukocyte esterase
   c. Serum creatinine 1.0 mg/dL
   d. Serum sodium 140 mEq/L, chloride 120 mEq/L, bicarbonate 13 mEq/L
   e. Serum potassium 6.2 mEq/L

Vignette 5

A 3-year-old girl presents to your office with a history of urinary tract infection without fever. Mom reports that her urine "smells bad" and that she complains of urgency and dysuria. Mom reports that she can hold her urine "forever" and seems to wet herself a few minutes after she voids. She has a hard large bowel movement every third day and frequently reports belly pain. Findings on physical examination include a temperature of 36.5°C, respiratory rate of 30 breaths per minute, pulse of 110 beats per minute, and blood pressure of 100/60 mm Hg. Her abdomen is soft, but there is stool palpable in her colon. Her external genitalia appear erythematous and have an amine-like odor. There is urine and stool staining her underwear. A clean catch urinalysis reveals:

1. Specific gravity	1.030
2. pH	6.5
3. Protein	negative
4. Glucose	negative
5. Ketone	negative
6. Bilirubin	negative
7. Blood	positive

CLINICAL VIGNETTES

8.	Nitrite	positive
9.	Leukocyte esterase	positive
Micro:		
10.	RBCs	3 to 5/hpf
11.	WBCs	5 to 7/hpf
12.	RBC casts	0/hpf
13.	Other cells	Multiple epithelial cells

1. What is the likely diagnosis?
a. Lower Urinary tract infection (cystitis)
b. Pyelonephritis
c. Contaminated specimen
d. Vesicoureteral reflux
e. Sexually transmitted disease (child abuse concern)

2. It is critical to understand that not all complaints of dysuria in the child signify infection. The child presented is constipated and is a vaginal voider. She is afebrile on presentation and the urine is likely contaminated, hence the epithelial cells and red blood cells. What is the MOST APPROPRIATE treatment?
a. Empiric antibiotics while awaiting sensitivities
b. Renal ultrasound
c. Antifungal cream
d. Treat constipation and address voiding habits
e. Referral to social services

3. Her mother also reports that she wets the bed nightly; this has just started. The daughter toilet trained at 2.5 years and had been dry for 1 year. What is the best way to manage her bed wetting?
a. Start ddAVP
b. Give her a bed-wetting alarm
c. Start antibiotics
d. Reassurance
e. Timed voids and constipation management

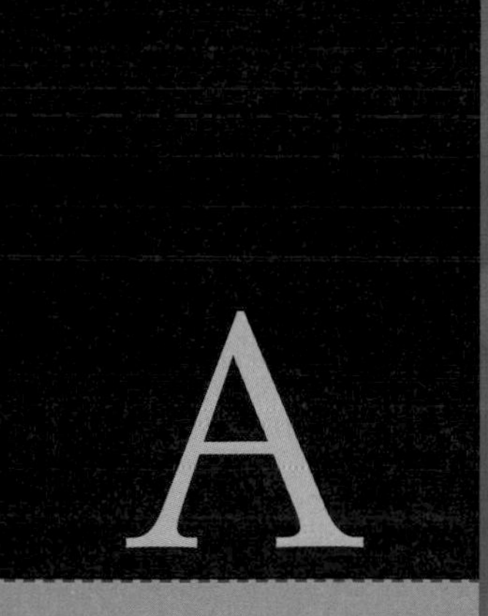

Answers

Vignette 1 Question 1
Answer D: The patient has clinical and laboratory evidence of glomerulonephritis, with the presence of red cell casts on urine microscopy, mild hypertension, edema, and slightly elevated creatinine. The best next test to order given this glomerulonephritic picture would be a C3 level to differentiate among the hypo- and normo-complementemic glomerulnephritides. Serum cholesterol may be considered if this patient had nephrotic syndrome, but his proteinuria was not severe (4+ on dipstick). His edema is more likely from salt and fluid retention. Serum IgA levels are not diagnostic, even for IgA nephropathy. ANA may be considered as a follow-up test if the C3 level is low. Urine osmolarity is not diagnostic for glomerulonephritis and would not be of value in furthering the investigation.

Vignette 1 Question 2
Answer B: PSGN is the most commonly acquired GN and typically presents in early school-age children, 1 to 4 weeks following a strep infection. It is associated with a low C3 level and positive ASO test. SLE is also associated with low C3 levels but may have low C4 as well. Also, SLE is less common in early school age children and in boys. HSP nephritis, IgA nephropathy, and typical HUS are not associated with low C3 levels. HSP often has other vasculitic findings, while HUS is associated with thrombocytopenia and hemolytic anemia.

Vignette 1 Question 3
Answer C: Diuretic use: The most common sequela of PSGN is hypertension, which is thought to be secondary to salt and fluid retention. Therefore, dietary salt and fluid restriction or use of diuretics may help with the edema and hypertension. Antibiotic therapy may be indicated if the patient has not been treated for his original (presumed) streptococcal infection, but more so to prevent rheumatic fever than disease progression. Even prompt treatment of streptococcal pharyngitis does not prevent the nephritis. Immunosuppression is not typically provided in limited cases of PSGN. A high-protein diet would not lessen the degree of proteinuria.

Vignette 2 Question 1
Answer B: This child has swelling due to the loss of protein in his urine; he has nephrotic syndrome. This explains the low serum albumin of 1.8, associated with the loss of albumin in his urine. The serum calcium is low because of the low serum albumin; however, if adjusted for the low serum albumin, this value would be normal at 8.7 mg/dL. Low oncotic pressure in the vasculature, results in fluid leakage into the interstitium, causing total body fluid overload, a decrease in the serum sodium, and also decreased perfusion of the kidneys and slight elevation in creatinine. Nephrotic patients do not typically suffer from severe acidosis, because most are able to appropriately acidify their urine.

Vignette 2 Question 2
Answer A: Most children who present with typical symptoms of nephrotic syndrome have minimal change disease (MCD). Symptoms which would be less typical for this diagnosis include significant hematuria (including gross hematuria), significant hypertension, older age groups (late adolescence), significantly increased creatinine level, and low C3 levels. FSGS often presents with nephrotic syndrome, but is more typical in older children. SLE may also present with nephrotic syndrome, but is typically seen in older adolescent females. HSP nephritis often has other vasculitic findings (rash, abdominal pain, joint involvement), while interstitial nephritis does not present with nephrotic syndrome.

Vignette 2 Question 3
Answer E: One of the more serious complications of nephrotic syndrome is spontaneous bacterial peritonitis. This patient has findings of bacterial peritonitis with fever, abdominal pain, and tenderness with palpation. Nephrotic patients are at increased risk of peritonitis from *Streptococus Pneumonial*, in addition to gastrointestinal flora, so antibiotic coverage should address both possibilities and include vancomycin. An ultrasound is indicated to confirm the presence of ascites (and in preparation for possible paracentesis), but should not be restricted to the RUQ (cholecystitis). This patient is also intravascularly depleted, with elevated heart rate (though some of this may be from the fever) and low blood pressure but increased weight overall. Fluid has been shifted from the vascular space into the interstitium, making him appear total body overloaded but intravascularly depleted. These patients benefit from intravascular colloid, like albumin, but do not require blood transfusions; typically the hemoglobin is elevated from intravascular contraction. Fluid should not be restricted, but preferably the patient should be provided fluid that will remain primarily in the intravascular space. Last, although IV steroids may be needed eventually for this patient's underlying disorder if he cannot tolerate oral medications, he has been doing well recently, so certainly steroid therapy is not what is needed most urgently.

Vignette 3 Question 1
Answer B: A VCUG would only be indicated to evaluate for the presence of vesicoureteral reflux or other specific anatomical

abnormalities of the bladder. With no previous history of febrile UTIs and the fact that this is a girl (making posterior urethral valves impossible), a VCUG is not indicated in this case. The other studies, however, are all indicated in the evaluation for a possible renal concentrating defect or metabolic abnormality as an etiology for the growth deficiency.

Vignette 3 Question 2
Answer E: The serum electrolytes reveal a hyperchloremic, non-gap metabolic acidosis. In the absence of diarrhea, this is indicative of renal tubular acidosis, especially with a urine pH >5.5. Diabetes insipidus (both nephrogenic and central) are ruled out by the normal urine osmolarity and, to some degree, the low serum sodium. The renal ultrasound shows no evidence of dysplasia of either kidney. There is trace glucosuria but in the presence of normoglycemia, diabetes mellitus is extremely unlikely, even more so if there are no ketones in the urine.

Vignette 3 Question 3
Answer A: In the setting of suspected RTA, determination of the type of RTA (mainly 1, 2, or 4) is essential for treatment and prognosis. Type 4 RTA is associated with hyperkalemia and often occurs in the setting of urinary obstruction; the low serum potassium is not explained by this potential diagnosis. Catheterization is unnecessary unless a sterile sample is required for suspected urinary tract infection. Calculating the urine anion gap helps discern between Type 1 and Type 2 RTA. Type 1 (distal) RTA is associated with a positive urine anion gap [(Na + K)—Cl], as there is a failure to produce ammonium (NH_4^+) distally and therefore less urinary chloride. In this scenario, there is already some indication that this may be Type 2 (proximal) RTA, as there is trace glucose and protein on urinalysis. Other findings in Type 2 RTA include low serum phosphorus (from urine losses) and increased urine potassium excretion. A DDAVP test is useful for determining if central DI is present. A serum lithium level may assist in the setting of suspected acquired nephrogenic DI. Elevated hemoglobin A1C may be seen with poorly controlled diabetes; however the serum glucose was normal.

Vignette 4 Question 1
Answer C: The diagnosis of posterior urethral valves is suggested by the decreased number of wet diapers and the palpable lower abdominal mass, which is likely his distended bladder. He is clinically dehydrated, as is often the case with the infant with late presentation of valves. A secondary urinary tract infection may also be present based on his presentation, but the underlying problem is the posterior urethral valves. Pyloric stenosis is a consideration, but the absence of a history of emesis or a palpable epigastric mass makes this diagnosis much less likely. UPJ obstruction also presents as an abdominal mass, but typically in the upper abdomen, and does not explain his fever and dehydrated appearance.

Vignette 4 Question 2
Answer A: With the suspicion of an obstructed urinary tract, a renal ultrasound would be indicated next and possibly desired before placement of a Foley catheter, as any findings of obstruction may then be altered. Placement of a Foley catheter would assist in bypassing any obstruction. VCUG will likely be indicated in this patient to confirm posterior urethral valves, but not as the first step in management evaluation. Cystoscopy also will likely be needed for potential surgical correction of the obstructing valves, but is also not the most appropriate immediate next step. Lasix renogram would potentially be useful for suspected obstructions proximal to the bladder. A karyotype is indicated only if there is an issue with ambiguity of the genitalia.

Vignette 4 Question 3
Answer E: In the setting of urinary tract obstruction, Type 4 renal tubular acidosis (RTA) may be present. All RTAs are notable for decreased urinary excretion of acid, causing an elevated urine pH and a hyperchloremic, normal gap metabolic acidosis. However, Type 4 RTA is typically associated with hyperkalemia. Also, with an unresolved obstruction, the serum creatinine is often elevated, as seen in postrenal injury. Boys with posterior urethral valves may have high-grades of VUR and be susceptible to UTIs. Given the patient's age, he requires hospitalization and evaluation for his urinary tract infection as well as management of his electrolytes and correction of his (presumed) posterior urethral valves.

Vignette 5 Question 1
Answer C: This is likely a contaminated specimen given the number of epithelial cells present. A clean catch urine is appropriate for toilet trained individuals but the clinical exam in this case suggests vaginal voiding (vulvovaginitis) which can result in a contaminated specimen. The "amine-like" odor is from vaginal pooling of urine, not a sexually transmitted disease.

Vignette 5 Question 2
Answer D: The most appropriate treatment option is to address the underlying condition. The physician must understand the voiding habits and toileting habits. Constipation should be addressed and a discussion must be had regarding appropriate toileting posture and voiding interval. Antibiotics are not indicated. There is no history of fever and the urinalysis is likely contaminated. Antifungal creams can actually make symptoms worse in the pre-pubertal female and do not treat the underlying cause (vaginal voiding). Renal ultrasound is not recommended at this point, though the urinalysis should be repeated after the symptoms are addressed. If hematuria is persistent or if fever develops, imaging should be performed.

Vignette 5 Question 3
Answer E: Timed voids and constipation management are the mainstay of therapy in this patient with secondary nocturnal enuresis. Treating the constipation and decreasing the sensitivity of the bladder during the day will lead to improved continence at night. She is still quite young and is not a candidate for medical or behavioral therapy at this point. However, simple reassurance without addressing the contributing factors to her symptoms will delay any clinical improvement.

Chapter

18 Genetic Disorders

Paula Goldenberg • Bradley S. Marino

Structural birth defects are categorized as minor or major. Minor birth defects such as skin tags, inner epicanthal folds, and rudimentary polydactyly are of little physiologic significance. Approximately 15% of newborn infants have at least one minor anomaly; 0.5% of infants have three or more minor anomalies. In contrast, major birth defects such as cleft palate, myelomeningocele, and congenital heart disease have an adverse effect on the infant. Major birth defects occur in 2% to 3% of all newborns. The probability of having a major birth defect increases as the number of minor anomalies present increases (Table 18-1). Birth defects can be caused by environmental or genetic factors. Genetic defects may be chromosomal, single gene, imprinting, cytogenetic, or multifactorial disorders.

ENVIRONMENTAL FACTORS

Environmental factors are known to cause at least 10% of all birth defects. **Teratogens** are environmental agents that cause congenital developmental anomalies by interfering with embryonic or fetal organogenesis or growth. Exposure to a teratogen before implantation (days 7 to 10 postconception) can either have no effect or can result in loss of the embryo. To disrupt organogenesis, a teratogenic exposure typically occurs before 12 weeks' gestation. Any teratogenic exposure after 12 weeks' gestation predominantly affects growth and central nervous system development.

Teratogens include intra-uterine infections, high-dosage radiation, maternal metabolic disorders, mechanical forces, and drugs. The most common maternal metabolic disorder that has teratogenic potential is diabetes mellitus; 10% of infants of diabetic mothers have a birth defect. Abnormal intrauterine forces such as uterine fibroids, breech positioning, congenital uterine anomalies, or oligohydramnios may cause fetal constraint, resulting in club foot or hip dysplasia. Table 18-2 lists the most common teratogenic drugs and their effects.

GENETIC FACTORS

Genetic disorders can be classified as disorders of single genes, chromosomes, imprinting, and molecular cytogenetics. Advances in molecular genetics (single gene disorders) and molecular cytogenetics (submicroscopic deletions and duplications) have blurred the distinction among these categories.

SINGLE-GENE DISORDERS

Normal human cells have 46 chromosomes (22 pairs of autosomes and 1 pair of sex chromosomes). Chromosomes contain genes, which occur in pairs at a single locus or site on specific chromosomes. These paired genes, called **alleles**, determine the genotype of an individual at that locus. If the genes at a specific locus are identical, the individual is **homozygous**; if they are different, the individual is **heterozygous**. More than 3,000 different single-gene disorders have been described and are classified by their mode of inheritance (autosomal dominant, autosomal recessive, or X-linked).

AUTOSOMAL DOMINANT DISORDERS

Autosomal dominant disorders are expressed after alteration of only one gene in the pair (often coding for a structural protein). Homozygous disease states of autosomal dominant disorders are rare and are usually severe or lethal. A mutant gene is inherited from one parent with the same condition. The risk for the affected parents' offspring is 50% for each pregnancy. Sometimes an individual is the first person in a family to display a trait due to spontaneous mutation. When a spontaneous mutation has occurred in a fetus, the risk of recurrence in a subsequent pregnancy is slightly higher than the chance of the spontaneous mutation occurring de novo, due to the rare

TABLE 18-1 Incidence of Major Anomalies in the Presence of Minor Anomalies

Number of Minor	Incidence of Major Anomalies (%)
0	<1
1	1
2	3
3	20

TABLE 18-2 Common Teratogenic Drugs

Drug	Results
Warfarin (Coumadin)	Hypoplastic nasal bridge, chondrodysplasia punctata
Ethanol	Fetal alcohol syndrome, microcephaly, CHD (septal defects, patent ductus arteriosus)
Isotretinoin (Accutane)	Facial and ear anomalies, CHD
Lithium	CHD (Ebstein anomaly, atrial septal defect)
Penicillamine	Cutis laxa syndrome
Phenytoin (Dilantin)	Hypoplastic nails, intrauterine growth retardation, cleft lip and palate
Radioactive iodine	Congenital goiter, hypothyroidism
Diethylstilbestrol	Vaginal adenocarcinoma during adolescence
Streptomycin	Deafness
Testosterone-like drugs	Virilization of female
Tetracycline	Dental enamel hypoplasia, altered bone growth
Thalidomide	Phocomelia, CHD (TOF, septal defects)
Trimethadione	Typical facies, CHD (TOF, TGA, HLHS)
Valproate	Spina bifida

CHD, congenital heart disease; HLHS, hypoplastic left heart syndrome; TGA, transpositions of the great arteries; TOF, tetralogy of fallot.

possibility of gonadal mosaicism. Autosomal dominant genes often cause conditions that manifest themselves with varying degrees of severity among affected individuals, a phenomenon known as **variable expressivity** or **variable penetrance**. Table 18-3 lists some important autosomal dominant diseases. Other chapters discuss some of these diseases in detail.

AUTOSOMAL RECESSIVE DISORDERS

Autosomal recessive disorders are only expressed after alteration of both the maternal and paternal genes of a gene pair (often coding for an enzyme). Because half of the normal enzyme activity is adequate under most circumstances, a person with only one mutant gene is not affected, whereas individuals who are homozygous for a defective gene have the disorder. Both parents of a child with an autosomal recessive disorder are usually heterozygous for that gene, and each child of such a couple has a 25% risk of inheriting the disorder. Table 18-4 lists the more common autosomal recessive disorders.

Most inborn errors of metabolism, with the exception of ornithine transcarbamylase (OTC) deficiency, are autosomal recessive disorders. Inborn errors of metabolism are discussed later in this chapter.

TABLE 18-3 Examples of Autosomal Dominant Diseases

Autosomal Dominant Disease	Frequency	Chromosome	Gene	Comments
Achondroplasia	1:25,000	4p	FGFR3	80% new mutations; proximal limb shortening
Adult polycystic kidney disease	1:1,200	16p	PKD1/PKD2	Renal cysts, intracranial aneurysm
Hereditary angioedema	1:10,000	11q	C1NH	Deficiency of C1 esterase inhibitor; episodic edema
Hereditary spherocytosis	1:5,000	8p, 14q	ANK1	See Chapter 11; some variants autosomal recessive
Marfan syndrome	1:20,000	15q	FBN1	Aortic root dilatation, tall stature
Neurofibromatosis	1:3,000	2p, 17q, 22q	NF1/NF2	50% new mutations; café au lait spots
Protein C deficiency	1:15,000	2q	Multiple genes	Hypercoagulable state
Tuberous sclerosis	1:30,000	9q, 16p	TSC1, TSC2	"Ash-leaf" spots; seizures
von Willebrand disease	1:100	12p	Multiple genes	See Chapter 11

p, short arm of chromosome; q, long arm of chromosome.

TABLE 18-4 Examples of Autosomal Recessive Diseases

Autosomal Recessive Disease	Frequency	Chromosome	Gene	Comments
Congenital adrenal hyperplasia	1:5,000 to 1:15,000; 1,700 in Yupik Eskimos	6p	CYP21A2,CYP17, CYP11A1, ACTHR	
Cystic fibrosis	1:2,000 (Caucasians)	7q, 19q	CFTR	See Chapter 8
Galactosemia disorder	1:60,000	9p	GALT	Carbohydrate metabolism
Gaucher disease	1:2,500 (Ashkenazi Jews)	1q	GBA	Lysosomal storage disorder
Infantile polycystic kidney	1:14,000	6p (or 16p = PKD1, TSC2)	PKD3	Renal and hepatic cysts, hypertension
Phenylketonuria	1:14,000	12q	PAH	Amino acid metabolism disorder
Sickle cell disease	1:625 (African Americans)	11p	HBB	See Chapter 11
Tay-Sachs disease	1:3,000 (Ashkenazi Jews)	15q	HEXA	Lysosomal storage disorder
Wilson disease	1:200,000	13q	ATP7B	Defective copper excretion

p, short arm of chromosome; q, long arm of chromosome.

X-LINKED DISORDERS

X-linked disorders, which are usually recessive, occur when a male inherits a mutant gene on the X chromosome from his mother. The affected male, termed **hemizygous** for the gene, has only a single X chromosome and, therefore, a single set of X-linked genes. The mother of the affected individual is heterozygous for that gene, because she has both a normal X chromosome and a mutant one. She may be asymptomatic or demonstrate mild symptoms of the disorder due to lyonization, in which only one X chromosome is transcriptionally active in each cell. Recurrence risk for X-linked disorders differs depending on which parent has the abnormal gene. An affected father will pass the defective X chromosome on to his daughters, who are carriers for the disorder; his sons will not be affected. A mother with an abnormal X chromosome is a carrier, and there is a 50% chance she will pass the abnormal chromosome to her progeny. Daughters who receive the abnormal X chromosome will be carriers for the disease, and sons will have the disease. Table 18-5 lists the most common X-linked disorders.

CHROMOSOMAL DISORDERS

Chromosomal disorders are responsible for pregnancy loss, congenital malformation, and mental retardation. Although more than 50% of first-trimester pregnancy losses are due to chromosomal imbalances, only 0.6% of newborn infants have chromosomal abnormalities. Most chromosomal defects arise de novo during gametogenesis, so that an infant can be conceived with a chromosomal abnormality without any prior family history. Chromosomal abnormalities can also be passed from parent to offspring. In such cases, there is often a family history of multiple spontaneous abortions or a higher-than-chance frequency of children with chromosomal problems.

TABLE 18-5 Examples of X-Linked Diseases

X-Linked Disease	Frequency	Comments
Bruton agammaglobulinemia	1:100,000	Absence of immunoglobulins; recurrent infections
Chronic granulomatous disease	1:1,000,000	Defective killing by phagocytes; recurrent infections
Color blindness	1:100,000	
Duchenne muscular dystrophy	1:3,600	Proximal muscle weakness; Gower sign
Glucose-6-phosphate dehydrogenase	1:10 (African Americans)	Oxidant-induced hemolytic anemia deficiency
Hemophilias A and B	1:10,000	See Chapter 11
Lesch-Nyhan syndrome	1:100,000	Purine metabolism disorder; self-mutilation
Ornithine transcarbamylase deficiency	—	Urea cycle disorder; hyperammonemia

Disorders of chromosome number may involve autosomes or sex chromosomes. Birth defects caused by autosomal abnormalities are generally more severe than those caused by sex chromosome abnormalities. Numeric defects of the autosomes include trisomy of chromosomes 21, 18, and 13. Examples of sex chromosome numerical abnormalities are Turner syndrome (45, X) and Klinefelter syndrome (47, XXY).

Chromosomal copy number abnormalities may be investigated by karyotype (aneuploidy, translocations), FISH (single locus DNA probes), or microarray which contains hundreds to a million submicroscopic DNA probes. Indications for obtaining chromosomal studies include: confirmation of a suspected chromosomal syndrome; multiple organ system malformations; significant developmental delay or mental retardation without an alternate explanation; short stature or extremely delayed menarche in girls; infertility or a history of multiple spontaneous abortions; ambiguous genitalia; or advanced maternal age. Fetal chromosomal or molecular testing may be accomplished through amniocentesis or chorionic villus sampling.

AUTOSOMAL TRISOMIES

Trisomy 21 (Down Syndrome)

Down syndrome is the most common genetic syndrome in humans, with an incidence of 1 per 700 live births. The risk of Down syndrome increases with advancing maternal age. The risk of having an infant with Down syndrome is 1:365 for mothers 35 years of age and 1:25 for those 45 or older. Of children with Down syndrome, 95% have three copies of chromosome 21 [trisomy 21 (47, +21)], which results typically from chromosomal nondisjunction during maternal meiosis. Four percent of Down syndrome patients have a Robertsonian unbalanced translocation of a third chromosome 21 attached to another autosome (46 total chromosomes). Many Robertsonian translocation cases are familial, meaning that one of the parents has a balanced translocation involving the long (q) arm of chromosome 21 attached to the long arm of another autosome. One percent of children with Down syndrome have chromosomal mosaicism, with some cells having two number 21 chromosomes (46 total chromosomes) and some cells having trisomy 21 (47 total chromosomes). The mosaicism results from a mitotic division error that occurred during embryonic development.

Common dysmorphic facial features include brachycephaly (flat occiput), flat facial profile, upslanted palpebral fissures, small ears, flat nasal bridge with epicanthal folds, and a small mouth with a protruding tongue. Anomalies of the hand include single palmar crease (simian creases), short, broad hands (brachydactyly) with an incurved fifth finger (clinodactyly) and hypoplastic middle phalanx, and an excessive gap between the first and second toes ("sandal sign"). Other features include short stature, generalized hypotonia, cardiac defects (endocardial cushion defects and septal defects are seen in 50% of cases), gastrointestinal anomalies (duodenal atresia and Hirschsprung disease), hypothyroidism, and mental retardation (IQ range 35 to 65). Leukemia is 20 times more common in children with trisomy 21 than in the general population. During the third and fourth decades, an Alzheimer-like dementia can develop. With improved medical, educational, and vocational management, life expectancy for patients with Down syndrome now extends well into adulthood.

Trisomy 18 (Edwards Syndrome)

Trisomy 18 occurs in 1 per 3,000 live births. Eighty percent of cases are the result of meiotic nondisjunction, which is associated with advanced maternal age. The remaining 20% may be partial (involving only a portion of the chromosome) or mosaic, caused by mitotic nondisjunction in the zygote. Chromosome translocation as the cause of trisomy 18 is extremely rare, and its presence should prompt karyotyping of the parents to exclude a balanced translocation. Clinical manifestations of trisomy 18 are shown in Table 18-6. The prognosis for patients with trisomy 18 is extremely poor: 50% die before reaching 2 months of age, and 90% to 95% die by 1 year of age.

Trisomy 13 (Patau Syndrome)

Trisomy 13 occurs in 1 per 8,000 live births but constitutes 1% of all spontaneous abortions. Approximately 75% of surviving

TABLE 18-6 Key Features of Trisomy 13 and Trisomy 18

	Trisomy 13	Trisomy 18
Head and neck	Microcephaly with sloping forehead	Prominent occiput
	Cutis aplasia of scalp	Narrow bifrontal diameter of forehead
	Microphthalmia	Low-set, malformed ears
	Cleft lip and palate	Micrognathia
Chest and abdomen	Congenital heart disease (VSD, ASD, PDA	Congenital heart disease (VSD, ASD, PDA)
	Omphalocele	Short sternum
Extremities	Clenched hands with overlapping fingers	Clenched hands with overlapping fingers
	Polydactyly	Rocker-bottom feet
	Polycystic kidney or other renal defects	Horseshoe kidney
Other	Cryptorchidism Agenesis of corpus callosum	Lack of subcutaneous fat

ASD, atrial septal defect; PDA, patent ductus arteriosus; VSD, ventricular septal defect.

cases are the result of meiotic nondisjunction, though the increased risk with advanced maternal age is much less than that for trisomy 21. Twenty percent of children with trisomy 13 have an unbalanced translocation of an additional chromosome 13 attached to another chromosome. Twenty percent of translocation cases are familial, meaning that one of the parents has a balanced translocation involving one chromosome 13 and another chromosome. The remaining 5% of children with trisomy 13 have mosaicism; some cells have 46 chromosomes with a normal karyotype, and some cells have 47 chromosomes with trisomy 13. The mosaicism results from a mitotic division error that occurs during embryonic development. Clinical manifestations of trisomy 13 are shown in Table 18-6. Prognosis for patients with trisomy 13 is extremely poor: 50% die before reaching 1 month of age, and 90% die by 1 year of age.

SEX CHROMOSOME ABNORMALITIES

Sex chromosome anomalies involve abnormalities in the number or structure of the X or Y chromosomes or both.

Turner Syndrome

Turner syndrome occurs in 1 per 5,000 live births. Approximately 98% of fetuses with Turner syndrome expire in utero; only 2% are born. Therefore, the recurrence risk for parents who have a child with Turner syndrome is no higher than that of the general population.

Several genotypes can cause the Turner phenotype. In 60% of cases, the karyotype is 45, X, in which the female lacks an X chromosome. Another 15% of individuals are mosaics with a genotype of 45, X/46, XX; 45, X/46, XX/47, XXX; or 45, X/46, XY. Mosaic individuals may have fewer physical stigmata of Turner syndrome. In the remaining 25% of cases, there are two X chromosomes but the short (p) arm of one of the X chromosomes is missing.

Clinical Manifestations

Dysmorphic features include lymphedema of the hands and feet, a shield-shaped chest, widely spaced hypoplastic nipples, a webbed neck, low hairline, cubitus valgus (increased carrying angle), short stature, and multiple pigmented nevi. Additional abnormalities include gonadal dysgenesis, gonadoblastoma, renal anomalies, congenital heart disease, autoimmune thyroiditis, and learning disabilities. Gonadal dysgenesis, present in 100% of patients, is associated with primary amenorrhea and lack of pubertal development due to loss of ovarian hormones. The gonads are appropriately infantile at birth but regress during childhood and develop into "streak" ovaries by puberty. In mosaics with a Y chromosome in one of their cell lines, gonadoblastoma is common. Therefore, prophylactic gonadectomy is necessary in these patients. Renal anomalies, usually duplicated collecting system or horseshoe kidney, occur in 40% of those with Turner syndrome. Congenital heart disease occurs in 20% of patients; common defects include coarctation of the aorta, aortic stenosis, and bicuspid aortic valve. As a consequence of having only one functional X chromosome, females with Turner syndrome display the same frequency of sex-linked disorders as males. The diagnosis is made by karyotype and fluorescent in-situ hybridization. Because of their mosaicism, some girls suspected of having Turner syndrome have a 46, XX karyotype in the peripheral blood, and a skin biopsy may be necessary to make the diagnosis.

Short stature has been successfully treated using human growth hormone. Secondary sexual characteristics develop after estrogen and progesterone administration. As mentioned earlier, gonadectomy is indicated in patients with dysgenetic gonads and the presence of a Y chromosome. With the rare exception of a few mosaics, women with Turner syndrome cannot become pregnant.

Klinefelter Syndrome

Klinefelter syndrome, caused by an extra X chromosome in males, affects 1 in 500 newborn males, 20% of aspermic adult men, and 1 in 250 men more than 6 ft tall. The karyotype is 47, XXY in 80% of cases and mosaic (XY/XXY) in 20%. Recurrence risk is the same as the initial risk in the general population.

Clinical Manifestations

The physical stigmata of Klinefelter syndrome are not obvious until puberty, at which time males are incompletely masculinized. They have a female body habitus with decreased body hair, gynecomastia, and small phallus and testes. Infertility results from hypospermia or aspermia. Affected males are usually taller than average relative to their families and their arm span can be greater than their height. There is an increased incidence of learning difficulties, but the average IQ is 98. Gonadotropin levels are usually elevated because of inadequate testosterone levels. Men with Klinefelter syndrome have a 20-fold increased incidence of breast cancer.

Testosterone therapy during adolescence may improve secondary sexual characteristics and prevent gynecomastia.

IMPRINTING DISORDERS

Imprinting refers to different phenotypes resulting from the same genotype, depending on whether the abnormal chromosome is inherited from the mother or father. **Uniparental disomy** is the term used when both chromosomes of a pair have been inherited from only one parent. Prader-Willi and Angelman syndromes are examples of imprinting, and some cases are also examples of uniparental disomy.

Prader-Willi Syndrome

Prader-Willi syndrome occurs in 1 per 15,000 newborns and is associated with a region of the long arm of chromosome 15 (15q11–13). Approximately 70% of those affected have a chromosome deletion in the paternally derived chromosome 15 and a normal maternal chromosome 15. Another 20% to 25% have normal-appearing chromosomes with two copies of maternal chromosome 15. This is known as **uniparental maternal disomy**, and the syndrome results from the lack of a paternal copy of chromosome 15. The remaining affected newborns have abnormalities of imprinting due to translocations narrowing the region. The recurrent risk for parents of an affected child is 1 in 100, unless the chromosome 15 deletion results from a parental translocation, which is extremely rare. The disorder is sporadic.

Clinical Manifestations

Dysmorphisms include narrow bifrontal diameter, almond-shaped eyes, a down-turned mouth, and small hands and feet. Short stature and hypogonadotropic hypogonadism with small genitalia and incomplete puberty are seen. These children suffer from severe hypotonia, which is associated with feeding difficulties and failure to thrive in infancy. By several years of age, these children develop an uncontrollable appetite that leads to severe central obesity. These children eat constantly unless food is locked away. Obesity-related obstructive sleep apnea and cardiorespiratory complications (Pickwickian syndrome) may develop. There is mild mental retardation with characteristic impulse-control problems.

For the average patient, strict dietary control is attempted but difficult to enforce. Although those affected can live normal life spans, complications of obesity such as obstructive sleep apnea and diabetes mellitus often lead to earlier death.

Angelman Syndrome

Approximately 60% of patients with Angelman syndrome have a microdeletion on the maternal chromosome 15 (deletion of 15q11–13) and a normal paternal chromosome 15. Five percent of cases result from **uniparental paternal disomy**, where two normal copies of paternally derived chromosome 15 are inherited. Five percent result from imprinting center mutations, and 5% are caused by a single gene mutation (UBE3A). Ten percent to 25% result from small subtelomeric deletions or translocations, or are of unknown etiology.

Clinical Manifestations

Dysmorphisms seen in Angelman syndrome include maxillary hypoplasia, large mouth, prognathism, and short stature. Patients are severely mentally retarded, with impaired or absent speech and inappropriate paroxysms of laughter. Jerky arm movements, ataxic gait, and tiptoe walk result in marionette-like movements, leading to its designation as the "happy puppet" syndrome. Most patients have seizures.

MOLECULAR CYTOGENIC DISORDERS

FRAGILE X SYNDROME

Fragile X, an X-linked form of mental retardation that occurs in 1 in 3,000 males, is an example of a trinucleotide repeat disorder. The gene involved, called FMR-1, is active in brain and sperm. In normal individuals, the DNA trinucleotide CGG is normally repeated about 6 to 54 times at the start of this gene. Those affected with fragile X have over 200 CGG repeats. The disorder received its name because a cytogenetically detectable breakage occurs at a specific fragile site on the X chromosome. Currently, Southern blot analysis and polymerase chain reaction (PCR) are used to determine the number of CGG repeats.

Clinical Manifestations

Individuals with Fragile X syndrome may have macrosomia at birth, macroorchidism due to testicular edema, dysmorphic facial features (large jaw and large ears), perseverative speech, and mental retardation (90% of affected males have an IQ between 20 and 49). Some males with fragile X syndrome have mental retardation as the sole manifestation. Up to 6% of patients with autism have Fragile X syndrome. There is no known treatment for Fragile X.

Female carriers of the fragile X chromosome may have a subnormal IQ or learning disabilities. Women with premutation (54 to 200 repeats) are at risk for premature ovarian failure. Males with premutation are at risk for Fragile X-associated tremor/ataxia syndrome, a neurodegenerative disorder.

CHROMOSOME 22Q11 DELETION SYNDROME

Microdeletion of 22q11.2 has been found in 90% of children with DiGeorge syndrome, in 70% of children with velocardiofacial syndrome, and in 15% of children with isolated conotruncal cardiac defects. Although the descriptive names of the above-mentioned disorders are still in use, the more general term **22q11.2 deletion syndrome** more appropriately encompasses the spectrum of abnormalities found in these children. Its prevalence in the general population is 1 per 4,000 live births. The deletion can be inherited (8% to 28% of cases), but more typically occurs as a de novo event. However, if a parent has the deletion, the risk to each child is 50%. The microdeletion can be detected using fluorescent in situ hybridization (FISH) probes or microarray.

Clinical Manifestations

Classic cardiac features of this spectrum of disorders include conotruncal defects such as tetralogy of Fallot, interrupted aortic arch, and vascular rings. Other common findings are absent thymus, hypocalcemic hypoparathyroidism, T-cell mediated immune deficiency, and palate abnormalities. These children usually have feeding difficulties, cognitive disabilities, and behavioral and speech disorders.

CHARGE SYNDROME

CHARGE is an acronym for a syndromic association of features including **C**oloboma of the retina or iris; ***H***eart abnormalities; ***A***tresia of the choanae; ***R***etarded growth; ***G***enital hypoplasia in males; and ***E***ar abnormalities that can include deafness and inner ear anomalies. Fifty percent of individuals with CHARGE syndrome can have a characteristic "hockey stick" palmar crease. CHARGE syndrome is caused by a point mutation in the gene *CHD7*.

OTHER MALFORMATIONS AND ASSOCIATIONS

Some syndromes without a detectable chromosomal abnormality have clinical features that suggest a chromosomal disorder. These syndromes often enter into the differential diagnosis of a suspected genetic disorder.

- **VATER** refers to the nonrandom association of ***V***ertebral and ***A***nal anomalies, ***T***racheoesophageal fistula with ***E***sophageal atresia, and ***R***adial or ***R***enal abnormalities.
- **Fetal alcohol syndrome** results from exposure to significant levels of serum alcohol during the prenatal period. Typical findings include short palpebral fissures, smooth philtrum, and thin upper lip. Affected infants may also have hypotonia, poor growth, developmental delay, congenital heart disease, and renal anomalies.

METABOLIC DISORDERS

APPROACH TO METABOLIC DISORDERS

Although individual metabolic disorders are rare, collectively they are responsible for significant morbidity and mortality. Inborn errors of metabolism are genetic diseases that occur when a defective protein disrupts a metabolic pathway at a specific step.

Precursors and toxic metabolites of excess precursors accumulate, and products needed for normal metabolism are deficient. Certain ethnic groups are at increased risk for specific metabolic errors.

Clinical presentation and age at onset vary. Urea cycle defects and organic acidemias present early in life with acute metabolic decompensation. Fatty acid oxidation and carbohydrate metabolism disorders usually present with lethargy, encephalopathy, and hypoglycemia after low carbohydrate intake or fasting. Lysosomal storage disorders are characterized by progressive hepatomegaly, splenomegaly, and, occasionally, neurologic deterioration. Findings that should increase suspicion for an inborn error of metabolism include emesis and acidosis after initiation of feeding, unusual odor of urine or sweat, hepatosplenomegaly, hyperammonemia, early infant death, failure to thrive, developmental regression, mental retardation, and seizures. Several important disorders are discussed here.

CARBOHYDRATE METABOLISM DISORDERS

Galactosemia

Galactosemia, the most common error of carbohydrate metabolism, is caused by a deficiency of the enzyme galactose-1-phosphate uridyltransferase, resulting in impaired conversion of galactose-1-phosphate to glucose-1-phosphate (which can undergo glycolysis). Galactose-1-phosphate accumulates in the liver, kidneys, and brain. The disorder occurs in 1 of 40,000 live births, and inheritance is autosomal recessive.

Clinical Manifestations

Clinical manifestations are noted within a few days to weeks after birth. Initial symptoms include evidence of liver failure (hepatomegaly, direct hyperbilirubinemia, disordered coagulation), renal dysfunction (acidosis, glycosuria, aminoaciduria), emesis, anorexia, and poor growth. Cataracts may develop by 2 months of age in untreated children. Infants with galactosemia are at increased risk of *Escherichia coli* sepsis. Older children can have severe learning disabilities, whether or not they were treated in infancy. Affected females have a high incidence of premature ovarian failure. Detecting reduced levels of erythrocyte galactose-1-phosphate uridyltransferase is diagnostic. Laboratory findings include a direct hyperbilirubinemia, elevated serum aminotransferase, prolonged prothrombin and partial thromboplastin times, hypoglycemia, and aminoaciduria. Galactose in the urine is detected by a positive reaction for reducing substances and no reaction with glucose oxidase on urine test strips.

Treatment

All formulas and foods containing galactose (including lactose-containing formulas and breast milk) must be eliminated from the infant's diet. Lactose free soy-based formulas should be substituted.

GLYCOGEN STORAGE DISEASES

Glycogen is a highly branched polymer of glucose that is stored in liver and muscle. Glycogen storage diseases (GSDs) are a group of conditions that result from deficiency of enzymes involved in glycogen synthesis or breakdown. Because many different enzymes are involved in glycogen metabolism, the clinical manifestations of the GSDs are variable. Typical manifestations include growth failure, hepatomegaly, and fasting hypoglycemia. The most common GSDs are **type I, von Gierke disease and type V, McArdle disease**. All are autosomal recessive disorders. Treatment is designed to prevent hypoglycemia while avoiding storage of even more glycogen in the liver.

AMINO ACID METABOLISM DISORDERS

Phenylketonuria

Phenylketonuria (PKU), the most common of these disorders, occurs in 1 in 10,000 live births. PKU results from a deficiency of phenylalanine hydroxylase, the enzyme that converts phenylalanine to tyrosine. With normal phenylalanine intake, patients develop high serum concentrations of toxic metabolites such as phenylacetic acid and phenyllactic acid.

Clinical Manifestations

Unlike most amino acid disorders, symptoms of untreated PKU develop gradually with progressive IQ loss during infancy. Neurologic manifestations include moderate to severe mental retardation, microcephaly, hypertonia, tremors, and behavioral problems. Tyrosine is needed for the production of melanin, so the block in the conversion of phenylalanine to tyrosine results in a light complexion. The patient's urine smells mouse-like from phenylacetic acid secretion.

Treatment

Prevention of mental retardation in PKU is achieved by early and lifelong dietary restriction of phenylalanine. All states include PKU detection in mandatory newborn screens. Women with PKU must decrease phenylalanine intake during pregnancy to avoid increasing their risk of having a child with microcephaly, mental retardation, and congenital heart disease.

Homocystinuria

Homocystinuria is caused by a defect in the amino acid metabolic pathway that converts methionine to cysteine and serine. The incidence of the cystathionine synthase deficiency is 1 in 100,000 live births. The neonatal screen used by most states detects increased methionine levels in the blood.

Clinical Manifestations

There are no symptoms in infancy. Clinical manifestations observed during childhood include a Marfan-like body habitus (long thin limbs and digits, scoliosis, sternal deformities, and osteoporosis), downward-dislocated eye lenses, mild to moderate mental retardation (60%), and vascular thromboses that result in childhood stroke, pulmonary embolism, or myocardial infarction.

Treatment

Dietary management is extremely difficult because restriction of sulfhydryl groups leads to a very low-protein, foul-tasting diet. Approximately 50% of patients respond to large dosages of pyridoxine.

Ornithine Transcarbamylase Deficiency

Ornithine transcarbamylase (OTC) deficiency, a urea cycle defect, is one of the few inborn errors of metabolism with X-linked inheritance. Amino acid catabolism produces free ammonia that is detoxified to urea through a series of reactions known as the **urea cycle**. In the urea cycle, ornithine joins with carbamoylphosphate through the action of OTC to form citrulline within the mitochondria. When OTC levels are less than 20% of normal, the nitrogen-containing moiety in ornithine cannot be quickly converted to urea for excretion and instead forms ammonia, which results in severe hyperammonemia when the patient consumes protein. Milder forms of the condition are seen in heterozygous females and in some affected males.

Clinical Manifestations

Within 24 to 48 hours after the initiation of protein-containing feedings, the newborn becomes progressively lethargic and may develop coma or seizures as the serum ammonia level rises. Female carriers may develop headaches and emesis after protein meals and manifest mental retardation and learning disabilities. Diagnosis is aided by measuring the level of orotic acid, a by-product of carbamoylphosphate metabolism, in the urine.

Treatment

Treatment centers on an extremely low-protein diet and the exploitation of alternative pathways for nitrogen excretion using benzoic acid and phenylacetate. Early intervention may minimize deleterious effects, but management is complex and extremely difficult for parents to maintain.

LYSOSOMAL STORAGE DISORDERS

Deficiency of a lysosomal enzyme causes its substrate to accumulate in lysosomes of tissues that degrade it, creating a characteristic clinical picture. These "storage" diseases are classified as mucopolysaccharidoses (e.g., Hurler, Hunter, and Sanfilippo syndromes), lipidoses (e.g., Niemann-Pick, Krabbe, Gaucher, and Tay-Sachs diseases), or mucolipidoses (e.g., fucosidosis and mannosidosis), depending on the nature of the stored material.

Hurler Syndrome

Deficiency of α-iduronidase leads to accumulation of the dermatan and heparan sulfates in tissues and their excretion in urine. Typical features include coarse facies, corneal clouding, exaggerated kyphosis, hepatosplenomegaly, umbilical hernia, and congenital heart disease. Developmental regression begins in the first year of life. Most children with Hurler syndrome die in early adolescence; the disease course and survival may be improved with stem cell transplant or enzyme replacement therapy.

Pompe Disease

A glycogen storage disease, Pompe disease is caused by deficiency of acid maltase that results in lysosomal accumulation of glycogen in muscle. It is characterized by profound hypotonia and extreme hypertrophic cardiomyopathy. Cognition is normal. The infantile form is usually fatal, due to cardiorespiratory failure, by 1 year of age. Early diagnosis and enzyme replacement therapy can be life saving.

Gaucher Disease

Gaucher disease is caused by deficiency of the enzyme β-glucosidase, leading to the accumulation of glucocerebroside. The classic form does not involve the central nervous system. Patients characteristically have hepatomegaly and splenomegaly. Storage of glucocerebroside in the bone marrow leads to anemia, leukopenia, thrombocytopenia, and recurrent episodes of bone pain. Radiologic changes include an Erlenmeyer flask shape of the distal femur. A low enzyme level in the white blood cells confirms the diagnosis. Recombinant enzyme therapy improves most symptoms.

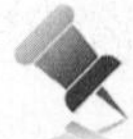

KEY POINTS

ENVIRONMENTAL FACTORS

- Environmental factors account for 10% of birth defects.
- Infectious agents, high-dose radiation, maternal metabolic disorders (e.g., diabetes, PKU), mechanical forces and drugs can all cause birth defects.
- A teratogenic exposure before 12 weeks' gestation affects organogenesis and tissue morphogenesis, whereas an exposure thereafter usually retards fetal growth and affects central nervous system development.

GENETIC FACTORS

- Single-gene defects are classified by their mode of inheritance as autosomal dominant, autosomal recessive, and X-linked disorders.
- Defective genes in autosomal dominant disorders typically encode structural proteins, whereas those in autosomal recessive disorders encode enzymes.
- In variable penetrance, there may be variable expression of a defective gene with variable degree of severity in affected individuals.
- Most inborn errors of metabolism are autosomal recessive disorders, with the exception of ornithine transcarbamylase deficiency (OTC) and some mitochondrial disorders.

CHROMOSOMAL DISORDERS

- Approximately 50% of first-trimester spontaneous abortions have chromosomal abnormalities.
- Birth defects caused by autosomal anomalies are generally more severe than those caused by sex chromosome anomalies.
- Indications for chromosomal studies (karyotype, FISH, microarray) include confirmation of a suspected chromosomal syndrome, multiple organ system malformations, significant developmental delay or cognitive impairment not otherwise explained, short stature or extremely delayed menarche in girls, infertility or a history of multiple spontaneous abortions, ambiguous genitalia, or advanced maternal age.

METABOLIC DISORDERS

- Decompensation from inborn errors of metabolism can be preceded by introduction of certain foods, changes in frequency of feeding or fasting states.
- Age of presentation with decompensation can be helpful in considering inborn errors in the differential. Severe, newborn illness may be associated with galactosemia, and ornithine transcarbamylase deficiency (OTC is X-linked).
- Early identification of Hurler syndrome, Gaucher's disease, and Pompe's disease would allow for enzyme replacement therapy and/or stem cell transplant (Hurler).

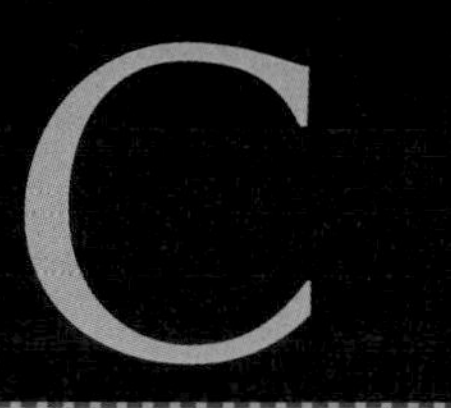

C Clinical Vignettes

Vignette 1

You are called to the full-term nursery to evaluate an infant with dysmorphic features. The infant is the product of a full-term pregnancy born via SVD to a 23-year-old G_1P_0 mother. The infant has brachycephaly, midface hypoplasia, epicanthal folds, upslanting palpebral fissures, small low-set rotated ears, a small mouth, and micrognathia with protruding tongue.

1. What other finding might support a clinical diagnosis when examining this infants' hands and feet?
   a. Hockey stick palmar crease
   b. Single palmar crease
   c. Rocker bottom feet
   d. Clenched hands with overlapping fingers
   e. Polydactyly

2. Which of the following tests would confirm the diagnosis and elucidate the recurrence risk for these parents?
   a. Chromosome 21 FISH for Down syndrome
   b. CHD7 sequencing for CHARGE syndrome
   c. 22q11 FISH studies for 22q11 deletion syndrome
   d. Karyotype
   e. State newborn screening

3. Beyond the findings above, the physical examination of this infant is completely unremarkable. In addition to CBC with differential, renal ultrasound, and statewide newborn screen, which of the following should be obtained while waiting for genetic test results, based on clinical suspicion?
   a. Head ultrasound to evaluate for brain anomalies
   b. Swallow study to evaluate for TE fistula
   c. Echocardiogram to evaluate for congenital heart disease
   d. Conjugated bilirubin for biliary anomalies
   e. Spinal ultrasound to evaluate for dysraphism

4. If there is an associated congenital heart anomaly, which of the following is most likely to be present?
   a. Complete AV canal (AVSD)
   b. Transposition of the great arteries (TGA)
   c. Coarctation of the aorta
   d. Ebstein anomaly
   e. Supravalvular aortic stenosis

5. Which of the following conditions is NOT a frequently noted comorbidity in individuals with Down syndrome?
   a. Hirschprung disease
   b. Alzheimer-like dementia
   c. Leukemia
   d. Hypothyroidism
   e. Hyperphagia

6. The karyotype results for this infant suggest an unbalanced 14q21q translocation with duplication of material on chromosome 21. Study of parental blood karyotype finds that this mother is a balanced carrier of this translocation. What would you expect would be the risk of this couple having another child with Down syndrome?
   a. Approximately the same as the general population risk
   b. Dependent on maternal age
   c. Slightly higher than the general population risk, to account for gonadal mosaicism
   d. Much higher than the general population risk

Vignette 2

During a 2-year well child examination, you note a male with hyperactivity, motor and speech delay, and autistic features. His pregnant mother mentions that she is concerned as her brother and her maternal uncle both have mental retardation, and these individuals behaved similarly as preschoolers. Physical examination is remarkable for large ears, and the child is nonverbal with hand-flapping behavior.

1. Which of the following tests is most likely to reveal this child's diagnosis?
   a. Karyotype
   b. DNA microarray
   c. FISH
   d. Southern blot for CGG repeats
   e. Serum amino acids and urine organic acids
   f. Methylation PCR for Prader-Willi/Angelman

2. If this testing is positive, what is the recurrence risk in the upcoming pregnancy?
   a. 50% in male newborns
   b. 50%in female newborns
   c. 100% in male newborns
   d. 50% in all newborns
   e. 25% in all newborns

Vignette 3

You are caring for infants in the neonatal intensive care unit (NICU). You receive a STAT page to a delivery room to resuscitate a term newborn full-term male with cyanosis. His color does not improve with intubation. His chest radiograph is notable for absent thymus. Echocardiogram reveals truncus arteriosus. You suspect a genetic diagnosis and following stabilization send the appropriate testing.

1. What electrolyte is especially important to follow in managing this infant?
   - **a.** Potassium
   - **b.** Magnesium
   - **c.** Glucose
   - **d.** Phosphorus
   - **e.** Calcium

Vignette 4

You are caring for "feeders and growers" in the NICU. One infant girl has very low muscle tone and requires nasograstric-tube feeding, as she cannot feed from a bottle. The feeding team has tried "everything" with no success, and a gastrostomy tube is being considered. While prerounding, you notice she has upslanting almond-shaped eyes and small hands and feet.

1. Which of the following would be the most likely diagnosis in this infant?
   - **a.** Down syndrome (Trisomy 21)
   - **b.** Angelman syndrome
   - **c.** Prader-Willi syndrome
   - **d.** 22q11.2 deletion syndrome
   - **e.** Pompe disease

2. What is the most likely inheritance of this syndrome in this patient?
   - **a.** Maternal deletion of 15q11-13
   - **b.** Paternal deletion of 15q11-13
   - **c.** Mutation of imprinting center
   - **d.** Maternal uniparental disomy
   - **e.** Paternal uniparental disomy

A Answers

Vignette 1 Question 1
Answer B: Single palmar crease (simian crease), a horizontal crease extending across the palm, is associated with Down syndrome. A superior palmar crease shaped like a hockey stick is present in 50% of individuals with CHARGE syndrome. Rocker bottom feet are a feature of Trisomy 18 syndrome. Clenched hands with overlapping fingers are eatures of both Trisomy 13 and 18 syndromes. Polydactyly is a feature of Trisomy 13 syndrome. Of note, unaffected newborns may also have single palmar creases.

Vignette 1 Question 2
Answer D: Karyotyping will confirm the diagnosis and provide information regarding the likelihood of these parents having another affected child. The patient in this vignette has multiple features of Down syndrome. A karyotype is indicated to assess for unbalanced translocations, which are more common when the mother is young and are associated with increased risk of recurrence. A chromosome 21 FISH would detect trisomy 21 duplication but not unbalanced translocations. Answers B and C test for conditions other than Down syndrome, as noted. State newborn screening varies from region to region but typically includes screening for hypothyroidism, metabolic disorders, congenital adrenal hypoplasia, and sickle cell disease.

Vignette 1 Question 3
Answer C: The septal defects most commonly associated with Down syndrome may not be discernible via auscultation in the newborn period. Congenital brain anomalies are commonly found in infants with Trisomy 13. A swallow study would be appropriate in an infant with VACTERL syndrome. Biliary anomalies are common in infants with Alagille syndrome. There is no increased association of dysraphisms with Down syndrome.

Vignette 1 Question 4
Answer A: Endocardial cushion defects are common in infants with Down syndrome. Fifty percent of infants with Down syndrome may have a complete AV canal. TGA is rarely found in syndromic conditions but may be noted in cases of prenatal trimethadione exposures. Coarctation of the aorta is commonly found in girls with Turner syndrome. Ebstein anomaly is associated with prenatal lithium exposure. Supravalvular aortic stenosis is more common in patients with Williams syndrome (7q11.23 deletion).

Vignette 1 Question 5
Answer E: Hyperphagia (excessive eating) is typically associated with Prader-Willi syndrome. The other conditions listed are known possible comorbidities of Down syndrome.

Vignette 1 Question 6
Answer D: Since one of the parents is a carrier of a balanced Robertsonian translocation, the risk of having another child with Down syndrome is greatly increased, about 10% overall. The risk for full trisomy 21 depends on maternal age (Answer B); however this infant has an unbalanced translocation. In this scenario, the mother's balanced carrier status was confirmed on karyotype from peripheral blood, so there is no gonadal mosaicism.

Vignette 2 Question 1
Answer D: The most likely diagnosis is Fragile X syndrome. Fragile X is the most common X-linked cause of mental retardation. It is also the most common genetic cause of autism. This patient's mother is describing X-linked inheritance in her family; both she and her mother are carriers of this disease. Fragile X syndrome is detected with >200 CGG repeats on Southern Blot or PCR testing. It would not be detected on karyotype, microarray, FISH, metabolic studies, or methylation PCR for Prader-Willi/Angelman, any of which may be employed in evaluating a child with developmental delay. Individuals with Angelman syndrome can have autistic features; however, Angelman is typically sporadic.

Vignette 2 Question 2
Answer A: Newborn boys of a mother who is a carrier of Fragile X syndrome have a 50% risk of Fragile X syndrome, as they either inherit the affected X chromosome or a normal X chromosome from their mother. Newborn girls have a 50% risk of being carriers. Parents with autosomal dominant disorders such as 22q11 deletion syndrome have a 50% risk of recurrence in all male and female pregnancies. In autosomal dominant disorders, the progeny can either inherit the normal allele or mutant allele from an affected parent. Autosomal recessive disorders, such as galactosemia, have a 25% risk of recurrence in all pregnancies, where each parent carries a mutant allele with a normal allele, and the affected child inherits both mutant alleles.

Vignette 3 Question 1
Answer E: This patient has a conotruncal heart defect (truncus arteriosus) and did not have a visible thymus on chest radiograph. These

two conditions lead to high suspicion for 22q11.2 deletion syndrome. Individuals with 22q11.2 deletion syndrome can have hypoparathyroidism leading to hypocalcemia, especially in the newborn period as they are weaning off maternal calcium support. The magnesium level may also be affected (low), and phosphorus may be high due to low parathyroid levels. Hypocalcemia would put this critically ill infant at risk for tonic seizures and possibly heart failure. The appropriate genetic testing to send for this infant is 22q11 FISH or microarray.

Vignette 4 Question 1

Answer C: The correct answer is Prader-Willi syndrome, associated with extreme hypotonia and feeding problems in the newborn period and these physical characteristic features. Individuals with Down syndrome may have upslanting palpebral fissures and brachydactyly (short fingers), but their palms are normally sized. The extremely low muscle tone and dysmorphic features described in this patient are not consistent with Angelman or 22q11.2 deletion syndrome. Pompe disease can be associated with extreme hypotonia, but this is typically due to progressive glycogen deposition, so is not present in the newborn period. Additionally, individuals with Pompe disease do not typically have dysmorphic features.

Vignette 4 Question 2

Answer B: Prader-Willi is an epigenetic disorder. It may be inherited via paternal deletion (70%), maternal uniparental disomy (UPD; 20% to 25%), or translocation involving the imprinting center (5%). Maternal deletions (60%) and paternal UPD (5%) in this same genetic region result in Angelman syndrome, as do imprinting center mutations.

Chapter

19 Ophthalmology

Constance West • Melanie Bradley • Katie S. Fine • Bradley S. Marino

VISION SCREENING

Vision screening in children is critical because the young eye is part of a dynamic system that may be quickly damaged by visual deprivation. The development of normal vision requires the production of *clear retinal images* and *proper eye alignment*. Table 19-1 lists the American Association of Pediatric Ophthalmology and Strabismus's recommendations for eye examination, vision screening, and referral. Children older than 8 years can be screened according to adult guidelines. Patients with a history of prematurity, intrauterine infection, CNS disease, or family history of ocular disease are at higher risk for eye pathology and require more extensive follow-up by a pediatric ophthalmologist.

STRABISMUS

Strabismus, or misalignment of the eyes, occurs in approximately 4% of children. When strabismus occurs in a child younger than 4 to 6 years, the child's brain may begin to "suppress" the image from the deviating eye, resulting in amblyopia. Amblyopia is found in the majority of patients with esotropia, and sometimes with exotropia or vertical deviations. Certain neurologic diseases are associated with an especially high incidence of strabismus, including cerebral palsy, Down syndrome, hydrocephalus, and brain tumors. Unilateral visual deprivation (e.g., ptosis) may also be associated with or lead to strabismus.

CLINICAL MANIFESTATIONS

The deviating eye of a patient with strabismus may turn inward (esotropia), outward (exotropia), upward, or downward. Diagnosis is made using the corneal light reflex and cover tests. (Note: With one eye covered, the patient fixes vision on an object. When the obscured eye is quickly uncovered, no eye movement should be detectable. The test is repeated on the other side. If eye drift is noted when either eye is uncovered, this is considered a positive cover test.)

TREATMENT

The most important consequences of untreated strabismus, aside from the cosmetic deformity, are **amblyopia** (discussed later in the chapter) and reduced stereopsis (depth perception). Treatment is aimed at eliminating or preventing amblyopia, realigning the eyes, and addressing any underlying/predisposing condition (if present). Some causes of strabismus respond to corrective lenses, occlusion, and/or atropine penalization, but usually surgery is needed as well. **Early medical and surgical intervention results in an improved chance for establishing normal acuity and alignment.**

AMBLYOPIA

Amblyopia, literally meaning "dull sight," describes the development of reduced vision in an otherwise normal eye. The condition occurs in 2% to 5% of the general population. Children are most susceptible between birth and 7 years of age. The earlier amblyopia develops, the more severe the visual defect. Strabismic amblyopia (about one-third of cases) is caused by suppression of retinal images from a misaligned eye. Anisometropic amblyopia (unequal refractive errors in the two eyes) causes a blurred retinal image in one eye and is responsible for amblyopia about a third of the time. The remaining cases are mixed mechanism and associated with both strabismus and anisometropia. Visual deprivation amblyopia due to opacities of the visual axis (e.g., corneal opacity, cataracts) is the least common cause of amblyopia. Other risk factors include premature birth and a family history of amblyopia or strabismus.

CLINICAL MANIFESTATIONS

Subnormal vision is the only sign of amblyopia. Untreated amblyopia leads to permanent vision loss and diminished stereopsis.

TREATMENT

The first step in treating amblyopia involves correcting any refractive errors with glasses. Visual opacities such as cataracts, if present, should be removed. Proper alignment must be restored. Finally, **occlusion** of the better-seeing eye forces visual development of the affected eye and the visual centers in the brain corresponding with that eye. Early intervention is crucial to promote normal vision; **beyond 8 years of age, treatment is usually unlikely to be successful**.

TABLE 19-1 Pediatric Eye Exam and Vision Screening Recommendations from the American Association of Pediatric Ophthalmology and Strabismus

Age	Method	Indications for Referral
Newborn	Red reflexes	Absent, white, dull, opacity, or asymmetric
	External inspection	Structural abnormality
	Pupil examination	Irregular shape, unequal size, poor or unequal reaction
3 to 6 months	Fix and follow to light or toy	Failure to fix and follow in a cooperative infant
	Red reflexes	Absent, white, dull, opacity, or asymmetric
	External inspection	Structural abnormality
	Pupil examination	Irregular shape, unequal size, poor or unequal reaction
6 to 12 months and until child is able to cooperate for verbal visual acuity	Fix and follow with each eye	Failure to fix and follow
	Alternate occlusion	Failure to object equally to covering each eye
	Corneal light reflex	Asymmetric or displaced
	Red reflexes	Absent, white, dull, opacity, or asymmetric
	External inspection	Structural abnormality
	Pupil examination	Irregular shape, unequal size, poor or unequal reaction
3 and 4 years	Visual acuity[a] (monocular)	20/50 or worse, or 2 lines of difference between the eyes
	Corneal light reflection/cover–uncover	Asymmetric/ocular refixation movements
	Red reflexes	Absent, white, dull, opacity, or asymmetric
	External inspection	Structural abnormality
	Pupil examination	Irregular shape, unequal size, poor or unequal reaction
5 years	Visual acuity[a] (monocular)	20/40 or worse, or 2 lines of difference between the eyes
	All other tests and referral indications are as in age 3 and 4 years	
Every 1 to 2 years after age 5	Visual acuity[a] (monocular)	20/30 or worse, or 2 lines of difference between the eyes
	All other tests and referral indications are as in age 3 and 4 years	

Note: These recommendations are based on panel consensus from the American Association of Pediatric Ophthalmology and Strabismus, updated 2007.
[a]Figures, letters, tumbling E or optotypes, Lea symbols (Good-Lite, Elgin, IL), vision-testing machines.

LEUKOCORIA

Leukocoria (white pupil or absence of the red reflex) in an infant or child may be caused by a number of entities, ranging from isolated ocular abnormalities to life-threatening systemic disease (Color Plate 26). All cases of leukocoria require prompt ophthalmologic referral.

DIFFERENTIAL DIAGNOSIS

Retinoblastoma, the most common intraocular malignancy of childhood, is a life-threatening cause of leukocoria. The disease occurs in approximately 1 in 20,000 live births, resulting in 300 new cases in the United States each year. The associated genetic defect is found on the q14 band of chromosome 13. Untreated retinoblastoma leads to death from brain and visceral metastasis in almost all cases.

Cataracts (opacities of the crystalline lens) occur in 1 of every 250 newborns, thus making cataracts the most common cause of leukocoria. They may be congenital or acquired and may be unilateral or bilateral. Cataracts are often genetically determined but may result from metabolic diseases or intrauterine infections.

Retinopathy of prematurity (ROP) is a retinal vascular disease of premature infants that can also lead to leukocoria. Risk factors include birth weight less than 1,500 g, gestational age less than 30 weeks, mechanical ventilation, and need for supplemental oxygen.

Other causes of leukocoria include congenital glaucoma and ocular toxocariasis (a parasitic infection most frequently acquired in infancy or young childhood).

CLINICAL MANIFESTATIONS

Leukocoria is detectable by routine screening of the **red reflex** in all neonates. Infants at high risk for retinoblastoma (positive family history in a first- or second-degree relative) or the development of ROP should be examined by an experienced ophthalmologist.

TREATMENT

Successful therapy combines treatment of the underlying condition with attention to associated amblyopia. Treatment of retinoblastoma may include **enucleation** (removal of the eye), chemotherapy, radiation therapy, and/or cryotherapy. Small or localized tumors may not require enucleation. Prognosis is directly related to the size of the tumor at diagnosis, and cure rates approach 90%. If retinoblastoma is not bilateral at presentation, the patient should be closely followed because 20% will develop another tumor in the previously unaffected eye.

Unilateral or bilateral congenital cataracts may be surgically removed. The visual prognosis for children requiring cataract extraction is not as good as that seen in adults because amblyopia or associated ocular abnormalities may limit the ultimate level of visual acuity. Congenital cataracts that are not removed by 2 to 3 months of age result in significant, usually irreversible, amblyopia.

Most cases of ROP regress spontaneously; however, laser ablation of the retina or cryotherapy performed at an intermediate stage of ROP reduces progression to retinal detachment and scarring. Infants with treated or regressed ROP remain at risk for the development of amblyopia, strabismus, myopia, and visual impairment. Some premature infants with periventricular leukomalacia develop central visual loss and may have difficulty with special orientation and other complex visual tasks.

NASOLACRIMAL DUCT OBSTRUCTION

Congenital nasolacrimal duct obstruction (dacryostenosis), a common cause of overflow tearing, occurs in about a quarter of neonates. Obstruction is usually caused by failure of the distal membranous end of the nasolacrimal duct to open.

CLINICAL MANIFESTATIONS

Chronic tearing in the absence of conjunctival injection is the hallmark of nasolacrimal duct obstruction. The presence of mucopurulent discharge and tenderness over the medial aspect of the lower lid suggests superimposed infection of the nasolacrimal sac (dacryocystitis). Less common causes of excess tearing in infancy include chronic irritation from allergens and infantile glaucoma.

Congenital nasolacrimal duct obstruction causes tearing with some mattering on the lashes, while infantile glaucoma is associated with corneal clouding, photophobia, and limbal conjunctival injection. Buphthalmos (increased corneal diameter accompanying infantile glaucoma) is a later finding in infantile glaucoma; evaluation by an ophthalmologist is warranted if there is any concern about infantile glaucoma.

TREATMENT

Treatment varies according to the severity of symptoms. The obstruction resolves spontaneously by 1 year of age in 96% of infants. Referral to an ophthalmologist is indicated if symptoms persist. **Probing** of the nasolacrimal duct system is performed at 12 to 15 months of age unless severe symptoms warrant earlier intervention. Superimposed dacryocystitis should be treated with warm compresses, nasolacrimal massage, and systemic antibiotics (i.e., a first-generation cephalosporin) in select cases.

OPHTHALMIA NEONATORUM

Ophthalmia neonatorum refers to conjunctivitis occurring within the first month of life. Any ocular discharge in the neonate requires evaluation because tears are usually absent in the first few weeks of life.

DIFFERENTIAL DIAGNOSIS

Common causes of ophthalmia neonatorum include chemical irritation, *Chlamydia trachomatis*, and *Neisseria gonorrhoeae*. Chemical conjunctivitis can be caused by birth trauma or by antibiotic prophylaxis given at birth to prevent gonococcal infection. Less common infectious causes, including herpes simplex virus (HSV), *Staphylococcus aureus*, *Haemophilus influenzae*, and *Pseudomonas aeruginosa*, typically manifest after the first week of life. Nasolacrimal duct obstruction should be considered in older neonates with persistent conjunctival discharge.

CLINICAL MANIFESTATIONS

Infants usually present with eyelid edema, conjunctival hyperemia, and ocular discharge. Age at onset and clinical features may suggest the diagnosis, but appropriate laboratory evaluation is required (Table 19-2).

TREATMENT AND PREVENTION

Infants with suspected gonococcal, HSV, or *P. aeruginosa* conjunctivitis should be referred to an ophthalmologist. Infants with conjunctivitis related to other causes require referral if signs worsen or symptoms persist after 3 days of treatment. Parents and their sexual partners should be treated for *Chlamydia* and gonococcal infections in the usual manner.

The incidence of neonatal conjunctivitis has decreased dramatically since the introduction of ocular prophylaxis with silver nitrate. **Erythromycin**, effective against both C. *trachomatis* and *N. gonorrhoeae*, currently is preferred.

INFECTIOUS CONJUNCTIVITIS

After the newborn period, infectious conjunctivitis (**pink eye**) is very common in childhood and may be bacterial or viral in origin. The infection causes inflammation in the conjunctiva, which overlies the sclera. Adenovirus in particular is a frequent cause of viral conjunctivitis.

DIFFERENTIAL DIAGNOSIS

Inflammation of the conjunctiva may be precipitated by exposure to allergens, toxins, chemicals, or irritants. Some systemic diseases may also have "red eyes" as part of the presentation.

Corneal abrasions may present with a red, painful, tearing eye that is sensitive to light. Examination of the eye with a blue-filtered light following instillation of **fluorescein** reveals the denuded area. Corneal abrasions are treated with eye patching (to decrease pain and promote healing) and topical antibiotics. Most heal within 24 hours.

CLINICAL MANIFESTATIONS

Table 19-3 compares and contrasts the clinical manifestations of viral, bacterial, and allergic conjunctivitis.

■ **TABLE 19-2** Distinguishing Features of Ophthalmia Neonatorum

Features	Chemical	*N. Gonorrhoeae*	*C. Trachomatis*
Age at onset	24 hours	2–4 days	4–10 days
Clinical features	Bilateral Serous discharge Conjunctival hyperemia	Bilateral Purulent discharge Marked eyelid edema	Unilateral or bilateral Mucopurulent discharge Conjunctival hyperemia
Complications	Self-limited	Sepsis Meningitis Arthritis Corneal ulceration Blindness	Corneal scarring Pneumonia
Diagnosis	Exclude serious causes	Conjunctival culture on chocolate or Thayer-Martin agar	Conjunctival *Chlamydia* culture; direct immunofluorescence antibody test
Treatment	None	Topical erythromycin; intravenous ceftriaxone Treat parents	Oral plus topical erythromycin; treat parent

■ **TABLE 19-3** Comparison of Viral, Bacterial, and Allergic Conjunctivitis

Symptom	Viral	Bacterial	Allergic
Pain	Mild	Mild to moderate	None
Discharge	Clear Mild to copious Prone to crusting	Mucopurulent Mild to copious Definite crusting	Clear Mild to moderate No crusting
Itching	Usually absent	Absent	Present
Injection	Diffuse	Diffuse	Diffuse
Vision	Normal	Normal	Normal
Possible etiologies	Adenovirus, ECHO virus, coxsackievirus	*Haemophilus influenzae, Streptococcus pneumoniaem, Neisseria gonorrhoeae*	Seasonal pollen or other allergen exposure

TREATMENT

In practice, most cases of infectious conjunctivitis are treated with a trial of antibiotic drops or ointment for 5 to 7 days. Choices include polymyxin-bacitracin, trimethoprim-polymyxin B, sodium sulfacetamide, erythromycin, or ofloxacin. Refractory cases require culture results to guide therapy. Although both viral and most bacterial conjunctivitis are usually self-limited diseases, antibiotics limit infectivity and decrease disease duration by approximately 2 days. (Notable exceptions include *Neisseria gonorrhoeae* conjunctivitis, which must be treated with parenteral ceftriaxone, and *Haemophilus influenzae* conjunctivitis that occurs in conjunction with same-sided otitis media, which must be treated with appropriate oral agents.)

Antibiotic drops that contain steroids (to decrease inflammation) must **not** be given if HSV-1 is thought to be the cause of the infection because there is an increased risk of more severe disease and visual impairment.

HORDEOLUM AND CHALAZION (STYES)

A **hordeolum** is an acute infection of the meibomian glands (internal hordeolum) or the sebaceous glands surrounding the eyelash follicle (external hordeolum). *Staphylococcus aureus* is the usual culprit. Localized tender swelling progresses to a point, which ruptures to the outside. Treatment involves warm compresses; the value of ophthalmic antibiotics is questionable. Occasionally, incision and drainage or systemic antibiotics may be indicated if an acute cellulitis develops.

Chalazions are areas of sterile lipogranulomatous reaction within the meibomian glands in the tarsal plate that may progressively enlarge. The affected area is typically firm but nontender. Excision may be required for cosmetic purposes or if the area becomes irritated and produces a mass effect. The condition may be chronic and recurrent; good lid hygiene can reduce the risk of recurrence.

PERIORBITAL CELLULITIS

Periorbital (preseptal) cellulitis is caused by bacterial infection of the eyelids and surrounding skin anterior to the orbital septum, a fibrous band that separates the subcutaneous lid from the orbit itself.

PATHOGENESIS

Bacteria gain access to the area around the eye through breaks in the skin (*Staphylococcus aureus*, group A *streptococcus*), hematogenous dissemination (*Streptococcus pneumoniae, Haemophilus influenzae*), insect bites, or via extension from infected sinuses or other upper respiratory structures (*S. pneumoniae, H. influenzae, Moraxella catarrhalis*). Both the Hib vaccine and the pneumococcal conjugate vaccine have contributed to a measurable decline in the incidence of periorbital infections.

DIFFERENTIAL DIAGNOSIS

Orbital cellulitis, in which the infection extends posterior to the orbital septum, is an emergency. Severe pain with eye movement, proptosis, vision changes, and decreased ocular mobility accompany this disease. A CT scan should be considered to confirm the diagnosis, identify any coinfected structures (e.g., sinuses), and delineate extension. Associated orbital abscesses sometimes require surgical drainage. Empirical parenteral antibiotic therapy should provide coverage against *S. aureus, S. pyogenes, S. pneumoniae, H. influenzae, M. catarrhalis*, and anaerobic bacteria found in the upper respiratory tract. Suggested regimens include cefuroxime (with clindamycin added if anaerobic infection is suspected) or ampicillin/sulbactam. Periorbital edema and erythema that accompany orbital cellulitis may be slow to resolve. When the patient appears recovered, he or she may be released with oral antibiotics to complete a 3-week course. Brain abscesses, meningitis, and cavernous sinus thrombosis are infrequent but serious complications of orbital cellulitis.

Other causes of a swollen eyelid include trauma, edema, allergies, and tumor.

CLINICAL MANIFESTATIONS

In periorbital cellulitis, the skin around the eye is indurated, warm, and tender, although there is no true eye pain. Fever is variably present in cases of localized skin trauma. In the young child with hematogenous seeding or extension as the source, the fever is generally quite high, with rapid progression of the swelling. The physical examination may reveal sinus tenderness, sore throat, or a point of entry on the skin. It is important to mark the area of induration to assist in documenting subsequent resolution (or lack thereof). Any child with signs or symptoms consistent with meningitis (Chapter 10) should receive a lumbar puncture.

TREATMENT

Intravenous antibiotics should begin as soon as possible and be continued until resolution of induration. For periorbital cellulitis that follows a break in the skin, a penicillinase-resistant penicillin or a first-generation cephalosporin is appropriate. Vancomycin may be required depending on local resistance patterns. Cefuroxime is the antibiotic of choice in other cases; occasionally, a third-generation cephalosporin is used to prevent extension to the meninges in the young child. The patient may be released with oral antibiotics to complete a 10-day course when symptoms abate.

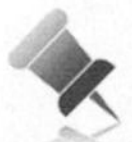

KEY POINTS

- Screening for strabismus by means of cover testing should be included in every pediatric health maintenance examination. Early recognition and treatment offer the best chance for avoiding permanent visual abnormalities.
- Amblyopia represents a common and potentially reversible cause of vision loss in children. Strabismus is the most common cause of amblyopia in children. Successful treatment depends on early recognition and referral for occlusion therapy and elimination of predisposing conditions.
- The most common cause of leukocoria is a congenital cataract. All cases of leukocoria require prompt ophthalmologic referral.
- All infants at high risk for retinopathy of prematurity should be seen by an ophthalmologist before discharge from the nursery.
- Retinoblastoma should be diagnosed early and treated aggressively to secure a favorable outcome.
- Nasolacrimal duct obstruction is a common cause of tearing in infants and neonates and typically resolves spontaneously. Referral is indicated if symptoms persist beyond 9 to 12 months of age and for infants with recurrent dacryocystitis.
- Conjunctivitis in the neonate may represent chemical irritation or acquired infection. *Chlamydia trachomatis* and *Neisseria gonorrhoeae* are the most common infectious agents.
- Conjunctivitis in the older child can be caused by infectious agents (bacteria, viruses) as well as systemic disease, irritants, and allergen exposure.
- Corneal abrasions may be diagnosed by examining the surface of an eye that has been exposed to fluorescein drops under a blue-filter light.
- Orbital cellulitis, characterized by (a combination of) eye pain, decreased mobility, vision changes, and proptosis, is a true emergency. Surgical drainage of associated abscesses may be required. Periorbital cellulitis may originate from a break in the skin, hematogenous spread, or by extension of respiratory or sinus bacteria.

C Clinical Vignettes

Vignette 1

A 4-year-old male who has not seen a doctor since 6 months of age presents to your office. His parents have refused all vaccinations. He was referred to you by his prekindergarten program when he failed his vision screening. You confirm that on the Snellen test, the child has 20/20 vision in the right eye and 20/80 vision in the left. The corneal light reflexes are asymmetric.

1. Which of the following is most likely to be abnormal in this patient?
   a. Red reflexes
   b. Fundoscopic examination
   c. Conjunctival culture
   d. Cover/uncover test
   e. Fluorescein examination

2. Given the patient's physical findings and screening results, which of the following is the most likely diagnosis?
   a. Isolated strabismus
   b. Isolated amblyopia
   c. Strabismic amblyopia
   d. Anisometropic amblyopia
   e. Visual deprivation amblyopia

3. The parents are concerned about the possibility of strabismus in their 1-month-old infant, since he occasionally looks "cross-eyed." The pregnancy was full-term, and there were no pre- or perinatal complications. The grandmother is babysitting the infant in her home at the moment. The patient's 1-month-old sibling should be referred to a pediatric ophthalmologist to evaluate for strabismus at what age if the corneal light reflexes continue to display occasional asymmetry?
   a. Now
   b. 2 months of age
   c. 4 months of age
   d. 6 months of age
   e. 9 months of age

Vignette 2

You are seeing a new baby for hospital follow-up. The patient is the product of a full-term pregnancy and vaginal delivery without complications. Weight, length, tone, and primitive reflexes are appropriate for gestational age. In response to your questioning, the parents respond that the baby does fix his gaze on their faces when they get close to him. A normal red reflex is present on the left. No red reflex is noted on the right; in fact, the pupil appears white.

1. Which of the following is the most likely cause of this patient's abnormal eye examination?
   a. Congenital cataract
   b. Optic neuritis
   c. Retinoblastoma
   d. Ocular toxocariasis
   e. Retinopathy of prematurity

2. A congenital cataract is confirmed in this neonate. After consulting with the pediatric ophthalmologist, who recommends surgical extraction, they still have grave concerns about the administration of anesthesia to an infant so young. They propose waiting until the child is older to remove the cataract. Which of the following represents your best advice to these parents?
   a. The cataract should be removed as soon as possible.
   b. The cataract should be removed by 3 months of age.
   c. The cataract should be removed by 6 months of age.
   d. The cataract does not need to be removed because the infant is likely already blind in the affected eye.
   e. Removal of the cataract in a timely manner will result in unaffected vision.

Vignette 3

A 4-year-old female is brought to your office in February for an acute care visit. A medical student who has already seen and examined the patient presents his history and physical examination findings. Yesterday her caretaker was called by her daycare to pick her up because she had "pink eye." The history is significant for 4 days of mild clear nasal discharge without itching, an infrequent, moist cough without associated increased work of breathing, and absence of fever. She is otherwise acting well. Her mother notes that her eyes do not seem to bother her even though they are slightly red, but she did wake up with some crusting this morning. She seems to be tearing more than usual but the parent has not noted any pus from the eyes. The physical examination reveals stable vital signs, a clear chest, mildly erythematous nasal turbinates, normal oropharynx, and moderate symmetric bilateral conjunctival injection associated with some clear tearing.

1. This patient's history and physical examination are most consistent with infection with which of the following organisms?
   a. Haemophilus influenzae
   b. Adenovirus
   c. Neisseria gonorrhoeae
   d. Chlamydia trachomatis
   e. Staphylococcus aureus

2. You confirm the history and physical examination findings, noting as well that the left tympanic membrane is opaque, erythematous, hypomobile, and bulging with displacement and blunting of the cone of light. Upon questioning, the mother tells you that the child has had only one previous ear infection (age 2 years) which cleared with "the pink, good-tasting medicine." Her physician did not note any fluid in the ear at her most recent health maintenance visit 2 months ago. What is the standard treatment for this child's condition?
   a. Intramuscular ceftriaxone once a day for 3 consecutive days
   b. No treatment is necessary.
   c. Oral amoxicillin-clavulanic acid
   d. Topical (ophthalmic) gentamicin drops
   e. Topical (ophthalmic) Tobradex drops

3. After discussing the likely etiology and treatment with the mother, she expresses concern about her 6-week-old infant, who is asleep in a carrier on the floor. She has noted increased tearing from the right eye since the age of 3 weeks. The tearing is clear. She denies any redness of the white part of the eye. Fever and cough are absent. The drainage does not appear to cause any discomfort in the patient, even in sunlight, although there is some scant crusting in the morning. The mother has not tried any oral medications or drops for the condition. Physical examination of the infant reveals moderate clear discharge from the right eye without conjunctival injection, absence of tenderness over the medial aspect of the lower lid, and a clear red reflex. This infant's discharge is most consistent with which of the following conditions?
   a. Dacryostenosis
   b. Dacryocystitis
   c. Chemical conjunctivitis
   d. Ophthalmia neonatorum
   e. Infantile glaucoma

A Answers

Vignette 1 Question 1

Answer D: In this patient, the spot of light reflecting off from one eye is not in the same place as the spot in the other eye. The term for this finding is "asymmetric corneal light reflexes." This finding is present when one eye is deviated, with esotropia (toward the nose) more common than exotropia (outward deviation). Red reflexes will likely be normal; if the child had a cataract in one eye, he would essentially be blind in that eye and would not test at 20/80. The fundoscopic examination would also likely be normal. If there is no conjunctival injection or discharge, a culture will not be helpful. Fluorescein examination is indicated in cases of suspected corneal abrasion, which presents with the sudden onset of severe pain and difficulty opening the affected eye.

Vignette 1 Question 2

Answer C: As this patient has not been seen since 6 months of age, it is as yet unclear whether the amblyopia is due to strabismus or to the refractive error in the left eye. While refractive errors and strabismus each cause about a third of cases of amblyopia, the deviation (strabismus) and "dull sight" in the affected eye point toward strabismic amblyopia as the most likely cause. Isolated strabismus would present with asymmetric corneal light reflexes, a positive cover/uncover test, and normal vision in each eye. Isolated amblyopia is rare without an underlying cause. Anisometropic amblyopia is characterized by unequal refractive errors in the two eyes. The eye with poor vision results in blurring of the image delivered to the visual cortex. While this child has a greater refractive difference than would be expected for his age, the presence of strabismus has probably resulted in partial suppression of the image from the deviated eye, rather than an underlying (primary) refractive error. Visual deprivation amblyopia is caused by an opacity in the visual axis, such as a congenital cataract.

Vignette 1 Question 3

Answer D: Intermittent slight eye deviation is normal in young infants. The American Academy of Ophthalmology recommends referral to an ophthalmologist if the strabismus is still present at 6 months of age. However, if the strabismus is severe and sustained, the infant would be referred sooner. Strabismus in the older sibling increases the infant's risk. Other risk factors which would increase the risk of pathology affecting sight include prematurity, congenital infections, and central nervous system disease.

Vignette 2 Question 1

Answer A: While most of the conditions listed about can result in leukocoria ("white pupil"), congenital cataract is the most common. They may be genetic in origin or due to metabolic disease or an intrauterine infection. This patient's finding is unilateral, but congenital cataracts can occur in both eyes. If not identified and removed early, cataracts lead to blindness. Retinoblastoma is much less common than congenital cataract but much more severe, in that it is a life-threatening malignancy and must be treated promptly. Recurrence in the second eye is common. Optic neuritis (inflammation of the optic nerve) does not cause leukocoria. In many (but not all) cases, fundoscopic examination will reveal a swollen optic disc. This disorder is rare in newborns but is associated with multiple sclerosis in adults. Infection with *Toxoplasma gondii* can result in cataracts, as can congenital rubella. Retinopathy of prematurity is unlikely to be the cause of this child's leukocoria given that the baby was born at term.

Vignette 2 Question 2

Answer A: The cataract should be removed as soon as possible. The infant is not blind in the affected eye, but will develop severe and irreversible amblyopia if the opacity is not removed before 2 months of age. Even with prompt removal of the cataract, visual acuity is generally poorer in children postextraction than in adults with late-onset cataracts.

Vignette 3 Question 1

Answer B: Viral conjunctivitis is generally characterized by mild or no pain, clear discharge without itching or other signs of allergy on physical examination, minimal crusting, bilateral injection, and the presence of other upper respiratory symptoms. *Haemophilus influenzae* and *Neisseria gonorrhoeae* are bacterial infections that can occur in older children, although the former and *Streptococcus pneumoniae* are more common as etiologic agents in young children beyond infancy. *Neisseria gonorrhoeae* and *Chlamydia trachomatis* are common causes of ophthalmia neonatorum, although the longstanding practice of instillation of erythromycin in eyes of newborns has decreased the incidence of both substantially.

Vignette 3 Question 2

Answer C: The presence of an associated ear infection changes doesn't necessarily indicate that the conjunctivitis is not viral in origin; however, it raises the possibility that the causative agent is

Haemophilus influenzae. Infection with this bacteria is usually associated with unilateral conjunctivitis of the same-sided eye and significantly more ocular purulence; however, *H. influenzae* cannot be ruled out. Therefore, this patient should be treated with amoxicillin-clavulanic acid. Amoxicillin alone is ineffective against *H. influenzae*, even at high doses. Intramuscular ceftriaxone would be appropriate if the child's otitis media does not respond to two rounds of antibiotics. Eye drops alone would not resolve this infection. However, eye drops are appropriate if the infection is thought to be viral. Studies have demonstrated that ophthalmic antibiotics decrease infectivity and decrease the duration of the condition by about 2 days, on average. This may be due to the flushing mechanism of installation of the drops. Most physicians would not use Tobradex (tobramycin-dexamethasone), on the off-chance that the infection is caused by HSV. Even though there are no associated skin lesions, the dexamethasone is unnecessary in this instance because the child has no significant eye pain. Withholding treatment is not appropriate in this case.

Vignette 3 Question 3

Answer A: The infant's history suggests dacryostenosis, or nasolacrimal duct obstruction, which occurs in up to 25% of typical infants. In such cases, the distal end of the nasolacrimal duct is either too small to accommodate eye secretions or still covered with membranous tissue. The vast majority of cases resolved by 12 months of age. Those which do not are addressed thereafter with probing by an ophthalmologist to fully open the distal end of the duct. Dacryocystitis is defined as infection of the nasolacrimal sac and may occur in conjunction with underlying obstruction. Hallmark findings include mucopurulent discharge with tenderness and possibly a palpable firmness along the medial aspect of the lower lid. Dacryocystitis is treated with systemic (oral) antibiotics, warm compresses, and nasolacrimal massage (although the value of this procedure is currently under investigation). Chemical conjunctivitis is unlikely given the absence of installation of drops. The infant is older than 30 days of age, so ophthalmia neonatorum cannot be the diagnosis. Infantile glaucoma presents with chronic, clear, excessive tearing which may be unilateral. This patient does not have corneal clouding or photophobia, which generally accompany glaucoma at some point. However, the parent should be educated to look for photophobia and clouding of the pupil and seek medical follow-up if appreciated. In addition, the discharge should lessen as the infant grows and the ductal passage opens and/or enlarges. If this is not the case, the patient should be referred to a pediatric ophthalmologist.

Chapter 20

Emergency Medicine: The Critically Ill and Injured Child

Brad Sobolewski • Jackie Grupp-Phelan • Bradley S. Marino

The critically ill or injured child must be evaluated rapidly to minimize morbidity and mortality. Whether presenting to the physician's office, local clinic, community hospital, or to the emergency department at a tertiary care center, the patient should be stabilized by administering basic life-support and pediatric advanced life support measures recommended by the American Heart Association. Once the patient is clinically stable, a problem list can be generated and the cause of the child's symptoms can be determined.

In 2010, the American Heart Association issued updated guidelines for basic life support, cardiopulmonary resuscitation, and emergency cardiovascular care. Prior to the updated guidelines the initial assessment of a critically ill patient followed the sequence of airway, breathing, and circulation. Presently, the American Heart Association recommends that the assessment of circulation occur prior to that of airway and breathing. This is based on a comprehensive review of the literature on adult and pediatric resuscitation. As a result the concept of hands-only CPR was introduced for the lay rescuer. In adults, bystander CPR with compressions only has been associated with a positive impact on survival in out of hospital cardiac arrest. However, conventional CPR (compressions with rescue breaths) remains the superior method in children.

DIFFERENTIAL DIAGNOSIS

Regardless of this paradigm shift in resuscitation, it is important to note that the majority of cases of pediatric cardiac arrest result from progressive respiratory failure or shock rather than a primary cardiac cause. Ninety percent of cases of pediatric cardiopulmonary arrest result from respiratory (45%), cardiac (25%), and primary central nervous system (20%) etiologies. Table 20-1 delineates the differential diagnoses of cardiopulmonary arrest in children.

CLINICAL MANIFESTATIONS AND TREATMENT

PRIMARY SURVEY

The **primary assessment** (Fig. 20-1) involves evaluation of Circulation, Airway, Breathing, Disability, and Exposure. The aim of the primary assessment is to identify life-threatening conditions and begin cardiopulmonary resuscitation (CPR), if necessary (Table 20-2).

CARDIOPULMONARY RESUSCITATION

Cardiopulmonary arrest is defined as the absence of a pulse in the large arteries of an unconscious patient who is not breathing. To assess the need for CPR first check to see if the patient is responsive to verbal or physical stimuli. If the patient is breathing regularly they do not need CPR. Chldren in respiratory distress will often assume a position of comfort that they should be allowed to maintain if possible. In the unresponsive child health care providers should take no longer than 10 seconds to check for a pulse. Palpate the brachial pulse in infants, and the femoral or carotid pulse in children. If there is no pulse, or if you encounter a patient who is not breathing (or merely gasping), this patient is in cardiopulmonary arrest, and you should initiate CPR, starting with chest compressions.

The goal of CPR is to provide high-quality chest compressions that generate blood flow to vital organs. High-quality compressions require a rescuer to push hard and fast at a rate of at least 100 compressions per minute. Effective compressions are administered with a force sufficient to depress the chest to a depth at least one-third the anterior–posterior diameter of the chest. This equates to a depth of 1.5 in (4 cm) in infants, and 2 in (5 cm) in children. After the initial set of compressions the

TABLE 20-1 The Differential Diagnosis of Cardiopulmonary Arrest in Children

Respiratory	Encephalitis
Upper airway obstruction (e.g., croup, epiglottitis, foreign body, laryngospasm, congenital anomalies, aspiration, bacterial tracheitis, neck trauma, thermal or chemical burns, retropharyngeal abscess, peritonsillar abscess)	Acute hydrocephalus
	Head or spinal cord trauma
	Seizure
	Tumor
Lower airway obstruction (e.g., foreign body, pneumonia, reactive airway disease, bronchiolitis, congenital anomalies)	Hypoxic-ischemic injury
	Gastrointestinal
	Abdominal trauma
Ventilation-perfusion mismatch (e.g., pneumonia, pulmonary edema, tension pneumothorax, hemothorax, chronic lung disease)	Bowel perforation or obstruction
	Peritonitis
Diffusion abnormality across the alveolus (e.g., ARDS)	Hypovolemic dehydration
	Metabolic
Massive pulmonary embolism	Diabetic ketoacidosis
Respiratory muscle failure (e.g., botulism, Guillain-Barré syndrome)	Addison disease
	Hyperthyroidism
Central hypoventilation (e.g., primary apnea, depression of the respiratory center of the brainstem)	Hypoglycemia
	Hyperkalemia
Cardiac	Hypocalcemia
Congenital heart disease (e.g., lesions with ductal-dependent systemic blood flow)	Hyponatremia
	Multisystem
Arrhythmia	Sudden infant death syndrome
Myocarditis	Drug intoxication[a]
Pericarditis	Trauma
Cardiac tamponade	Anaphylaxis
Congestive heart failure	Hypothermia
Myocardial trauma	Septic shock
Central Nervous System	***Renal***
Meningitis	Acute and chronic renal failure

[a]Narcotics, tricyclic antidepressants, barbiturates, benzodiazepines, calcium channel blocker, β-blocker.

airway is then opened using the head tilt chin lift maneuver and two rescue breaths are then administered, assuring that chest rise is visualized. A compression-to-ventilation ratio of 30:2 is appropriate for the lone rescuer, whereas a ratio of 15:2 can be used if two rescuers are present. It is important to remember that fatigue during CPR can lead to ineffective chest compressions. Rotate the role of chest compressions every 2 minutes. Minimize interruptions to chest compressions whenever possible, as coronary perfusion pressure may rapidly decline during delays.

CIRCULATION

Circulation is assessed by evaluating pulses (central and peripheral), capillary refill, and blood pressure. **In children, heart rate is the most sensitive measure of intravascular volume status.** Capillary refill is the most sensitive measure of adequate circulation. Blood pressure fluctuations are an insensitive indicator, because hypotension is a late finding in hypovolemia. Cardiopulmonary monitors are helpful to determine the electrical activity of the heart and to provide continuous feedback on the patient's cardiopulmonary status.

AIRWAY

The goals of **airway** management are to recognize and relieve obstruction, promote adequate gas exchange, and prevent aspiration of gastric contents. The airway is assessed and, if necessary, secured as follows:

- Immobilize the cervical spine if there is a possibility of spinal cord injury.
- Open the airway via the jaw-thrust or chin-lift maneuver and relieve any obstruction caused by the tongue or soft tissues of the neck.

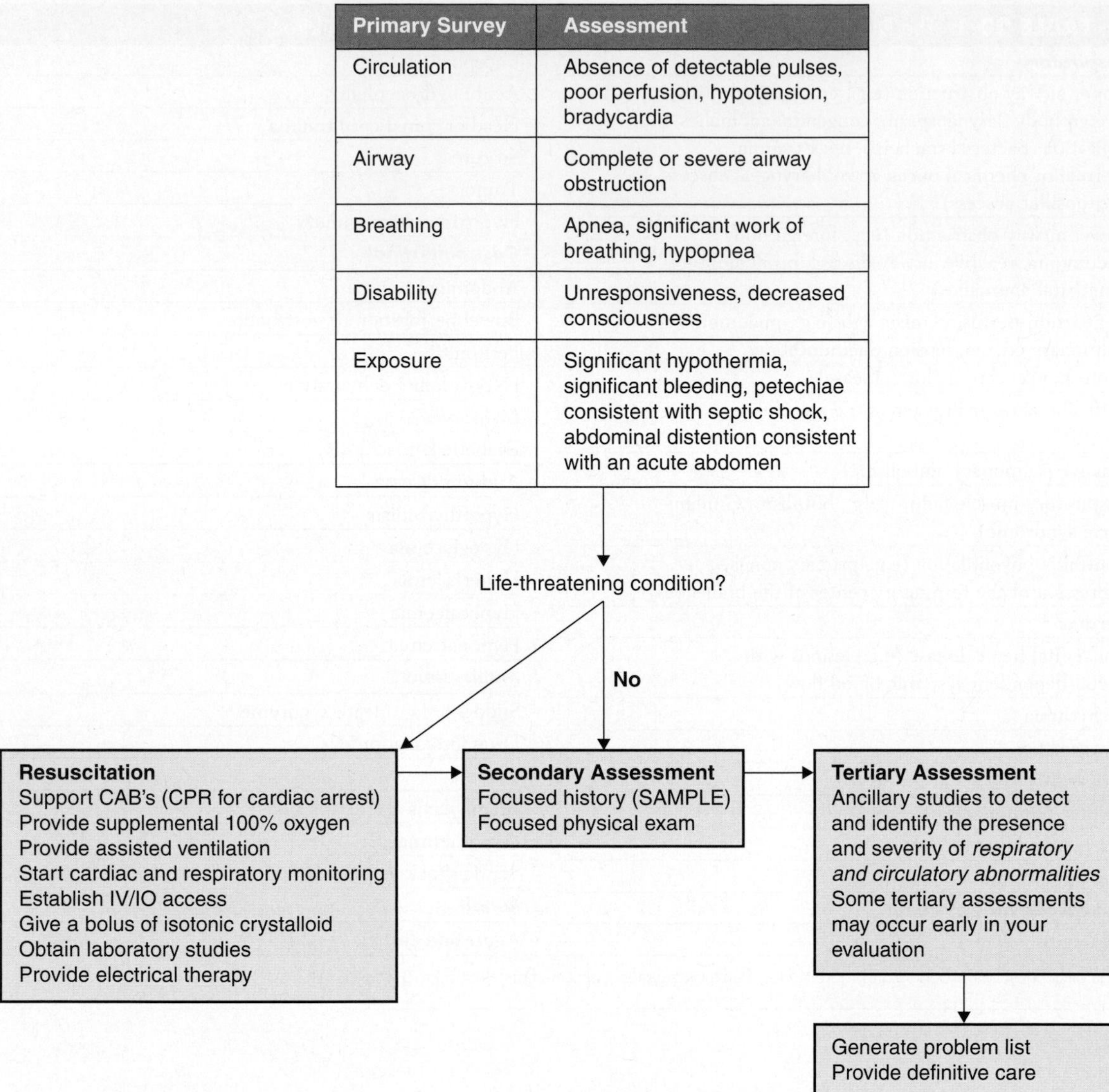

Primary Survey	Assessment
Circulation	Absence of detectable pulses, poor perfusion, hypotension, bradycardia
Airway	Complete or severe airway obstruction
Breathing	Apnea, significant work of breathing, hypopnea
Disability	Unresponsiveness, decreased consciousness
Exposure	Significant hypothermia, significant bleeding, petechiae consistent with septic shock, abdominal distention consistent with an acute abdomen

Life-threatening condition?
No
Resuscitation
Support CAB's (CPR for cardiac arrest)
Provide supplemental 100% oxygen
Provide assisted ventilation
Start cardiac and respiratory monitoring
Establish IV/IO access
Give a bolus of isotonic crystalloid
Obtain laboratory studies
Provide electrical therapy
Secondary Assessment
Focused history (SAMPLE)
Focused physical exam
Tertiary Assessment
Ancillary studies to detect and identify the presence and severity of respiratory and circulatory abnormalities
Some tertiary assessments may occur early in your evaluation
Generate problem list
Provide definitive care

Figure 20-1 • Algorithm of the initial assessment of the pediatric patient.

(Modified from Nichols DG, Yaster M, Lappe DG, et al. Golden Hour: The Handbook of Advanced Pediatric Life Support. St. Louis, MO: Mosby Yearbook;1991:2,128.)

- Clear the airway (suction the nose and mouth as indicated).
- Remove any visualized foreign body if the patient cannot cough or vocalize.
- Place an oral or a nasopharyngeal airway, if indicated.
- Provide 100% oxygen via nasal cannula, face mask, nonrebreather mask, or bag valve mask.
- Assist ventilation (e.g., bag mask ventilation), if indicated.

BREATHING

Once an airway is established, air exchange should be evaluated. Examination of chest wall movement will reveal the presence and effectiveness of spontaneous respirations. If spontaneous respiration is present with adequate oxygenation and ventilation, intubation is not indicated. If respiratory effort or chest wall excursion is not adequate, or if the airway cannot be easily maintained endotracheal tube placement is necessary. Both cuffed and uncuffed endotracheal tubes are appropriate for intubating infants and children. Cuffed endotracheal tubes may decrease the risk of aspiration, and in circumstances where poor lung compliance or high airway resistance are present, a cuffed endotracheal tube may be preferable.

- The size of the uncuffed endotracheal tube should equal 4 + (age in years ÷ 4)
- The size of the cuffed endotracheal tube should equal 3.5 + (age in years ÷ 4)

Though helpful, these calculations are less accurate estimates of endotracheal tube size than length-based resuscitation tapes, especially for children less than 35 kg.

TABLE 20-2 Basic CPR in Infants and Children

Infant (Below 12 mo of age)	Child (Age 1 y to adolescent)	Adolescent and Adult
Check for responsiveness Unresponsive if no breathing or only gasping		
CIRCULATION **Health care providers check for pulse for no more than 10 s**		
Brachial or femoral	Carotid	
If pulseless, begin chest compressions **Rate of approximately 100/min** **Allow complete recoil between compressions**		
Landmark: Just below the nipple line Technique: **1 rescuer:** 2 fingers OR **2 rescuers:** 2 thumbs, with hands encircling chest Depth: 1.5 in (4 cm) or at least one third the anterior–posterior diameter of the chest	Landmark: Center of the chest, between nipples Technique: 2 hands: Heel of 1 hand with second on top OR 1 hand: heel of hand only Depth: 2 in (5 cm) or at least one-third the anterior–posterior diameter of the chest	Landmark: Center of the chest, between nipples Technique: 2 hands: heel of one hand, other hand on top Depth: at least 2 in (5 cm)
AIRWAY		
Position patient supine Head tilt-chin lift (jaw thrust for suspected trauma)		
If airway obstructed with foreign body and patient is unable to breathe or talk		
Back blows and chest compressions	Abdominal thrusts (Heimlich maneuver)	
BREATHING		
2 rescue breaths after compressions		
Mouth to nose	Mouth to mouth	
Compression:Ventilation ratio		
30:2 (1 rescuer) 15:2 (2 rescuers)		30:2
If pulse present and no compressions required		
15–20 breaths per minute OR 8–10 breaths per minute with an advanced airway in place. Breaths are asynchronous with chest compressions		10–12 breaths per minute OR 8–10 breaths per minute with an advanced airway in place. Breaths are asynchronous with chest compressions
DEFIBRILLATION (AED) Minimize interruptions to compressions before and after shock Resume CPR with compressions immediately after each shock		
Less than 1 y of age Insufficient evidence to recommend for or against the use of an AED. A manual defibrillator is preferred if available	*1–8 y old* Use attenuated dose if a pediatric system is availabe. Use adult system if pediatric system is *not* available	*8 y old—Adult* Use standard adult AED with pad-cable system

Blood oxygenation (via pulse oximetry or arterial blood gas measurement) and blood CO_2 level (by arterial or venous blood gas measurement) should be assessed to help guide respiratory management. To avoid hyperoxia, titrate oxygen administration to maintain the oxyhemoglobin saturation ≥94%.

Neonatal intubation is traditionally performed without premedication, but intubation of the infant or child is undertaken with premedication in the following **rapid-sequence** fashion, which should only be performed by providers proficient in the evaluation and management of the pediatric airway:

1. Preoxygenate with 100% oxygen.
2. Administer a vagolytic drug (atropine) in children less than 1 year of age. Ideally it should be administered at least 3 to 5 minutes prior to the sedative and paralytic.
3. Administer a sedative, hypnotic, and/or opioid drug (e.g., etomidate, ketamine, versed, fentanyl).
4. Administer a paralyzing dose of a neuromuscular blocking agent (e.g., succinylcholine [depolarizing agent], or rocuronium or vecuronium [nondepolarizing agents]).
5. Assess the patient for apnea, jaw relaxation, and loss of muscle tone following fasciculation.
6. Intubate the trachea under direct visualization.
7. Confirm correct placement of the endotracheal tube using at least two methods (auscultation, chest rise and fall, end tidal CO_2 detector, mist in the tube).

Applying cricoid pressure during rapid sequence intubation is no longer universally recommended as there is insufficient evidence that it will prevent aspiration of gastric contents during intubation in children. Do not continue to use cricoid pressure if it interferes with ventilation or airway visualization. In the unconscious patient premedication is not indicated. In the child with septic shock do not use etomidate when performing rapid sequence intubation, as it can cause adrenal suppression, and is associated with a higher mortality rate. Rarely, a patient cannot be intubated or ventilated with a bag and mask, and an emergency needle cricothyrotomy is required to establish an airway.

DISABILITY

A rapid screening neurologic examination is performed to note pupillary response, level of consciousness, and localizing findings. It is important to consider the patient's behavior in the context of normal childhood development. If possible, allowing the child to remain in the arms of a parent can improve the ability to get an accurate examination. When encountering medically complex children with special needs be sure to ask caregivers about their child's adaptive behaviors and specific concerns related to their medical history.

EXPOSURE

Because of children's large surface-to-body mass ratio, they cool rapidly, and passive heat loss can be problematic. Careful attention should be provided to patients with burns, or those with fevers as they can lose body heat rapidly. Children exposed to toxins with remnants of those substances on their clothing and/or skin should be appropriately decontaminated to reduce the risk of chemical exposure to medical providers and other patients.

VASCULAR ACCESS

Vascular access is critical for resuscitative fluid and drug administration during cardiopulmonary resuscitation and is outlined in Figure 20-2. If hypotension due to hemorrhage is suspected, gaining proximal control of the hemorrhage and volume resuscitation with type O-negative blood is vital. Optimally, a full set of screening tests (including complete blood count, arterial and/or venous blood gas, electrolyte and chemistry panel, and blood glucose) is obtained at the time of vascular access. If difficultly obtaining intravenous access is suspected, obtaining labortaory studies can be deferred if obtaining those studies might jeopardize the ability to successfully place the IV. If ingestion is a possibility, serum and urine toxicology and acetaminophen and salicylate levels may be obtained.

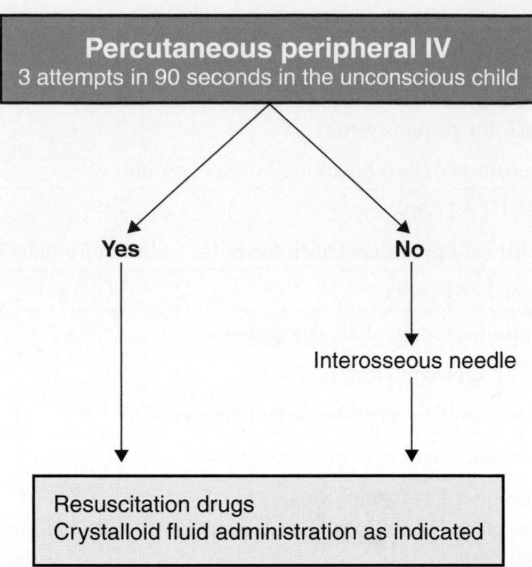

Figure 20-2 • Vascular access management during cardiopulmonary resuscitation.

SECONDARY ASSESSMENT

After completion of the primary assessment and appropriate interventions to stabilize the child, the **secondary assessment** should be performed. The components of the secondary assessment are the focused history and physical examination. The **SAMPLE** mnemonic may be utilized to identify important aspects of the child's history and presenting complaint (**S**igns and Symptoms; **A**llergies; **M**edications; **P**ast medical history; **L**ast meal; **E**vents leading up to the injury and/or illness). The clinician should attempt to gain information that might help explain impaired respiratory, cardiovascular, or neurologic function. A thorough head-to-toe physical examination follows. The severity of the child's illness or injury should determine the extent of the physical examination.

TERTIARY ASSESSMENT

The **tertiary assessment** consists of ancillary studies to detect and identify the presence and severity of *respiratory* and *circulatory abnormalities*. The term *tertiary* does not mean these are performed third. The timing of tertiary tests is dictated by the clinical situation. Ancillary studies that may assist with the assessment of cardiorespiratory abnormalities include: arterial blood gas, arterial lactate, venous blood gas, central venous oxygen saturation, hemoglobin concentration, oxyhemoglobin saturation via pulse oximetry, invasive arterial pressure monitoring, mixed venous pressure monitoring, exhaled CO_2 monitoring, chest X-ray, echocardiography, and peak expiratory flow rate.

SHOCK

Shock is a syndrome characterized by the inability of the circulatory system to provide adequate delivery of oxygen and nutrients to meet the metabolic demands of the body tissues and vital organs. Children, especially neonates, will initially try to compensate by becoming tachycardic and increasing systemic vascular resistance through peripheral vasoconstriction. Hypotension, a late finding, leads to cellular hypoperfusion, metabolic acidosis, and cellular death. Three relationships explain hypotension in shock:

- **Stroke volume** is determined by preload (ventricular end diastolic volume), afterload (systemic vascular resistance), and myocardial contractility
- **Cardiac output** = stroke volume × heart rate
- **Blood pressure** = cardiac output × systemic vascular resistance

Shock may be compensated, decompensated, or irreversible. In **compensated shock**, homeostatic mechanisms maintain essential organ perfusion by increasing heart rate and systemic vascular resistance in an effort to preserve cardiac output and perfusion pressure respectively. Blood pressure, urine output, and cardiac function may all be normal. In **decompensated shock**, compensatory mechanisms fail and patients become hypotensive because of ischemia, endothelial injury, and the elaboration of toxic materials. Signs of inadequate end-organ perfusion include depressed mental status, tachypnea, decreased urine output, weak central pulses, mottled or gray skin color, and metabolic acidosis. In infants and children **hypotension is defined by systolic blood pressure.** The following values represent the estimated fifth percentile for systolic blood pressure in children of various ages. Any value systolic blood pressure less than the following is considered hypotension:

- <50 mm Hg in term neonates (0 to 28 days)
- <70 mm Hg in infants (1 month to 12 months)
- <70 mm Hg + (2 × age in years) in children 1 to 10 years
- <90 mm Hg in children ≥10 years of age

Eventually, cellular function deteriorates and multiorgan system dysfunction results. When this process has caused irreparable functional loss in essential organs, a terminal or **irreversible** shock state is reached. It is important to note that shock evolves along a continuum, and **a patient in decompensated shock can progress to cardiopulmonary arrest in minutes.**

Shock can be categorized into hypovolemic, cardiogenic, distributive, and obstructive types. Specific etiologies are outlined in Table 20-3.

1. **Hypovolemic shock** is the most common type of shock in children and is due to decreased intravascular volume, which results in decreased venous return and myocardial preload. Because of the reduction in myocardial preload, there is a resultant decrease in stroke volume, cardiac output, and blood pressure. Pulses are often weak and capillary refill is prolonged in patients with this form of shock.
2. **Cardiogenic shock** is the result of "pump failure." Inadequate stroke volume, whether due to poor contractility, or arrhythmias result in diminished cardiac output and hypotension. In the patient with tachyarrhythmias (SVT, VT), therapeutic decisions are based on whether the patient is hemodynamically stable or unstable.

TABLE 20-3 The Etiologies of Shock
Hypovolemic
Water and electrolyte losses (diarrhea, emesis)
Inadequate fluid intake
Osmotic diuresis (e.g., diabetic ketoacidosis)
Hemorrhage (internal and external)
Plasma losses ("third spacing" or capillary leak)
Burns
Cardiogenic
Congenital heart disease
Myocarditis
Ischemic heart disease
Cardiomyopathies (inherited or acquired abnormality of ventricular function)
Arrhythmia
Myocardial traumatic injury
Poisoning or drug toxicity (e.g., β-blocker, calcium channel blocker ingestion, chemotherapy)
Distributive
Anaphylaxis
Neurologic injury (head or spinal cord)
Septic shock
Obstructive
Cardiac tamponade
Tension pneumothorax
Massive pulmonary embolism
Congenital heart lesions with ductal-dependent systemic blood flow

Supraventricular Tachycardia (SVT): narrow QRS complex (≤0.09 s)

- Hemodynamically stable: Vagal maneuvers and adenosine.
- Hemodynamically unstable or SVT refractory to medications: Synchronized cardioversion 0.5 to 1 J/kg; if initial cardioversion is unsuccessful increase to 2 J/kg. Sedate if possible prior to cardioversion, but do not delay cardioversion.

Ventricular Tachycardia (VT) or Ventricular Fibrillation (VF): wide QRS complex (≥0.09 s)

- Hemodynamically stable VT: Amiodarone or procainamide, and treat hypomagnesemia and/or hypokalemia. Multiple antiarrhythmic drugs should not be used simultaneously because of the risk of conduction abnormalities and hypotension. If medication therapy does not convert the VT, synchronized cardioversion 0.5 to 1 J/kg may be utilized; if initial cardioversion is unsuccessful increase to 2 J/kg.

- VF/pulseless VT: Provide CPR until the defibrillator is ready to deliver unsynchronized cardioversion at 2 J/kg followed by immediate resumption of CPR for 2 minutes. If a shockable rhythm persists shock again at 4 J/kg. Administer epinephrine 0.01 mg/kg (0.1 mL/kg of the 1:10,000 concentration) every 3 to 5 minutes.

Patients with asystole or pulseless electrical activity require 2 minutes of CPR and administration of epinephrine, and an additional 2 minutes of CPR with a new rhythm and pulse check. It is important to consider the reversible causes of pulseless arrest in children, the so-called H's and T's. They include hypovolemia, hypoxia, hydrogen ion (acidosis), hypoglycemia, hypo/hyperkalemia, hypothermia, tension pneumothorax, tamponade (cardiac), toxins, thrombosis (pulmonary or coronary).

For a full discussion of drug physiology, indications, dosage, route of administration, effects, and side effects, see the American Academy of Pediatrics and American Heart Association *Pediatric Advanced Life Support Provider Manual.* Table 20-4 describes the indications and effects of each drug.

3. **Distributive shock** results from an abnormality in vasomotor tone that leads to maldistribution of a normal circulatory volume and a state of relative hypovolemia. Because of peripheral pooling, preload is reduced, causing a decrease in stroke volume, cardiac output, and blood pressure. Systemic vascular resistance is also decreased due

TABLE 20-4 Drugs Used in Pediatric Cardiorespiratory Resuscitation

Drug	Indication	Action
Adenosine	Supraventricular tachycardia	Adenosine stimulates electrical adenosine receptors in the heart and causes temporary atrioventricular node conduction block and interrupts reentry circuits that involve the AV node.
Amiodarone	Atrial (refractory SVT) and ventricular arrhythmias (refractory VF, refractory pulseless VT, hemodynamically stable VT)	Amiodarone blocks Na, K, and Ca channels and β-receptors in the myocardium, as well as α- and β-receptors in the vascular periphery. Amiodarone slows atrioventricular (AV) conduction, prolongs the AV refractory period and QT interval, and slows ventricular conduction (widens the QRS complex).
Atropine	Bradycardia and AV block	Atropine is a parasympatholytic drug that increases heart rate, conduction through the AV node, and cardiac output by blocking vagal stimulation.
Calcium (calcium gluconate or calcium chloride)	Hypocalcemia, hyperkalemia, hypermagnesemia, and calcium channel blocker overdose	Routine administartion in cardiac arrest provides no benefit. Calcium increases myocardial contractility, increases ventricular excitability, and increases conduction velocity through the myocardium.
Dextrose (glucose)	Hypoglycemia	Glucose administration increases blood glucose level.
Epinephrine	Asystole, bradycardia, pulseless arrest, VT/VF, shock	The α-adrenergic-mediated vasoconstriction of epinephrine increases systemic vascular resistance, aortic diastolic pressure, and coronary perfusion. It also increases chronotropy, and inotropy through β1-adrenergic receptor stimulation. The increased heart rate and stroke volume increase cardiac output. The increased cardiac output and systemic vascular resistance increase blood pressure.
Lidocaine	Pulseless VT/VF, VT with pulse	Lidocaine decreases ventricular automaticity and supresses ventricular arrhythmias. Not as effective as amiodarone to produce return of spontaneous circulation or survical to hospital admission after VF arrest.
Procainamide	SVT, atrial flutter, VT (with pulses)	Procainamide prolongs the refractory period of the atria and ventricles and decreases conduction velocities in the atrium, bundle of His, and ventricle.
Sodium bicarbonate	Severe refractory metabolic acidosis and/or hyperkalemia, sodium channel blocker overdose (e.g., tricyclic antidepressant)	Routine administration is not recommended in cardiac arrest. Sodium bicarbonate increases blood pH.

Drugs that can be given by endotracheal tube include lidocaine, atropine, naloxone hydrochloride, and epinephrine (high dose).
AV, atrioventricular; SVT, supraventricular tachycardia; VF, ventricular fibrillation; VT, ventricular tachycardia.

to vasomotor dysfunction. Because both systemic vascular resistance and cardiac output are reduced, severe hypotension results. **Septic shock**, a cause of distributive shock, results when certain pathogens infect the blood. The early compensated stage of septic shock is characterized by decreased systemic vascular resistance where patients may have bounding pulses, whereas in the late decompensated phase, hypovolemia from third spacing and pump failure due to myocardial depression becomes more apparent. Early administration of broad spectrum antibiotics and intravenous fluids is critical in patients with suspected sepsis. **Anaphylactic shock** is a form of distributive shock that is precipitated by exposure to allergens. It is defined as a rapidly developing illness involving the skin, mucosal tissue, or both and respiratory compromise, hypotension, or both. Cutaneous symptoms are present in more than 90% of cases of anaphylaxis. A third type of distributive shock is **neurogenic (spinal) shock** which occurs after a spinal cord or central nervous system injury. These patients often have both bradycardia and hypotension, in contrast to the tachycardia and hypotension seen in order forms of shock because the sympathetic tract has been disrupted.

4. **Obstructive shock** is a condition of impaired cardiac output caused by physical obstruction of blood flow into or out of the heart. Cardiac tamponade and tension pneumothorax cause obstruction of blood flow into the heart, while pulmonary embolism and congenital heart disease lesions with ductal-dependent systemic blood flow produce obstruction of blood flow out of the heart. Lesions that obstruct blood flow into the heart decrease preload stroke volume and cardiac output. Lesions that obstruct blood flow out of the heart may cause myocardial pump failure, secondary cardiogenic shock, and decreased stroke volume and cardiac output.

CLINICAL MANIFESTATIONS

History and Physical Examination

The history should focus on potential causes of shock. Hypovolemic shock is likely if there is a history of vomiting, diarrhea, polyuria, burns, trauma, surgery, gastrointestinal bleeding, intestinal obstruction, long periods in the sun, or pancreatitis. A history of congenital heart disease, arrhythmias, or chemotherapy (doxorubicin) administration may point to cardiogenic shock. Distributive shock should be contemplated when there is a history of fevers, toxic ingestion, anaphylaxis, or head or spinal cord injury. In addition, any immunocompromised patient who presents with a history of fever and is ill-appearing may be in septic shock.

Serial vital signs are critical in the diagnosis and management of children with shock. In early "warm" compensated septic shock, vasodilation, warm extremities, tachycardia, a widened pulse pressure, and adequate urine output are seen. In contrast, symptoms of hypovolemic, cardiogenic, and late "cold" uncompensated septic shock include vasoconstriction, tachycardia, cold extremities, poor peripheral pulses, altered consciousness, pallor, sweating, ileus, and oliguria. The use of serial vital sign reports in the electronic medical record are an important means by which to detect downward trends in hemodynamic parameters. Automatic alarms or prompts provided by the electronic record to highlight worrisome trends are useful as well.

DIAGNOSTIC EVALUATION

During the stabilization period, the clinician must attempt to categorize the potential etiology of shock based on the patient's history, exam, and initial ancillary studies. All patients with shock should be placed on a cardiac monitor regardless of their oxygen saturation on pulse oximetry. The degree of tachycardia is the best determinant of the level of intravascular depletion or vasomotor abnormality. Hypotension is a late finding and occurs only after 40% to 45% of the intravascular volume has been depleted. Diagnostic tests are obtained on the basis of the specific causes suspected.

TREATMENT

The treatment of shock is aimed at ensuring perfusion of critical vascular beds (coronary, cerebral, hepatic, renal) and preventing or correcting metabolic abnormalities arising from cellular hypoperfusion. All patients in shock should receive supplemental oxygen as a part of their initial therapy as management of hypoxia reduces the level of metabolic acidosis. Correcting metabolic acidosis results in better cellular function, better myocardial performance, and decreased systemic and pulmonary vascular resistance.

Hypovolemic shock is treated with normal saline or lactated Ringer's solution administered in 20 mL/kg boluses up to (and in some cases beyond) a total of 60 mL/kg until hemodynamic status normalizes. If hemorrhage is the cause of the hypovolemia, type O-negative, cross-matched whole blood or packed red cells may be given. In cardiogenic shock resulting from a congenital heart defect, surgery, a catheter-based interventional procedure (e.g., balloon angioplasty or valvuloplasty, balloon atrial septostomy), or inotropic support may be indicated. Children with severe ischemic injury to the heart, dilated cardiomyopathy, or myocarditis may ultimately need a heart transplant. In distributive shock due to anaphylaxis, intramuscular epinephrine, intravenous fluids, intravenous steroids, diphenhydramine, and albuterol nebulizers are employed. Sometimes intubation for laryngospasm and vasopressors for intractable hypotension are needed. Septic shock is treated with fluids, vasopressors, and broad-spectrum antibiotics. Antibiotics are considered a resuscitation medication for septic shock. Pneumothorax is treated by needle or chest tube decompression (removal) of the air from the pleural space. Pericardial tamponade is treated by pericardiocentesis. Neonates with lesions with ductal-dependent systemic blood flow should be started on prostaglandin (PGE_1) therapy as soon as possible to maintain ductal patency and systemic blood flow.

THE CRITICALLY INJURED CHILD

Injuries and accidents are the leading cause of morbidity and mortality for children and adolescents. Motor vehicle associated injuries are the most common cause of death of children of all ages, whether the child is a passenger or struck by a moving vehicle. Blunt injury mechanisms predominate, and it should be presumed that multiple injuries are present until proven otherwise.

CLINICAL MANIFESTATIONS

History and Physical Examination

The priorities of assessing children who are seriously injured are similar to adults. However, because of their size, developmental immaturity, larger head to body mass ratio and unique physiology the causes and mechanisms of injury in children can vary widely. Most serious pediatric injuries are due to blunt trauma, often involving the brain. Apnea, hypoventilation, and hypoxia are five times more common than hypovolemia in seriously injured children.

Children have a smaller body mass, less fat and connective tissue, and a proportionately larger head. These physiologic characteristics result in greater force transmission to internal organs. This results in a high frequency of intraabdominal and traumatic brain injuries. Conversely, the child's skeleton is incompletely calcified and more elastic than that of an adult. Internal injuries may be present even when fractures are not.

Common Mechanisms of and Patterns of Injury

Children involved in motor vehicle accidents can suffer serious injuries even when properly restrained. These injuries include chest and abdominal injuries, as well as lower spine fractures as a result of forward flexion of the spine against the lap belt, with compression of the lumbar vertebrae. Unrestrained children are at risk for multiple injuries, including head and neck injuries.

Children struck by a motor vehicle have different injury patterns than adults. Whereas adults may be struck on the lower extremities, children are shorter, and thus the vehicle's bumper may strike their head, chest, or abdomen causing multiple injuries.

Bike helmets can greatly reduce the number of serious head injuries in children involved in bicycle accidents. Helmeted children can still suffer upper extremity fractures, lacerations, and internal abdominal injuries should their abdomen strike the handlebars.

Children who fall from a height can suffer a multitude of injuries depending on the height of the fall and the surface of impact. Children who fall from a low height often suffer upper extremity injuries because they brace themselves against impact by extending their arms. Children falling from a moderate to high height can sustain head and neck injuries, as well as multiple fractures of their upper and lower extremities.

The Abused Child

Injuries as a result of child abuse are a leading cause of mortality in children less than 1 year of age. It is important to be suspicious of child abuse if the patterns of injury do not match the child's developmental age and the mechanism of injury. Special attention should be paid to inconsistencies in the medical history such as vague details, a delay in seeking care, or discrepancies between the given history and the degree of injury. Findings on physical exam and diagnostic evaluation suggestive of child abuse, especially in infants and small children include intracranial bleeding and retinal hemorrhages which are often caused by an adult shaking the child, trauma to the genital or perianal area, evidence of multiple old fractures in various stages of healing, fractures of long bones in children less than 3 years of age, and bizarrely patterned injuries such as cigarette burns, whip or ligature marks, or sharply demarcated burns. Please see Chapter 21 for more information on the diagnosis and treatment of the abused child.

DIAGNOSTIC EVALUATION

Injured children should ideally be evaluated and managed at a specialized facility with experienced personnel and specialized equipment and resources for pediatric patients. Critically injured children should be transferred to a level one trauma facility as soon as they are stabilized.

Head Injuries

Head injuries in children are one of the most common presenting complaints to the emergency department. Given the frequency of head injuries, please see the section on Closed Head Injuries later in this chapter.

Cervical Spine Injuries

In multiply injured children, or in those that have been injured during a fall careful attention should be paid to maintaining immobilization of the cervical spine. Children should be placed in an appropriately sized semirigid collar. The cervical spine should continue to be immobilized during attempts to intubate at all times.

Thoracic Injuries

Penetrating trauma to the thorax is much less common in children than in adults. Nevertheless, careful auscultation of the lungs can reveal decreased or absent breath sounds, suggesting the presence of a pneumothorax, hemothorax, or pulmonary contusion. Muffled heart sounds are characteristic of a pericardial effusion. Tension physiology occurs when the mediastinal structures are pushed to the opposite side of the thorax by a rapidly expanding pneumothorax resulting in the rapid development of obstructive decompensated shock. During the initial assessment of children with multiple injuries a chest X-ray should be obtained to evaluate for pneumothorax, hemothorax, or widened mediastinum (suggesting an aortic dissection) prior to allowing the child to leave the trauma bay for additional studies, such as computed tomography (CT).

Abdominal Injuries

Children with blunt abdominal injuries who are conscious are often frightened both by the events surrounding their injury, and their presence in the emergency department. Obtaining an accurate examination of the abdomen can therefore be difficult. Avoid deep painful palpation of the abdomen initially. Carefully inspect the surface of the abdomen for bruising, especially characteristic patterns caused by a car's seat belt or a bicycle's handlebars. Children who have sustained blunt abdominal trauma and are hypotensive should be rapidly assessed as they have significant odds of having internal injuries. Focused Assessment Sonography in Trauma (FAST) is a technique utilizing ultrasound to identify intraabdominal or pericardial blood. In the hemodynamically stable child with significant abdominal pain a contrast CT of the abdomen and pelvis is indicated. CT scans can identify solid organ injuries, which require operative repair far less frequently than equivalent injuries in adults. Less easily identified by CT scan, but equally important to consider are injuries to the pancreas and small intestine (particularly the duodenum). Rupture of a hollow viscus requires immediate operative intervention. Conversely, a hematoma of the duodenum can present with delayed symptoms of abdominal pain and vomiting, and may not be recognized on initial imaging studies.

Laboratory screening studies can be used in order to assess children with suspected blunt abdominal trauma, but without significant pain in order to reduce their exposure to the ionizing radiation of CT scans. The presence of anemia on complete blood count (hematocrit <30%), hematuria on urinalysis (>5 red blood cells per high-power field), or elevated liver transaminases (serum aspartate aminotransferase concentration more than 200 U/L or serum alanine aminotransferase concentration more than 125 U/L) increases the odds of an intraabdominal injury being detected on a subsequent CT scan. Children with any of these abnormal lab values should be assessed by contrast CT scan of the abdomen and pelvis. Elevated pancreatic enzymes (amylase >125 IU/L) may indicate intraabdominal injury, but is not specific for pancreatic injury. Obtaining baseline values for amylase and lipase can be helpful when assessing subsequent symptoms. Finally, patients that have suffered a femur fracture also have increased odds of having an intraabdominal injury.

Suspected Child Abuse

Injured children who are suspected to have been abused should undergo evaluation at a specialized pediatric facility with access to trained personnel and social services. Children younger than 2 years of age cannot give a reliable history of physical injuries and thus should undergo a radiographic skeletal survey looking for fractures. CT of the brain to identify skull fractures or intracranial bleeding is the test of choice for children who have sustained head trauma, especially those that have been forcefully shaken. An examination of the fundi by an ophthalmologist is also essential in order to assess for the presence of retinal hemorrhages. Abnormal laboratory studies, similar to those obtained in selected cases of blunt abdominal trauma, can indicate the presence of solid organ abdominal injuries. Please see Chapter 21 for more information on the diagnosis and treatment of the abused child.

TREATMENT

The management of critically injured children should occur at a facility with specialized personnel and resources. Critically injured hypotensive children have an extremely high risk of imminent mortality. Hemorrhagic shock is initially treated with 20 mL/kg of normal saline boluses. Up to three boluses total should be given in order to improve hemodynamic status. However, administration of blood products should be considered if the child is actively bleeding, or if three normal saline boluses fail to improve the child's circulatory status. It is important to note that **children with acute blood loss will not become frankly hypotensive until they have lost approximately 40% to 45% of their circulating blood volume.** Children with lesser degrees of hemorrhage will present with signs and symptoms of compensated hypovolemic shock.

Orotracheal intubation under direct laryngoscopy is the preferred method of airway management. Rapid sequence intubation may be required. Tube thoracotomy is indicated in children with pneumothorax or hemothorax. Remember to maintain cervical spine immobilization at all times. A surgeon trained in the management of pediatric injuries should be consulted as soon as possible in suspected intraabdominal injuries. An unstable pelvis should be wrapped with a sheet or appropriate pneumatic device in order to prevent continued extravasation of blood. Obvious long bone injuries should be splinted and immobilized.

Children with head injuries and suspected intracranial bleeding should undergo prompt evaluation and management including a neurological exam, assessment of the GCS, and a CT scan of the head. See the following section for more information on treatment for head injuries.

Head Trauma

Acute head trauma is the most common cause of pediatric death and disability in the developed world. Head injuries in children most often result from motor vehicle accidents, bicycle mishaps, falls, or child abuse. Males are twice as likely as females to sustain significant head trauma. Recovery from a head injury depends on the severity of the initial injury and factors contributing to secondary neuronal injury such as hypotension and hypoxia. Severe injury is often associated with behavioral changes, motor impairment, and memory problems. Approximately 10% of children hospitalized for a traumatic brain injury have a seizure, and 35% of these patients will subsequently develop a seizure disorder.

A **concussion** is defined as a brief alteration or loss of consciousness following relatively mild head trauma. Brain injury is undetectable, and the neurologic examination returns to normal within hours. In contrast, **cerebral contusions** represent a direct injury to the brain itself. **Diffuse axonal injury** results from shearing forces on the white matter of the brain that occur with rapid deceleration of the head. It is frequently followed by brain edema, further disruption of blood flow, inflammation, and ischemia. Brain hemorrhages that occur secondary to trauma are typically epidural or subdural (Table 20-5; Fig. 20-3). Some severe brain injuries may also result in subarachnoid injury and bleeding into the CSF.

CLINICAL MANIFESTATIONS

History

Severe brain injury may occur in the absence of external signs of trauma. The source of injury should be described by the child and caretaker separately whenever possible; a history that is not consistent with a given injury is suggestive of child abuse. Reports of vomiting, severe headache, and mental status changes strongly suggest increased intracranial pressure. Confusion, loss of consciousness, amnesia, seizures, and visual impairment may also be present after significant injury.

Physical Examination

It is crucial to get an accurate neurological exam, and to assess the child's mental status. Signs and symptoms of a serious head injury include lethargy, decreased level of consciousness, behavioral changes, vomiting, abnormal pupil exam, and posturing. These symptoms occur because of elevated intracranial pressure, which if unchecked, can lead to herniation. The combination of

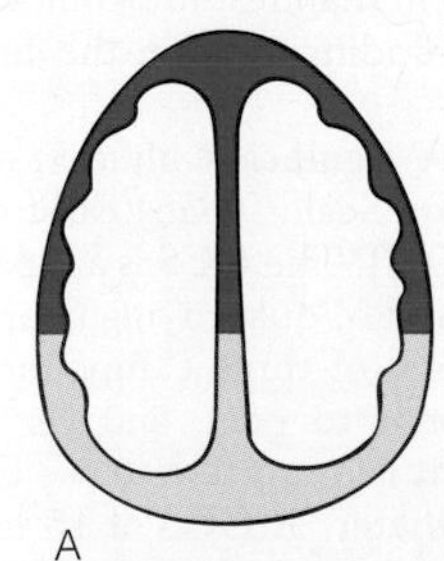

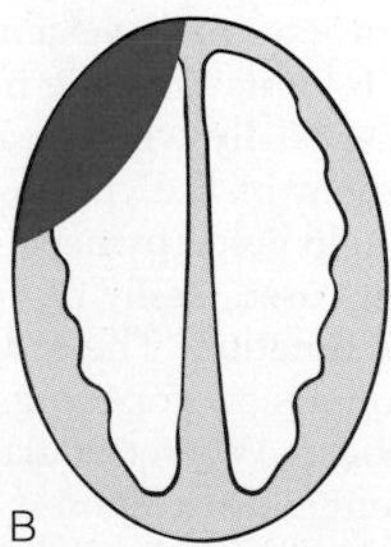

Figure 20-3 • (A) Subdural and (B) epidural brain hemorrhages.

TABLE 20-5 Differentiating Acute Subdural and Epidural Bleeds

	Subdural	Epidural
Location	Between the dura and arachnoid layers	Between the skull and the dura
Symmetry	Usually bilateral	Usually unilateral
Etiology	Rupture of bridging cortical veins or subdural veins	Rupture of middle meningeal artery or vein
Typical injury	Direct trauma or shaking	Direct trauma in the temporal area
Consciousness	Intact but altered	Impaired-lucid-impaired
Common associated findings	Seizures, retinal hemorrhages	Ipsilateral pupillary dilatation, papilledema, contralateral hemiparesis
Appearance on CT with contrast	Crescentic	Biconcave
Prognosis	High morbidity; low mortality	High mortality; low morbidity
Complications	Herniation	Skull fracture; uncal herniation

bradycardia, hypertension, and irregular respirations are known as **Cushing's triad**, and are indicative of increased intracranial pressure which may be as a result of intracranial hemorrhage or swelling or brain tissues after trauma. Patients with these three findings are at risk for imminent herniation. Cranial nerve function, especially pupil size and reactivity, may help localize the injury. Papilledema may be evident on visualization of the fundus. A patient with a head injury and unequal pupils may be herniating, as the brain tissue is pushed below the tentorium and exerting pressure on the third cranial nerve.

It is also important to look for signs of a **basilar skull fracture** on physical exam, including hemotympanum, or CSF rhinorrhea or otorrhea. and diffuse bruising around the eyes (raccoon eyes), or postauricular (Battle's sign) bruising. Palpate the entire skull for depressions or step-offs, which are concerning for depressed skull fractures. Infants with open fontanelles and cranial sutures may tolerate rises in intracranial pressure better and may have more subtle symptoms. Look for bulging of the anterior fontanelle and widened cranial sutures in addition to the aforementioned signs and symptoms.

Sensory and motor function is difficult to assess in the patient with impaired mental status, who may respond minimally even to noxious stimuli. Deep tendon and pathologic reflexes should be assessed in all patients. Serial neurologic examinations track evolving lesions and response to interventions.

Falls in which the child strikes the side or back of their head may be associated with a higher rate of intracranial bleeding. Almost all children who present with intracranial hemorrhage requiring neurosurgical intervention will manifest in significant symptoms, or have abnormal exam findings within the first 4 to 6 hours after the initial injury.

Especially when dealing with more significant injuries, assessment of the child's Glasgow Coma Scale (GCS) early on can help guide management (Table 20-6). The GCS is a rapid, widely used, easily reproducible method of quantifying neurologic function. The score is a sum total of three components including eye opening, motor response to pain, and verbal response. When calculating the GCS it is important to use the patient's best response for each parameter. A GCS of 15 is a perfect score, and indicates a patient who is awake, alert, and cooperative. Three is the minimum score, and is indicative of deep coma or death. A GCS of 13 to 15 is indicative of a mild traumatic brain injury, 9 to 12 a moderate injury, and ≤8 or less a severe injury. Patients with GCS ≤8 following head trauma are at risk for severe morbidity and death and generally require immediate intervention.

Patients with head injuries should receive a primary survey as soon as possible. Moderate to severe injury may result in altered breathing and the need for respiratory support. The GCS should be calculated to help guide initial therapy.

DIAGNOSTIC EVALUATION

Cervical spine films are indicated for any patient with significant head trauma to rule out cervical injury. A **CT scan of the head** is indicated in children who have lost consciousness for greater than 5 seconds or have an abnormal neurologic exam or altered mental status, a palpable skull fracture, a severe mechanism of injury, and multiple episodes of vomiting following the initial injury. The primary goal of obtaining a head CT is to identify intracranial bleeding (subdural or epidural hematoma, or subarachnoid bleeding). Children who present without loss of consciousness, have not vomited, and have a normal neurologic exam can be safely observed without need for head CT. New evidence suggests that the risk of radiation exposure to immature tissues may be greater than that of adults. As such, efforts should be made in order to avoid exposing children to excess ionizing radiation from CT scans whenever possible. In patients who have sustained mild trauma, have a normal examination, and have a history of a brief alteration or loss of consciousness with subsequent return to normal mental status, the decision regarding imaging is made by the examining physician. A CT of the brain is of little or no benefit in children with mild injury and no loss of consciousness.

TREATMENT

Specific treatment depends on the severity of the injury. Patients with suspected head or neck injury should be positioned on a back board with appropriate cervical spine immobilization in the field. Early consultation with a pediatric

TABLE 20-6 Coma Scales

	Score	Older Children and Adults	Infants and Young Children
Eye opening	4	Spontaneous	
	3	To voice	
	2	To pain	
	1	None	
Best motor response	6	Obeys commands	Obeys commands, normal spontaneous movements for age
	5	Localizes to pain	
	4	Normal flexion withdrawal	
	3	Abnormal flexion (decorticate)	
	2	Extension (decerebrate)	
	1	None (flaccid)	
Verbal response	5	Oriented	Smiles, oriented to sounds, follows objects, interacts
	4	Disoriented, converses	Cries but consolable, inappropriate interactions
	3	Inappropriate words	Inconsistently consolable and moans, makes vocal sounds only
	2	Incomprehensible sounds	Inconsolable restless, agitated
	1	None	None

Adapted from American College of Surgeons. Advanced Trauma Life Support for Doctors Student Course Manual. 7th Ed, American College of Surgeons; 2004.

neurosurgeon may be necessary in order to consider invasive intracranial pressure monitoring in patients with severe head trauma. Those with severe injury and GCS ≤8 generally require intubation.

Hypotension is uncommon in isolated head trauma, but associated injuries may lead to shock (hypovolemic shock from hemorrhage; neurogenic shock from spinal cord injury; cardiogenic shock from myocardial contusion). In traumatic brain injuries the combination of hypoxia and hypovolemia can result in significantly reduced oxygen delivery to the brain and be devastating. Efforts should be focused on assuring adequate central nervous system perfusion and oxygenation. Infants with open cranial sutures and fontanelles can not only tolerate greater increases in intracranial pressure but also have worse outcomes than older children with similar traumatic brain injuries. In contrast to older children and adults, infants can become hypotensive solely from intracranial hemorrhage.

The goal of supportive therapy is to optimize the **cerebral perfusion pressure**, which is the difference between the mean arterial pressure and the intracranial pressure. **Cerebral edema** is the most significant complication in the acute period. Normal oxygenation, normoglycemia, hyperosmolality, and elevation of the head of the bed are recommended to minimize intracranial hypertension and secondary brain injury. Mild hyperventilation, which reduces cerebral blood flow, is used to decrease intracranial pressure during the initial phase of therapy. Patients with evidence of impending herniation should be vigorously hyperventilated and given an osmotic agent such as mannitol and/or furosemide to decrease intracranial pressure acutely. Patients with evidence of significant cerebral edema require intracranial pressure monitoring with a subdural bolt or intraventricular catheter.

Patients with moderate injury and/or a declining GCS should be admitted to the hospital for further observation, serial neurologic examinations, and intervention as needed. Children with mild trauma should be observed in the hospital or at home with a reliable, competent caregiver for at least 24 hours. Any evidence of persistent headache, confusion, irritability, behavior changes, or visual disturbances should prompt further medical attention and workup.

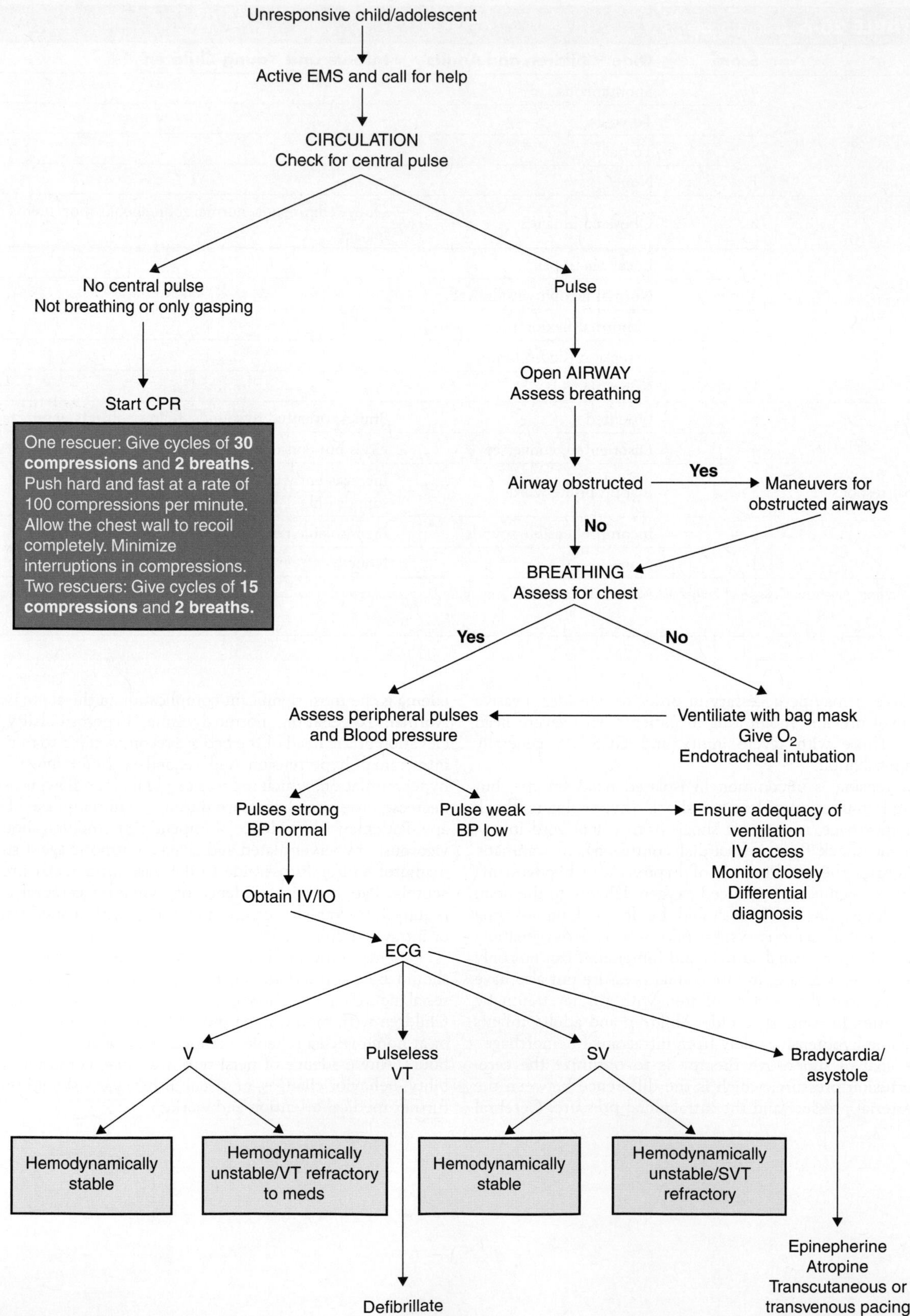

Figure 20-4 • Management of the unresponsive child or adolescent.

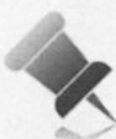

KEY POINTS

- No matter what the cause of cardiopulmonary arrest, the algorithms outlined for pediatric basic and advanced cardiac life support should be followed. A primary assessment (**C**irculation, **A**irway, **B**reathing, **D**isability, **E**xposure) should be performed, followed by resuscitative measures, if necessary.
- Approximately half of the causes of pediatric arrest are due to respiratory arrest, which can be brought about by upper airway obstruction, lower airway obstruction, restrictive lung disease, or any etiology that results in inadequate gas exchange.
- Management of the unresponsive child or adolescent is shown in Figure 20-4.
- If resuscitation does not establish cardiac output, the following mechanical or metabolic causes should be investigated: hypothermia, tension pneumothorax, hemothorax, cardiac tamponade, profound hypovolemia, profound metabolic imbalance, toxic ingestion, and closed head injury.
- Determine the category of shock and whether the patient has early or late manifestations.
- Hypovolemic shock accounts for most cases of shock in children.
- In hypovolemic shock, hypotension is a late finding, and the degree of tachycardia is the most sensitive measure of intravascular fluid status.
- In septic shock, antibiotics are a resuscitation medication and their administration should not be delayed.
- A patient in decompensated shock can progress to cardiopulmonary arrest in minutes.
- Children with acute blood loss will not become frankly hypotensive until they have lost approximately 40% to 45% of their circulating blood volume.
- When obtaining labs during the evaluation of a hemodynamically stable child with blunt abdominal trauma the presence of anemia on complete blood count, hematuria on urinalysis, or elevated liver transaminases increases the odds of an intraabdominal injury being detected on a subsequent CT scan.
- A CT scan of the head is indicated to evaluate for intracranial hemorrhage following head trauma in children who have lost consciousness for greater than 5 seconds or have an abnormal neurologic exam or altered mental status, a palpable skull fracture, a severe mechanism of injury, and multiple episodes of vomiting following the initial injury.
- Children can suffer multiple injuries during accidents involving motor vehicles. Paying careful attention to the mechanism of injury can aid clinicians in their evaluation.

C Clinical Vignettes

Vignette 1

While you are working at a community pediatric clinic, a patient's mother calls for help from an adjacent examination room. You are the first medical professional to enter the room and see a 2-month-old infant lying motionless on the table. He is not breathing spontaneously. He has no pulses. You determine that this unresponsive pulseless child is in cardiopulmonary arrest.

1. What is the correct ratio of chest compressions to rescue breaths for the lone rescuer in pediatric CPR?
   a. 3:1
   b. 10:1
   c. 15:2
   d. 30:2
   e. 60:2

2. Which of the following is the most appropriate anatomic location and vessel for the assessment of central pulses in this patient?
   a. The wrist/radial arteries
   b. The upper arm/brachial arteries
   c. The neck/carotid arteries
   d. The groin/femoral arteries
   e. The feet/dorsalis pedis

3. Which of the following is the most common cause of pediatric cardiopulmonary arrest?
   a. Cardiac arrhythmias
   b. Metabolic abnormalities
   c. Overwhelming infections
   d. Trauma
   e. Respiratory problems

Vignette 2

A previously healthy 4-year-old male presents to the emergency department with a 2-day history of vomiting and diarrhea. He has no significant past medical history, attends preschool, and his immunizations are up to date. On physical examination he is ill-appearing, with strong central pulses but weak peripheral pulses. His heart rate is 180 beats per minute, and his blood pressure is 94/68 mm Hg. He is breathing comfortably at a rate of 16 breaths per minute. His abdomen is soft and nontender with no palpable masses or organomegaly. His oral mucous membranes and lips are dry. His skin is pale and has decreased turgor. You are concerned that this patient is dehydrated.

1. Which of the following is the earliest physical finding associated with intravascular volume depletion in children?
   a. Capillary refill
   b. Mental status
   c. Blood pressure
   d. Heart rate
   e. Urine output

2. You note that this patient is in compensated hypovolemic shock. In this patient, the definition of hypotension would consist of a systolic blood pressure less than which of the following?
   a. 60 mm Hg
   b. 72 mm Hg
   c. 78 mm Hg
   d. 86 mm Hg
   e. 90 mm Hg

3. The patient's nurse places a peripheral intravenous catheter in this 15-kg, 4-year-old male and requests orders for fluid type and rate. Which of the following is the most appropriate initial choice (both fluid and amount) for volume resuscitation in this patient?
   a. Packed red blood cells 150 mL
   b. Lactated Ringers 30 mL
   c. Normal saline (0.9% sodium chloride solution) 300 mL
   d. ½ Normal saline (0.045% sodium chloride solution) 300 mL
   e. 3% Normal saline 45 mL

Vignette 3

A 2-year-old girl presents to the emergency department with a 3-day history of fevers and vomiting. Her mother notes that she laid her daughter down for a nap earlier in the day, and that she slept longer than usual and was difficult to arouse. On physical examination, she is listless and responds only to vigorous stimuli. She has weak central pulses and no notable peripheral pulses. Her heart rate is 200 beats per minute. Her blood pressure is 65/40 mm Hg. She is making grunting noises with each breath, is breathing at a rate of approximately 25 breaths per minute, and has subcostal retractions. Her skin is pale with mottling of her limbs. She also has a rash on her lower extremities that has the appearance of bruises.

1. All but which of the following should be included in the emergency management of this child?
   a. Administer 100% oxygen.
   b. Obtain a focused history from her mother.

c. Place the patient on cardiac monitors and continuous pulse oximetry.
d. Place a central venous catheter.
e. Administer a broad-spectrum intravenous antibiotic.

2. Given your history, physical examination, and initial laboratory results, you suspect that this patient is in septic shock. Despite aggressive administration of intravenous fluids, her blood pressure does not improve. All but which of the following factors are thought to account for the hypotension resulting from septic shock?
   a. Increased preload
   b. Decreased systemic vascular resistance
   c. Myocardial pump failure
   d. Decreased stroke volume
   e. Decreased cardiac output

3. The patient's respiratory status worsens despite the administration of 100% oxygen by bag valve mask. The decision is made to proceed with rapid sequence intubation. What is the appropriate size for a cuffed endotracheal tube in this 2-year-old patient?
   a. 4.0
   b. 4.5
   c. 5.0
   d. 5.5
   e. 6.0

Vignette 4

You are evaluating a 10-year-old male who was struck by a car going at 30 mph while riding his bicycle. He was not wearing a helmet. On physical examination, he has strong central and peripheral pulses. His heart rate is 110 beats per minute, and he is breathing spontaneously. His blood pressure is normal. There is a large hematoma on his forehead. His eyes open in response to painful stimuli, and his pupils are equal and reactive to light. He vocalizes by incomprehensibly moaning. When you pinch his right arm, he attempts to push your arm away and appears to be moving all four extremities. His abdomen is soft and nontender. He has an obvious deformity of the distal left lower extremity (tibia).

1. All but which of the following are appropriate immediate interventions in this patient?
   a. Immobilize the cervical spine in a semirigid collar
   b. Obtain IV access
   c. Splint and immobilize the injured extremity
   d. Transfuse with O negative packed red blood cells
   e. Administer supplemental oxygen

2. What is this patient's Glasgow Coma Scale score?
   a. 7
   b. 9
   c. 11
   d. 13
   e. 15

3. The patient develops irregular breathing. He no longer opens his eyes to stimuli, and his limbs are extended. He does not vocalize. His pupils are unequal, with the left being fixed and dilated. His heart rate is 54 beats per minute, and his blood pressure is 154/82 mm Hg. Which of the following is the most likely reason for this patient's clinical deterioration?
   a. Hemorrhage from an intraabdominal injury
   b. Seizures induced by his recent head trauma
   c. Brain herniation
   d. Uncontrolled bleeding from a fractured lower extremity
   e. Tension pneumothorax

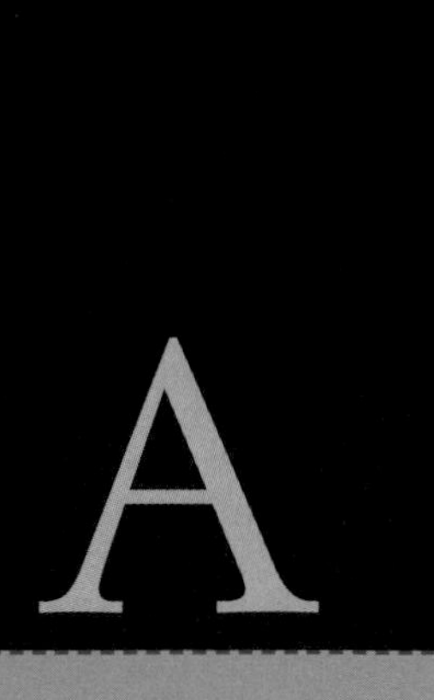

Answers

Vignette 1 Question 1

Answer D: The goal of CPR is to provide high-quality chest compressions that generate blood flow to vital organs at a rate of at least 100 compressions per minute. The American Heart Association recommends alternating chest compressions with rescue breaths in children in cardiorespiratory arrest. For the lone rescuer, a compression-to-ventilation rate of 30:2 is recommended. Since even a brief interruption of compressions can result in loss of coronary perfusion pressure, an increased ratio of compressions to breaths is recommended when providing CPR as a lone rescuer. The ratio of 15:2 is appropriate if at least two providers are present. None of the other options are recommended in pediatric CPR.

Vignette 1 Question 2

Answer B: The most appropriate place to palpate for central pulses in a small infant are the brachial arteries. Even experienced health care providers often cannot reliably feel the carotid or femoral pulses in an infant this age and size. The radial artery and dorsalis pedis are both examples of anatomic locations for the assessment of peripheral, rather than central, pulses.

Vignette 1 Question 3

Answer E: In adults, cardiac etiologies are the most common causes of arrest. In contrast, 45% of pediatric arrests result from initial respiratory compromise progressing to respiratory failure/arrest, which compromises coronary perfusion and oxygenation and results in full cardiopulmonary arrest.

Vignette 2 Question 1

Answer D: In children, heart rate is the most sensitive measure of intravascular volume status. Capillary refill is the most sensitive measure of adequate circulation. Mental status can be an important indicator of dehydration but is more variable than other indices. Urine output is difficult to quantify outside the hospital, where output is measured by strict diaper weights or a Foley catheter. Blood pressure fluctuations are an insensitive indicator of intravascular volume status; children are able to preserve normal to near-normal blood pressure relatively longer than adults. Hypotension is a late and ominous finding in hypovolemic shock indicating decompensation and impending arrest.

Vignette 2 Question 2

Answer C: The patient in this vignette is 4 years old. Therefore, he would be hypotensive if his systolic blood pressure were less than 78 mm Hg. In patients between the ages of 1 and 10 years, hypotension can be estimated as a systolic blood pressure of less than 70 mm Hg + (2 × age in years). Term neonates (infants 0 to 28 days old) are hypotensive if the systolic blood pressure is less than 60 mm Hg. Infants 1 to 12 months of age are hypotensive below a systolic blood pressure of 70 mm Hg. Patients older than 10 years of age are hypotensive if their systolic blood pressure falls below 90 mm Hg.

Vignette 2 Question 3

Answer C: Crystalloid solutions, including normal saline and lactated Ringers, are the most appropriate fluid choices in hypovolemic shock. The initial fluid bolus is 20 mL/kg, which equals approximately 25% of the typical intravascular fluid volume. Of the available choices answer C, 300 mL of normal saline, is the most appropriate answer. A patient who is simply dehydrated but not losing blood (either internally or externally, as in trauma) does not need blood products. While lactated Ringers is an appropriate choice, 30 mL is an inadequate volume for resuscitation of a 15-kg patient in hypovolemic shock. Administration hypotonic (1/2 normal saline) or hypertonic (3% normal saline) solutions will result in significant, possibly life-threatening electrolyte abnormalities.

Vignette 3 Question 1

Answer D: This patient is in decompensated shock as defined by her systolic blood pressure that is less than the estimated fifth percentile for a 2-year-old patient [70 + (age × 2)]. Early on, the etiology of shock is often uncertain. Immediate management centers on maximizing oxygen delivery to essential tissues. This includes administering 100% oxygen and assisting ventilation with a bag valve mask when appropriate. This particular patient has signs of respiratory distress, manifested by grunting and retractions, which are signs of increased work of breathing.

It is also important to place this patient on monitors as soon as possible, as the information provided (heart rate and oxyhemoglobin saturation) are vital pieces of information that will help you assess the impact of administered therapies. That being said, electrical activity picked up by the heart monitor does not always translate into cardiac muscle activity, so direct evaluation of the patient cannot be ignored.

Though the etiology of this patient's shock is not yet certain, the history of fever and bruising of the lower extremities suggests the possibility of septic shock. The bruises may be representative of purpura fulminans, a condition manifested by cutaneous bruising and widespread coagulopathy following infection by certain bacterial pathogens. Antibiotics are a resuscitation medication in patients with suspected septic shock, and their administration should not be delayed.

A focused history can help establish an etiology for the patient's illness and can guide therapies. In addition to questions from the SAMPLE mnemonic (*signs* and *symptoms*, *allergies*, *medications*, *past* medical history, *last* meal, *events* leading to illness), immunization history is important in patients with possible sepsis.

Establishing IV access as soon as possible will allow prompt administration of resuscitative therapies. Though a central venous catheter allows for rapid administration of isotonic fluids and medicines, as well as the monitoring of hemodynamic function, placement of a central venous catheter in children is technically difficult and not immediately necessary in this case. Attempts should first be made to place a peripheral IV, followed by interosseous access if peripheral IVs are unsuccessful.

Vignette 3 Question 2

Answer A: Septic shock is a form of distributive shock caused by the deleterious effects of pathogens that have invaded the bloodstream. Vasomotor dysfunction results in decreased peripheral vascular resistance. Capillary leak occurs, and intravascular fluids are maldistributed and pool in peripheral tissues. Because of peripheral pooling, preload is reduced, causing a decrease in stroke volume, cardiac output, and blood pressure. The early compensated stage of septic shock is characterized by decreased systemic vascular resistance (distributive shock), in which patients may have bounding pulses. Late decompensated shock involves significant hypovolemia from third spacing, and pump failure due to myocardial depression becomes more apparent.

Vignette 3 Question 3

Answer A: The correct size for a cuffed endotracheal tube in this patient is 4.0. The size of a cuffed endotracheal tube should equal 3.5 + (age in years / 4). The size of an uncuffed endotracheal tube is estimated by 4 + (age in years / 4). It is appropriate to intubate using either a cuffed or uncuffed endotracheal tube in pediatric patients; however, a cuffed tube may decrease the risk of aspiration of gastric contents and is preferred in patients with poor lung compliance. It is important to note that length-based resuscitation tapes (like the Broselow tape) are more accurate in patients less than 35 kg. In practice, one ET tube is made available in the estimated size, as well as 1 larger and 1 smaller.

Vignette 4 Question 1

Answer D: This patient has multiple injuries. Bicyclists struck by a moving vehicle are at risk for injuries to the brain and cervical spine. The cervical spine should be immobilized with a semirigid collar to protect against further injury in the absence of reliable examination and radiographic findings. It is appropriate to obtain intravenous access as soon as possible in order to obtain helpful laboratory studies and to administer medications and fluids. Splinting and immobilizing injured limbs with suspected fractures can reduce pain and mitigate further hemorrhage from long bone fractures. Though this patient is breathing on his own, he does have examination findings suggesting a closed head injury, including his depressed mental status and bruising to his scalp. The injured brain is sensitive to hypoxia and hypovolemia. Supplemental oxygen will certainly not harm this patient. A transfusion of red blood cells is not immediately necessary in this patient, as he is not hypotensive and has no obvious active internal or external hemorrhaging. Though it is possible to exsanguinate from a femur fracture, skeletal injuries to the distal appendicular skeleton rarely lead to hemorrhagic shock unless an overlying major artery has been injured. Administration of isotonic crystalloid is appropriate as the initial fluid therapy.

Vignette 4 Question 2

Answer B: This patient has a GCS of 9. He opens his eyes to painful stimuli, which is worth 2 points for the eye score. He attempts to push the examiner's hand away, netting 5 points for best motor response. Finally, he is moaning. These incomprehensible sounds yield a score of 2 on the verbal assessment. A GCS of 9 indicates that this patient has at least a moderate traumatic brain injury.

Vignette 4 Question 3

Answer C: This patient has suffered from cerebral herniation (uncal), a severe complication of traumatic brain injury. He has Cushing's signs, which include bradycardia, hypertension, and irregular breathing. These are thought to occur due to pressure exerted on the brainstem by herniating cerebral tissue. Uncontrolled hemorrhage from various injuries would likely lead to hypotension, rather than hypertension as seen in this patient. Though seizures can manifest with abnormal vital signs and posturing, the unequal pupils are more suggestive of herniation. A tension pneumothorax presents with decompensated obstructive shock, characterized by absent breath sounds in the affected hyperinflated hemithorax, a deviated trachea, hypoxia, and hypotension. Treatment consists of immediate needle decompression.

Chapter 21

Poisoning, Burns, and Injury Prevention

William Tsai • Katie S. Fine

Nowhere does the old adage "an ounce of prevention is worth a pound of cure" resonate more true than in pediatrics. As a group, injuries are the most significant cause of morbidity and mortality in children and adolescents. When an untoward event occurs, timely evaluation and treatment may limit disability and preserve quality of life.

ACUTE POISONING

EPIDEMIOLOGY

Poisoning is one of the more common pediatric medical emergencies, resulting in over a million emergency department visits per year. Children **younger than 6 years** of age account for over half of all cases of poisonous ingestion. These are more likely to involve only one substance and usually denote **accidental** ingestion, although abuse by caretakers must be considered. **Adolescents** account for a smaller percentage; such ingestions are often **intentional**, represent a suicide attempt or gesture, and may involve multiple substances. Recreational drug use in this population may also lead to unintentional but fatal overdoses. Intentional ingestions are more likely to require medical intervention and result in death.

CLINICAL MANIFESTATIONS

The history should include the substance and amount ingested, time elapsed since ingestion, early symptoms, subsequent behavior, and any attempts at treatment. In unknown ingestions, it is important to elicit potential exposures to prescription medications, cosmetics, cleaning products, over-the-counter cold medicines, pesticides, and vitamins. The physical examination begins with the primary survey to evaluate the need for emergency cardiopulmonary support (Chapter 20). Other findings which aid in diagnosis include rapid evaluation of temperature and other vital signs, mental status, odors on the breath/skin/clothing, pupil size and reactivity, and skin color and feel. The characteristic clinical manifestations and treatments of the most common poisonings in children are listed in Table 21-1.

DIFFERENTIAL DIAGNOSIS

The possibility of toxicologic ingestion should be considered in any patient presenting with acute-onset illness involving multiple organ systems, including altered mental status, acute behavior changes, respiratory compromise, seizures, arrhythmias, and/or coma.

DIAGNOSTIC EVALUATION

Initial screening studies include assessment of oxygen saturation, dextrose-stick, electrocardiogram, serum electrolytes and osmolarity, and a venous blood gas to determine pH, PCO_2, bicarbonate level, and base deficit/excess. Blood and urine toxicology screens are often helpful, but specific substances may not be detected on routine laboratory screens (e.g., iron, organophosphates).

TREATMENT

Parents should be instructed to immediately call 911 or their local poison control center. The American Academy of Pediatrics has recently reaffirmed its recommendation that syrup of ipecac no longer routinely be kept at home or given by parents following accidental ingestions.

Patients who present in unstable condition must be evaluated and treated according to the ABCDEs discussed in Chapter 20. With regard to ingestions, the "D" in the mnemonic may stand for: **d**extrose (as several commonly ingested agents precipitate hypoglycemia); empiric **d**rug treatment (relating to possible antidotes or cardiac stabilizers, etc.); and appropriate **d**econtamination. Treatment decisions should be based on the estimated maximal potential dose ingested.

Activated charcoal is the favored method of gastric decontamination in most pediatric poisonings. It is administered by mouth or nasogastric tube and minimizes absorption by binding the substance and hastening its elimination. Activated charcoal is ineffective in ingestions with alcohol, hydrocarbons, iron, and lithium. **Whole bowel irrigation** is an option for ingestions involving iron; the procedure is usually undertaken

TABLE 21-1 Signs, Symptoms, and Treatment of Specific Pediatric Poisonings

Substance[a]	Clinical Manifestations	Suggested Labs[b]	Antidote/Treatment
Acetaminophen	May be initially asymptomatic. Nausea/vomiting, anorexia; may progress over days to jaundice, abdominal pain, liver failure	Serum acetaminophen level 4–24 hrs after ingestion[c]; (late) serum hepatic transaminases (↑), prothrombin time (↑)	A: Oral *N*-acetylcysteine (most effective within 8–10 hrs of ingestion) 140 mg/kg PO × 1, then 70 mg/kg PO q 4 hrs × 17 doses; Intravenous *N*-acetylcysteine 300 mg/kg over 21 hrs T: Activated charcoal (w/in 4 hrs)
Anticholinergic agents (atropine, scopolamine, first-generation antihistamines)	"Mad as a hatter, red as a beet, blind as a bat, hot as a hare, dry as a bone"; drowsiness, delirium, hallucinations, seizure; skin flushing; fused dilated pupils; fever, cardiac dysrhythmias; dry mouth, speech and swallowing difficulties, nausea, vomiting	Drug screen	A: Physostigmine in select cases of severe anticholinergic signs and symptoms T: Activated charcoal/cathartic; whole bowel irrigation for sustained-release preparations; benzodiazepines for agitation and seizure control
Carbon monoxide	Lethargy, irritability, confusion, dizziness, headache; nausea; irregular breathing, cyanosis; palpitations; progression to coma, death	Blood carboxyhemoglobin levels; blood gas (metabolic acidosis with normal PaO_2)	A: Oxygen T: Normobaric oxygen 100% until asymptomatic and carboxyhemoglobin level ≤5%; hyperbaric oxygen if available for severe poisoning
Ethanol[d] (wine/beer/liquor; also found in cold preparations and mouthwash)	Lethargy, CNS depression, nausea/vomiting, ataxia, respiratory depression, coma, hypotension, hypothermia (in young children)	Serum ethanol level, blood glucose (↓), electrolytes (↓ potassium), blood pH (↓), ↑ osmolal gap	A: None T: Supportive care, glucose if needed, correction of electrolytes, parenteral fluids
Ethylene glycol (radiator fluid, de-icing solution)	Anorexia, vomiting, lethargy, respiratory/cardiovascular collapse	Serum ethylene glycol level; ↑ osmolal gap; arterial blood gas monitoring (metabolic acidosis); serum electrolytes (↑ anion gap); serum calcium (↓); urinalysis (calcium oxalate crystals)	A: None T: Fomepizole (preferred) or ethanol to prevent metabolism; sodium bicarbonate to correct metabolic acidosis; hemodialysis
Hydrocarbons (in fuels, household cleaners, polishes, and other solvents)	Tachypnea, coughing, respiratory distress, cyanosis, fever (aspiration); nausea/vomiting, gastrointestinal discomfort (oral ingestion); mental status changes	Arterial blood gas monitoring, chest X-ray (initial and 4–6 hrs after exposure)	A: None T: Avoid gastric emptying.[e] Prevent aspiration, which results in chemical pneumonitis and possibly proliferative alveolar thickening and chronic lung function abnormalities. Supportive respiratory care
Ibuprofen	Nausea/vomiting, anorexia, stomach pain; gastrointestinal bleeding (obvious or occult) Massive ingestion: mental status changes/stupor/coma; seizures	Serum ibuprofen level 4 hrs after ingestion;[f] serum transaminase levels (↑), alkaline phosphatase (↑); metabolic acidosis with ↑ anion gap	A: None T: Activated charcoal/cathartic; respiratory support/seizure control

■ **TABLE 21-1** (continued) Signs, Symptoms, and Treatment of Specific Pediatric Poisonings

Substance[a]	**Clinical Manifestations**	**Suggested Labs**[b]	**Antidote/Treatment**
Methanol (in windshield washer fluid; toxic in very small amounts; toxicity related to formation of formic acid)	Nausea/vomiting, inebriation; ↑ minute ventilation to offset metabolic acidosis as methanol is metabolized; ocular findings 18–24 hrs after ingestion (blurred vision, optic disc hyperemia/edema)	Serum methanol level; arterial blood gases (severe metabolic acidosis); ↑ osmolal gap	A: None T: Fomepoizole (preferred) or ethanol to block metabolism; sodium bicarbonate for metabolic acidosis; folate to hasten formic acid elimination (cofactor therapy); hemodialysis in severe cases
Iron	Nausea/vomiting, diarrhea, gastrointestinal blood loss, acute liver failure, seizures, shock, coma	Serum iron level (3–5 hrs post ingestion), serum pH (↓), glucose (↑), bilirubin and liver function tests (↑), PT (prolonged), WBC (↑); abdominal radiograph (radiopaque material)	A: Deferoxamine chelation T: Whole bowel irrigation; dialysis (late, severe)
Organophosphates (insecticides)	SLUDGE (salivation, lacrimation, urination, defecation, gastric cramping, emesis); small but reactive pupils; sweating; muscle fasciculations; confusion; coma	Plasma or red blood cell cholinesterase activity (↓)	A: Atropine sulfate followed by pralidoxime chloride T: Activated charcoal (if ingested)
Opiates	Bradycardia, hypotension, decreased respiratory rate, pinpoint pupils, somnolence, coma	Toxicologic screen (urine and serum)	A: Naloxone[g] T: Gastrointestinal decontamination if appropriate; respiratory support
Salicylates (aspirin, anti-diarrheal medications	Hyperpnea/tachypnea (respiratory alkalosis/metabolic acidosis), fever, nausea, vomiting, dehydration, tinnitus, agitation, seizures	Blood gas (↑pH, ↓PCO2, ↓bicarbonate), glucose (↑), electrolytes (↓potassium), PT and PTT (prolonged), serum salicylate level	A: None T: Gastric emptying/activated charcoal,[h] alkalinization of the serum to increase renal excretion and prevent entry into CNS; correct hypokalemia which inhibits salicylate excretion; fluid/electrolyte management; hemodialysis in severe cases
Sympathomimetic agents (**decongestants**; also amphetamines, cocaine)	Tachycardia, hypertension, fever, large but reactive pupils, sweating, agitation, delirium/psychosis, seizures	Electrolytes (↓potassium), blood glucose (↑), EKG	A: None T: Activated charcoal/cathartics; sedatives for severe agitation
Theophylline	Tachycardia, hypotension, tachypnea, vomiting, agitation, seizures	Serum theophylline level (every 2–4 hrs), blood glucose (↑), potassium (↓), pH (↓), calcium (↑), phosphate (↓), EKG	A: None T: Activated charcoal/whole bowel decontamination; hemodialysis in severe ingestions

continues

■ **TABLE 21-1** (continued) Signs, Symptoms, and Treatment of Specific Pediatric Poisonings

Substance[a]	Clinical Manifestations	Suggested Labs[b]	Antidote/Treatment
Tricyclic antidepressants	Anticholinergic effects as above; tachycardia, hypertension progressing to hypotension, confusion, drowsiness, dry mucous membranes, dilated but responsive pupils, agitation, seizures, coma, dysrhythmias[i]	ECG (prolonged PR interval, widened QRS complex, prolongation of the QT interval, AV block, ventricular arrhythmias); these effects may be delayed	A: None T: Activated charcoal; sodium bicarbonate (blood alkalinization) for conduction abnormalities; all patients with tricyclic antidepressant ingestions should be admitted and monitored in an intensive care unit

[a]Substances in bold represent the most common pediatric toxicologic emergencies.
[b]All patients with suspected ingestions should receive serum and urine toxicology screens because ingestion of multiple substances is common, especially in intentional poisonings.
[c]An accepted nomogram exists for predicting the severity of the toxicity based on a blood acetaminophen measurement taken at least 4 hours after ingestion.
[d]Physicians should have a high suspicion of co-ingestions in adolescents with ethanol intoxication. The clinical manifestations of co-ingestion of a central nervous system stimulant may be attenuated, whereas ingestion with a depressant may potentiate the effects of alcohol.
[e]Some specific exceptions.
[f]An accepted nomogram exists for predicting the severity of the toxicity based on a blood ibuprofen measurement taken 4 hrs. after ingestion.
[g]Naloxone administration may result in withdrawal symptoms (tachypnea, tachycardia, sweating, agitation, seizures) in chronic users.
[h]Aspirin ingestion causes delayed gastric emptying, so GI decontamination plays a significant role.

following activated charcoal administration as well. Hemodialysis is beneficial for selected ingestions to prevent life-threatening complications.

Gastric lavage is no longer recommended in the management of poisoned patients. If used, it is generally only effective if performed in the first hour after ingestion or when the compound ingested slows gastric emptying (aspirin, tricyclic antidepressants). Gastric lavage is contraindicated in patients who are vomiting and those thought to have ingested corrosive/caustic substances, hydrocarbons, or agents known to cause neurologic depression (increasing the risk of an unprotected airway).

CONCUSSION

The latest definition of concussion, which resulted from a large multidisciplinary symposium in Zurich in 2008, defines concussion as collection of abnormal functional processes affecting the brain precipitated by head (face/neck) trauma. Features typically include immediate impairment of short-term memory, which is often short-lived and resolves without intervention; symptoms which vary in severity and may include loss of consciousness; and the absence of structural changes on imaging studies. The use of sport-specific helmets has been shown to reduce the risk of concussion in some sports, but does not eliminate that risk entirely. Children and adolescents, with their developing brains, may be at increased risk over the adult population for more severe or lingering impairment.

EPIDEMIOLOGY

High school football has the highest rate of concussion (when corrected for "time in play"). Soccer has the second highest rate; lacrosse is third. For non-school-based sports clubs, rates of concussion are highest in ice hockey. The average age of concussion is slowly falling, likely due to the increase in organized competitive sports in middle childhood.

CLINICAL MANIFESTATIONS

History

Signs and symptoms of concussion may be physical (headache, nausea/vomiting, problems with balance or vision); cognitive (difficulty concentrating, forgetfulness, confusion, and feeling "out of it" mentally); emotional (irritability, depression); and sleep/wakefulness disruptions. Amnesia for events immediately before and after the injury is very common. Loss of consciousness is less common but, when present, may represent more severe neurologic involvement.

Physical Exam

The physical examination is identical to that for any head trauma victim. The examiner should look for evidence of external trauma, including scalp lacerations, contusions, skull depressions indicating possible depressed skull fracture, hemotympanum, and drainage from the ears/nose. Vision should be evaluated and balance assessed. A complete neurologic examination, followed by screening tests to identify cognitive impairment, is essential.

DIAGNOSTIC EVALUATION

Several tools exist to evaluate the degree of an athlete's cognitive impairment on the field. The most widely used is the Sports Concussion Assessment Tool 2. It consists of questions designed to elicit information about the patient's self-reported symptoms, signs of loss of conscious, Glascow coma score, anterograde and retrograde amnesia, cognitive processes, and balance and coordination (reprinted at http://aappolicy.aappublications.org/cgi/reprint/pediatrics;126/3/597). Research regarding coordination of SCAT2 score with severity of concussion is ongoing.

As previously mentioned, concussion is primarily a functional process rather than a structural one. Neuroimaging is not routinely indicated but should be considered in patients with loss of consciousness, abnormal/not improving Glascow coma scores, suspected depressed skull fracture, neck pain, irritability, poor coordination/balance, and/or severe headache. Computed tomography (CT) is the initial study of choice. Patients with persistent symptoms are monitored with serial neuropsychiatric testing to document improvement/resolution of impairment.

TREATMENT

The cornerstones of treatment are *physical and cognitive rest*. Physical exertion is prohibited until the athlete is asymptomatic at rest for a proscribed period (see below). Activities requiring concentration such as reading, doing homework, and working on the computer may worsen symptoms.

"Return to play" recommendations are guided by symptoms as well as the severity of the initial impairment. "Asymptomatic," as mentioned above, includes both the absence of physical pain and return to preinjury cognitive levels. The majority of athletes are asymptomatic within a week of the injury. A stepwise increase in physical exertion is recommended; any return of symptoms results in increased restriction until the athlete is again asymptomatic. Light aerobic activity is followed by sport-specific training, noncontact drills, and finally contact practice, if applicable. Athletes who return to play too soon are at risk for severe neurologic morbidity and possible mortality due to a subsequent blow to the head while still symptomatic ("second impact syndrome").

DROWNING

Drowning is a frequent cause of morbidity and mortality in the pediatric population. More than 1,400 pediatric drownings were reported in the United States in 2008. **Near drowning** is defined as survival for a period of time after suffocation by water immersion. Incidence peaks in the older infant/toddler age group and again in adolescence. Rates are twice as high in blacks and three times higher in boys. **Bathtubs** are the most common site of drowning in the first year of life. Large buckets and residential pools are particularly dangerous for toddlers, whereas natural water sources account for most adolescent injuries.

Reliable predictors of outcome include water temperature, time of submersion, presence of aspiration (and pulmonary parenchymal injury), and effectiveness of early resuscitation efforts. Submersion for more than 5 minutes in warm water associated with significant aspiration and minimal response to initial cardiopulmonary resuscitation (CPR) virtually always results in major disability or death.

All patients with a history of near drowning should be evaluated with serial chest radiographs and blood gas measurements for 24 hours. Those with hypoxemia and mental status changes require aggressive respiratory and circulatory support.

Toddlers and young children must be supervised at all times while in the bathtub or around pools or other bodies of water. Residential and commercial swimming pools should be fenced in (with unscalable fences) and have locked gates. Isolation fencing (fencing limited to the immediate pool area) is more effective at preventing accidental drowning than perimeter property fencing. CPR training is available to parents through the American Heart Association and many area hospitals. Learning to swim is an important preventive measure but does not take the place of close supervision.

FOREIGN BODY ASPIRATION

The natural curiosity of children coupled with the toddler's tendency to put everything in the mouth make **foreign body aspiration** a frequent occurrence in the pediatric population. Aspiration is the accidental inspiration of foreign material into the respiratory tract. Most objects and foodstuffs are immediately expelled from the trachea by coughing. Unfortunately, foreign bodies that lodge in the upper or lower respiratory tract are more problematic.

EPIDEMIOLOGY

The highest incidence of foreign body aspiration is noted in children 6 to 30 months old. Aspiration into the lower airways is much more common than tracheal obstruction. While the angle of the right main stem bronchus in adults favors right-sided aspiration, no such propensity exists in young children given the symmetric bronchial angles in this age group. Many children do not have fully erupted second molars until age 30 months; inappropriate food choices include nuts, popcorn, hot dogs, hard vegetables, meat with bones, and seeds. Food, coins, and small toys constitute the most commonly aspirated objects. Inadequate supervision and pediatric anatomy result in increased risk.

DIFFERENTIAL DIAGNOSIS

Patients who experience partial obstruction or obstruction of a distal airway may present up to a week after the initial event with no witnessed episode of choking. Wheezing and respiratory distress may be mistaken for asthma; pneumonia is a consideration when breath sounds are decreased. Of note, findings on auscultation in cases of foreign body aspiration are localized to one side of the chest only. This classic triad of cough, wheezing, and decreased breath sounds are, however, not always present. Chronic foreign body aspiration should be considered in patients with recurrent focal pneumonias and/or lung abscesses.

CLINICAL MANIFESTATIONS

Following an initial episode of choking and coughing, many children may be asymptomatic for a period of time. When symptoms occur, presentation varies depending on where the foreign body lodges in the respiratory tree (Table 21-2). If the obstruction is **complete**, the chest radiograph demonstrates significant one-sided atelectasis, and the heart is drawn toward the affected lung throughout the entire respiratory cycle. However, a **partial** obstruction allows air to enter during inspiration, where it becomes trapped (ball-valve obstruction). In these cases, the inspiratory film may appear normal, but the expiration radiograph will show a hyperinflated obstructed lung with mediastinal shift away from the blockage (Fig. 21-1). In less obvious cases, lateral decubitus chest films or flouroscopy may detect subtle unilateral hyperinflation and enhance diagnosis. Lateral radiographs of the neck may demonstrate subglottic densities of tissue inflammation.

TREATMENT

Airway intervention is contraindicated in the child in the field who is actively coughing, crying, or speaking. If the airway is compromised, the choking response protocol (abdominal thrusts) is the same for children as for adults. For infants, back thumps

TABLE 21-2 Signs and Symptoms of Foreign Body Aspiration

Location of Obstruction	Associated Signs and Symptoms
Total tracheal obstruction	Acute asphyxia, severe retractions with poor chest wall movement
Extrathoracic, partial	Inspiratory and expiratory stridor, retractions
Intrathoracic, partial	Expiratory wheeze; frequently inspiratory stridor as well
Main stem bronchus	Cough and expiratory wheeze; may be blood-tinged sputum
Lobar/segmental bronchus	Decreased breath sounds over affected lobe; wheezing, rhonchi

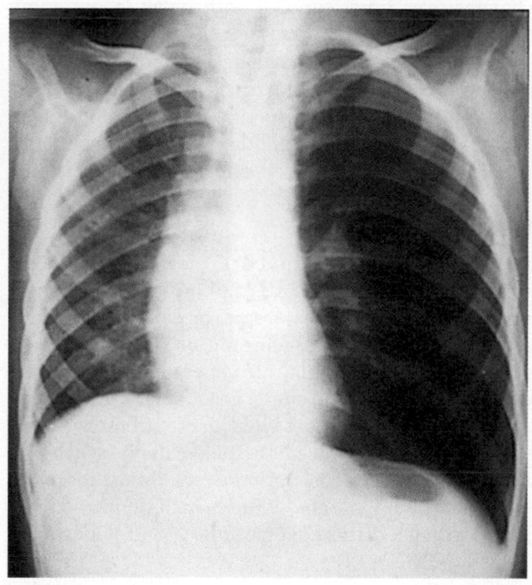

Figure 21-1 • Expiratory film in foreign body aspiration with partial obstruction; the obstructed left lung is hyperinflated, whereas the heart and mediastinum are shifted to the right.

and chest thrusts are alternated, with the infant's body angled slightly head-down.

Foreign bodies must be removed from the airway to alleviate symptoms. **Rigid bronchoscopy** is the treatment of choice. Thereafter, prognosis depends on the degree of lung damage, which is directly related to time interval to diagnosis. Most patients recover quickly with minimal sequelae.

BURNS

Burns are the third leading cause of death in children, behind motor vehicle accidents and drowning. An estimated 15% to 25% of burns are the result of **abuse**. Fortunately, the great majority of burns are not life threatening. Patients who survive severe burns are often left with significant scarring and disability.

EPIDEMIOLOGY

The great majority of burns are **scald** injuries, resulting from contact with hot liquids. These may occur in association with spillage of hot food or drinks or be due to bathing injuries. Scald burns that end in demarcated lines without associated splash marks suggest abuse. **Contact** burns are the next most common and result from direct contact with a hot surface (iron, stove). Contact burns due to cigarettes are the most common burn injury in abused children. **Flame** burns are less frequent but result in a high mortality rate due to associated smoke inhalation injury. Typical scenarios for an **electrical** burn involve a young child putting conductive material into a wall socket or an infant sucking on the connected end of an extension cord. **Chemical burns** result from exposure to strong acidic or alkaline material.

RISK FACTORS

Boys and children younger than 4 years of age, particularly those with disabilities, are at the greatest risk for burn injury.

CLINICAL MANIFESTATIONS

Clinical severity is based on affected body surface area and depth. Partial-thickness burns are divided into first- and second-degree burns. **First-degree** burns involve only the epidermis; the skin is red, dry, and tender but does not blister. First-degree burns usually heal within a week with no residual scarring. **Second-degree** burns may be superficial (less than half the depth of the dermis) or deep (involving most of the dermis but leaving appendages such as sweat glands and hair follicles intact). Superficial partial-thickness burns are often caused by scald injuries. They are painful and exhibit blisters and/or weeping but generally resolve in a few weeks with little scarring. Deep second-degree injuries may or may not be painful. They result in significant scarring and may require skin grafting. **Third-degree burns** extend into the subcutaneous tissue and are nontender due to sensory nervous tissue loss.

Specific injury sites and patterns are characteristic of abuse (Fig. 21-2).

TREATMENT

Burned areas should be placed immediately in lukewarm water or covered with wet gauze or cloth. Minor burns (superficial burns involving 10% of the total body surface area or less) respond to gentle cleansing, **silver sulfadiazine** (an antimicrobial agent), and daily dressing changes until reepithelialization occurs. Burns that are severe, circumferential, extensive (more than 10% to 15% of the body), or that involve the face, hands, perineum, or feet require more

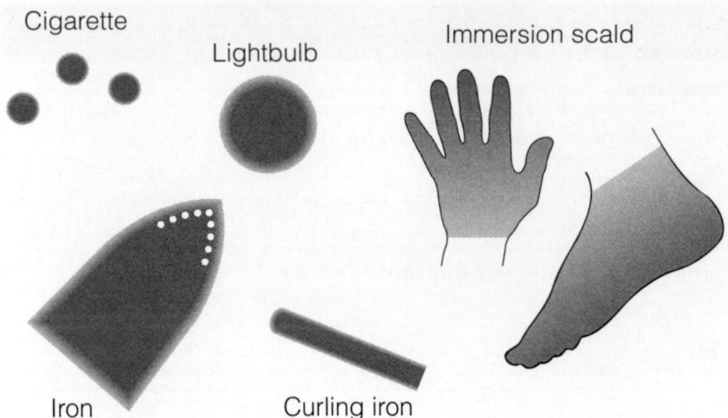

Figure 21-2 • Burn injury patterns consistent with abuse.

specialized care. Treatment includes appropriate management of airway, breathing, and circulation issues; effective electrolyte and fluid therapy to account for increased fluid loss; specialized nutritional support; prevention of infection; pain management; excision and skin grafting; optimization of cosmetic recovery; and early mobility and rehabilitation.

CHILD ABUSE AND NEGLECT

Injuries intentionally perpetrated by a caretaker that result in morbidity or mortality constitute **physical abuse**. **Sexual abuse** is defined as the involvement of a child in any activity meant to provide sexual gratification to an adult. Failure to provide a child with appropriate food, clothing, medical care, schooling, and a safe environment constitutes **neglect**.

EPIDEMIOLOGY

Almost half the children who are brought for medical attention as a result of physical abuse are below 1 year of age; the great majority is preschool aged. It is estimated that upto 10% of emergency room injury visits involving children younger than 5 years result from abuse. Parents, the mother's boyfriend, and stepparents are the most frequent perpetrators. Reports of abuse that increase in number and severity of injury over time are highly correlated with increased mortality.

Reports of sexual abuse have increased over the past decade. The abuse may occur at any age. Relatives and family acquaintances account for most cases; molestation by strangers is uncommon. In 80% of reports, the victims are girls; most are abused by stepfathers, fathers, or other male family members. Male sexual abuse is probably underrecognized.

Neglect results in more deaths than physical and sexual abuse combined. It is the most common cause of failure to thrive in developed nations.

RISK FACTORS

Abuse and neglect occur at all socioeconomic levels but are more prevalent among the poor. Children with special needs (mental retardation, cerebral palsy, prematurity, chronic illness) and those younger than 3 years of age are at particular risk. Caretakers who have themselves suffered abuse, who are alcohol or substance abusers, or who are under extreme stress are more likely to abuse or neglect.

DIFFERENTIAL DIAGNOSIS

Most cases of suspected abuse are subsequently substantiated by child protective services. Care should be taken to differentiate bruises from Mongolian spots, which commonly occur in the buttocks area. Occasionally, osteogenesis imperfecta has been mistaken for abuse. Skin conditions such as bullous impetigo may mimic cigarette burns or other forms of abuse. Children with extensive bruising should undergo coagulation studies to rule out hematologic abnormalities (von Willebrand, etc.).

CLINICAL MANIFESTATIONS

History

An injury that is **inconsistent with the stated history**, or **a history that changes over time**, coupled with **delay in obtaining appropriate medical care** strongly suggests abuse. Age-inappropriate sexual behavior and knowledge are consistent with sexual abuse. Victims of physical or sexual abuse may act out by abusing others, attempting suicide, running away, or engaging in high-risk behaviors. Abuse places children at an increased risk for poor school performance, low self-esteem, and depression.

Physical Examination

Growth parameters are often stunted in neglacted children. As with burns, the location and pattern of injury may strongly suggest abuse (Fig. 21-3). Bruises, burns, or lacerations in different stages of healing occur in chronic or repeated abuse. Bruises associated with normal play are generally limited to the shins and elbows. Bruises on the chest, head, neck, or abdomen and bruises on a nonambulatory child are extremely suspicious. Vigorous shaking may lead to **shaken baby syndrome** (SBS), which results from acceleration/deceleration forces to the head. Virtually pathognomoic injuries include intracranial (subdural) hemorrhage, diffuse axonal injury, and widespread

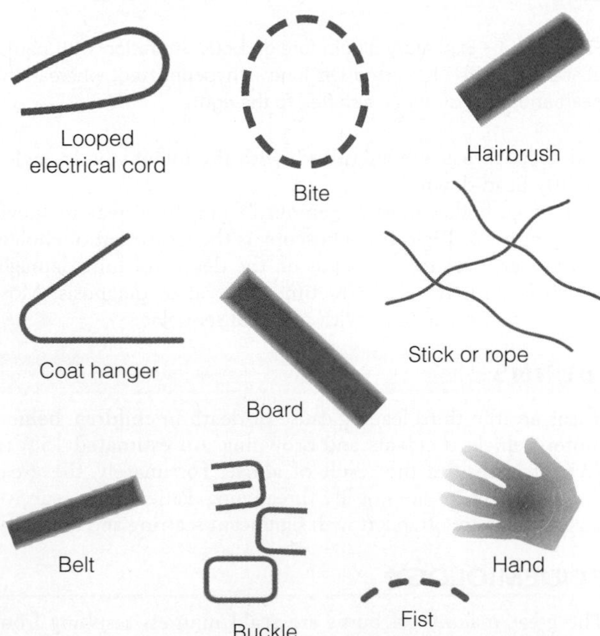

Figure 21-3 • Body marks consistent with abuse.

retinal hemorrhages, which may result in permanent vision loss. SBS has the highest mortality rate of any reported form of child abuse. Falls from beds, changing tables, cribs, counters, or toilet seats do not cause the injuries seen in SBS.

DIAGNOSTIC EVALUATION

A skeletal survey and bone scan reveal areas of past injury that may not be evident on physical examination. Fractures which are highly specific for abuse include bilateral fractures, bucket handle fractures, metaphyseal chip fractures, and fractures of the (especially posterior) ribs, scapula, sternum, or spinous processes. Fractures that occur before ambulation are usually inflicted. CT scans will reveal **intracranial injuries, which in infants are highly suggestive of abuse**; 95% of intracranial injuries and two thirds of all head injuries in infants are due to abuse. When sexual abuse is suspected, rectal, oral, vaginal, and urethral specimens should be examined for *Neisseria gonorrhoeae*, *Chlamydia trachomatis*, and other sexually transmitted diseases. Other studies include blood tests for syphilis and human immunodeficiency virus.

TREATMENT/PREVENTION

Health care workers are **required by law** to report any suspicion of child abuse or neglect to state protection agencies. Victims should be immediately removed from their homes and placed in protective custody. Many family intervention programs that focus on social support, nursing staff visits, and parenting skills are being evaluated across the country in an attempt to provide children with safer home environments. Pediatricians can aid in preventing child abuse by providing parents with realistic expectations for their child's behavior at each health maintenance appointment. It is also important to recognize when the family and/or caregiver experiences an acute crisis or social isolation; referral for supportive services may make a significant difference in the home environment of the child.

SUDDEN INFANT DEATH SYNDROME

By definition, sudden infant death syndrome (**SIDS**) is the unexpected death of an infant less than 1 year of age for which the etiology remains unclear despite a thorough history and postmortem evaluation. It is the leading cause of death in children between 1 month and 1 year of age. The cause of SIDS remains unproven but is thought to be related to delayed maturation of brainstem respiratory or cardiovascular control and arousal mechanisms.

RISK FACTORS

Although multiple factors have been associated with an increased risk for SIDS, none has proven prognostic value (Table 21-3). Incidence peaks between 3 and 5 months of age. More cases are reported during the winter months.

DIFFERENTIAL DIAGNOSIS

Cases that initially appear to be SIDS may in fact result from infection, congenital heart disease, metabolic disorders, seizures, accidental trauma, or abuse.

Apparent life-threatening events (ALTEs) are characterized by choking, gagging, or apnea in combination with changes in color (cyanosis) and muscle tone that resolve spontaneously or with care gives stimulation (i.e., picking up The infant). They understandably are extremely frightening to the caregiver. A differential diagnosis list is found in Table 21-4.

PREVENTION

Infants should be placed on their backs while sleeping. Contrary to popular belief, 24-hour home apnea monitoring does not decrease the risk of sudden infant death syndrome (SIDS). Use of monitors should be reserved for infants with documented episodes of apnea, bradycardia, or desaturation.

TABLE 21-3 SIDS: Risk Factors

Prone Sleeping Position[a]
Child/birth factors
Male gender
Low birthweight/intrauterine growth restriction[a]
Prematurity[a]
Multiple gestation
African American or American Indian race
Maternal factors
Maternal smoking during pregnancy[a]
Young maternal age
Lower socioeconomic status
Higher parity
Single parenthood
Fewer years of maternal education
Environmental factors
Soft bedding
Potentially obstructive materials in the bed

[a]Factors with highest risk.

TABLE 21-4 Differential Diagnosis of ALTEs

Idiopathic (apnea of infancy)
Infection
Respiratory
Respiratory syncytial virus
Pertussis
Systemic
Sepsis
Meningitis
Metabolic disease
Gastroesophageal reflux
Aspiration
Seizures
Cardiac arrhythmias
Abuse

KEY POINTS

- Along with a careful history, information gathered from vital signs, physical examination, and early laboratory data may suggest the substance ingested by conforming to a specific toxidrome (see Table 21-1).
- Concussions should be treated with physical and cognitive rest. Return-to-play recommendations are guided by symptoms as well as the severity of the initial impairment.
- After an initial episode of coughing and/or choking, the patient with foreign body aspiration may be asymptomatic for up to several days. Physical examination findings in a patient with foreign body aspiration are generally localized to one side of the chest.
- Child neglect is the most common cause of failure to thrive in developed countries.
- An injury that is inconsistent with the history, a history that changes over time, and a delay in seeking appropriate medical care all strongly suggest abuse.
- Shaken baby syndrome includes intracranial bleeding, diffuse axonal injury, and retinal hemorrhages. Intracranial injuries in the absence of substantiated major trauma (i.e, motor vechicle collision) are virtually pathognomonic of abuse in infants.
- Babies should be put to sleep on their backs (supine).
- The use of a home apnea monitor does not decrease an infant's risk of sudden infant death syndrome.

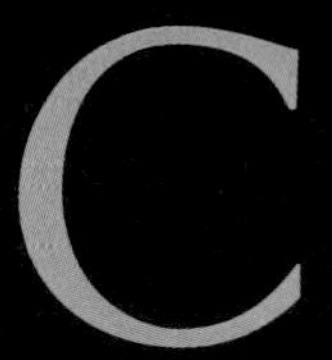

Clinical Vignettes

Vignette 1

A 4-year-old male is brought to the emergency department with the chief complaint of altered mental status. The parents note that their child has become increasingly sleepy over the last hour and is now unresponsive. The EMS team reports that he responds to deep sternal rub and that his saturations are 100% on room air. There is no history of seizure disorder. On physical examination, heart rate is 40 beats per minute, respiratory rate 7 breaths per minute, and blood pressure is 50/30 mm Hg. The child has sonorous breathing, stirs to deep painful stimulus, and has pinpoint pupils. The rest of his physical examination is normal. A rapid bedside glucose is 140 mg/dL. You suspect drug overdose. While waiting for establishment of an intravenous line, further history is obtained from the child's grandmother. On questioning, she states that several medications are accessible at home. These include oxycodone ibuprofen, acetaminophen, decongestants, and aspirin. They are located in a pillbox, and she doesn't recall locking it away this morning.

1. Ingestion of which of the following medications is most likely to cause this patient's constellation of symptoms?
   a. Oxycodone
   b. Ibuprofen
   c. Acetaminophen
   d. Decongestants
   e. Aspirin

2. Which of the following tests would most likely confirm the diagnosis?
   a. Complete blood count
   b. Arterial blood gas
   c. Serum osmolarity
   d. Prothrombin time
   e. Urine drug screen

3. While in the resuscitation room, the child becomes apneic and is unresponsive to painful stimuli. In addition to providing appropriate respiratory support, which of the following is the best immediate treatment for this patient?
   a. Flumazenil
   b. Digibind
   c. Naloxone
   d. Physostigmine
   e. Fomepizole

4. Anticipatory guidance aimed at decreasing the frequency of accidental ingestions at home includes all of the following except:
   a. placing household cleaning supplies out of reach of children
   b. keeping medication in a lockbox
   c. use of child-proof caps and blister packs
   d. keeping syrup of ipecac at home
   e. the use of poison control centers

Vignette 2

A 2-year-old female is brought to the emergency department with the chief complaint of difficulty breathing. She was in her high chair eating and suddenly started coughing and sputtering. The parents called EMS, and she was brought to the emergency department. She has no significant past medical history. On physical examination, her vital signs are normal except that she is tachypneic and coughing. Pulse oximetry reads 100% on room air. On auscultation, she has diffuse wheezes over the right hemithorax. The remainder of the physical examination is normal.

1. Which of the following tests would most likely confirm the diagnosis?
   a. Chest radiographs with decubitus views
   b. Arterial blood gas
   c. Peak flow measurements
   d. Contrast esophagram
   e. Chest ultrasound

2. Chest radiographs demonstrate unilateral hyperinflation in the right middle lobe, suggesting airway foreign body. Which of the following is the best definitive treatment for this patient?
   a. Intubation and flexible bronchoscopy
   b. Bronchodilator therapy
   c. Rigid bronchscopy in the operating room
   d. Heimlich maneuver
   e. Flexible layrngoscopy under conscious sedation

3. In this patient with airway foreign body for a brief period of time, which of the following is the most likely prognosis regarding lung function?
   a. Bronchiectasis and emphysema of the affected lobe
   b. Quick recovery, minimal sequelae
   c. Recurrent pneumonias
   d. Chronic asthma
   e. Exercise intolerance

Vignette 3

A 6-month-old male is brought to the emergency department with increasing sleepiness. His mother states that after returning home from work, she noticed the baby was initially irritable and has since become somnolent. The mother's boyfriend, who was caring for the infant, had stated to the mother that the baby was crying a lot and wouldn't take a bottle. The mother brought the child in because he has stopped feeding altogether. He was a premature baby at 30 weeks' gestation and has known gastroesophageal reflux. On physical examination, the vital signs are normal but he is difficult to arouse. His back and buttocks have bluish discolorations that look like bruises. The mother, when questioned, has no explanation for the discolorations—they appear new to her. You begin to suspect child abuse.

1. Following intial stabilization, your best response to your suspicion at this time consists of which of the following?
   - **a.** Refer the patient to their pediatrician for more in-depth workup.
   - **b.** Perform a skeletal survey and, if negative, discharge home.
   - **c.** Document concern in the medical record and fax immediately to the child's pediatrician.
   - **d.** Interview the boyfriend and mother separately and determine the likelihood of abuse.
   - **e.** Report your suspicion to state protective agencies.

2. Which of the following is not a risk factor for pediatric abuse or neglect?
   - **a.** Low socioeconomic status
   - **b.** Child with history of prematurity
   - **c.** Extreme caregiver stress
   - **d.** Male caregiver gender
   - **e.** Child with history of chronic illness

3. Which of the following tests is the most appropriate diagnostic study following initial stabilization of this patient?
   - **a.** Head computed tomography (CT)
   - **b.** Skeletal survey
   - **c.** Fundoscopic examination
   - **d.** Nuclear medicine bone scan
   - **e.** Chest radiograph

Vignette 4

A 3-month-old female is brought to your office. Earlier that morning, the mother called 911 due to a cyanotic spell. Soon after a feeding, the mother heard gasping and returned to the baby's room. The infant was awake and struggling but appeared unable to breathe. The mother noted circumoral cyanosis. On further questioning, she reports that the baby seemed stiff but did not have any shaking movements. She was frightened that the baby might die; however, by the time EMS arrived, the child appeared well. EMS declined to transport the infant to the hospital. At your office, the baby has a normal physical examination.

1. Which of the following findings in the above vignette does not support the diagnosis of apparent life-threatening event (ALTE)?
   - **a.** Color change
   - **b.** Frightening to the observer
   - **c.** Change in muscle tone
   - **d.** Gasping respirations
   - **e.** Event occurs after feeding

2. Which of the following diagnoses below is not typically included in the differential diagnosis for ALTE?
   - **a.** Infantile colic
   - **b.** Gastroesophageal reflux
   - **c.** Congenital heart disease
   - **d.** Child abuse
   - **e.** Seizures

3. The mother states that her nephew died of sudden infant death syndrome (SIDS) a few years ago, and she is worried the same may happen with her infant. She requests a home apnea monitor. Which of the following represents the most appropriate response?
   - **a.** Use of a home apnea monitor at night decreases the risk of SIDS.
   - **b.** Use of a 24-hour home apnea monitor does not decrease the incidence of SIDS.
   - **c.** Placing the infant prone in the crib is more effective than home apnea monitoring.
   - **d.** 24-hour home apnea monitoring only reduces the risk of SIDS in children without prior medical problems.
   - **e.** 24-hour home apnea monitoring should only be used in conjunction with medical supervision and prescription medications such as caffeine.

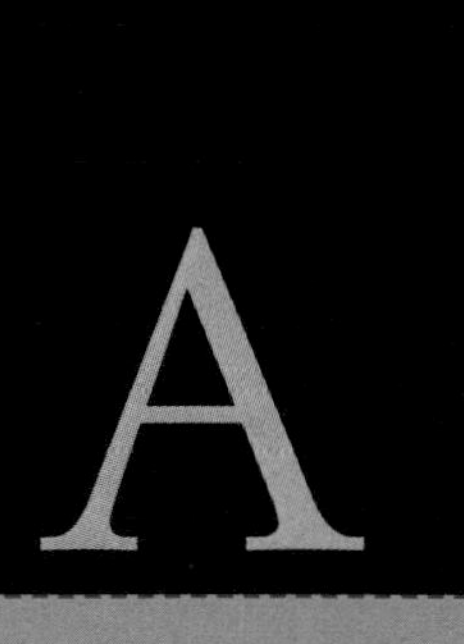

Answers

Vignette 1 Question 1

Answer A: *Oxycodone* is an opiate agonist that binds to opiate receptors in the central nervous system (CNS), causing inhibition of ascending pain pathways and producing generalized CNS depression. Overdose of opiates produces the clinical constellation portrayed: generalized CNS depression, hemodynamic compromise, and miosis. *Acetaminophen* overdose results from acute ingestion of more than 150 mg/kg. The patient is typically asymptomatic over the first 24 to 48 hours. Gastrointestinal symptoms such as abdominal pain and vomiting manifest later. Thereafter, serum hepatic enzyme levels begin to rise. Finally, in severe ingestions, liver failure ensues with prolongation of the prothrombin time, elevation of ammonia, and the development of cerebral edema and hepatic encephalopathy. Overdose with *ibuprofen*, a nonsteroidal anti-inflammatory drug (NSAID), results in gastrointestinal irritation. Over the short term, decreased mental status is not a feature of NSAID overdose. *Decongestants* such as pseudoephedrine have side effects quite opposite from those of opiate overdose; excessive ingestion produces agitation, hypertension, tachycardia, seizures, and mydriasis. *Aspirin* toxicity causes hyperpnea/tachypnea, fever, nausea and vomiting, agitation, and seizures. Older children may report tinnitus. Depressed mental status is a late finding.

Vignette 1 Question 2

Answer E: Standard toxicology results for urine drug screens include detection of opiates, benzodiazepines, and THC (the active chemical in marijuana). These screens are easy to obtain, and the results are rapidly available. A complete blood count is not helpful in confirming the diagnosis of opiate toxicity. It may have utility in determining alternate diagnoses in patients with altered mental status. The arterial blood gas may be helpful in evaluating a patient with suspected aspirin toxicity. The classical blood gas finding in salicylate toxicity is a mixed respiratory alkalosis with a concomitant metabolic acidosis. In opiate toxicity, the arterial blood gas may show hypoventilation, but this is not specific and can occur in other disorders with depressed mental status. Measurement of serum osmolarity assists in the diagnosis of ethylene glycol toxicity. In this type of ingestion, an osmolar gap can be calculated, suggesting the diagnosis. Opiate toxicity does not influence the osmolar gap. The prothrombin time is prolonged in liver failure as a consequence of acetaminophen toxicity. This is a late finding and not present in opiate toxicity.

Vignette 1 Question 3

Answer C: Naloxone is the antidote for acute opiate toxicity. It competes with and displaces opiates from opiate receptor sites. The onset of action is rapid, reversing respiratory and mental status depression within seconds of intravenous administration. Naloxone may also be given subcutaneously or instilled into an endotracheal tube. The effects are short lived, and patients frequently require multiple boluses or the institution of a continuous drip. In patients who are chronic opiate users, administration of naloxone may result in symptoms of drug withdrawal and should be given with caution. Flumazenil is used for benzodiazepine overdose and works quickly after intravenous administration. It has no use in cases of opiate intoxication. Digibind is the antidote for acute digoxin poisoning. Physostigmine is used to reverse the effects of organophosphate poisoning. Its mechanism of action involves stopping the hydrolysis of acetylcholine at the neuromuscular junction, thus preserving synaptic transmission at the neuromuscular junction. Fomepizole is used in ethylene glycol poisoning. It serves as a competive substrate that interferes with the metabolism of ethylene glycol, thereby limiting the production of the toxic metabolite.

Vignette 1 Question 4

Answer D: The American Academy of Pediatrics has recommended that syrup of ipecac no longer routinely be kept at home. There is no evidence to suggest its use is beneficial and it is contraindicated in children who have or may have depressed mental status. Inaccessibility of cleaning supplies, the use of medication lock boxes, the use of childproof caps and blister packages, and the notification and advice of poison control centers in acute poisoning are important measures in decreasing the number and morbidity of severe poisonings.

Vignette 2 Question 1

Answer A: In cases of suspected foreign body aspiration, a chest radiograph with lateral decubitus views would be most helpful in establishing the diagnosis of airway foreign body. While most airway foreign bodies are not radio-opaque, indirect findings such as areas of atelectasis/hyperinflation on chest radiograph may increase diagnostic certainty. The decubitus views will demonstrate dependent areas of lung which remain hyperinflated, signifying areas of ball-valve-type obstruction. Alternatively, expiratory views may be taken to localize areas of hyperinflation. Although a normal lateral decubitus chest radiograph does not fully rule out airway foreign body, it is the best answer in the case above. Bilateral decubitus lung radiographs are more sensitive than expiratory films, and easier to obtain in young children. The arterial blood gas will help determine the respiratory status of the patient but will not elucidate its etiology. Peak flow measurements do not differentiate air trapping from a *reactive airways* component versus an *airway foreign body*. Contrast esophograms are not useful in the diagnosis of airway foreign body but are performed when vascular rings or slings are considered in the differential of respiratory distress. While chest sonography may sometimes detect lung atelectasis, its sensitivity is quite limited. Chest ultrasonography is unable to differentiate hyperinflated lung from normal lung tissue.

Vignette 2 Question 2

Answer C: In cases of suspected airway foreign body, removal should be attempted by rigid bronchoscopy in the operating room. While flexible laryngoscopy and bronchoscopy may aid in diagnosis, the utility in treatment (i.e., foreign body removal) is quiet limited. Therefore, rigid bronchoscopy is the treatment of choice. Airway intervention in the field is contraindicated in the child who is actively crying, coughing, or speaking. The operating room is a more controlled environment for children who require semiurgent airway control. Bronchodilator therapy may ameliorate any airway reactive component, if present, but is not a definitive therapy. The Heimlich maneuver may be performed in the field in a patient who has complete obstruction of the trachea but is not appropriate in the patient above.

Vignette 2 Question 3

Answer B: The prognosis of patients with airway foreign bodies depends on the amount of lung damage sustained. This is usually a function of the time duration the foreign body has been in the airway. The longer an object remains in the airway, the longer the chronic inflammatory response has a chance to damage the airway. In this case, the acute presentation and prompt removal would most likely result in a rapid recovery and minimal complications. Bronchiectasis is often encountered in patients with cystic fibrosis complicated by hemoptysis. However, it may also present in cases of long-standing airway foreign body. Emphysema is very rare in children in the absence of conditions predisposing to air-leak syndromes. On occasion, a child with an airway foreign body may be diagnosed with pneumonia more than once before the foreign body is suspected and removed. When an airway foreign body is removed before major lung pathology develops, reactive lung disease and exercise intolerance are not associated complications.

Vignette 3 Question 1

Answer E: Health care workers who suspect that a pediatric patient has been the subject of abuse and/or neglect are required by law to notify state protective agencies of their concerns. The suspicion does not have to be substantiated. Suspicious injuries, stories that are inconsistent with a child's development abilities (e.g., a broken arm or leg in a child who is not yet mobile) or histories which change over time should be reported. Cases of suspected child abuse should be reported to the appropriate state authorities immediately; discharging the child home for subsequent follow-up with the pediatrician is inappropriate. The skeletal survey may be normal even in cases of severe child abuse, and the decision to refer should not rely on findings of this test. Finally, repeated interviews and interrogations of the caregivers should be carried out by the proper state authorities; this is not within the purview of the treating clinician.

Vignette 3 Question 2

Answer D: Abuse is perpetuated at all socioeconomic levels but is more prevalent at lower socioeconomic levels. Children with special needs (mental retardation, cerebral palsy, prematurity, and chronic illness) are also at increased risk. Caretakers who have themselves suffered abuse, who are alcohol or substance abusers, or who are under extreme stress are more likely to abuse or neglect. There is no known increased risk of child abuse based on male caregiver gender.

Vignette 3 Question 3

Answer A: While all the above tests are beneficial in both the diagnosis and baseline documentation of child abuse, CT of the head is the best initial test in this scenario. In a child with suspected abuse and depressed mental status, consideration should be given to intracranial hemorrhage. In shaken baby syndrome, pathognomonic injuries include subdural hemorrhage, retinal hemorrhages, and characteristic fractures such as posterior rib fractures. The prompt identification of intracranial injury is necessary in affecting the appropriate treatment plan of this infant. The skeletal survey, ophthalmologic exam, nuclear medicine bone scan, and the chest radiograph are helpful in the diagnosis and management of children with suspected abuse, but evaluation for intracranial hematoma by head CT should take precedence.

Vignette 4 Question 1

Answer E: ALTE's are characterized by choking, gagging, or apnea in concert with changes in color and muscle tone. In addition, the event must be frightening to the observer. While these events may occur in relation to feedings, this is not part of the definition.

Vignette 4 Question 2

Answer A: Infantile colic is characterized by excessive, inconsolable crying in an infant without underlying pathology or identifiable need. It occurs most commonly between the ages of 3 weeks and 3 months. Color changes, choking, gagging, and changes in muscle tone are not present. While the symptoms of colic may be distressing, they are generally exhausting rather than acutely frightening to the observer. The presence of any of the findings seen in ALTE should make one question the diagnosis of colic. Gagging associated with gastroesophageal reflux may occur in relation to feedings and can produce symptoms of ALTE. Congenital heart disease may cause cyanosis and difficulty feeding (such as increased work of breathing) that may result in gagging or choking along with apnea. Infants who have sustained intracranial hemorrhage from child abuse may manifest with seizures or apnea. Seizure disorder, with changes in muscle tone and cyanosis, is an important part of the differential diagnosis; a neurologic workup should be considered in infants with ALTE.

Vignette 4 Question 3

Answer B: Twenty-four-hour home apnea monitoring has not been shown to reduce the incidence of SIDS in healthy children. Use should be reserved for infants with documented episodes of apnea, bradycardia, or desaturation. Prone sleeping position has been associated with an increased incidence of SIDS; infants should be placed on their backs to sleep. There is also no evidence to suggest 24-hour home apnea monitoring in concert with medication such as caffeine decreases the incidence of SIDS.

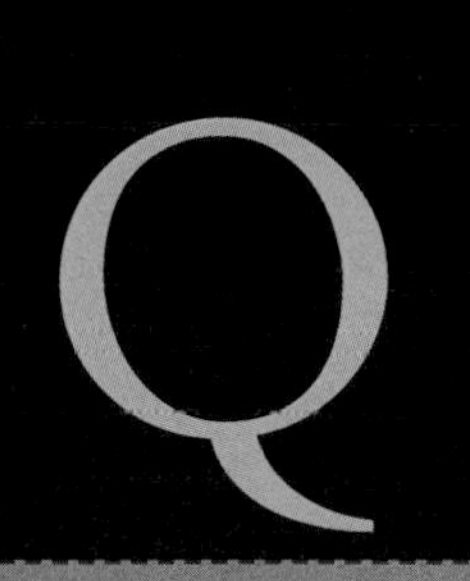

Questions

1. A 2-year-old female child presents with VT, severe ventricular dysfunction, hypotension, and metabolic acidosis. The patient is cardioverted into ventricular fibrillation which degenerates into asystole. What is the most appropriate indication for using intravenous epinephrine in this patient?
   - **a.** Ventricular ectopy
   - **b.** Asystole
   - **c.** Severe refractory metabolic acidosis and/or hyperkalemia
   - **d.** Bradycardia
   - **e.** Supraventricular tachycardia

2. A 16-year-old female patient presents with short stature and no secondary sexual characteristics. What diagnosis must be considered?
   - **a.** Turner syndrome
   - **b.** Isolated growth hormone deficiency
   - **c.** Cushing disease
   - **d.** Familial short stature
   - **e.** Addison disease

3. Galactosemia, a disorder of carbohydrate metabolism, is inherited in an autosomal recessive fashion. What is the risk of galactosemia in a child whose parents are both carriers for the disorder?
   - **a.** 100%
   - **b.** 75%
   - **c.** 50%
   - **d.** 25%
   - **e.** 0%

4. Which of the following statements is true regarding children with sickle cell disease?
   - **a.** Vaccinations are not required because they receive penicillin prophylaxis.
   - **b.** Gallstones typically develop before the age of 3 years.
   - **c.** Episodes of dactylitis should be treated with antibiotics.
   - **d.** Hydroxyurea maintenance therapy decreases the number and severity of vasoocclusive crises.
   - **e.** Acute chest syndrome requires only supportive care.

5. A mother brings her 5-year-old son to your office in New Mexico for his regular health maintenance visit. A quick review of the patient's chart reveals that he and his family are strict vegans (i.e., they eat no animal products of any kind). Their house is very small, so all the children spend a good deal of time outside. The mother states that her son eats plenty of dark green vegetables and iron-fortified grains. She does not believe in providing supplemental vitamins and minerals. This child is most at risk for nutritional deficiency involving which of the following?
   - **a.** Vitamin B_{12}
   - **b.** Vitamin B_6
   - **c.** Niacin
   - **d.** Riboflavin
   - **e.** Vitamin D

6. A 6-year-old boy presents with a newly appreciated heart murmur. He is asymptomatic, with normal growth and development and normal exercise tolerance. On examination, S1 and S2 are normal; a II/VI low-frequency midsystolic murmur is heard at the left lower sternal border. His pulses are normal. The most likely diagnosis is
   - **a.** bicuspid aortic valve
   - **b.** Still's murmur
   - **c.** ventricular septal defect
   - **d.** atrial septal defect
   - **e.** coarctation of the aorta

7. You are called to the delivery room for a routine birth. The infant cries when the cord is cut. You examine the child under the warmer and notice that when he stops crying, his chest heaves and he turns blue. You are unable to pass the NG tube through the nose for suctioning. Which condition is most likely causing this infant's respiratory distress?
   - **a.** Choanal atresia or stenosis
   - **b.** Vocal cord paralysis
   - **c.** Subglottic stenosis
   - **d.** Recurrent laryngeal nerve damage
   - **e.** Laryngeal web

8. A 3-year-old girl is diagnosed with new-onset insulin-dependent diabetes mellitus. Which of the following laboratory findings is consistent with diabetic ketoacidosis?
   - **a.** Hypoglycemia
   - **b.** Hypercarbia
   - **c.** Ketones in urine
   - **d.** Increased venous blood pH
   - **e.** Decreased BUN

9. During a male newborn examination, the testes are not palpable in the scrotal sacs. One testis is palpable high in the right inguinal canal and cannot be gently manipulated into the anatomically correct position. The left testis is not palpable but is discovered in the abdomen after consultation with a pediatric urologist and an abdominal ultrasound. In counseling the parents, which one of these statements regarding cryptorchidism is true?

a. More than 99% of males have bilateral descended testes at age 1 year.
b. Impaired sperm production is not a concern if neither testis descends.
c. Malignant degeneration is not a risk factor for testes which do not descend as long as they are placed within the scrotal sac through surgery by 1 year of age.
d. This infant is no more likely than his peers to manifest an inguinal hernia.
e. Microphallus is a common associated condition.

10. A 5-year-old boy presents with a waddling limp and has had a stiff right hip for the last 2 months. He has minimal complaints of pain. Which of the following is the most likely diagnosis?

a. Legg-Calvé-Perthes disease
b. slipped capital femoral epiphysis
c. toddler's fracture
d. septic arthritis
e. juvenile idiopathic arthritis

11. A 17-year-old young girl on oral contraceptive therapy for regulation of her menstrual periods presents with a 1-week history of left leg pain and swelling. Evaluation with a Doppler ultrasound reveals absence of flow in the left femoral and popliteal veins. The clot extends proximally to the left external iliac vein. The most important potential complication that one should be cautious about in this girl is

a. venous insufficiency
b. limb overgrowth
c. pulmonary embolism
d. edema
e. gangrene

12. A woman with a seizure disorder under medical management wants to conceive a child. Her risk of having a child with a neural tube defect is greatest if her gestational medical regimen includes which of the following?

a. Phenobarbital
b. Phenytoin
c. Ethosuximide
d. Carbamazepine
e. Primidone

13. A 2-month-old infant presents to your emergency department with a heart rate of 220 beats per minute, pulses, and adequate perfusion. After giving the infant oxygen, you note abnormal P waves and a narrow QRS (≤0.08 seconds) on the cardiac monitor. Which of the following is the best course of action?

a. Administer IV/IO epinephrine
b. Administer IV adenosine by rapid bolus
c. Administer IV calcium chloride
d. Administer IV atropine by rapid bolus
e. Administer IV sodium bicarbonate

14. A 3-month-old infant presents with a history of abnormal movements that his parents think might be seizures. You observe an episode of recurrent rhythmic flexor-extensor spasms that repeat about 30 times before subsiding. The EEG shows hypsarrhythmia, and a Wood lamp exam is positive for several flat, hypopigmented macules scattered over the skin surface. This child's infantile spasms are most likely a result of which of the following underlying disorders?

a. Von Recklinghausen disease
b. Tuberous sclerosis
c. Von Hippel-Lindau disease
d. Sturge-Weber disease
e. Bilateral acoustic neurofibromatosis

15. A 21-month-old girl arrives at your clinic in May with a vaccination record that indicates that she has received 3 DTaP doses, 3 HiB doses, 3 IPV doses, 3 pneumococcal conjugate vaccine doses, 2 hepatitis A vaccine doses, and 3 hepatitis B vaccine doses. Which of the following should be administered at this visit?

a. DTaP, Hib, IPV, varicella
b. DTaP, Hib, pneumococcal conjugate vaccine, MMR, and varicella
c. DTaP, hepatitis A, IPV, pneumococcal conjugate vaccine
d. DTaP, hepatitis B, MMR, and varicella
e. DTaP, hepatitis A, IPV, MMR, and varicella

16. The mother of a 30-month-old boy is concerned that the child's speech is "garbled." The child uses "ma-ma" and "da-da" appropriately. He uses about 30 other words, but most of them are mispronounced (for instance, "boo" instead of "blue"). The boy's aunt, uncle, and cousins came to visit for a weekend and were unable to understand more than half of what he said. Examination of the ears reveals normal canals with translucent, mobile tympanic membranes and visible landmarks. Which of the following evaluations for speech delay should be performed first?

a. Receptive language testing
b. Phonetic testing
c. Dysfluency evaluation
d. Tympanogram testing
e. Audiologic (hearing) assessment

17. A 13-year-old girl presents with recurrent abdominal pain over the last 3 months. She has missed a total of 8 days of school. There is no associated fever, weight loss, gastrointestinal bleeding, and the pain does not occur in relation to meals or awaken her from sleep. There is diffuse abdominal tenderness but no other abnormal findings on examination. Which approach is likely to help in the diagnosis and management of her condition?

a. Abdominal CT scan with contrast
b. Upper and lower endoscopy and biopsies
c. Explaining the likely etiology of her symptoms using a biopsychosocial model and symptomatic therapy
d. A diet history and a diet elimination trial
e. Referral to a psychiatrist

18. A newborn male child has a flat facial profile, upslanted palpebral fissures, epicanthal folds, a small mouth with a protruding tongue, small genitalia, and simian creases on his hands. Which of the following chromosomal disorders is most likely in this child?

a. Trisomy 21
b. Trisomy 18
c. Trisomy 13

d. Klinefelter syndrome
e. Turner syndrome

19. At a 2-year well-child visit, you collect information that your patient lives in a very old rental home with peeling paint. Both the capillary (screening) and venous blood lead measurements are 50 μg/dL. The patient has a history of constipation but is otherwise asymptomatic. Which of the following courses of action is most appropriate?
    a. Initiate chelation therapy in a lead-free environment within 48 hours.
    b. Redraw the blood lead level in 1 week and test all siblings; treat if ≥50 μg/dL.
    c. Optimize calcium and iron intake and repeat the blood lead level in 1 month; treat if ≥50 μg/dL.
    d. Refer the family to a lead-removal company; repeat the blood lead level 1 month after decontamination of the home, and treat if ≥50 μg/dL.
    e. Refer the case to child protective services for parental neglect.

20. A young couple is in your office for their prenatal visit, and you are discussing infant feeding. The father states that he prefers that the mother breastfeed the baby. The mother is hesitant to commit to breastfeeding because she plans on returning to full-time employment 6 weeks after the child is born. Neither her mother nor her sisters chose to breastfeed. She is concerned that human breast milk may not provide all the nutrients that the child needs, and she believes formula is a more complete nutritional source for infants. She is willing to consider exclusive breastfeeding based on the American Academy of Pediatrics recommendation. If her baby is exclusively breastfed, when should the child begin receiving oral vitamin D supplementation?
    a. Never
    b. Within the first several days
    c. Age 2 months
    d. Age 4 months
    e. Age 6 months

21. A 12-year-old female patient presents with fever, night sweats, weight loss, fatigue, anorexia, and painless, rubbery, cervical lymphadenopathy. What is the most common presentation of Hodgkin disease?
    a. Fever, night sweats, and/or weight loss of >10% in the preceding 6 months (i.e., "B" symptoms)
    b. Mediastinal lymphadenopathy
    c. Painless, rubbery, cervical lymphadenopathy
    d. Pruritus
    e. Extreme fatigue and anorexia

22. Which of the following medication groupings is most appropriate for a patient 12 years old with persistent asthma who has failed to achieve well-controlled asthma while receiving Step 2 treatment?
    a. None
    b. A daily low-dose inhaled corticosteroid
    c. A daily medium-dose inhaled corticosteroid and a long-acting inhaled β2-agonist
    d. A daily low-dose inhaled corticosteroid and a long-acting β-agonist
    e. A daily medium-dose inhaled corticosteroid and nedocromil

23. Crops of papular, vesicular, pustular lesions starting on the trunk and spreading to the extremities, in addition to small, irregular red spots with central gray or bluish-white specks that appear on the buccal mucosa, is the classic description of which of the following infections?
    a. Measles
    b. Erythema infectiosum (fifth disease)
    c. Roseola infantum
    d. Zoster (shingles)
    e. Rubella
    f. Hand-foot-mouth disease
    g. chickenpox

24. A 20-month-old boy who was treated with high-dose amoxicillin (90 mg/kg/day) for acute otitis media 3 weeks ago now presents with acute-onset ear pain, a bulging, erythematous right tympanic membrane, and decreased mobility on pneumatic otoscopy examination. Which of the following is the most appropriate antibiotic choice for this child?
    a. Azithromycin
    b. Amoxicillin-clavulanate
    c. Erythromycin
    d. Trimethoprim-sulfamethoxazole
    e. Dicloxacillin

25. Which of the following is considered a risk factor for neonatal respiratory distress syndrome?
    a. Neonatal sepsis
    b. Poorly controlled maternal diabetes
    c. Maternal preeclampsia
    d. Neural tube defects
    e. Trisomy 21

26. A mildly febrile 6-year-old patient presents to your office with dysuria and urinary frequency and urgency. She has a history of one prior UTI about 8 months ago. You obtain a dipstick urinalysis and send a urine culture. The dipstick is positive for nitrites and leukocyte esterase. Which of the following is the most appropriate course of action at this time?
    a. Await culture results and tailor therapy based on bacterial sensitivities.
    b. Begin empiric amoxicillin.
    c. Begin empiric amoxicillin and schedule the child for a renal ultrasound within the next 6 weeks.
    d. Begin empiric amoxicillin and schedule the child for a renal ultrasound and voiding cystourethrogram within the next 6 weeks.
    e. Admit the child to the hospital for IV ampicillin and gentamycin and schedule a DMSA scan.

27. A 3-month-old infant presents with cyanosis and an echocardiogram reveals that the child has tetralogy of Fallot. What four associated lesions describe tetralogy of Fallot?
    a. Ventricular septal defect, overriding aorta, pulmonary stenosis, right ventricular hypertrophy
    b. Ventricular septal defect, atrial septal defect, pulmonary stenosis, right ventricular hypertrophy
    c. Ventricular septal defect, atrial septal defect, aortic stenosis, right ventricular hypertrophy
    d. Ventricular septal defect, coarctation of the aorta, aortic stenosis, right ventricular hypertrophy
    e. Ventricular septal defect, mitral valve prolapse, pulmonary stenosis, left ventricular hypertrophy

28. A 3-year-old boy with a known diagnosis of factor XI deficiency presents to the emergency department with uncontrolled bleeding from a lip laceration following a fall. The most appropriate product that can be used for factor replacement in this child prior to suturing is

a. cryoprecipitate
b. granulocyte infusions
c. fresh frozen plasma (FFP)
d. platelet transfusion
e. DDAVP

29. At the health maintenance visit for a 12-year-old male, you note that he has entered his pubertal height growth spurt. The patient's mother asks about what changes her son should be expecting in his body over the next several years. As part of your review, you mention that the most typical sequence of pubertal events in males is which of the following?

a. Peak height velocity, pubarche, penile enlargement, testicular enlargement
b. Peak height velocity, testicular enlargement, penile enlargement, pubarche
c. Testicular enlargement, pubarche, penile enlargement, peak height velocity
d. Testicular enlargement, peak height velocity, penile enlargement, pubarche
e. Pubarche, testicular enlargement, peak height velocity, penile enlargement

30. A 4-year-old child with known asthma presents to the emergency department with a chief complaint of wheezing for the past 8 hours. On examination, he is alert and cooperative, mildly tachypneic, has diffuse loud expiratory wheeze, and has a pulse oximetry reading of 89% while breathing room air. He has already taken 3 albuterol aerosols at home in the past hour. He is unchanged after receiving another albuterol inhalation treatment in the emergency department. Appropriate next management would include

a. supplemental oxygen
b. albuterol inhalation
c. ipratropium bromide inhalation
d. oral corticosteroids
e. all of the above

31. A previously healthy 3-year-old boy presents with a history of fever and diarrhea for the past 2 days. The fever has not responded to ibuprofen, and his urine output has decreased today. On examination, he is alert, has a temperature of 101° F, has a heart rate of 115 beats per minute, has a blood pressure of 105/60 mm Hg, and has mild diffuse abdominal tenderness. The serum electrolytes are normal, but his BUN is 60 mg/dL and his serum creatinine is 1.8 mg/dL. The complete blood count is normal. Urinalysis shows 1+ protein, small blood, and occasional hyaline casts. The kidney ultrasound is normal. Which of the following statements regarding his acute renal failure is most accurate?

a. It is due to hemolytic-uremic syndrome.
b. It is due to pyelonephritis.
c. It is due to interstitial nephritis.
d. It is due to the use of ibuprofen in a dehydrated state.
e. It is due to urinary tract obstruction.

32. A 14-year-old girl presents with several weeks of profound fatigue, intermittent low-grade fevers, a facial rash, and joint pain. The rash recently worsened markedly after sun exposure. On physical examination, she has a malar rash extending over the bridge of the nose (but sparing the nasolabial folds), painless oral ulcers, and painful limitation of movement in her wrists and finger joints. On laboratory testing, her WBC is 3,500/mm^3, Hgb is 9.5 g/dL, and platelet count is 120,000/mm^3. A urinalysis shows 15 to 19 RBC/hpf and an elevated protein of 100 mg/dL. Which of the following tests will most likely be positive?

a. Antinuclear antibody (ANA)
b. Rheumatoid factor (RF)
c. Anti-double-stranded DNA (dsDNA) antibody
d. Anti-Smith (Sm) antibody
e. Anti-Ro (SS-A) antibody

33. A 3-month-old female infant presents to your emergency department unresponsive and with fever, tachypnea, bradycardia, and hypotension. What order should you follow in your initial assessment?

a. Airway, breathing, circulation, disability, exposure
b. Breathing, airway, circulation, disability, exposure
c. Circulation, airway, breathing, exposure, disability
d. Exposure, breathing, airway, circulation, disability
e. Exposure, airway, breathing, circulation, disability

34. A 4-year-old male child presents with abrupt-onset petechiae and ecchymoses. Other than the skin findings, the child appears well and is hemodynamically stable. No splenomegaly is noted. A complete blood count reveals a normal white blood cell count, a normal hematocrit, and a platelet count of 12,000/mm^3. Large platelets are seen on the peripheral smear. No premature white cell forms are seen on peripheral smear. The parent reports that the child had a viral illness 2 weeks before presentation. Which of the following is the *most* likely diagnosis?

a. Isoimmune thrombocytopenia
b. Leukemia
c. Sepsis
d. Immune thrombocytopenic purpura
e. Hypersplenism

35. A child presents with a reduced number of CD3+ T cells, an increased number of B lymphocytes that are mildly abnormal in function, has a conotruncal heart lesion, hypoplastic thymus, and hypocalcemia. Which of the following chromosomal disorders is most likely in this child?

a. Zellweger syndrome
b. Microdeletion of 22q11.2
c. Trisomy 13
d. Gaucher disease
e. Wilson disease

36. A 4-month-old, former 30-week premature infant is seen in late October for well-child care. His mother is concerned about the transfusions that the infant required during her course in the neonatal intensive care unit and wishes to restrict her exposure to blood products. Referral for administration of which of the following would be most appropriate to limit her risk of severe bronchiolitis?

a. Ribavirin
b. Nasal influenza vaccine
c. Injected influenza vaccine
d. IV RespiGam
e. IM palivizumab

37. The mother of a 2-month-old infant brings her daughter to your office during the summer for her regular health maintenance visit. The child is cared for by her maternal grandmother 3 days a week while the mother is at work. The infant is exclusively fed a cow milk–based commercial formula when she is with the mother; the grandmother believes that the child should also receive juice diluted with water due to the warm weather. Which of the following represents the most appropriate dietary counseling regarding this infant's diet?

a. Formula-fed infants at this age require free water supplementation during warm months to maintain optimal hydration.
b. Formula-fed infants at this age require glucose supplementation during the warm months to maintain optimal caloric intake.
c. Formula-fed infants do not require any additional vitamin, mineral, caloric, or fluid supplementation beyond their formula for the first 6 months of life.
d. Dilution of this infant's formula with water or juice on the days that she is with the maternal grandmother is unnecessary but harmless.
e. This infant should be switched to a soy protein–based formula.

38. No red reflex is seen on funduscopic examination of a newborn. Which of the following is the most likely diagnosis?

a. Retinoblastoma
b. Leukocoria
c. Congenital cataract
d. Congenital glaucoma
e. Toxocariasis

39. A 5-year-old boy is brought to your office complaining of progressive fatigue, weakness, and nausea over the past few months. He was a model student, but he is now having trouble in school and displaying frequent outbursts, the last of which resulted in his being sent home for hitting another child. Initial lab results show mild hypoglycemia, hyponatremia, and hyperkalemia. The child is diagnosed with adrenal insufficiency and treated appropriately; however, his behavior continues to worsen, and he begins to have difficulty walking and speaking. Which of the following is the most likely etiology of his behavior problems?

a. Tay-Sachs disease
b. Gaucher disease
c. Niemann-Pick disease
d. Adrenoleukodystrophy
e. Rett syndrome

40. An 8-year-old girl thought to have attention-deficit disorder (inattentive-type) undergoes EEG testing and is found to have a 3-Hz spike-and-wave pattern. Results of the EEG, coupled with videotaping of episodes of the patient's "inattention," lead to a diagnosis of childhood absence epilepsy. Which of the following is most appropriate for initial treatment of the child's disorder?

a. Methylphenidate
b. Carbamazepine
c. ACTH
d. Ethosuximide
e. Phenobarbital

41. A child presents with lymphedema of the hands and feet, a shield-shaped chest, widely spaced hypoplastic nipples, short stature, and multiple pigmented nevi. In addition, she had a coarctation of the aorta that was repaired and has renal disease. Her parents continue to be worried that there is something in addition to her heart condition that is causing failure to thrive. Which of the following chromosomal disorders is most likely in this child?

a. Trisomy 21
b. Trisomy 18
c. Trisomy 13
d. Klinefelter syndrome
e. Turner syndrome

42. A 14-year-old patient familiar to the emergency room staff due to multiple visits in the last 3 months is brought in by her mother for ingestion of an unknown number of acetaminophen tablets. The mother states that she keeps all the medicines in the house locked up because "this is just the sort of thing my daughter would do to me." She saw the girl stuffing something into her bedside drawer while she was passing the girl's room and discovered a bottle marked "acetaminophen 500 mg, 250 tablets." Only 4 tablets remained in the bottle. The mother did not believe that her daughter took the tablets until she began vomiting about an hour later. The girl refuses to speak in her mother's presence but eventually admits that she took "many tablets" about 4:00 p.m. (3 hours ago). Which of the following is recommended as an antidote for this patient's ingestion?

a. Atropine sulfate
b. Hemodialysis
c. Whole bowel irrigation
d. Oral *N*-acetyl cysteine
e. Activated charcoal

43. Which of the following scenarios is consistent with abuse rather than accidental injury?

a. A 30-month-old child with a bucket handle fracture
b. A 12-month-old infant with a rib fracture
c. A 6-month-old infant with retinal hemorrhages in the absence of signs of external head trauma
d. Abdominal bruises in a 9-month-old infant
e. All of the above

44. A 2-year-old presents with painless rectal bleeding. The hemoglobin is 9 g/dL. Capillary refill remains normal. The best next step to positively identify the cause of bleeding is

a. Colonoscopy
b. Transfusion with packed red blood cells
c. Meckel diverticulum scan
d. Gastric lavage
e. Stool culture

45. A 3-week-old male infant presents to the emergency department with 24-hour history of vomiting and poor feeding. He is found to be hypotensive and hypoglycemic. His serum electrolyte values are as follows: Na 121 mmol/L, K 6.9 mmol/L, CO_2 20 mmol/L, chloride 105 mmol/L, BUN 17 mg/dL, creatinine 0.7 mg/dL, and glucose 36 mg/dL. He receives 20 mL/kg NS fluid bolus and 2 mL/kg dextrose 25. What other life-saving intervention should this infant receive?

a. IV azithromycin
b. IV bicarbonate
c. IV hydrocortisone
d. IV albumin
e. IV calcium

46. A 7-year-old girl presents with a 3-week history of dozens of asymptomatic red, scaly 5 to 10 mm plaques appearing on the trunk. When the scales are pulled off, they bleed. Her nails are pitted. The most appropriate laboratory test is

a. A bacterial culture of the red plaques
b. A fungal culture of the red plaques
c. A throat culture
d. A Tzanck smear
e. A complete blood count

47. An 8-year-old patient of yours with attention-deficit/hyperactivity disorder is experiencing unacceptable adverse effects due to his stimulant medication. You have prescribed immediate- and extended-release preparations of two separate agents in the past. You believe that the patient may benefit from switching to a nonstimulant medication. Which of the following medications approved for the treatment of attention-deficit/hyperactivity disorder is classified as a nonstimulant?

a. Oral atomoxetine
b. Oral lisdexamfetamine
c. Oral methylphenidate
d. Oral dextroamphetamine
e. Oral mixed amphetamine salts

48. A 9-month-old girl presents with a 3-day history of fever to 103° F (39.4° C). This morning, the girl developed a rash. On physical examination, the girl is afebrile and has an erythematous, maculopapular rash over her trunk, arms, and legs. Which of the following is the most likely cause of this patient's illness?

a. Human parvovirus B19
b. Measles
c. Human herpesvirus 6
d. Chickenpox
e. Group A β-hemolytic streptococci

49. A 2-year-old child is brought to the emergency department following a brief (<2 minutes) generalized seizure. Initial vitals include a temperature of 102.9° F. Following the history, physical examination, and laboratory studies, you determine that the patient has had a febrile seizure. The parents are appropriately concerned and have a number of questions. You would be correct in telling them which of the following?

a. Children who experience a single febrile seizure have no greater risk of subsequently developing epilepsy than children who have not experienced a febrile seizure.
b. The morbidity and mortality associated with febrile seizures is extremely high.
c. At least half of patients who experience an initial febrile seizure will experience seizures with subsequent episodes of fever.
d. Patients who have experienced a single febrile seizure should be placed on preventative anticonvulsant medication.
e. Febrile seizures are usually associated with intracranial infections.

50. A 3-year-old boy presents with an elbow hemarthrosis after falling on his elbow. There is no history of spontaneous bleeding. There is no history of epistaxis, gingival bleeding, or cutaneous bruising. The child's maternal grandfather had frequent spontaneous bleeding and hemarthroses after trauma on multiple occasions. Laboratory results revealed a prolonged PTT, normal PT, and a platelet count of 150,000/mm^3. The factor VIII coagulant activity (VIII:c) is low and the factor IX level is normal. What is the *most* likely diagnosis?

a. Idiopathic thrombocytopenic purpura
b. Von Willebrand disease
c. Vitamin K deficiency
d. Hemophilia A
e. Liver disease

51. A 10-week-old boy is brought to the emergency department by his mother with a history of failure to thrive and poor feeding. He occasionally vomits small amounts of formula. His birth weight, length, and head circumference were at the 50th percentile; however, his weight has dropped to the 10th percentile and his length to between 25th and 40th percentiles. His vital signs are normal, and the physical exam is otherwise unrevealing. Venous blood gas and electrolyte study results include pH 7.32, sodium 134 mEq/L, potassium 4.5 mEq/L, chloride 106 mEq/L, and bicarbonate 10 mEq/L. Which of the following diagnoses is the most likely?

a. Inborn error of metabolism
b. Renal tubular acidosis
c. Pyloric stenosis
d. Chronic diarrhea
e. Cystic fibrosis

52. A 2-year-old girl presents with a swollen left knee, limping, and morning stiffness in the left knee of 3 months' duration. On physical examination, there is a left knee joint effusion, synovial thickening, and limitation of movement. In addition, the left leg is longer than the right and there is atrophy of the quadriceps. The remainder of the review of systems and physical examination is normal. On laboratory testing, a complete blood count is normal. An antinuclear antibody (ANA) test is positive at a titer of 1:320. This child is at most risk for which of the following sequelae/complications?

a. Glomerulonephritis
b. Hemolytic anemia
c. Chronic, nongranulomatous anterior uveitis (iridocyclitis)
d. Acute anterior uveitis (iridocyclitis)
e. Rheumatic heart disease

53. A 9-year-old boy diagnosed with pneumonia 2 days ago presents to the emergency department via ambulance in respiratory distress. His past medical history is noncontributory, and he is at low risk for contracting tuberculosis. He is hypoxic and requires oxygen. A STAT portable chest radiograph reveals a large right-sided pleural effusion, which shifts in the decubitus position. Fluid is obtained via thoracentesis for Gram stain and culture. Which of the following is the most likely pathogen responsible for this boy's pneumonia?

a. Staphylococcus aureus
b. Nontypeable Haemophilus influenzae
c. Chlamydophila pneumoniae
d. Klebsiella pneumoniae
e. Mycoplasma pneumoniae

54. During a routine annual physical examination, a 9-year-old previously healthy girl has a blood pressure of 140/75 mm Hg in all four extremities. The physical examination is otherwise completely normal, except for obesity. The family history is positive for hypertension in the father and paternal uncle. The blood pressure remains in the 140/70 mm Hg range on two repeat examinations performed 1 week apart, using a cuff that is appropriate for her obesity. The urinalysis, serum electrolytes, and serum creatinine levels are normal. Which of the following is the most appropriate next step in the management of this patient?

a. Reassure the patient that her blood pressure is normal for her size.
b. Advise observation, with repeat blood pressure checks every month.

c. Advise an immediate evaluation by a nephrologist and cardiologist.
d. Advise a regimen of weight reduction and regular exercise.
e. Advice a regimen of diuretic therapy.

55. A parent brings her 12-week-old child to your office because he has a scaly facial rash. The boy was exclusively breastfed for 8 weeks but was switched to commercial cow milk–based formula about a month ago when his mother went back to work. She has been putting lotion on the rash, but it has not helped. The child's birth weight was at the 50th percentile but has now dropped toward the 25th percentile line. The physical examination reveals an eczematous rash over both cheeks. The stool is guaiac-positive but not grossly bloody. Based on the history and physical examination, you suspect that the patient may be allergic to cow milk protein. Which of the following is the best next step in the management of this patient?

a. Recommend that the mother see her obstetrician about medication to help her begin lactating again.
b. Switch the patient from cow milk–based formula to whole cow's milk.
c. Switch the patient from cow milk–based formula to soy formula.
d. Switch the patient from cow milk–based formula to a protein hydrolysate formula.
e. Begin parenteral alimentation to permit total bowel rest.

56. A 16-year-old male is brought to your office by his mother, who insists that you perform a urine drug screen on her son. You begin by interviewing the mother and the young man together, but explain to the parent that you will also be conducting part of the interview and the physical examination without her present in the room. She states that she will only agree to let you speak with him alone if you agree to discuss with her any high-risk behaviors that he admits to engaging in. Concerning patient confidentiality in regard to adolescents, you are required by law to inform the parent of this minor of which of the following?

a. Use of marijuana
b. Suicidal ideation
c. Petty theft
d. Consensual sexual relations with another minor of the opposite gender
e. Consensual sexual relations with another minor of the same gender

57. You see a 4-year-old child for declining school performance and behavior problems. His mother notes that he is a poor sleeper. He snores loudly and often gasps in his sleep. Sometimes she sleeps with him because she is afraid he will stop breathing. You note a slight fall off the growth curve and very large tonsils. A neck film demonstrates large adenoids as well. The child's insurance company will not pay to have the tonsils and adenoids removed unless you can prove they are causing him significant health problems. Which test is the most likely to give you that information?

a. Bronchoscopy
b. Overnight pulse oximetry monitoring
c. Polysomnography
d. Fluoroscopy
e. Overnight EEG monitoring

58. An infant who was discharged from the hospital on day-of-life presents to your office 3 days later for follow-up. The mother did not receive prenatal care. You notice bilateral purulent discharge from the eyes. There is marked eyelid edema and conjunctival swelling (chemosis). What is the most likely pathologic agent?

a. Chlamydia trachomatis
b. Neisseria gonorrhoeae
c. Group B *Streptococcus*
d. Toxoplasma gondii
e. Treponema pallidum

59. An unresponsive adolescent patient is brought to the emergency department with suspected ingestion of an unknown substance. EMS received a call from the hotel room where the youth was found, but no one else was there when they arrived. The patient is on 100% inspired oxygen and has required several bouts of positive pressure ventilation in the ambulance. On exam, the patient has a heart rate of 55, blood pressure 85/50, pinpoint pupils, and track lines on his left arm. Along with ongoing cardiovascular and respiratory support, which of the following should be administered to this patient?

a. Pralidoxime chloride
b. Physostigmine
c. Naloxone
d. Atropine sulfate
e. Desferrioxamine

60. A 15-month-old boy is brought to the emergency department with a fever and difficulty breathing. Right-sided wheezing is noted on the physical examination. The patient does not improve with aerosolized nebulizer treatment. An inspiratory chest radiograph is normal; however, the expiratory film demonstrates right-sided hyperinflation, with mediastinal shift to the left. This patient's respiratory symptoms are most likely due to which of the following?

a. Pneumonia
b. Foreign body aspiration
c. Pneumothorax
d. Empyema
e. Viral upper respiratory infection

61. You are seeing an 18-month-old boy who is new to your practice. His father is concerned about his child's development in relation to his two older brothers. The boy avoids eye contact and does not respond to efforts to engage him in reciprocal play such as peek-a-boo and patty cake games. He does not generate spontaneous language but can repeat certain words if spoken to him over and over. He spends a lot of time by himself rocking back and forth and becomes very agitated if this activity is interrupted. Which of the following conditions is most consistent with this child's reported behaviors?

a. Down syndrome
b. Hearing impairment
c. Autism
d. Attention-deficit/hyperactivity disorder
e. Asperger syndrome

62. An 8-year-old boy is referred to the emergency department by his pediatrician for a chief complaint of weakness. The weakness has been slowly progressive over the last several weeks. A review of symptoms reveals a history of constipation, polyuria, and polydipsia. The child is on no medications, and past medical history is noncontributory. In the primary physician's office, the patient had a serum potassium measurement of 2.8 mEq/L. A blood pressure measurement in the emergency department is normal for age, height, and gender. Urine electrolyte studies reveal an elevated urine potassium value. Which of the following conditions is the most likely cause of this patient's hypokalemia?

a. Excessive sweating
b. Renal tubular acidosis
c. Anorexia nervosa
d. Cushing syndrome
e. Renovascular disease

63. A 2-week-old female infant presents with generalized hypotonia, duodenal atresia, and hypothyroidism. What other structural defect is she most likely to have?

a. Malrotation
b. Endocardial cushion defects
c. Cleft palate
d. Renal disease
e. Sensorineural hearing loss

64. Which of the following condition(s) is (are) often associated with polyhydramnios?

a. Duodenal atresia
b. Tracheoesophageal fistula
c. Congenital hydrocephalus with myelomeningocele
d. Renal agenesis
e. A, B, and C

65. A 3-year-old boy presents with violent episodes of intermittent colicky pain, emesis, and blood per rectum. A tubular mass is palpated in the right lower quadrant. The abdominal radiograph reveals a dearth of air in the right lower quadrant and air-fluid levels consistent with ileus. Which of the following procedures will best assist in diagnosis and treatment?

a. Esophagogastroduodenoscopy
b. Rectal biopsy
c. Air contrast or double contrast enema
d. Stool culture
e. Colonoscopy

66. An 18-month-old female child presents with blood-streaked stool. The stool is grossly positive on occult blood testing. Which of the following diagnoses is most likely?

a. Anal fissure
b. Peptic ulcer disease
c. Mallory-Weiss tear
d. Inflammatory bowel disease
e. Necrotizing enterocolitis

67. A 4-year-old boy was seen by his pediatrician for fever and abdominal pain. The pain began after a sledding accident the day before his visit in which he fell on his right side. His mother noticed that his abdomen appeared distended today, particularly on the right side. In the pediatrician's office, he is noted to be hypertensive and has gross hematuria. What is the most likely diagnosis?

a. Pyelonephritis
b. Liver contusion
c. Renal contusion
d. Wilms tumor
e. Neuroblastoma

68. You are called to evaluate a newborn with an apparent foot deformity. On close examination, you note adduction of the forefoot, inversion of the foot, and plantar flexion at the ankle that is relatively fixed. Which of the following is true of this patient's condition?

a. This clinical picture is most consistent with metatarsus adductus.
b. This deformity will respond to stretching exercises.
c. This deformity will correct spontaneously when the child is able to bear weight.
d. This deformity will require surgical repair.
e. This deformity may be associated with other congenital malformations.

69. A 12-year-old boy with Crohn disease for 2 years is seen with an acute exacerbation. He is complaining of abdominal pain and diarrhea and has right lower quadrant fullness. The most effective approach in this acute setting is which of the following?

a. Perform a colonoscopy for cancer surveillance.
b. Obtain a stool culture to exclude acute infectious colitis and imaging studies to evaluate for abscess or fistula.
c. Initiate therapy with mercaptopurine or azathioprine.
d. Perform a capsule endoscopy.
e. Start biologic therapy with anti-TNF alpha antibody.

70. A 3-year-old girl periodically experiences swelling around her lips and breaks out in hives when she eats the snacks provided at daycare. Which of the following is the most appropriate for determining whether the child's symptoms are due to food allergies?

a. Skin prick testing to foods
b. Food-specific IgE levels
c. Skin prick testing to foods followed by double-blind placebo-controlled food challenges
d. Open-label food challenges
e. Endoscopy

71. An 11-year-old girl is referred to your office following an abnormal screen for scoliosis. You diagnose idiopathic scoliosis on exam using Adam's forward bending test. Subsequent radiographs reveal a lateral curvature of 35°. The patient is premenarchal. You refer the patient to an orthopedic surgeon and counsel the parent that the specialist will probably recommend

a. external bracing
b. follow-up radiographs every 6 months
c. stretching exercises
d. surgical fixation
e. no intervention

72. A child in the emergency department has point tenderness over the proximal tibia and an appropriate history of trauma. The radiograph shows a fracture through the growth plate that extends into the epiphysis and joint space. This type of fracture would be characterized as which of the following?

a. Salter-Harris Type I
b. Salter-Harris Type II
c. Salter-Harris Type III
d. Salter-Harris Type IV
e. Salter-Harris Type V

73. A 4-year-old Caucasian boy presents for evaluation of persistent jaundice. The family reports that the boy had neonatal jaundice on the first day of life and was treated with phototherapy. He has always had mild icterus, but has had increased icterus at times, especially following other mild illnesses, such as ear infections and colds. There is a family history of his father and paternal grandmother having undergone splenectomy. On examination, the boy has mild scleral icterus, and his spleen is palpable about 3 cm below the left costal margin. The laboratory evaluation reveals a total bilirubin of 1.9 mg/dL (unconjugated fraction is 1.5 mg/dL), normal liver transaminases, hemoglobin of 11.2 gm/dL, a normal MCV, and an elevated reticulocyte count of 8%. An osmotic fragility test is performed and demonstrates positive results. What is the most likely diagnosis?

a. Iron-deficiency anemia
b. Hereditary spherocytosis
c. Acute blood loss
d. Acute leukemia
e. Sickle cell disease

74. An adolescent comes to you with a chief complaint of painless vaginal discharge. You note projection of the breast areola as a secondary mound above the contour of the breast and pubic hair of adult texture and color with no spread to the medial surface of the thighs. This patient's examination is most consistent with which Tanner stage of development?

a. Stage I
b. Stage II
c. Stage III
d. Stage IV
e. Stage V

75. Which of the following statements about acute myeloid leukemia (AML) is true?

a. The preferred treatment for all types of AML is bone marrow transplant.
b. Chemotherapy used for AML is more intense than that used for ALL.
c. Hyperleukocytosis is not a problem with AML.
d. Patients with Down syndrome and AML have a worse prognosis.
e. Secondary AML has a good response to therapy.

76. A 13-year-old male patient presents with intermittent abdominal pain, diarrhea, weight loss, and growth failure and is noted on colonoscopy to have inflammatory skip lesions throughout the colon with rectal sparing. Which of the following statements is true?

a. Ulcerative colitis typically is characterized by rectal sparing.
b. Ulcerative colitis typically is characterized by skip lesions.
c. Crohn disease typically is characterized by transmural disease.
d. Ulcerative colitis typically is associated with growth failure.
e. Ulcerative colitis typically is associated with perianal disease.

77. You are moonlighting in the pediatric emergency department when a 10-year-old male arrives by ambulance with lethargy, confusion, dizziness, and a severe headache. His parents and maternal grandmother are in the adult emergency department with less severe but similar symptoms. The emergency medical technicians report that they were called by the police who found the family sleeping in their car with the engine running at their Christmas tree stand. Carbon monoxide poisoning is suspected. Which of the following should be the first step in the evaluation and management of this patient?

a. Obtain an EKG
b. Draw an arterial blood gas
c. Draw a blood carboxyhemoglobin level
d. Administer 100% oxygen
e. Stabilize the patient for transfer to a hyperbaric oxygen chamber

78. A 5-year-old girl presents to the emergency department with a 12-hour history of fever and respiratory distress. On physical examination, the girl appears toxic, is drooling, and leaning forward with her chin extended. She has a temperature of 104° F (40° C) and a respiratory rate of 32 breaths per minute. Which of the following is the most likely diagnosis?

a. Epiglottitis
b. Croup
c. Bacterial pneumonia
d. Diphtheria
e. Anaphylaxis

79. In response to your question concerning guns in the home during a routine adolescent health maintenance visit, the mother of the patient tells you that her husband, the boy's stepfather, keeps a loaded handgun in the bed table drawer for protection. You would be correct in telling this family that an adolescent who lives in a home with a gun

a. is less likely than peers who do not live with guns to die from homicide.
b. is less likely than peers who do not live with guns to commit suicide.
c. is mature enough to use good safety precautions, so storing the handgun separately from the ammunition is unnecessary.
d. has a 10-fold greater risk of dying from suicide than peers who do not live in homes with guns.
e. is less likely than peers who do not live with guns to be shot during a domestic dispute.

80. You are seeing a new patient for a health maintenance visit. The child is able to tell you his age and gender and speaks in five-to-eight-word sentences. His grandmother tells you that he is able to pedal a tricycle. He can perform a broad jump when the behavior is modeled and is able to copy a circle. However, he cannot yet balance on one foot or copy a cross. You record that the patient's developmental achievement is consistent with his age. Which of the following most closely correlates with this child's age in years?

a. 2 years
b. 3 years
c. 4 years
d. 5 years
e. 6 years

81. A child weighing 27 kg with a history of vomiting for 36 hours is judged to be 10% dehydrated based on vital signs and physical examination. The serum sodium measurement is 134 mEq/L. An initial 540-mL bolus of normal saline results in stabilization of the heart rate and improved capillary refill. Which of the following is the most appropriate parenteral fluid choice for the next 8 hours?

a. D_5 0.2 normal saline with 20 mEq/L KCl (added after urination) at 120 mL/hr
b. D_5 0.2 normal saline with 20 mEq/L KCl (added after urination) at 180 mL/hr
c. D_5 0.2 normal saline with 20 mEq/L KCl (added after urination) at 220 mL/hr
d. D_5 0.45 normal saline with 20 mEq/L KCl (added after urination) at 220 mL/hr
e. D_5 0.45 normal saline with 20 mEq/L KCl (added after urination) at 180 mL/hr

82. An 8-year-old boy presents with growth failure and vague abdominal pain. The abdomen is distended. There is no perianal disease, abdominal mass, or tenderness. The next set of diagnostic tests should include

a. CBC, CRP, tissue transglutaminase assay
b. CT scan of the abdomen
c. urinalysis, sweat chloride, laparotomy
d. colonoscopy, upper endoscopy
e. stool culture for ova and parasites

83. A 3-year-old boy presents to the pediatrician with fever, pallor, anorexia, joint pain, petechiae, and hepatosplenomegaly. Which of the following is the most likely diagnosis?

a. Acute lymphoblastic leukemia
b. Acute myelogenous leukemia
c. Juvenile chronic myelogenous leukemia
d. Aplastic anemia
e. Osteosarcoma

84. A 16-year-old girl who is 2 years postmenarche presents with mildly uneven shoulders and a small degree of one-sided rib prominence. Radiographs reveal a 25° scoliosis. Which of the following represents the best treatment?

a. Posterior spinal fusion
b. Intensive physical therapy
c. Scoliosis bracing
d. Spinal manipulation
e. Observation with repeat X-ray in 1 year

85. A 5-year-old boy who returned from a camping trip to his grandparents' farm in Virginia develops a fever of 103° F, a headache, vomiting, and an erythematous, macular rash on his wrists and ankles. On physical examination, he is moderately tachycardic with otherwise stable vital signs and no focal signs of infection. A CBC reveals a normal WBC count and differential and normal hemoglobin. However, the boy's platelet count is 65,000/mm^3. Serum electrolytes are normal. Blood cultures and immunofluorescent studies are sent. Which of the following is the most appropriate next course of action?

a. Discharge home on amoxicillin with close follow-up and reliable caregivers
b. Discharge home on amoxicillin-clavulanic acid with close follow-up and reliable caregivers
c. Hospitalization for observation pending further test results
d. Hospitalization for intravenous doxycycline and cefotaxime
e. Hospitalization for intravenous doxycycline

86. A 5-year-old boy presents with painful swelling of the hand and feet since the day before. Since earlier today, he has palpable purpura on the lower extremities, and also developed intermittent, colicky midabdominal pain. Prior to these events, he had a cold for 1 week. He did not have fevers and overall is well appearing. On physical examination, he has normal vital signs. He has palpable purpura on the lower extremities and buttocks. He has scrotal swelling. His hand and feet are puffy, and he has pain with movement of the ankle joints. His abdominal examination is unremarkable. A complete blood count shows normal results with a platelet count of 350,000/mm^3. Which of the following laboratory tests is most often abnormal in this disease process?

a. Antinuclear antibody (ANA)
b. Antineutrophil cytoplasmic antibody (ANCA)
c. Complement C3 and C4 levels
d. Urinalysis
e. Serum creatinine

87. A 12-month-old male infant presents with a hemoglobin of 7.5 and a hematocrit of 22%. The mean corpuscular volume is 65 and the adjusted reticulocyte count is 1.0%. What is the *most* likely cause of anemia in this child?

a. Iron-deficiency anemia
b. Anemia of chronic disease
c. Transient erythrocytopenia of childhood
d. Thalassemia syndrome
e. Parvovirus B19 aplastic crisis

88. A 12-year-old male adolescent presents with a 1-month history of fever, weight loss, fatigue, and pain and localized swelling of the midproximal femur. Which of the following is the most likely diagnosis?

a. Ewing sarcoma
b. Osteosarcoma
c. Chronic osteomyelitis
d. Benign bone tumor
e. Eosinophilic granuloma

89. You are examining a 3-year-old girl at her well-child visit. While she is staring at her stuffed cow in your hands, you quickly cover her right eye with an index card. When the index card is removed seconds later, you notice that the right eye "drifts" back toward the center. This reaction in response to the cover test indicates what abnormal condition?

a. Strabismus
b. Amblyopia
c. Leukocoria
d. Retinoblastoma
e. Nasolacrimal duct obstruction

90. A 14-year-old girl is brought to your office by her mother because she is complaining of "seeing double." The history is significant for headaches that waken the patient from sleep in the morning but are relieved by vomiting. On physical examination, you note that she is unable to abduct either eye. Lower extremity reflexes are slightly exaggerated. Which of the following physical signs is most likely to be present in this patient?

a. Hypotension
b. Papilledema
c. Tachycardia
d. Patency of the anterior fontanelle
e. Erythema migrans

91. A previously healthy 4-year-old girl presents with a history of diarrhea and vomiting for the past 3 days and decreased urine output for the past 12 hours. On examination, she has a heart rate of 120 beats per minute, blood pressure of 105/65 mm Hg, and no edema. The blood tests reveal serum sodium of 128 mEq/L, potassium 5.6 mEq/L, bicarbonate 12 mEq/L, BUN 55 mg/dL, and creatinine 1.6 mg/dL. The urine tests reveal a fractional excretion of sodium of 0.1. The kidney ultrasound is normal. Which of the following constitutes the most appropriate immediate management of this child's acute renal failure?

a. Intravenous normal saline bolus to correct the renal hypoperfusion
b. Intravenous bicarbonate to correct the metabolic acidosis
c. Intravenous furosemide to correct the fluid overload

d. Intravenous antibiotics to correct the infectious gastroenteritis
e. Initiation of dialysis to correct the acute renal failure

92. A very tired mother brings her 6-week-old infant to your office because "he screams for hours and hours a day and nothing makes him stop." His parent describes the crying spells as occurring daily and lasting several hours, usually through the late afternoon and early evening. Nothing seems to console the child during these episodes. While he is crying, the infant often pulls his knees to his abdomen as if he is in pain. Other than the crying spells, the child is asymptomatic. He feeds well and moves his bowels regularly. The child's weight, length, and head circumference are normal, and his physical examination is normal. This patient's history and physical examination are most consistent with which of the following conditions?

a. Feeding intolerance
b. Cow milk protein allergy
c. Intussusception
d. Hirschsprung disease
e. Colic

93. A newborn infant has a slight hip click on hip examination. Which of the following risk factors would most strongly support further evaluation?

a. Female patient
b. First born
c. Torticollis
d. Metatarsus adductus
e. Breech presentation or family history of developmental dysplasia of the hip

94. A 14-year-old patient in your practice with anorexia nervosa has fallen to 80% of her ideal body weight for height and gender. She has not menstruated in 9 months. She has postural hypotension and a low heart rate. Which of the following murmurs is most likely to be present on this patient's cardiac examination?

a. A midsystolic click, followed by a murmur
b. A fixed split S_2
c. A vibratory holosystolic murmur in both axilla
d. A third heart sound
e. A nonspecific ejection murmur at the base of the heart

95. You are offering preventive counseling to the parent of a 12-month-old child at a health maintenance visit. The child weighs 18 lb. You would be correct in informing the parent that this child should be

a. restrained in a rear-facing infant car seat in the back seat of the car until he has reached 2 years of age
b. restrained in a forward-facing infant car seat in the back seat of the car since he is now ≥1 year of age
c. restrained in a rear-facing infant car seat in the front seat of the car until he has reached 20 lb in weight
d. restrained in a forward-facing infant car seat in the front seat of the car since he is now ≥1 year of age
e. restrained in a forward-facing booster seat in the back seat of the car since he is now ≥1 year of age

96. A 4-week-old male infant born at term presents with emesis, dehydration, and poor weight gain. The pediatrician evaluating the child palpates an olive-sized mass in the child's epigastrium. She believes the infant may have pyloric stenosis. Which of the following clinical presentations is most consistent with pyloric stenosis?

a. Projectile nonbilious emesis
b. Bilious emesis
c. Bloody diarrhea
d. Violent episodes of intermittent colicky pain and emesis
e. Right lower quadrant abdominal pain

97. A 5-year-old boy presents to the emergency department with complaints of dizziness and confusion. Three days before presentation, he developed a low-grade fever and vomited twice. Since then, the fever and vomiting have resolved, but the patient has passed 8 to 10 loose, foul-smelling stools per day. The boy's mother has been afraid to give him anything but water or diluted juice due to his history of vomiting. Deep tendon reflexes are diminished throughout. This patient's ataxia and confusion are most likely due to which of the following electrolyte imbalances?

a. Hypomagnesemia
b. Hyperkalemia
c. Metabolic alkalosis
d. Hypochloremia
e. Hyponatremia

98. A 13-year-old male presents to the office with short stature. Growth data demonstrates that he has been growing between the third and fifth percentile at a steady rate since age 4 years. His father started shaving at age 17 and completed his growth at age 19 years. What examination and workup would support the diagnosis of constitutional delay of growth and puberty?

a. Acne and axillary hair, Tanner III pubic hair, testicular volume 12 cc, bone age 14 years, TSH 1.5 (0.5 to 4.8), IGF-I 340 (152 to 540)
b. No axillary hair, Tanner I pubic hair, testicular volume 4 cc, bone age 11 years, TSH 12 (0.5 to 4.8), IGF-I 200 (152 to 540)
c. Scant axillary hair, Tanner II pubic hair, testicular volume 5 cc, bone age 11 years, TSH 2.1 (0.5 to 4.8), IGF-I 420 (152 to 540)
d. No axillary hair, Tanner I pubic hair, testicular volume 4 cc, bone age 11 years, TSH 3.1 (0.5 to 4.8), IGF-I 62 (152 to 540)

99. A 24-month-old male in your office for his regular health maintenance visit has the following results on screening tests: hemoglobin 9.6 g/dL; capillary blood lead level 16 mcg/dL. He lives in Section 8 housing in poor repair built before 1960. Which of the following is the most appropriate next course of action?

a. Counsel the family regarding lead removal and recheck the level in 6 months.
b. Refer the family to the local governmental lead-management agency.
c. Obtain a venous lead level for confirmation.
d. Start the patient on oral succimer on an outpatient basis.
e. Obtain neurodevelopmental testing for the patient.

100. A 10-year-old girl presents with linear streaks of thickened and indurated skin on the right arm and trunk. The linear streak on the right arm has a longitudinal orientation and extends from the upper arm to the dorsal aspect of the hand, whereas the linear streak on the trunk is transversely oriented. The lesions are surrounded by a halo of erythema with a violaceous appearance. The central portion is hyperpigmented and thickened. Which of the following complications is this child most likely to develop?

a. Esophageal dysfunction
b. Pulmonary fibrosis
c. Contracture of the right elbow
d. Raynaud phenomenon
e. Digital necrosis

A Answers

1. b (Chapter 20)
Epinephrine is used for asystole, bradycardia, and/or pulseless VT or ventricular fibrillation. Epinephrine increases systemic vascular resistance, chronotropy, and inotropy, thereby increasing cardiac output and systolic and diastolic blood pressure. By increasing systolic blood pressure, cerebral blood flow is increased; by increasing diastolic blood pressure, coronary perfusion is increased. Epinephrine may change fine ventricular fibrillation to coarse ventricular fibrillation and promote successful defibrillation.

2. a (Chapter 18)
Turner syndrome is relatively common, with an incidence of 1 in 2,500. Female patients present with short stature and delayed puberty caused by primary ovarian failure. Other stigmata, including webbed neck, a low hairline, and increased carrying angle, may not be present. Patients with Cushing syndrome present with other physical characteristics, including moon facies, buffalo hump, and abdominal striae. In isolated growth hormone deficiency and familial short stature, patients do not have delayed puberty. Patients with Addison disease present with fatigue, weakness, nausea, and vomiting. In the acute setting, they may present with cardiovascular shock.

3. d (Chapter 18)
The child has a 25% chance of acquiring the autosomal recessive disorder. Because each parent is a carrier for the disorder, each parent has one normal allele and one mutant allele. The probability of the child receiving an affected allele is 0.5 from each parent. Therefore, the child has a 25% risk (0.5×0.5).

4. d (Chapter 11)
Hydroxyurea maintenance therapy has been shown to reduce the number and severity of vaso-occlusive crises in individuals with sickle cell disease. Children with sickle cell disease, like all children, require all routine childhood vaccinations. Despite penicillin prophylaxis, children with sickle cell disease are still at high risk of sepsis caused by *Streptococcus pneumoniae*. These children require both the pneumococcal conjugate vaccine (7-valent) during infancy and the pneumococcal polysaccharide vaccine (23-valent) at 4 to 6 years of age. Gallstones typically develop during adolescence as a result of chronic hemolysis. Dactylitis, or hand-foot syndrome, is the earliest manifestation of vaso-occlusive disease. It is caused by avascular necrosis of the metacarpal and metatarsal bones and requires analgesics, not antibiotics. Acute chest syndrome requires both supportive care (supplemental oxygen, red blood cell transfusions) and antibiotics.

5. a (Chapter 4)
Children with vegan diets are at risk for vitamin B_{12} deficiency, iron deficiency, and, if exposed to inadequate sunlight, vitamin D deficiency as well. A child who lives in New Mexico and spends a lot of time outdoors can be assumed to have adequate vitamin D levels. Calcium is unlikely to be a concern if the child is indeed eating many dark green, leafy vegetables. Finally, the boy is fed iron-fortified grains regularly, so unless a screening hematocrit is low, iron stores are likely sufficient. Vitamins B_{12} and B_6, niacin, and riboflavin are all B vitamins. Of these, vitamin B_{12} is found only in foods of animal origin, so vegans in particular are at risk for deficiency of this substance.

6. b (Chapter 7)
Functional or "innocent" murmurs are heard in up to 80% of children at some point and represent normal blood flow through a structurally normal heart. They are accentuated by increased cardiac output (i.e., during exercise, with fever, or with anemia). A Still's murmur is the most common innocent murmur. It has a low-pitched, vibratory quality and is heard best in the supine position. A bicuspid aortic valve is associated with an S2 click. If stenosis or regurgitation is present, an associated murmur will be heard. The murmur of a ventricular septal defect is higher frequency and occurs throughout systole. Small VSDs may have pronounced murmurs and a thrill and not uncommonly undergo spontaneous closure during the first 2 years of life. An atrial septal defect is characterized by fixed and wide splitting of S2, due to delayed closure of the pulmonary valve. A soft systolic ejection murmur may be present, due to increased flow across the pulmonary valve. The hallmark findings in coarctation of the aorta are discrepant pulses and blood pressures in the upper and lower extremities. A systolic ejection murmur may be present at the left upper sternal border. Continuous murmurs may also be present across the chest or back, if collateral arteries are present.

7. a (Chapter 2)
Upper airway obstruction in the neonate can result from all the conditions listed. However, the child does not turn blue when crying (mouth breathing). Inability to pass the NG tube in this clinical setting is virtually diagnostic of choanal atresia or significant stenosis. There is no communication between the nose and pharynx, and thus no air flow. Bilateral choanal atresia is an emergency. This patient will likely require endotracheal intubation and surgery to correct the defect. Vocal cord paralysis may result from recurrent laryngeal nerve damage during delivery. If this were the case, the infant should have a soft, hoarse cry, and stridor might be noted. Subglottic stenosis

and laryngeal web would also result in stridor. In all three of these conditions, passage of the NG tube would not be impeded.

8. c (Chapter 14)

The child with diabetic ketoacidosis (DKA) usually exhibits some combination of polyuria, polydipsia, fatigue, headache, nausea, emesis, and abdominal pain. When DKA occurs, ketones are formed in the blood and cleared in the urine. Hyperglycemia, and not hypoglycemia, is typical. Primary metabolic acidosis with secondary respiratory alkalosis is noted (decreased venous blood pH and hypocarbia). Dehydration results in an elevated BUN level. When DKA is present, the patient's total body potassium is depleted from significant potassium loss in the osmotic diuresis. However, serum potassium measurements at presentation may appear high, low, or normal.

9. a (Chapter 2,17)

Although >99% of males have bilateral descended testes by 12 months of age, testes that do not descend on their own by 3 to 6 months of age are unlikely to do so. Testes that remain outside the scrotum develop ultrastructural changes and impaired sperm production resulting in possible infertility. There is also an increased risk of malignancy, even after the testis is surgically relocated (and even in the contralateral testis). Ninety percent of patients with cryptorchidism also have inguinal hernias. Cryptorchidism may occur as an isolated defect or be part of a genetic syndrome; however, there is no known increase in the risk of microphallus in these patients.

10. a (Chapter 16)

Legg-Calvé-Perthes (LCP) disease. Although LCP can have associated hip or knee pain, it is commonly known as "the painless limp." The peak age of onset is 3 to 8 years. Slipped capital femoral epiphysis (SCFE) is incorrect because the peak age range of this disorder is peripubertal, approximately ages 8 to 14 years. SCFE typically has pain associated. A "toddler's fracture" is a nondisplaced fracture of the tibia in children aged 2 to 4 years which is often not appreciated on plain films at presentation. Most heal within 4 weeks, and any associated limp would disappear within 2 months. Septic arthritis is usually acute in presentation and has associated pain, fever, inability to walk, and elevations of C-reactive protein and erythrocyte sedimentation rate. Juvenile idiopathic arthritis (JIA) rarely presents in the hip; the most common location is the knees. Morning stiffness is a common complaint with JIA.

11. c (Chapter 11)

Pulmonary embolism (PE) is a potentially fatal complication of deep vein thrombosis (DVT). The classic signs and symptoms of PE include sudden chest pain, dyspnea, anxiety, and cyanosis. Hemoptysis is uncommon. A helical CT (spiral CT) or a ventilation/perfusion (V/Q) scan is the recommended diagnostic study. While small emboli can be managed by anticoagulation therapy and close monitoring, massive PE may require thrombolytic therapy with recombinant tissue plasminogen activator (r-tPA) or thrombectomy. Venous insufficiency is also a common complication noted after DVT but is not a significant issue in the acute setting. Limb overgrowth, edema, and gangrene from a venous ulcer are all potential complications of DVT.

12. d (Chapter 2)

Women who are taking carbamazepine or valproic acid are at an increased risk of producing a child with a neural tube defect if they are treated with this drug during their pregnancies. The mechanism for this is unclear. The other anticonvulsants listed do not increase the risk for neural tube defects specifically, although they may be associated with a higher risk for other birth defects. Other drugs which do increase the risk of neural tube defects include aminopterin, pyrimethamine, trimethoprim, sulfasalazine, methotrexate, phenothiazines, and cyclophosphamide.

13. b (Chapter 20)

With probable supraventricular tachycardia, the best course of action listed is to administer IV adenosine by rapid bolus to temporarily block the AV node and interrupt the likely reentrant circuit causing the SVT. In a hemodynamically unstable patient, synchronized cardioversion 0.5 to 1.0 J/kg is recommended with an increase to 2 J/kg if initial cardioversion is unsuccessful. The use of epinephrine is indicated in cases of asystole, bradycardia, pulseless VT, or VF. The use of atropine is indicated in cases of bradycardia and atrioventricular block. Calcium may be used for hypocalcemia, hyperkalemia, hypermagnesemia, and calcium channel blocker overdose. Sodium bicarbonate may be used if the infant is acidotic secondary to decreased perfusion and oxygen delivery to the tissues.

14. b (Chapter 15)

Infantile spasms typically present between 2 and 7 months of age and may be idiopathic or associated with other neurologic or developmental diseases. Hypsarrhythmia, characterized by widespread random, high-voltage slow waves and spikes that spread to all cortical areas, is the characteristic EEG finding in infantile seizures. All children with infantile seizures should receive a Wood lamp exam to determine whether ash-leaf spots, the lesions described here, are present. Ash-leaf spots are the earliest manifestation of tuberous sclerosis, a neurocutaneous disease which may present with infantile spasms. Von Recklinghausen disease and bilateral acoustic neurofibromatosis are forms of neurofibromatosis. Café-au-lait spots, which are hyperpigmented, are seen in these diseases. Von Hippel-Lindau disease presents primarily in adults. Infants with Sturge-Weber may have seizures, but the port wine stain is present at birth and is the primary skin lesion.

15. b (Chapter 1)

She needs a fourth dose of DTaP, a fourth dose of HiB, and a fourth dose of pneumococcal conjugate vaccine. She needs the MMR and varicella vaccines unless there is a reliable history that she has had chickenpox. She has already completed the required vaccination courses for hepatitis A and hepatitis B. Three doses of IPV are appropriate for her age.

16. e (Chapter 1,15)

Speech delay is the most common developmental concern raised by parents. As many as 15% of children have some sort of speech/language delay at one time or another during the preschool years. Any child with suspected language delay should receive a full audiologic assessment, followed by referral to a speech pathologist for further workup and treatment (if indicated). The most common cause of mild-to-moderate hearing loss in young children is otitis media with effusion, but this child has clear, mobile tympanic membranes, so a tympanogram is unnecessary. Evaluation of the boy's ability to understand and produce language, as well as speak fluently, is part of a comprehensive speech assessment following the hearing test.

17. c (Chapter 9)

Functional abdominal pain is best treated with a biopsychosocial model. Medical treatment might include acid reduction therapy for pain associated with dyspepsia, antispasmodic agents, smooth muscle relaxants, or low doses of tricyclic psychotropic agents for pain or nonstimulating laxatives or antidiarrheals for pain associated with altered bowel pattern. A CT scan and endoscopy are unlikely to identify abnormalities based on the history and physical examination. A diet history and elimination diet are unlikely to provide additional insight since the pain is not related to meals. Psychiatric referral is premature and sends the message that there is only an emotional component to these symptoms.

18. a (Chapter 18)

The clinical description is that of a patient with trisomy 21 or Down syndrome. Common dysmorphic facial features include flat facial profile, upslanted palpebral fissures, a flat nasal bridge with epicanthal folds, a small mouth with a protruding tongue, micrognathia, and short ears with downfolding earlobes. Other dysmorphic features are excess skin on the back of the neck, microcephaly, a flat occiput (brachycephaly), short stature, a short sternum, small genitalia, and a gap between the first and second toes ("sandal gap toe"). Anomalies of the hand include single palmar creases (simian creases) and short, broad hands (brachydactyly) with fingers marked by an incurved fifth finger and a hypoplastic middle phalanx (clinodactyly). Features of trisomy 18 include hypertonia, microcephaly, corneal opacities, micrognathia, and rocker bottom feet. Features of trisomy 13 include microcephaly, occipital scalp defects, iris coloboma, microphthalmia, cleft lip and palate, and clenched hands. Boys with Klinefelter syndrome do not have physical features identifiable at birth that could lead to suspicion of the disorder. Girls with Turner syndrome have a webbed neck, low posterior hairline, wide-spaced nipples, cubitus valgus (wide carrying angle), and edema of the hands and feet.

19. a (Chapter 1)

Asymptomatic patients with blood lead levels >45 μg/dL require chelation within 48 hours. EDTA (edetate calcium-disodium) is an appropriate treatment for asymptomatic patients with blood lead levels between 45 and 69 μg/dL. It is administered in the hospital. Outpatient oral succimer is also an option in this patient. BAL (intramuscular dimercaprol) is added to EDTA when a patient's blood lead level reaches 70 μg/dL or greater. The family should be removed from the home while decontamination is taking place. Siblings of any patient with elevated lead levels should be tested, and nutritional therapy is certainly not contraindicated; however, patients with levels exceeding 45 μg/dL require chelation treatment per American Academy of Pediatrics and Centers for Disease Control recommendations.

20. b (Chapter 4)

Breastfed infants should receive oral vitamin D supplementation beginning in the first several days after birth to prevent rickets, a condition in which developing bone fails to mineralize due to inadequate 1,25-dihydroxycholecalciferol. Rickets is rare in breastfed infants but does occur. Dark-skinned infants and those exposed to limited sunlight in northern latitudes are particularly at risk. Rickets in breastfed infants becomes clinically and chemically evident in late infancy; rickets due solely to vitamin D deficiency begins to respond to supplementation within weeks. The American Academy of Pediatrics recommends exclusive breastfeeding during the first 6 months of life and continuation of breastfeeding during the second 6 months for optimal infant nutrition. Studies have shown that breastfed infants have a lower incidence of infections, including otitis media, pneumonia, sepsis, and meningitis. Breastfed infants are less likely to experience feeding difficulties associated with allergy (eczema) or intolerance (colic).

21. c (Chapter 18)

Although all of the choices are possible presentations of Hodgkin disease, choice *c* is the most common presentation, occurring in approximately 80% of patients. Approximately two thirds of patients will have mediastinal lymphadenopathy, and 20% to 30% will experience choice *b* symptoms. Pruritus, fatigue, and anorexia are also common presenting symptoms. The pruritus is often extremely difficult to control prior to diagnosis, but resolves very rapidly once chemotherapy begins. Patients will often have more than one of the presenting signs or symptoms listed here.

22. d (Chapter 8)

The preferred therapy regimen for a patient ≥12 years with persistent asthma (symptoms [before treatment] >2 days per week or waking with symptoms >2 nights per month, or use of an inhaled β-agonist >2 times per week) that is not well-controlled on Step 2 (low-dose inhaled steroids) is daily low-dose inhaled corticosteroid and a long-acting inhaled β2-agonist. Answer *a* is most appropriate for patients with intermittent asthma, who can control their sporadic symptoms with an inhaled β2-agonist as needed. Answer *b* is the preferred therapy for a patient with mild persistent asthma. Answer *c* is an acceptable Step 4 treatment. Nedocromil is an older drug and presumed mast cell membrane stabilizer that may be an alternative to low-dose inhaled corticosteroids in patients with mild persistent asthma.

23. a (Chapter 6)

Measles is caused by a paramyxovirus and characterized by malaise, high fever, cough, coryza, conjunctivitis, Koplik spots, and an erythematous maculopapular rash. Koplik spots are small, irregular red spots with central gray or bluish-white specks that appear on the buccal mucosa. Rubella is caused by rubella virus and is characterized by mild fever and erythematous maculopapular rash, with generalized lymphadenopathy, especially of the posterior auricular, cervical, and suboccipital nodes. Roseola infantum is caused by herpesvirus 6 and is characterized by high fever followed by a maculopapular rash that starts on the trunk and spreads to the periphery. The fever typically resolves as the rash appears. Erythema infectiosum is caused by parvovirus B19 and is characterized by marked erythema of the cheeks ("slapped cheek" appearance) and an erythematous, pruritic, maculopapular rash starting on the arms and spreading to the trunk and legs. Hand-foot-and-mouth disease is caused by coxsackie A virus and is characterized by ulcers on the tongue and oral mucosa and a maculopapular vesicular rash on the hands and feet. Chickenpox is caused by varicella-zoster virus and is characterized by fever and a pruritic papular, vesicular, pustular rash starting on the trunk and spreading to the extremities. The infected child is infectious until the last lesion is crusted over. Zoster, or shingles, is caused by reactivation of varicella-zoster virus from the dorsal root ganglion and is characterized by fever and painful pruritic crops of vesicles along a dermatomal distribution in an individual with previous varicella-zoster infection.

24. b (Chapter 10)

High-dose amoxicillin is the recommended first-line antibiotic treatment for acute otitis media. Children who have been treated with antibiotics within the past month are eligible for second-line therapy with amoxicillin-clavulanate, an oral second- or third-generation cephalosporin, or IM ceftriaxone. The most common bacteria that cause acute otitis media are *Streptococcus pneumoniae*, *Haemophilus influenzae*, and *Moraxella catarrhalis*. Azithromycin, erythromycin, and trimethoprim-sulfamethoxazole are minimally effective against β-lactamase-producing strains of *H. influenzae* or *M. catarrhalis*. Dicloxacillin is not active against gram-negative organisms such as *H. influenzae* and *M. catarrhalis*.

25. b (Chapter 2)
Infants with neonatal sepsis or pneumonia typically have normal surfactant production and do not benefit from surfactant replacement therapy. Preeclampsia is associated with acceleration of lung maturation and surfactant production. Full-term infants with neural tube defects have normal lung maturation. Newborns with trisomy 21 are at risk for pulmonary hypertension due to delayed development of the pulmonary vasculature, but typically have appropriate surfactant production. Infants of diabetic mothers, especially those with poor control, have delayed maturation of surfactant production and are at increased risk for neonatal respiratory distress syndrome at any gestational age.

26. d (Chapter 17)
A child with a suspected UTI and positive leukocyte esterase on dipstick urinalysis should be treated for presumptive UTI until culture results become available. Children older than 5 years of age with a recurrent UTI warrant further workup to rule out anatomic abnormalities (renal ultrasound) and vesicoureteral reflux (VCUG). A nontoxic-appearing child of this age does not need to be admitted to the hospital for treatment. On the other hand, empiric treatment should never be withheld in a febrile child with a suspected UTI and a dipstick urinalysis which is positive for leukocyte esterase.

27. a (Chapter 7)
The central feature of tetralogy of Fallot is a malaligned ventricular septal defect. The malalignment in the septum is characterized by an anteriorly displaced infundibulum (the septal muscle in the outlet area). This leads to subpulmonary narrowing and an aorta that appears to override the inferior portion of the septum. The amount of pulmonary stenosis (right ventricular outflow obstruction) varies in patients with TOF. Right ventricular outflow obstruction leads to right ventricular hypertrophy in these patients. Atrial septal defect, aortic stenosis, coarctation of the aorta, mitral valve prolapse, and left ventricular hypertrophy are not associated with tetralogy of Fallot. Left ventricular hypertrophy may be found in patients with coarctation of the aorta or aortic stenosis.

28. c (Chapter 11)
Fresh frozen plasma (FFP) is indicated for replacement of missing coagulation factors when the specific factor concentrate is unavailable. FFP is prepared by either separating the liquid portion of whole blood or by collecting the liquid portion of the blood by apheresis technology and freezing it within 8 hours of collection. FFP contains all of the normal coagulation factors and naturally occurring inhibitors of coagulation. Cryoprecipitate is a rich source of fibrinogen and clotting factors VIII and XIII. Granulocyte infusions are usually used in the neonate or infant with prolonged neutropenia and life-threatening sepsis. Platelet transfusions are effective in cases of thrombocytopenia or functional platelet defects. DDAVP is used in von Willebrand disease or mild hemophilia A patients.

29. c (Chapter 3)
The typical sequence of pubertal events in the male begins with testicular enlargement from the prepubertal size of about 2.5 mm in length. This is followed in rapid succession by pubic hair growth, penile enlargement, and maximal height growth velocity (approaching 9 cm/y).

30. e (Chapter 8)
A patient with an acute asthmatic episode who has already taken multiple dosages of albuterol at home should still receive a trial of another dose in the emergency department. Failure to respond to initial treatment and the presence of hypoxemia signal a moderate to severe acute asthma episode that will require more aggressive treatment. The addition of the anticholinergic agent ipratropium results in significant improvement in a large percentage of patients. The lack of response to initial treatment also is an indication to begin treatment with systemic corticosteroids to help relieve airway inflammation. Supplemental oxygen will help relieve the hypoxemia caused by ventilation perfusion mismatch and can also produce mild bronchodilation.

31. d (Chapter 17)
This patient displays the characteristic findings of acute renal failure due to the use of ibuprofen in a subject with decreased renal perfusion. He would be expected to have decreased renal perfusion based on symptoms and signs of mild to moderate dehydration (tachycardia, decreased urine output). In the presence of decreased renal perfusion, the intrarenal vasodilatory prostaglandins comprise a powerful mechanism for maintenance of glomerular filtration rate. Interference with this compensatory mechanism, by the use of nonsteroidal anti-inflammatory drugs as in this case, is a common mechanism that can precipitate intrinsic acute renal failure. This patient does not have hemolytic uremic syndrome since his complete blood count is normal (no hemolysis, thrombocytopenia, or schistocytes). He does not have any evidence for pyelonephritis (no costovertebral angle tenderness, no white blood cells in the urine, no bacteria in the urine). He does not display any clinical features characteristic of interstitial nephritis (no skin rashes, no white blood cells in the urine) or urinary tract obstruction (normal kidney ultrasound).

32. a (Chapter 13)
This child most likely has classical systemic lupus erythematosus given that she fulfills 6 out of 11 criteria for the classification for the condition: malar rash, photosensitivity, oral ulcers, arthritis, cytopenias, and active urine sediment. A positive ANA is present in essentially all patients with SLE; therefore, the correct answer is *a*. Anti-double-stranded DNA antibodies are present in up to 70% of patients with active SLE, anti-Smith antibodies in up to 50%, anti-Ro antibodies in up to 60%, and rheumatoid factor is rare in SLE. Anti-double-stranded DNA and anti-Smith antibodies are highly specific for SLE; therefore, its presence is highly suggestive of SLE.

33. a (Chapter 20)
The primary assessment is the initial evaluation of the critically ill or injured child when life-threatening problems are identified and prioritized. The proper order of the primary survey or initial assessment is airway, breathing, circulation, disability, and exposure. After the primary survey is complete, resuscitation should occur if the condition is life threatening. Once the life-threatening issues are addressed, the secondary survey should be performed.

34. d (Chapter 11)
The most likely diagnosis is immune thrombocytopenic purpura. Isoimmune thrombocytopenia is noted in newborns, not in children. Isoimmune IgG antibodies are produced against the fetal platelet when the fetal platelet crosses the placenta and has antigens that are not found on the maternal platelet. The maternal antibodies cross the placenta and attack the fetal platelets. Leukemia, sepsis, and hypersplenism may all cause thrombocytopenia in the child's age group, but are unlikely in this case. The white blood cell count is normal, and no immature white cells are seen on the peripheral smear. Sepsis is unlikely given that the child appears well and is

hemodynamically stable. Hypersplenism is unlikely when the spleen is normal on palpation.

35. b (Chapter 18)

Microdeletion of 22q11.2 has been found in 90% of children with DiGeorge syndrome, in 70% of children with velocardiofacial syndrome, and in 15% of children with isolated conotruncal cardiac defects. Although the above-mentioned names are still in use, the more general term *22q11.2 deletion syndrome* more appropriately encompasses the spectrum of abnormalities found in these children. Its prevalence in the general population is 1 per 4,000 live births. The deletion can be inherited (8% to 28% of cases), but more typically occurs as a de novo event. However, if a parent has the deletion, the risk to each child is 50%. The microdeletion can be detected using fluorescent in situ hybridization (FISH) probes. Classic cardiac features of this spectrum of disorders include conotruncal defects such as tetralogy of Fallot, interrupted aortic arch, and vascular rings. Other common findings are absent thymus, hypocalcemic hypoparathyroidism, T-cell-mediated immune deficiency, and palate abnormalities. These children usually have feeding difficulties, cognitive disabilities, and behavioral and speech disorders.

36. e (Chapter 10)

Palivizumab is an RSV monoclonal antibody approved for monthly injection during the winter months in infants at high risk for severe RSV disease. These include children younger than 24 months who are former premature infants or have chronic pulmonary disease (bronchopulmonary dysplasia) requiring oxygen therapy within the last 6 months. RespiGam is an intravenous polyclonal immunoglobulin with high RSV antibody concentration which is also appropriate for administration in children at high risk for complicated RSV infections; however, palivizumab is preferred because it is easier to administer and is not a blood product. Neither the nasal nor the injectable influenza vaccine is approved for infants younger than 6 months of age. Ribavirin is not appropriate for prophylactic use.

37. c (Chapter 4)

Formula-fed infants do not require supplementation with vitamins, minerals, additional caloric sources, or free water during the first 6 months of life, regardless of local climate. Dilution of the formula is potentially harmful to an infant under 6 months of age due to the inability of the immature kidney to fully dilute urine. If this infant is feeding well, growing appropriately, and tolerates the formula, there is no reason to switch to a soy protein-based formula at this time.

38. c (Chapter 2)

The absence of a red reflex on funduscopic examination (also called leukocoria, for "white pupil") calls for immediate consultation with a pediatric ophthalmologist. The most common cause is a congenital cataract, which may occur spontaneously, secondary to a genetic predisposition, or as a result of metabolic disease or intrauterine infection. Retinoblastoma, congenital glaucoma, and toxocariasis may also cause leukocoria but are much less common than congenital cataracts.

39. d (Chapter 15)

The child in the vignette is initially diagnosed with adrenal insufficiency, which can be associated with adrenoleukodystrophy. Treatment of the insufficiency does not help with the personality changes and declining cognitive faculties. His difficulty with walking is likely due to increasing spasticity. The first three disorders listed are all gray matter degenerative diseases which present earlier in life with hypotonia, mental retardation, and seizures. Rett syndrome is a disease of general cerebral atrophy which presents almost exclusively in girls early in the second year of life.

40. d (Chapter 15)

Absence seizures begin between ages 4 and 9 years and consist of brief episodes of staring associated with altered consciousness. The typical duration is 5 to 10 seconds. Often, the staring is accompanied by subtle clonic activity in the face or arms or simple automatisms (such as eye blinking, chewing, or perseverative motor activity). Absence seizures start and stop abruptly and have no postictal phase. Although brief, absence seizures can occur in clusters many times a day and interfere with learning and socialization. In a typical absence seizure, the EEG shows abrupt onset and offset of 3-per-second generalized symmetric spike and slow-wave complexes. In a child with untreated absence epilepsy, 3 to 5 minutes of hyperventilation will often precipitate a typical absence seizure. Ethosuximide has higher efficacy and a lower side-effect profile and is the preferred drug for treating absence epilepsy (vs. valproic acid). For children with partial-onset epilepsy, oxcarbazepine should be considered for initial monotherapy based on current efficacy evidence. Considering all factors, including cost, carbamazepine, valproic acid, topiramate, and phenytoin are other reasonable choices to treat partial-onset seizures. Methylphenidate is a stimulant medication which is often beneficial in the treatment of attention-deficit/hyperactivity disorder.

41. e (Chapter 18)

Turner syndrome occurs in 1 per 5,000 live births. Approximately 98% of fetuses with Turner syndrome expire in utero; only 2% are born. Therefore, the recurrence risk for parents who have a child with Turner syndrome is no higher than that of the general population. Dysmorphic features include lymphedema of the hands and feet, a shield-shaped chest, widely spaced hypoplastic nipples, a webbed neck, low hairline, cubitus valgus (increased carrying angle), short stature, and multiple pigmented nevi. Additional abnormalities include gonadal dysgenesis, gonadoblastoma, renal anomalies, congenital heart disease, autoimmune thyroiditis, and learning disabilities. Gonadal dysgenesis, present in 100% of patients, is associated with primary amenorrhea and lack of pubertal development due to loss of ovarian hormones. The gonads are appropriately infantile at birth but regress during childhood and develop into "streak" ovaries by puberty. In mosaics with a Y chromosome in one of their cell lines, gonadoblastoma is common. Therefore, prophylactic gonadectomy is necessary in these patients. Renal anomalies, usually duplicated collecting system or horseshoe kidney, occur in 40% of those with Turner syndrome. Congenital heart disease occurs in 20% of patients; common defects include coarctation of the aorta, aortic stenosis, and bicuspid aortic valve. As a consequence of having only one functional X chromosome, females with Turner syndrome display the same frequency of sex-linked disorders as males. The diagnosis is made by karyotype and fluorescent in situ hybridization. Because of their mosaicism, some girls suspected of having Turner syndrome have a 46,XX karyotype in the peripheral blood, and a skin biopsy may be necessary to make the diagnosis.

Short stature has been successfully treated using human growth hormone. Secondary sexual characteristics develop after estrogen and progesterone administration. As mentioned earlier, gonadectomy is indicated in patients with dysgenetic gonads and the presence of a Y chromosome. With the rare exception of a few mosaics, women with Turner syndrome cannot become pregnant.

42. d (Chapter 21)

Oral *N*-acetyl cysteine is the antidote for acetaminophen ingestion. It is most effective if administered within 8 to 10 hours of ingestion. Multiple doses are required. If the patient refuses, a nasogastric tube may be placed. The administration of *N*-acetyl cysteine should not be delayed until after the 4-hour acetaminophen level is drawn if the patient presents prior to this time. Activated charcoal may be beneficial if used within 4 hours of ingestion and is often followed by whole bowel irrigation, but neither of these is considered an antidote specific to acetaminophen poisoning. Neither hemodialysis nor atropine sulfate, which is used in cases of organophosphate poisoning, affects blood levels of acetaminophen.

43. e (Chapter 21)

Fractures which are highly specific for abuse include bilateral fractures, bucket handle fractures, metaphyseal chip fractures, and fractures of the (especially posterior) ribs, scapula, sternum, or spinous processes. Fractures that occur before ambulation are usually inflicted. Bruises on the chest, head, neck, or abdomen and bruises on a nonambulatory child are extremely suspicious for abuse. Vigorous shaking may lead to shaken baby syndrome (SBS), which results from acceleration/deceleration forces to the head. Virtually pathognomonic injuries include intracranial (subdural) hemorrhage, diffuse axonal injury, and widespread retinal hemorrhages, which may result in permanent vision loss. SBS has the highest mortality rate of any reported form of child abuse. Falls from beds, changing tables, cribs, counters, or toilet seats do not cause the injuries seen in SBS. Injuries in different stages of healing occur in chronic or repeated abuse.

44. c (Chapter 9)

Painless rectal bleeding sufficient to lower hemoglobin in a 2-year-old is a common presentation of Meckel diverticulum. A colonoscopy would not reveal this since the bleeding point is sufficiently proximal to the ileocecal valve. Transfusion is not needed at this time. However, close monitoring and the availability of packed red blood cells as proper management. Gastric lavage would likely not identify a source of bleeding since the most likely cause is distal to the ligament of Treitz. Bacterial colitis is usually associated with bloody diarrhea, not painless rectal bleeding.

45. c (Chapter 14)

This infant presents with classic clinical and biochemical evidence of adrenal crisis from congenital adrenal hyperplasia (21-hydroxylase deficiency). This classic presentation consists of hypotension, hypoglycemia, hyponatremia, hyperkalemia in a 2- to 6-week infant, typically male (females are usually identified in the newborn period with ambiguous genitalia). All emergency personnel should think of adrenal insufficiency when a child presents in this fashion. These infants need fluid, salt, dextrose, and stress dosing of hydrocortisone for survival. Answer *a* (azithromycin) is not a wide-spectrum antibiotic or one that is considered a drug of choice for sepsis in the infant. The infant's HCO_3 level is not low enough to warrant the consideration of IV bicarbonate. Albumin could help improve intravascular volume but would not add any additional therapeutic benefit beyond the fluid resuscitation that was already provided. Hypocalcemia is not generally present in patients with adrenal insufficiency. If the patient has cardiovascular issues related to hyperkalemia, calcium is a useful adjunct to stabilize the myocardium as the extracellular potassium level is lowered.

46. c (Chapter 6)

The patient described in the question has psoriasis. The scaly red plaques concentrated on her trunk demonstrate the Auspitz sign which is pinpoint bleeding when the scale is removed. Nail pitting is a common finding in patients with psoriasis. Psoriasis is a chronic disease but is often exacerbated by infection in many patients, particularly group A β-hemolytic *Streptococcus* (GAS) in genetically susceptible patients. In addition, GAS may be the precipitating factor in a subtype of psoriasis known as guttate psoriasis. Recognizing and treating streptococcal pharyngitis in guttate psoriasis may improve the patient's outcome. Patients with psoriasis are also directed to try and avoid exacerbating factors such as streptococcal infections.

Because this patient has psoriasis, a bacterial (a) or fungal (b) culture of the plaques would not be necessary and could be misleading if a skin contaminant was found. Tzanck smears (d) are used to look for multinucleated giant cells consistent with herpes viruses such as HSV-1 and -2 or varicella, neither of which is associated with psoriasis. A complete blood count (e) would not be necessary in patients with psoriasis and, if checked, should be normal.

47. a (Chapter 15)

The goal of pharmacologic therapy for ADHD is sustained symptom reduction throughout the day with a tolerable minimum of adverse effects. Atomoxetine is a highly specific norepinephrine reuptake inhibitor; its nonstimulant status sets it apart from the stimulants commonly used to treat ADHD (methylphenidate, dextroamphetamine, and mixed amphetamine salts). Unlike the psychostimulants, atomoxetine has a generally low incidence of side effects and low abuse potential. In the United States, atomoxetine carries a "black box" warning mandated by the FDA alerting physicians and patients due to an increased risk of suicidal ideation. Individuals with ADHD should continue to take their medications over the weekends and during holidays for good control of symptoms in academic and nonacademic settings. Pharmacologic intervention should be administered along with behavioral management and support for the patient and family in order to achieve the best possible outcome.

48. c (Chapter 10)

Roseola is a febrile illness caused by human herpesvirus 6. Children have elevated temperatures for 3 to 5 days, followed by a rash that develops after an abrupt defervescence. The rash consists of erythematous, maculopapular lesions that begin on the trunk and subsequently spread to the neck, face, and extremities.

The characteristic rash of erythema infectiosum (fifth disease; human parvovirus B19) is facial erythema giving a "slapped cheek" appearance, followed by spread to the extremities in a reticular pattern. Measles is a confluent, erythematous, maculopapular rash that starts on the head and progresses caudally. Children with measles have high fever and associated cough, coryza, and conjunctivitis. The rash of chickenpox begins as pruritic, erythematous macules that evolve to vesicles and later crust. As initial lesions resolve, new crops form so lesions in different stages are observed simultaneously. The rash of scarlet fever, caused by group A β-hemolytic streptococci, is an erythematous, "sandpaper-like" rash which first appears on the neck or trunk, spreads to the extremities, and may desquamate 10 to 14 days later. Fever and pharyngitis accompany the rash.

49. c (Chapter 15)

Febrile seizures are typically brief, generalized seizures with fever which occur in up to 5% of otherwise healthy children ages 6 months to 5 years. Febrile seizures, even when recurrent, are not considered epilepsy. However, children with febrile seizures have an increased risk of developing epilepsy. Between 2% and 7% of all children with febrile seizures develop epilepsy if followed to age 25 years. Overall, the morbidity and mortality associated with febrile seizures is extremely low. Only about a third of patients with an initial febrile seizure will experience recurrent febrile seizures. Anticonvulsant medication is not indicated in the vast majority of patients with initial or even recurrent febrile seizures. By definition, the diagnosis of febrile seizure excludes children with intracranial infection or prior history of nonfebrile seizure.

50. d (Chapter 11)

The most likely diagnosis is hemophilia A. Hemophilia A is an X-linked disorder that is caused by deficiency of factor VIII. Hemophilia B is also an X-linked disorder and is caused by factor IX deficiency. Hemophilias A and B are characterized by spontaneous or traumatic hemorrhages, which can be subcutaneous, intramuscular, or within joints (hemarthroses). Life-threatening internal hemorrhages may follow trauma or surgery. The PTT is prolonged, the PT is normal, and in hemophilia A the factor VIII coagulant activity (VIII:c) is decreased. Other than their factor replacement regimens, there is no distinguishable difference between hemophilias A and B. Idiopathic thrombocytopenic purpura is unlikely in this patient, since the platelet count is normal at 150,000. With no history of epistaxis, gingival bleeding, or cutaneous bruising, von Willebrand disease is unlikely. Hemarthroses are not typical for von Willebrand disease. Vitamin K deficiency occurs in the neonate who is exclusively breastfed and has not received prophylactic vitamin K injection after birth or in the child with significant fat malabsorption. In vitamin K deficiency and in liver disease, there is a prolonged PT and normal factor VIII coagulant activity. The most appropriate therapy for complications of hemophilia A is to infuse factor VIII concentrate.

51. a (Chapter 5)

This patient has a metabolic acidosis (pH $\leq$7.4) with an increased anion gap ($[134 + 4.5] - [106 + 10] = 22.5$, outside the normal range of 12 ± 4). Metabolic acidosis with an increased anion gap usually results from increased acid production (such as in diabetic ketoacidosis), decreased acid excretion (renal failure) or inborn errors of metabolism. Chronic diarrhea usually causes either normal anion gap acidosis or, less commonly, metabolic alkalosis. Pyloric stenosis also results in metabolic alkalosis (HCl loss via vomiting). Children with cystic fibrosis may exhibit alkalosis. Renal tubular acidosis results in a metabolic acidosis with a normal anion gap.

52. c (Chapter 13)

This child has a chronic arthritis as evidenced by the presence of joint swelling, limitation of movement, limping, and morning stiffness of more than 6 weeks' duration. Of note, pain is commonly absent in chronic arthritis (in contrast to acute arthritis or mechanical derangements). The most common cause of chronic arthritis in childhood is juvenile idiopathic arthritis (JIA). The involvement of less than five joints indicates oligoarticular JIA. About 70% of children with oligoarticular JIA have a positive antinuclear antibody test. A common complication is chronic, nongranulomatous anterior uveitis in up to 30% of individuals (c). This form of uveitis is asymptomatic but can lead to severe sequelae including blindness. For this reason, frequent surveillance slit-lamp examinations are indicated. These children are not at risk for the development of SLE and its complications (e.g., glomerulonephritis or hemolytic anemia). Acute anterior uveitis with conjunctival injection, severe pain, and photophobia occurs most commonly in patients with HLA-B27-associated disease but not in the context of oligoarticular JIA. Rheumatic heart disease is a consequence of acute rheumatic fever, but not of JIA.

53. a (Chapter 10)

Cases of suspected bacterial pneumonia that are complicated by large (compromising) pleural effusions (or pleural abscesses) are most likely caused by *Staphylococcus aureus*.

Streptococcus pneumoniae is the most common cause of bacterial pneumonia after infancy and can result in an effusion; however, the effusions seen with *S. pneumoniae* (and the other pathogens listed) are usually small.

Bilateral diffuse interstitial infiltrates are common in pneumonia due to *M. pneumoniae*. Focal abnormalities such as lobar consolidation and small effusions may occur. The effusions seen in pneumonia due to nontypeable *H. influenzae* are usually small. Diffuse interstitial infiltrates may be present in pneumonia due to *C. pneumoniae*. Pleuritis and small pleural effusions may occur. *Klebsiella pneumoniae* is an uncommon cause of lobar pneumonia in children. It may cause pneumonia in adults with underlying problems such as alcoholism, diabetes mellitus, and chronic obstructive pulmonary disease.

54. d (Chapter 17)

This patient most likely has primary essential hypertension. Given her obesity and family history, the hypertension is most likely to benefit from weight loss and exercise.

This patient has sustained hypertension. Reassurance or further observation is inappropriate, since the high blood pressure has already been verified with the appropriate technique. The kidney function is normal, so an underlying renal etiology is unlikely. The cardiac examination is normal and four extremity blood pressures are equally elevated, so an urgent cardiology evaluation is not needed. If the blood pressure is not controlled by exercise and weight loss, then this patient may benefit from diuretic therapy.

55. d (Chapter 4)

Feeding intolerance may lead to food aversion and failure to thrive; the most significant cause is cow milk protein intolerance or allergy. Allergy may be accompanied by eczema or wheezing. A severe local allergic reaction within the bowel results in colitis, indicated by anemia and/or obvious blood in the stools. Other possible nonspecific symptoms include vomiting, irritability, and abdominal distention. If there is no evidence of any underlying disease in formula-fed infants with characteristic symptoms, substitution of a protein hydrolysate formula is recommended. Soy formula is not an appropriate initial substitution because as many as 25% of children with cow milk protein allergy are also intolerant of soy protein. Whole cow milk should not be given to infants younger than 1 year of age and would contain the same offending protein. Parenteral alimentation is not indicated for protein intolerance but may be necessary following surgery for another gastrointestinal condition (intussusception, volvulus).

56. b (Chapter 3)

A portion of the adolescent health maintenance visit is dedicated to interviewing the parent and child together to evaluate family dynamics, explore past medical and family history, and gather nonsensitive health-related information. Additional time should be set aside to interview and evaluate the adolescent alone, which permits open discussion of more sensitive issues. Laws regarding confidentiality and consent vary from state to state, but in all cases, behaviors that represent a serious threat to the adolescent's health must be disclosed. These include being subjected to physical or sexual abuse and plans to harm oneself or others. That said, the physician can ask the patient's permission to disclose information to the parents when he or she deems it in the best interest of the child. For instance, patients may be willing to discuss issues related to their sexual behavior, drinking, or drug use with their parents in the presence of a supportive physician that they would never bring up at home. Depending on the state, adolescents below the age of 18 years can provide confidential consent for their own health care regarding (1) contraception, prenatal care, and sexually transmitted diseases and (2) issues related to mental health and/or substance abuse evaluation and treatment. In addition, various states grant "mature" or "emancipated" minors (those who have children, are married, are enlisted in the service, or are living apart from their parents) the right to consent to or decline health care.

57. c (Chapter 8)

Polysomnography is not always necessary to diagnose obstructive sleep apnea, but it is the gold standard. This test usually is performed in the hospital overnight and includes monitoring of the respiratory effort, airflow, oxygenation, sleep state, and heart rate. Bronchoscopy would show enlarged adenoids but does not measure airflow. Overnight EEG monitoring may be done in children who have central sleep apnea or are suspected of having certain types of seizures (nocturnal seizures). Pulse oximetry monitoring is performed as part of polysomnography. Fluoroscopy has no role in the diagnosis of obstructive sleep apnea.

58. b (Chapter 2,10,19)

Gonococcal ophthalmia neonatorum has an onset of symptoms at 2 to 4 days of age. Characteristic features include bilateral involvement, purulent discharge, marked eyelid edema, and chemosis. Diagnosis is suggested by Gram stain and confirmed on conjunctival culture plated on chocolate or Thayer-Martin agar. The infant must be treated with parenteral antibiotics to prevent blindness and other complications. The great majority of gonococcal eye infections are prevented by the instillation of silver nitrate or erythromycin in the neonatal nursery. Chlamydial infections of the eye usually present at 4 to 10 days of life with unilateral or bilateral mucopurulent discharge and conjunctival injection. Group B *Streptococcus* does not typically cause ophthalmia neonatorum, although it can cause sepsis and other complications in the neonatal period. Congenital toxoplasmosis can cause chorioretinitis that persists long term. Congenital syphilis does not have any characteristic findings on eye examination.

59. c (Chapter 21)

Based on presentation and physical examination, this patient most likely has overdosed (accidentally or intentionally) on a narcotic. Opiates cause bradycardia, hypotension, respiratory depression, somnolence, and pinpoint pupils. Naloxone is the antidote for opiate poisoning. Atropine and pralidoxime chloride are indicated for organophosphate poisoning. Physostigmine is used to counteract the effects of anticholinergic agents. Deferoxamine (desferrioxamine) chelation is beneficial in patients with iron ingestions. Since this patient is likely a chronic user of narcotics, the naloxone should be infused slowly and at a relatively low dose to decrease the likelihood of seizures.

60. b (Chapter 21)

Aspiration is the accidental inspiration of foreign material into the respiratory tract. Foreign body aspiration is most common in children 6 to 30 months old. Food, coins, and small toys constitute the most commonly aspirated objects. Aspiration into the lower airways is much more common than tracheal obstruction. While the angle of the right mainstem bronchus in adults favors right-sided aspiration, no such propensity exists in young children given the symmetric bronchial angles in this age group. Patients who do not acutely obstruct their airways may present up to a week after the initial event with no witnessed episode of choking. Wheezing and respiratory distress may be mistaken for asthma; pneumonia is a consideration when breath sounds are decreased. Of note, findings on auscultation in cases of foreign body aspiration are localized to one side of the chest only. In cases of complete obstruction, the chest radiograph demonstrates significant one-sided atelectasis, and the heart is drawn toward the affected lung throughout the entire respiratory cycle. However, a partial obstruction allows air to enter during inspiration, where it becomes trapped (ball-valve obstruction). In these cases, the inspiratory film may appear normal, but the expiration radiograph will show a hyperinflated obstructed lung with mediastinal shift away from the blockage. Lateral decubitus films should be obtained if a foreign body is suspected and expiratory studies are normal as the child is too young to expirate.

61. c (Chapter 15)

This patient exhibits behaviors that are consistent with the diagnosis of an autism spectrum disorder. He has impaired social interaction, does not communicate with others, and engages in repetitive, stereotypic behavior (rocking). Patients with Down syndrome have developmental delay but socialize with others and attempt to communicate at this age; their development is not described as deviant, as this patient's could be. A child with an isolated hearing impairment would communicate nonverbally but clearly and, depending on the severity, may be unable to repeat works spoken to him, as this child does. Although rocking and other self-stimulatory behaviors are found in developmentally normal children as well as those with autism and other disorders, its presence in this setting lends support for the diagnosis of autism spectrum disorder.

62. b (Chapter 5,17)

Normal serum potassium levels range from 3.5 to 5.5 mEq/L. This patient has symptomatic hypokalemia. The two studies which are most helpful in categorizing hypokalemia are patient blood pressure and urine potassium value. Both blood pressure and urine potassium levels are elevated in patients with Cushing syndrome and renovascular disease. Normotensive patients with decreased potassium levels may be anorexic or losing potassium from the skin or gastrointestinal track (e.g., laxative abuse). Renal tubular acidosis is the only condition listed for which one would expect the patient to have a normal blood pressure and elevated urine potassium measurement.

63. b (Chapter 18)

Functional and structural abnormalities in children with trisomy 21 include generalized hypotonia (obstructive sleep apnea), cardiac defects (endocardial cushion defects and septal defects are seen in 50% of cases), gastrointestinal anomalies (duodenal atresia and Hirschsprung disease), atlantoaxial instability, developmental delay, moderate mental retardation, and hypothyroidism. There is a higher frequency of leukemia in children with trisomy 21 than in the general population.

64. e (Chapter 2)

Congenital malformations causing fetal bowel obstruction frequently lead to polyhydramnios. Most tracheoesophageal fistulas are accompanied by esophageal atresia. Congenital or genetic defects that impair fetal swallowing also promote polyhydramnios. Therefore, hydrocephalus with myelomeningocele is also correct. Fetal urine production is a major contributor to amniotic fluid volume. Renal agenesis causes profound oligohydramnios or absence of amniotic fluid.

65. c (Chapter 9)

The history, physical examination, and abdominal radiograph are classic for a diagnosis of intussusception, the "telescoping" of a proximal segment of bowel into a more distal segment. In cases of intussusception, air or double-contrast enema demonstrates a coiled spring appearance to the bowel in the right lower quadrant. The contrast or air enema results in hydrostatic reduction of the intussusception in 75% of cases.

66. a (Chapter 9)
The most common cause of rectal bleeding in toddlers is an anal fissure. If there were significant upper GI tract bleeding from peptic ulcer disease or a Mallory-Weiss tear, the child would likely have melena instead of blood-streaked stool. Inflammatory bowel disease and necrotizing enterocolitis could both cause lower GI tract bleeding (hematochezia or blood-streaked stool) but are unlikely in an 18-month-old.

67. d (Chapter 12)
This is a classic presentation of Wilms tumor. Patients with Wilms tumor may come to medical attention after abdominal trauma. The trauma causes hemorrhage into the tumor, resulting in pain, abdominal distention, and hematuria. The patient may also have an associated anemia, depending on the degree of hemorrhage. Hypertension is frequently found in patients with Wilms tumor and resolves with treatment.

68. e (Chapter 16)
This clinical picture is most consistent with idiopathic talipes equinovarus. Dorsiflexion at the ankle is not possible in patients with this disorder. Metatarsus adductus, or in-toeing of the forefoot, is a less severe condition that often responds to regular passive stretching. Talipes equinovarus will result in a severe limp and foot ulcerations if correction is not achieved by the time the child begins to ambulate. Many but not all cases do require surgical repair; serial bracing or casting has enjoyed a revival of sorts in recent years. One in seven patients with talipes equinovarus will have an associated congenital malformation.

69. b (Chapter 9)
Evaluation for other conditions (e.g., bacterial colitis, *C. difficile* infection) is important before starting therapy directed against IBD. Similarly, complications of IBD may require antibiotics or surgery rather than anti-inflammatory drugs (e.g., prednisone). Cancer risk is somewhat increased in long-standing Crohn disease. Therapy with mercaptopurine and azathioprine will not provide symptom relief for weeks. Therapy with anti-TNF alpha antibody may be helpful but other options may be preferable and excluding an abscess is the first order of business. A capsule endoscopy is helpful for occult small intestinal disease but less likely to be the test of choice in an acute setting.

70. c (Chapter 13)
Food allergy is an IgE-mediated clinical response triggered by antigen-specific IgE bound to mast cells and basophils, resulting in cellular degranulation and the resultant immediate clinical response. While skin prick tests measure the wheal-and-flare response of food-specific IgE bound to skin mast cells, this response is frequently falsely positive. As such, a positive test has to be followed by the development of clinical symptoms in response to oral challenges to the implicated food (but not the placebo) via a double-blind placebo-controlled food challenge, a procedure that must be performed in a hospital/office setting equipped to respond to acute life-threatening anaphylaxis. Food-specific IgE levels can often be falsely positive and should not be used alone to diagnosis food allergy. Open-label food challenges are often helpful but are not used for definitive diagnosis. Finally, an endoscopy is useful to examine gastrointestinal anatomy and possible pathology but does not diagnose food allergy.

71. a (Chapter 16)
Scoliosis in a premenarchal female is likely to progress and should be treated aggressively. Curvature of 25° to 45° requires bracing to halt progression of the curve. If external bracing is not successful and the curve progresses to greater than 40° to 50°, surgery is required. Stretching exercises are not effective in the treatment of scoliosis.

72. c (Chapter 16)
A fracture through the growth plate that extends into the epiphysis and into the joint space is consistent with a Salter-Harris Type III fracture. If the fracture extended into the metaphysis only, this would constitute a Type II fracture. Fractures through both the metaphysis and epiphysis into the joint space are Type IV. Type I fractures occur along the growth plate only, whereas Type V fractures result from compression of the growth plate. Type III fractures such as the one described in the vignette may require open reduction and fixation but have a relatively good prognosis.

73. b (Chapter 11)
Based on the information provided, this patient most likely has hereditary spherocytosis (HS) which gives a positive result on the osmotic fragility test. Patients with HS have a history of neonatal jaundice, occurring usually in the first 24 hours of life. HS is caused by a defect in the red blood cell membrane proteins (spectrin, ankyrin, or band 3 protein). Inheritance is usually autosomal dominant, but 25% of cases are caused by new mutation or autosomal recessive forms. None of the other listed diagnoses would give positive results on the osmotic fragility test.

74. d (Chapter 3)
The examination described is most consistent with Tanner stage IV development (see Table 3-2). Stage III is characterized by enlargement and elevation of the breast and areola without separation of their contours, and pubic hair spread sparsely over the pubis which is less dark and curly than adult pubic hair. In stage V, the areola regresses to the general contour of the breast, and pubic hair is adult in texture and amount and has spread to the medial thighs.

75. b (Chapter 12)
The chemotherapy used in AML is more intense than that used in ALL, and the myelosuppression is severe. Patients require hospitalization for aggressive supportive care until they begin to show signs of count recovery. Hyperleukocytosis is more likely to by symptomatic in AML (and thus more likely to require treatment) than in ALL because AML blasts are larger and stickier than ALL blasts. Patients with Down syndrome and AML have an excellent overall survival rate, while secondary AML is extremely difficult to treat and outcomes are poor. Not all patients with AML will go on to bone marrow transplantation. Low-risk AML is treated with chemotherapy alone.

76. c (Chapter 9)
Crohn disease typically is associated with transmural inflammatory disease resulting in fistulae or stricture formation. Lesions may be found from the mouth to the anus but most commonly appear in the ileum and/or colon involvement with skip lesions, rectal sparing, segmental narrowing of the ileum (string sign), granuloma, perianal disease, and growth failure. Ulcerative colitis typically is characterized by rectal involvement, rectal bleeding, and diffuse superficial mucosal ulceration. Ulcerative colitis is associated with an increased the risk of colon cancer.

77. d (Chapter 21)
Carbon monoxide poisoning presents with lethargy, irritability, confusion, dizziness, headache, and nausea. Signs include irregular breathing, cyanosis, and mental status changes. Unconscious patients are

severely affected and have a high risk for death. Oxygen is considered an antidote for carbon monoxide poisoning; immediate administration of oxygen is indicated for affected patients. While all the other options listed should also be performed in this patient, the most immediate need is oxygen.

78. a (Chapter 10)

Epiglottitis consists of inflammation and edema of the epiglottis and aryepiglottic folds. Most cases occur during the winter months in children 3 to 5 years of age. Fever, sore throat, hoarseness, and progressive stridor develop over 1 to 2 days. On examination, the child appears toxic, drools, and leans forward to maximize airway patency. Epiglottitis is considered a life-threatening emergency because of the propensity of the swollen tissues to cause sudden and irreversible airway occlusion.

Children with croup typically experience the sudden onset of a hoarse voice, barky cough, and inspiratory stridor, which may progress to respiratory distress. Patients may have a prodrome consisting of low-grade fever and rhinorrhea 12 to 24 hours prior to the onset of stridor. Children with bacterial pneumonia may present with nonspecific constitutional complaints, including fever, irritability, vomiting, abdominal pain, and lethargy. Abrupt onset of fever, chills, dyspnea, and chest pain is typical. Drooling and other symptoms related to the upper airway are rarely present. The onset of diphtheria may be abrupt, with a low-grade fever, sore throat, mild pharyngeal injection, and development of a membrane on the tonsils. The membrane may extend to involve the nasopharynx and laryngotracheal areas. Due to the use of the diphtheria-tetanus-acellular pertussis vaccine, diphtheria is a rare disease in most areas of the world. Anaphylaxis is a life-threatening immunoglobulin E–mediated allergic reaction that may occur with foods, medicines, and other triggers. Children often present with respiratory distress, wheezing, pruritis, and hives.

79. d (Chapter 3)

Although guns are often bought with the intention of making a home safer, they actually increase the risk of gun death in family members living in the home. Adolescents who live in a home with a gun are three times more likely to die of homicide and 10 times more likely to commit suicide with a gun than their peers who live in homes without guns.

80. b (Chapter 1,15)

A 36-month-old child with typical development should be able to pedal a tricycle, broad jump, copy a circle, use five- to eight-word sentences, and know his or her own age and gender. Two-year-old children can jump with 2 feet off the floor and copy straight lines but cannot broad jump or copy circles. In contrast, 4-year-old children can generally balance on one foot, copy a cross, dress themselves, and wash and dry hands. At age 5 years, a child can skip with alternating feet, draw a person with six or more body parts, and name four colors. Six-year-olds can ride bikes and write their own names.

81. c (Chapter 5)

This child, judged to be 10% dehydrated, is 3,000 mL behind on fluids (3 kg). A total of 540 mL is subtracted from the deficit, leaving 2,460 mL to be given over the next 24 hours. Half of this is provided over the first 8 hours (1,230 mL at 153 mL/hr) along with maintenance fluids (67 mL/hr). The most appropriate fluid choice for a child this age is D_5 0.2 normal saline (with 20 mEq/L KCl to be added after the patient has urinated). If the child had hypernatremic dehydration, the deficit would need to be replaced over a longer period.

82. a (Chapter 9)

Both celiac disease and Crohn disease are possible. Anemia may be present with both. The tissue transglutaminase assay (IgA) should be elevated in celiac disease. Inflammatory markers such as elevated CRP and platelet count are often elevated in Crohn disease. Physical examination does not justify a CT scan next. A urinary tract infection, hydronephrosis, or cystic fibrosis may be the etiology of the complaint but a laparotomy is not yet indicated. Colonoscopy and upper endoscopy are not yet indicated but either or both may be in the next round of testing. Without a history of diarrhea, the symptoms and signs are unlikely due to bacterial or parasitic infection.

83. a (Chapter 12)

The leukemias account for the greatest percentage of childhood malignancies. Acute leukemias constitute 97% of all childhood leukemias and are divided into acute lymphocytic leukemia (ALL) and acute myelogenous leukemia (AML). ALL accounts for 75% of all childhood acute leukemias. A history of fever, pallor, anorexia, bone pain, lymphadenopathy, petechiae, and hepatosplenomegaly is consistent with ALL. Leukemic cell dissemination results in bone marrow failure, reticuloendothelial system infiltration, and penetration of sanctuary sites (CNS and testicles). Marrow infiltration results in crowding out of normal marrow blood cell precursors, which then results in anemia (pallor) and thrombocytopenia (petechiae). Infiltration of the reticuloendothelial system results in lymphadenopathy and hepatosplenomegaly. Bone pain is caused by expansion of the marrow cavity, destruction of cortical bone by leukemic cells, or metastatic tumor. Although fever and petechiae are consistent with aplastic anemia, bone pain, lymphadenopathy, and hepatosplenomegaly are not.

84. e (Chapter 16)

Observation is the best answer because this girl is skeletally mature and her curve is unlikely to progress significantly in the future. If no progression is seen in 1 year on radiograph, then minimal further follow-up would be indicated, and she should have an essentially normal spine in the future. Posterior spinal fusion is only indicated for scoliosis over 40° to 50° in skeletally mature patients. Intensive physical therapy has not been shown to alter the natural history of scoliosis. Bracing is only indicated for curves over 25° to 30° in patients who are still growing. Spinal manipulation has not been shown to effect scoliosis curve progression.

85. d (Chapter 10)

The boy's history and clinical picture are most consistent with Rocky Mountain spotted fever or ehrlichiosis. He is significantly ill (and vomiting) and should be admitted to the hospital. Both Rocky Mountain spotted fever and ehrlichiosis are rapidly progressive; treatment should be initiated immediately when these diseases are suspected. Delay in treatment can be fatal. Because this boy has no history of a tick bite and is sufficiently ill, empiric antibiotic treatment should include coverage for Rocky Mountain spotted fever and ehrlichiosis (doxycycline) and meningococcemia (cefotaxime or ceftriaxone).

86. d (Chapter 13)

Henoch-Schönlein purpura (HSP) is the most common vasculitis in childhood and the classic tetrad of findings consists of skin (purpura), joint (acute arthritis), gastrointestinal (abdominal pain, GI bleeding), and kidney disease. Approximately 20% of patients will have renal involvement early in the disease course, most often microscopic hematuria. Severe renal involvement with azotemia is rare (less than 5% of cases). Autoantibodies are negative. Even though HSP is an IgA-mediated immune complex disease, C3 and C4 levels are usually normal.

87. a (Chapter 11)
The adjusted reticulocyte count (ARC) = ([measured hematocrit]/[normal hematocrit for age]) × reticulocyte count. An ARC less than 2.0 suggests ineffective erythropoiesis, whereas an ARC greater than 2.0 signifies effective erythropoiesis. Anemia caused by a lack of production of red blood cells will therefore have an ARC less than 2.0, whereas anemias resulting from hemolysis or chronic blood loss will have an ARC greater than 2.0. The mean corpuscular volume (MCV) is used to describe the anemia as microcytic, macrocytic, or normocytic. All of the anemias noted in the question result from decreased red cell production and have an inadequate reticulocytosis (ARC $<$2.0). Decreased red cell production is due to either deficiency of hematopoietic precursors or bone marrow failure. The microcytic anemia described in the question is most likely due to iron deficiency, which is not only the most common microcytic anemia, but also the most common cause of anemia during childhood. It is most often seen between 6 and 24 months of age. Thalassemia syndromes are also microcytic anemias but are less common than iron-deficiency anemia. Anemia of chronic disease may be microcytic or normocytic. Transient erythrocytopenia of childhood is a normocytic anemia that is an acquired red cell aplasia. Parvovirus B19 aplastic crisis is a normocytic anemia that results from parvovirus B19 marrow suppression of erythropoietic precursors.

88. a (Chapter 12)
The clinical description is most consistent with Ewing sarcoma. Unlike osteosarcoma, Ewing sarcoma tends to involve systemic symptoms, such as fever, weight loss, and fatigue. Ewing sarcoma usually involves the diaphyseal portion of the long bones. The most common sites for Ewing sarcoma are the midproximal femur and the bones of the pelvis. The most common sites of osteosarcoma are the distal femur, proximal tibia, and proximal humerus. Benign bone tumors and eosinophilic granuloma are generally not painful. Chronic osteomyelitis may present with fever, pain, and localized swelling, but weight loss is unlikely.

89. a (Chapter 19)
A positive cover test is consistent with strabismus or misalignment of the eyes. This child is at risk for amblyopia (reduced vision in the affected eye) and loss of depth perception. She should be referred to a pediatric ophthalmologist for evaluation and treatment, which may include surgical realignment. Leukocoria describes a white pupil (i.e., absence of the red reflex). Retinoblastoma is a potential cause of leukocoria. Nasolacrimal duct obstruction occurs in infancy and presents with tearing.

90. b (Chapter 15)
In older patients with acute courses, the signs of hydrocephalus with increased intracranial pressure are relatively clear and include morning headache that improves after upright positioning or vomiting; irritability and/or lethargy; and papilledema and diplopia (CN VI palsy). Spasticity, clonus, and hyperreflexia most prominent in the legs are additional neurologic signs of hydrocephalus. The Cushing triad, consisting of hypertension, bradycardia, and slow irregular respirations, is a late and ominous sign of increased intracranial pressure implying imminent risk of brain herniation. Hypotension and tachycardia would not be expected. The anterior fontanelle typically closes prior to age 2 years. Erythema migrans is a rash associated with Lyme disease (Chapter 10); although Lyme disease can be associated with abducens nerve palsy, the presence of additional signs and symptoms of increased intracranial pressure on examination make this etiology more likely.

91. a (Chapter 17)
This patient displays the characteristic findings of prerenal acute renal failure due to decreased renal perfusion from dehydration. She has tachycardia, decreased urine output, and a low fractional excretion of sodium. Recognition and prompt treatment of prerenal failure is essential to prevent progression to intrinsic renal failure. The treatment of choice is restoration of renal perfusion by correcting the intravascular volume deficit with an intravenous bolus of normal saline. This will usually result in restoration of kidney function and urine output as well as correction of the acidosis and hyperkalemia.

The metabolic acidosis does not require urgent specific correction with bicarbonate. The patient does not display signs of significant fluid overload and therefore does not require furosemide (which may cause more harm than good in this situation). The gastroenteritis is most likely viral in etiology and does not require immediate antibiotic therapy. Dialysis would be indicated only if the patient had persistent fluid overload, hyperkalemia, or acidosis that is unresponsive to other medical therapies.

92. e (Chapter 4)
Colic is a syndrome of recurrent irritability that occurs most commonly in infants 3 weeks to 3 months of age. The episodes occur daily and persist for several hours, usually in the late afternoon or evening. During the attacks, the child draws the knees to the abdomen and cries inconsolably. The crying resolves as suddenly and spontaneously as it begins. Colic is often mistaken for cow milk protein allergy, although the latter typically occurs in slightly older infants and may involve bloody stools, an eczematous rash, poor growth, abdominal distention, and vomiting. Intussusception is rare in a child this young and is not temporally cyclical. Hirschsprung disease is unlikely as the child is stooling normally.

93. e (Chapter 16)
Breech presentation or family history of developmental dysplasia of the hip (DDH), either of which warrants a hip ultrasound. The remaining options are all minor risk factors for DDH.

94. a (Chapter 3)
As many as 40% of patients with anorexia nervosa develop mitral valve prolapse, evidenced by a midsystolic click and/or murmur. Other cardiac abnormalities (arrhythmias) can occur as a complication of anorexia but are less common. Anorexic patients will often present with bradycardia; however, bradycardia alone does not result in a click or murmur. A prolonged QTc interval may develop in patients who purge by vomiting (which is more common in bulimia) due to hypokalemia.

95. a (Chapter 1)
The routine use of seat belts and child car seats has been shown to be highly effective in reducing the incidence of severe injury and death in the pediatric population. All states require car seat restraint of passengers under 40 lb. Children who are 72 years of age or older may ride facing forward, whereas lighter/younger infants must face the rear. When a child passenger has reached the height/weight limit for his or her car seat (usually up to 40 lb), a booster seat should be employed. The child should be restrained in a booster seat until the standard lap belt fits correctly (across the chest and thighs) and the child is tall enough for the legs to bend at the knees with the feet hanging down. This usually does not occur until the child is 8 to 12 years old or approximately 57 inches in height. Because air bags are designed primarily for adults, children should always ride belted in the back seat.

96. a (Chapter 9)

Projectile nonbilious vomiting is the cardinal feature seen in virtually all patients with pyloric stenosis. Physical findings vary with the severity of the obstruction. The classic finding of an olive-sized, muscular, mobile, nontender mass in the epigastric area occurs in most cases. Dehydration and poor weight gain are common when the diagnosis is delayed. Hypokalemic, hypochloremic metabolic alkalosis with dehydration is seen secondary to persistent emesis in the most severe cases.

97. e (Chapter 5)

Children who lose electrolytes in their stool and are supplemented with free water very dilute juices are prone to the development of hyponatremia. Symptoms of hyponatremia include anorexia, nausea, confusion, and lethargy. The ataxia may be due to weakness or to lethargy. Hypomagnesemia is uncommon unless the patient has been receiving medication or parenteral nutrition. Hyperkalemia presents with symptoms of paresthesias and weakness but is less likely given the history of present illness. Patients with protracted vomiting and those who are being treated with loop or thiazide diuretics may develop metabolic alkalosis, but acidosis would be expected in this patient. This patient may indeed have hypochloremia, but it is unlikely to be the primary cause of his symptoms.

98. c (Chapter 14)

Scant axillary hair/Tanner II pubic hair, testicular volume 5 cc, and bone age of 11 years with normal screening labs describe a boy with prepubertal physical exam findings, a delayed bone age, and likely euthyroid with normal growth hormone screening parameters. Answer *a* is a more pubertal advanced boy with an advanced bone age. Answer *b* describes a boy with pubertal delay but with biochemical evidence of hypothyroidism. Answer *d* describes a boy with pubertal delay but with biochemical concerns that may suggest growth hormone deficiency.

99. c (Chapter 21)

Lead poisoning is an ideal condition for which to screen given its lack of early symptoms, its harmful effect on cognitive development at preclinical levels, and its amenability to treatment. Children ages 9 months to 6 years should be assessed for an increased risk of lead exposure with a questionnaire developed by the Centers for Disease Control (2001). Current recommendations vary depending on practice location, with most areas under universal screening coverage, which involves testing all children at the ages of 12 and 24 months. Research is under way to determine how to better define and target high-risk groups and decrease the number of tests performed on the general population. Many offices screen for elevated blood lead levels by performing a capillary micro-lead measurement. Any capillary blood level >10 μg/dL must be confirmed by a venous blood lead test due to a relatively high false positive rate. All elevated screening (capillary) blood tests should be confirmed with a venous sample before treatment is initiated unless the child is acutely symptomatic.

100. c (Chapter 13)

This child has linear scleroderma, a condition characterized by linear streaks of indurated and thickened skin and underlying soft tissues. Major sequelae include growth restriction and limitation of the affected areas. In this case, there is a high risk for the development of a right elbow contracture as the linear scleroderma extends over the elbow joint. The child is at very low risk for the development of systemic sclerosis, a condition in which internal organ disease, such as esophageal dysfunction, cardiopulmonary disease, severe Raynaud phenomenon, and peripheral arterial disease is commonly seen.

Index

Page numbers followed by *t* refer to tables; page numbers followed by *f* refer to figures.

AAP. *See* American Academy of Pediatrics (AAP)
Abdominal pain, 134–135, 141, 149, 151
ABO incompatibility, 31
Absence epilepsy, 276, 278
Absence seizures, 262*t*, 263
Abuse, 54, 56, 366. *See also* Child abuse; Substance use and abuse
Acanthosis nigricans, 243
ACE inhibitors. *See* Angiotensin-converting enzyme inhibitors
Acetaminophen, 144, 147, 195, 340, 355*t*, 365
Acetazolamide, 270, 277, 279
Achondroplasia, 287
Acid reflux. *See* Gastroesophageal reflux
Acid–base status, child's, 70, 72
Acidosis, 67–68, 67*t*, 302–303, 303*f*
ACIP-recommended vaccination, 45*f*
Acne vulgaris, 77–78, 78*f*–79*f*
Acquired nevi, 80
Acquired structural heart disease, 97–99
Activated charcoal, 354, 355*t*–357*t*
Acute cerebellar ataxia, 271, 277, 279
Acute chest syndrome, 189
Acute gastroenteritis (AGE), 176
Acute head trauma, 345
Acute hematogenous osteomyelitis (AHO), 290, 292
Acute hemolytic transfusion reactions, 199
Acute kidney injury (AKI), 305–307, 306*t*
Acute laryngotracheobronchitis, 158–159, 159*f*
Acute liver failure, 147
Acute lymphoblastic leukemia (ALL), 205–211, 206*f*–207*f*, 209*t*–210*t*, 220, 222
    poor prognostic factors for, 220, 222
Acute myeloid leukemia (AML), 202, 205–211, 206*f*–207*f*, 209*t*–210*t*
Acute otitis media (AOM), 155–156
Acute poisoning, 354–357, 355*f*–357*f*
Acute poststreptococcal glomerulonephritis (APGN), 301
Acute psychosis, 56
Acute renal failure (ARF), 305
Acute rheumatic fever (ARF), 157, 157*t*
Acute tubular necrosis (ATN), 305
Acyanotic congenital heart disease, 94–97, 94*f*, 96*f*–97*f*
Acyclovir, 74, 75, 167, 177, 268
Adalimumab, 85
Adapalene, 78
Adaptive development, 256, 257*t*
Adaptive immune system, 224
Addison disease, 65, 254
Adduction, 289, 291
Adenosine, 104, 105*f*, 341, 342*t*
    for supraventricular tachycardia, 109, 112
Adenovirus, 332–333, 334
ADHD. *See* Attention-deficit/hyperactivity disorder
Adolescent and Young Adult (AYA) oncology, 205
Adolescent medicine, 43–52
    eating disorders, 44–49, 49*t*
    office visit, 43–44, 44*t*
    sexual development/reproductive health, 44, 46*f*, 46*t*, 47*f*–48*f*
    substance use and abuse, 50–51, 50*t*–51*t*
    violence in adolescent population, 51–52
Adrenal dysfunction, 247–249, 248*f*
Adrenal insufficiency, 252, 254
Adrenoleukodystrophy, 260, 279
Ages and Stages Questionnaire (ASQ), 11
AIDS, 169–170
Airway films, 114
Airway foreign body, 363, 366
Airway management, 337–338
Airway obstruction, 114–127, 116*t*–121*t*, 122*f*, 123*t*–124*t*, 125*t*, 126*f*, 358–359, 359*f*, 359*t*
    in children, 127
AKI. *See* Acute kidney injury
Alagille syndrome (AGS), 147–148
Albendazole, 164
Albumin, 300
Albuterol, 122, 343
Albuterol plus ipratropium, 130, 132
Alcohol, 44*t*, 50*t*–51*t*, 51. *See also* Fetal alcohol syndrome
    ingestion, 56
Alkalinizing agent, 302
Alkalosis, 68
Alkylating agents, 208*t*–209*t*, 213
Allergic march, 239
Allergic reactions, 199
    to drugs, 80
Allergic rhinitis, 228, 237, 239
Allergic salute, 239
Allergic shiners, 239
Allergies, 58, 227–229
    eruptions secondary to, 79–80
    food, 229
Alloimmunization and delayed hemolytic transfusion reactions, 200
Allopurinol, 208, 211
α-fetoprotein, 273
Alpha interferon, 81
α-methyldopa, 190
α-thalassemia, 184–185, 184*t*, 201, 203
Alport syndrome, 301
Altered mental status, 363, 365
ALTEs. *See* Apparent life-threatening events
Ambiguous genitalia, 20
Amblyopia, 327
American Academy of Pediatrics (AAP), 11, 57, 258, 365
American Heart Association, 235, 336, 352, 358
Amino acid metabolism disorders, 321–322
Aminocaproic acid (Amicar), 196
Aminoglycosides, 154, 306
Aminotransferases, elevation of, 147
Amiodarone, 105*f*, 106, 106*f*–107*f*, 112, 341, 342*t*
Amitryptiline, 279
Amniotic fluid volume, abnormalities in, 22–25
Amoxicillin, 156, 157, 162, 172, 173, 176, 295, 298
Amoxicillin-clavulanic acid, 335
Amphetamines, 50*t*, 56, 356*t*

Ampicillin, 30, 136, 157, 163, 298
Ampicillin-sulbactam, 158, 162, 331
Amyloidosis, 240
Anabolic steroids, 50*t*
Analgesic overuse headache, 268
Anaphylactic shock, 343
Anemia, 146, 179–183, 180*t*–181*t*
  of inflammation, 185–186
  mechanism of, 201, 203
Anencephaly, 273
Aneurysms, of coronary artery, 98
Angelman syndrome, 320
Angioedema, 229
Angiotensin-converting enzyme (ACE) inhibitors, 95, 99, 305, 306*t*
Angiotensin receptor blockers, 307
Anion gap, 67, 67*t*, 70, 72
Anorexia nervosa, 44–49, 49*t*
  complication of, 53, 55
  DSM-IV criteria for, 55
  hospitalization, 53, 55
Antacid therapy, 139
Anthracyclines, 99, 210, 213
Anti-inflammatory drugs, 115, 157
Antiarrhythmic medications, 99, 100*t*
Antibiotics, 76, 78, 81, 98–99, 126, 136, 138*t*, 139–141, 140*t*, 208, 208*t*, 226, 268, 274, 285, 286, 287, 297, 300, 306*t*, 329, 330–331, 343, 352
  for infectious disease, 154, 155–157, 160, 162, 163–164, 169, 171–172
  prophylaxis, 273, 295–296, 329
Antibody deficiency syndromes, 225*t*
Anticholinergic agents, 125, 141, 273, 355*t*
Anticholinesterase agents, 271
Anticipatory guidance, 1–10
Anticoagulants, 106, 235
Anticoagulation therapy, 198–199
Anticonvulsants, 226, 261–262, 264, 268*t*, 270
Antidepressants, 270
Antidiarrheals, 135, 141, 164
Antiemetics, 141
Antiepileptic medications, 79, 272
Antifungal agents, 77, 154, 169
Antihistamines, 74, 76, 80, 228, 355*t*
Antimetabolites, 208*t*
Antinuclear antibody, 238, 240
Antinuclear cytoplasmic antibody (ANCA), 301
Antiparasitic agents, 154
Antipyretics, 74
Antiretrovirals, 169
Antispasmodic agents, 135
Antithymocyte globulin (ATG), 192
Antithyroid medications, 57, 247
Antitissue transglutaminase IgA, 149, 151
Antitumor antibiotics, 208*t*
Antitumor necrosis factor antibody, 146
Antivirals, 75, 154, 167
AOM. *See* Acute otitis media
Aorta, coarctation of, 96–97
Aortic arch, interrupted, 93–94, 93*f*
Aortic stenosis, 98
Aortic valve stenosis, 112
Apgar scores, 25, 27
APGN. *See* Acute poststreptococcal glomerulonephritis
Aplastic anemia, 192
Aplastic crisis, 189
Apnea, 109, 111, 160
  of infancy, 128*t*, 129
  obstructive, 115
Apparent life-threatening events (ALTEs), 128*t*, 129, 361
  diagnosis of, 364, 366
Appendicitis, 135–136
Appetite suppressants, 60
ARF. *See* Acute renal failure; Acute rheumatic fever
Arginine vasopressin, 243
Arrhythmias, 86, 100–106, 100*t*, 101*f*–107*f*
Arterial switch procedure, 110, 113
Arteriohepatic dysplasia. *See* Alagille syndrome (AGS)
Arteriovenous malformation (AVM), 270
Arthritis, septic, 286–287
ASD. *See* Atrial septal defect
Aseptic meningitis, 162
Asparaginase, 208*t*, 209
Asperger syndrome, 258
Aspiration syndromes, 128, 129
Aspirin, 68, 84, 98, 235, 356*t*–357*t*, 365
Asthma, 115, 116*t*–121*t*, 122*f*, 123*t*–124*t*, 132, 228–229
Asymmetric corneal light reflexes, 334
Asymmetric periflexural exanthem of childhood. *See* Unilateral thoracic exanthem
Ataxia, 271
Ataxia cerebral palsy, 260
Ataxia-telangiectasia, 271
ATN. *See* Acute tubular necrosis
Atomoxetine, 259
Atopic dermatitis, 227–228
Atrial fibrillation, 104, 104*f*, 106
Atrial flutter, 104, 104*f*
Atrial septal defect (ASD), 94
Atrial septostomy, 110, 113
Atrial tachycardia, 92
Atrioventricular canal defect, 95–96, 96*f*
Atropine, 102*f*, 340, 342*t*, 348*f*, 356*t*
Attention-deficit/hyperactivity disorder (ADHD), 259, 259*t*
Aura, 263
Auspitz sign, 78
Autism spectrum disorders (ASD), 11–13, 258–259, 258*t*
Autoimmue thyroiditis, 252, 254
Autoimmune disorders, 229–235, 230*t*–231*t*, 233*t*, 235*t*
Autoinflammatory disorders, 229–235, 230*t*–231*t*, 233*t*, 235*t*
Autosomal dominant disorders, 315–316, 316*t*
Autosomal recessive disorders, 316, 317*t*
Autosomal trisomies, 318–319, 318*t*
AV block, 101, 101*f*
AVM. *See* Arteriovenous malformation
Azathioprine, 146, 233
Azidothymidine, 191
Azithromycin, 53, 55, 126, 157, 160, 162, 169, 176
AZT. *See* Zidovudine

Baclofen, 260
Bacterial infections
  bacteremia, 155–170, 157*t*, 158*f*–159*f*, 161*t*–163*t*, 165*t*–166*t*, 166*f*
  endocarditis, 98–99
  skin manifestations of, 76–77
  vaginosis, 169
Bacterial vaginosis (BV), 55
Barlow maneuver, 291–292
Barlow provocative tests, 280, 281*f*
Basilar skull fracture, 346
Basophils, 193
Beckwith–Wiedemann syndrome, 216
Beclomethasone, 124
Benign familial hematuria, 302
Benzathine penicillin G, 157
Benzene, 192
Benzodiazepine, 264, 355*t*
Benzoic acid, 322
Benzoyl peroxide, 78, 79*f*
Beta-adrenergic agents, 160
Beta-agonists, 122, 124–125
Beta-blockers, 92, 97, 100*t*, 101, 105*f*, 106, 108, 112, 270
Beta thalassemia, 184–185, 184*t*, 202, 204
Beta$_2$-agonists, 116*t*–120*t*, 121*t*, 122, 123*t*–124*t*
Bicarbonate, 302
Bidirectional Glenn operation, 113
Bilateral adrenal hyperplasia, 249
Bilateral conductive hearing loss, cause of, 15, 16
Bilateral decubitus chest radiographs, 131, 133
Biliary atresia, 34
Bilirubin, 30
Birth defects. *See* Genetic disorders
Bisphosphonate infusion, 251
Bladder control, 308
Bleeding, gastrointestinal, 142–147, 143*t*, 145*f*, 146*t*
Bleomycin, 213

Blood. *See* Hematology
Blood products transfusion, 199–200
BMI. *See* Body mass index
Bochdalek hernia, 34
Body mass index (BMI), 57, 59
Bone infection, 285
Bone tumors, 206*f*–207*f*, 216–218, 220, 222
Bordetella pertussis, 175–176
Botulinum toxin, 260
Brachial arteries, 352
Bradyarrhythmias, 101, 101*f*, 102*f*
Brain hemorrhage, 345, 345*f*, 346*t*
Brain tumors, 206*f*–207*f*, 213–214, 213*t*–214*t*
Brainstem compression, 287
Breast milk jaundice, 30
Breastfeeding, 57, 58*t*, 62
Breathholding spells, 263
Breathing, evaluation of, 338–340
Bronchiectasis, 366
Bronchiolitis, 132, 159–160
Bronchodilators, 115, 122–125, 126
    therapy, 366
Bronchomalacia, 127
Bronchoscopy, 114
Brudzinski sign, 163
Bruises, from child abuse, 360–361, 360*f*
Bruton tyrosine kinase deficiency. *See* X-linked agammaglobulinemia
BT shunt, 113
Budesonide, 124
Bulimia nervosa, 44–49, 49*t*
Bullous impetigo, 76
Bupropion, 51
Burns, 359–360, 360*f*

C1 esterase inhibitor deficiency, 229
Calcineurin inhibitors, 304*t*
Calcitriol, 251
Calcium, 66–67
    disorders of, 250–251
Calcium channel blockers, 100*t*, 101, 108, 305
Calcium chloride, 342*t*
Calcium gluconate, 342*t*
    in treating hyperkalemia, 66, 70, 72
Cancer. *See* Oncology
Candidiasis, 169
Cannabis ingestion, 54, 56
Cantharidin, 75
Caput succedaneum, 20, 40
Carbamazepine, 147, 191, 244, 265*t*, 268*t*, 273, 278
Carbapenems, 154
Carbazazepine, 27*t*
Carbohydrate metabolism disorders, 321
Cardiogenic shock, 341, 343
Cardiology, 86–108
    acquired structural heart disease, 97–99
    acyanotic congenital heart disease, 94–97, 94*f*, 96*f*–97*f*
    arrhythmias, 86, 100–106, 100*t*, 101*f*–107*f*
    cyanotic congenital heart disease, 89–94, 90*f*, 91*f*–92*f*, 93*f*, 98*t*
    cyanotic neonate evaluation, 86–89, 88*t*
    functional heart disease, 86, 99
    heart murmurs, 86, 87*t*
Cardiomyopathies, 110, 112
Cardiopulmonary arrest, 336, 337*t*
Cardiopulmonary resuscitation (CPR), 336–337, 338*f*, 339*t*, 340*f*, 342*t*
Cataracts, 328
Cation exchange resin, administration of
    for managing hyperkalemia, 70, 72–73
CAVE, 281
Cavus, 289, 291
Cefazolin, 286
Cefotaxime, 162, 163, 171, 177, 287
Ceftriaxone, 53, 55, 156, 162, 163, 168, 169, 171–172, 176, 287, 330, 330*t*
Cefuroxime, 162, 172, 331
Celiac disease, 152
Cell-mediated immunity disorders, 224–225, 225*t*
Central nervous system tumors, 206*f*–207*f*, 213–214, 213*t*–214*t*
Cephalexin, 76
Cephalohematoma, 20
Cephalosporin, 76, 154, 158, 163, 168, 286–287, 298, 331
Cerebral edema, 242, 347
Cerebral palsy (CP), 259–260, 260*t*, 279
Cerebral perfusion pressure, 347
Cerebrospinal fluid, meningitis signs in, 163*t*
Cervical motion tenderness, 53, 56
Cervical spine films, 346
CF. *See* Cystic fibrosis
CGD. *See* Chronic granulomatous disease
Chalazion, 330
Chancre, 167
Chandelier sign. *See* Cervical motion tenderness
CHARGE syndrome, 320
CHD. *See* Congenital heart disease
Chemical conjunctivitis, 335
Chemotherapy, 57, 100*t*, 136, 138*t*, 139, 140*t*, 206, 207–211, 208*t*, 213–219, 214*t*, 217*t*, 329, 343
Chest radiograph, 363, 365–366. *See also* Radiograph
Chiari type II malformations, 273
Chickenpox. *See* Varicella
Child abuse, 344, 345, 360–361, 360*f*
Childhood, health supervision in, 2*t*–9*t*
Childhood Autism Rating Scales (CARS), 258
Childhood epilepsy syndromes, 263
Children
    acid–base status in, 70, 72
    developmental age, 14–15, 16
    fluid and hydration management, method for, 69, 71–72
Chlamydia trachomatis, 18, 168, 174, 176–177, 334
    first-line treatment for, 53, 55
    urine NAAT for, 53, 55
Chloramphenicol, 192
Chloroma, 207
Choanal atresia, 21, 38, 41, 114
Choking, 10, 16. *See also* Foreign body aspiration
Chordae, 20
Chromosomal disorders, 317–320, 318*t*
Chromosome 22q11 deletion syndrome, 89, 320
Chronic ataxias, 271
Chronic granulomatous disease (CGD), 227
Chronic kidney disease (CKD), 307–308
Chronic leukemias, 205
Chronic pulmonary hypertension, 127
Cimetidine, 75
Ciprofloxacin, 176
Circulation, assessment of, 337
Circumcision, 297
Cisplatinum, 208*t*, 216, 218
Citrate, 302
Clarithromycin, 162
Clavicle fracture, 21
    at birth, 38, 42
Clavulanic acid, 156, 162
Cleft palate, 33
Clindamycin, 76, 77, 78, 79*f*, 157, 162, 168, 331
Clinical Adaptive Test/Clinical Linguistic and Auditory Milestone Scale (CAT/CLAMS), 256
Clonidine, 263
Clostridium difficile, 139, 150, 151, 152, 164
Clotrimazole, 77*t*
Clubfoot. *See* Talipes equinovarus
Coagulation disorders, 196–199
Coarctation of the aorta, 96–97
    diagnosis of, 109, 111
    treatment side effects, 109, 111
Cocaine, 26*t*, 50*t*, 100*t*, 304*t*, 356*t*
Colic, 58
Colitis, 58, 139
Colonoscopy, for Crohn's disease, 150, 153
Combined immunodeficiency syndromes, 226
Common atrioventricular canal defect, 95–96

Common variable immunodeficiency (CVID), 226, 238, 239–240
Communicating hydrocephalus, 273–274
Compensated hypovolemic shock, 350, 352
Compensatory reticulocytosis, 203
Complement immunity disorders, 225*t*, 227
Complete airway obstruction, 358
Complete atrioventricular canal defect, 95–96, 96*f*
Complete AV canal (AVSD), 323, 325
Complete blood count (CBC), 55, 149, 151, 207, 220
Complex febrile seizures, 261
Complex partial seizures, 262*t*, 263, 278
Computed tomography (CT), 114
  for pseudotumor cerebri, 277, 279
Concussion, 345, 357–358
Conduction block. *See* AV block
Confidentiality, 54, 56
  of information, 43
Congenital adrenal hyperplasia, 111, 248–249, 248*f*
Congenital aganglionic megacolon. *See* Hirschsprung disease
Congenital cataract, 332, 334
Congenital clubfoot, foot deformity in, 289, 291
Congenital diaphragmatic hernia, 34
Congenital diarrhea, 152
Congenital heart disease (CHD), 86, 87, 88*t*, 89–97, 90*f*, 91*f*–92*f*, 93*f*, 94*f*, 96*f*–97*f*, 366
Congenital hypothyroidism, 246
Congenital megakaryocytic hypoplasia, 194
Congenital nasolacrimal duct obstruction, 329
Congenital nevi, 80, 80*f*
Congenital tracheal stenosis, 127
Congenital/perinatal infections, 22*t*–25*t*, 25
Conjugated hyperbilirubinemia, 34
Conjugated seven-valent pneumococcal vaccine, 155, 331
Conjunctivitis, 329–330, 330*t*
Connective tissue disorders, 234
Conotruncal heart defect, 324, 325–326
Constipation, 141–142
Constitutional delay, 244–245
Contaminated specimen, 312, 314
Corneal abrasion, 329
Coronary artery aneurysms, 98, 238, 240
Coronary artery disease, 99
Corpulmonale, 127
Corticosteroids, 80, 81, 116*t*–119*t*, 121*t*, 123*t*–124*t*, 125, 146, 158, 159, 199, 208*t*, 228, 235, 271, 304*t*
Cortisol, 248–249
Cough-variant asthma, 120
CP. *See* Cerebral palsy
CPR. *See* Cardiopulmonary resuscitation
Cradle cap, 19. *See also* Infantile seborrhea
Craniosynostosis, 274
Critical illness, emergency management of, 336–349, 338*f*, 340*f*, 341*t*
Critical pulmonary stenosis, 40
Critically injured child, 343–348
Crohn's disease, 144–147, 146*t*, 152
  intervention, 150, 153
  upper endoscopy and colonoscopy for, 150, 153
Cromolyn, 123*t*–124*t*, 228
Croup, 158–159, 159*f*
Cryoprecipitate, 199
Cryptorchidism, 20, 41, 297
Cryptosporidium, 141
Crystalloid solutions, 352
CT. *See* Computed tomography
Cushing disease, 245–246, 249
Cushing triad, 274, 346
Cushing's syndrome, 353
Cyanosis, 89
Cyanotic congenital heart disease, 89–94, 90*f*, 91*f*–92*f*, 93*f*
Cyanotic neonate, 86–89, 88*t*
Cyclophosphamide, 208*t*–209*t*, 211, 213, 216, 217, 233, 235, 300
Cyclosporine, 85, 192, 234
Cystic fibrosis (CF), 125–127, 125*t*, 126*f*, 130, 132
Cystitis, 297–298, 299*f*
Cytarabine, 208*t*, 211
Cytomegalovirus, 23*t*
Cytosine arabinoside, 210

D-penicillamine, 147
D-TGA. *See* D-transposition of great arteries
D-transposition of great arteries (D-TGA), 89–90, 90*f*
  intervention, 110, 113
  surgical intervention, 110, 113
Dacryocystitis, 335
Dacryostenosis, 333, 335. *See also* Nasolacrimal duct obstruction
Dactinomycin, 217*t*
Dactylitis, 240
Dapsone gel, 78
Daunomycin, 209
DDAVP. *See* Desmopressin acetate
DDH. *See* Developmental dysplasia of hip
Decompensated shock, 352–353
Decongestants, 228, 356*t*, 365
Deep vein thrombosis, 198–199
Deferasirox, 185
Deferoxamine, 185, 356*t*
Deformities, foot, 289, 291
Dehydration, 63–65, 64*t*, 111, 112, 139–141
Delayed hypersensitivity skin testing, 237–238, 239
Demeclocycline, 244
Dental caries, 10
Denver Developmental Screening Test II (Denver II), 11, 256
Dermatitis, 227–228, 234
Dermatology, 74–85
  acne vulgaris, 77–78, 78*f*–79*f*
  bacterial infections, 76–77
  eruptions secondary to allergic reactions, 79–80
  hyperpigmented lesions, 80, 80*f*
  infantile hemangiomas, 81
  presumed viral exanthems, 76, 76*f*
  psoriasis, 78–79
  superficial fungal infections, 77, 77*f*, 77*t*
  viral infection, 74–76, 75*f*
Dermatomyositis, 230*t*, 233–234
Desmopressin acetate (DDAVP), 71, 196, 244, 308
Development of poststreptococcal glomerulonephritis, 173, 175
Developmental delay, 256
Developmental dissociation, 256
Developmental dysplasia of hip (DDH), 280, 281*f*
  early osteoarthritis, 289, 292
  risk factors for, 289, 291
Developmental quotient (DQ), 256
Developmental shoulder dysplasia, 42
Dexamethasone, 249
Dextroamphetamine, 245, 259
Dextrose, 247, 342*t*, 354
Diabetes insipidus (DI), 243–244, 303–304
Diabetes mellitus, 241–243
Diabetic ketoacidosis (DKA), 241–242
Diamond-Blackfan anemia (DBA), 192
Diaper rash, 77
Diarrhea, 63, 139–141, 140*t*, 144, 163–164
  intermittent, 149, 151
Diazepam, 264
DIC. *See* Disseminated intravascular coagulation
Diet, 139. *See also* Nutrition
Diethylstilbestrol, 316*t*
Diffuse axonal injury, 345
DiGeorge syndrome, 224. *See also* Chromosome 22Q11 deletion syndrome
Digibind, 365
Digitalis, 100*t*, 105*f*
Digoxin, 66, 101, 104, 105*f*, 106, 112, 138*t*, 247

Dilated cardiomyopathy (DCM), 99, 110, 112
 diuretics for, 110, 112
 echocardiogram for, 110, 112
 intubation and positive pressure ventilation therapy, 110, 113
Diphenhydramine, 80, 229, 343
Diphtheria and tetanus toxoids and acellular pertussis (DTaP) vaccine, 12*f*
Diphyllobothrium latum, 191
Disseminated intravascular coagulation (DIC), 196
Distributive shock, 342–343
Diuretics, 66, 68, 95, 99, 110, 112, 157, 300, 304–305
 for hypertension, 310, 313
DKA. *See* Diabetic ketoacidosis
DMD. *See* Duchenne-type muscular dystrophy
Double bubble sign, 33
Down syndrome, 95, 258, 318, 325
Doxorubicin, 208*t*, 211, 216, 217–218, 343
Doxycycline, 78, 79*f*, 168–169, 171–172, 174, 176, 177
Drennan's sign, 293
Drowning, 10, 358
Drug use and abuse, 50–51, 50*t*–51*t*, 54, 56
Drugs, allergic reactions to, 80
DTaP vaccine. *See* Diphtheria and tetanus toxoids and acellular pertussis vaccine
Duchenne-type muscular dystrophy (DMD), 271, 279
Ductal-dependent pulmonary blood flow lesions, of cyanotic congenital heart disease, 90–92, 91*f*–92*f*
Ductal-dependent systemic blood flow lesions, of cyanotic congenital heart disease, 92–94, 93*f*
Ductal-independent mixing lesions, of cyanotic congenital heart disease, 89–90, 90*f*
Ductus arteriosus, 96, 97*f*
Duodenal atresia, 33–34
Dysequilibrium syndrome, 308
Dysfluency, 13, 256
Dyslipidemia, 60
Dystonia, 260
Dystrophin, 99

Early onset sepsis, 29–30
Early osteoarthritis, 289, 292
Eating disorders, 44–49, 49*t*
Ebstein anomaly, 92, 92*f*
EBV. *See* Epstein-Barr virus (EBV)
ECG. *See* Electrocardiogram
ECHO. *See* Echocardiogram (ECHO)
Echocardiogram (ECHO)
 for coarctation of the aorta, 109, 111
 for congenital heart disease, 323, 325
 for D-transposition of the great arteries (D-TGA), 110
 for dilated cardiomyopathy, 110, 112
Ecstasy, 50*t*
Eczema, 227–228, 239
Edrophonium chloride, 271
Edwards syndrome. *See* Trisomy 18
EEG. *See* Electroencephalogram
Eisenmenger syndrome, 95
Electrocardiogram (ECG)
 of hyperkalemia, 66, 66*f*
 of long QT syndrome, 104*f*
 for supraventricular tachycardia, 109, 112
 of Wolff-Parkinson-White syndrome, 103*f*
Electroencephalogram (EEG)
 of epilepsy, 262, 263
 for seizures, 276, 278
Electrolyte
 abnormality, 69, 71
 hypertonic saline infusion for correcting, deficit, 69, 71
 in infants, 69, 71
 management, 63–68
 requirements, 69, 71
Elevated 17-hydroxyprogesterone, 253, 255
Emergency management, 336–349
 primary assessment, 336–340, 338*f*, 339*t*, 340*f*
 secondary assessment, 342
 of shock, 341–343, 341*t*
 of status epilepticus, 264
 tertiary assessment, 340–341
Emesis, 63, 136–137, 138*t*
Emphysema, 366
Encephaloceles, 273
Encephalopathy, 264, 268, 269*t*, 305
Encopresis, 141
End-stage renal disease (ESRD), 295, 307
Endocarditis, 98–99
Endocrinology, 241–255
 adrenal dysfunction, 247–249, 248*f*
 calcium disorders, 250–251
 diabetes mellitus, 241–243
 puberty disorders, 249–250
 short stature, 244–246
 thyroid dysfunction, 246–247
 water regulation disorders, 243–244
Endotracheal tube, size of, 351, 353
Enteral therapy, 141
Enteritis, 139
Enterobius vermicularis, 164
Enthesitis-related arthritis (ERA), 231, 231*t*
Enucleation, 329
Enuresis, 308
Environmental factors, of genetic disorders, 315, 316*t*
Enzyme-linked immunosorbent assay (ELISA) test, 174, 177
Epididymitis, 297
Epidural brain hemorrhage, 345*f*, 346*t*
Epiglottitis, 158, 159*f*
Epilepsy syndromes, 262–264, 262*t*, 265*t*–267*t*
Epinephrine, 102*f*, 106, 107*f*, 111, 112, 125, 159, 229, 342–343, 342*t*, 348*f*
Epiphyseal fractures, 285*f*
Epstein-Barr virus (EBV), 157–158, 158*f*
Equinus, 289, 291
ERA. *See* Enthesitis-related arthritis
Erb palsy, 21, 42
Erythema infectiosum, 170
Erythema migrans, 171
Erythema multiforme, 79–80
Erythema nodosum, 164
Erythema toxicum, 19, 38, 40
Erythrocyte sedimentation rate (ESR), 149, 151, 238, 240, 290, 292
Erythromycin, 78, 79*f*, 138*t*, 157, 162, 164, 329, 330, 330*t*
Erythromycin estolate, 160
Esmolol, 105*f*
Esophagogastroduodenoscopy, for Crohn's disease, 150, 153
Essential hypertension, 304–305, 304*t*
Essential tremor, 263
Estrogen therapy, 319
Etanercept, 79, 85
Ethanol, 67*t*, 316*t*, 355*t*, 356*t*
Ethosuximide, 264, 266*t*, 268*t*, 276, 278
Ethylene glycol, 67*t*, 355*t*
Etoposide, 208*t*, 211, 217
Ewing sarcoma, 216–217, 220, 222
Exchange transfusion, 33
Extrapyramidal cerebral palsy, 260
Extremities, 21–22
Eye. *See* Ophthalmology

Failure to thrive (FTT), 58–59, 59*t*, 126
Famciclovir, 74
Familial Mediterranean Fever (FMF), 235
Familial short stature, 244–246
Fanconi anemia, 192
Fanconi syndrome, 302
Febrile reactions, 199
Febrile seizures, 261
Febrile transfusion reactions, 202, 204
Feeding, of infants, 57–60, 58*t*–60*t*
Felbamate, 268*t*
Female genitalia, 20
Fentanyl, 340
Fetal alcohol syndrome, 39, 42, 258, 320
Fever of unknown origin (FUO), 154–155
Fidaxomicin, 141
Fine motor, 256, 257*t*
First generation cephalosporins, 290, 292
Fitz-Hugh-Curtis syndrome, 168

5-aminosalicylic compounds, 146
Flecainide, 106
Flexible bronchoscopy, 133
Fluconazole, 169
Fludrocortisone, 249
Fluid and hydration management, 63–68
  maintenance needs, 69, 72
  method for, 69, 71
Fluid losses, 63
Fluid restriction, 244
Flumazenil, 365
Fluorescein, 329
Fluoride supplementation, 13, 16, 57
Fluoroquinolones, 154
Fluorosis, 13
Fluticasone, 124
Focal epilepsy, 262
Focal segmental glomerulosclerosis (FSGS), 299, 299*t*, 313
Focused Assessment Sonography in Trauma (FAST), 344
Folate, 183, 356*t*
Folic acid supplementation, 273
Folliculitis, 77
Fomepizole, 355*t*, 356*t*, 365
Fontan operation, 113
Food allergies, 229
Food and Drug Administration, 259, 264
Foot deformities, 280–281
  in congenital clubfoot, 289, 291
Foreign body aspiration, 358–359, 359*f*, 359*t*, 363, 365–366
Formoterol, 122
Fosphenytoin, 264, 267*t*, 278
Fracture, 283–285, 285*f*, 361
  clavicle, 21
Fragile X syndrome, 258, 320, 323, 325
Fresh frozen plasma, 199
Friedreich ataxia, 271, 279
Frozen plasma, 199
FSGS. *See* Focal segmental glomerulosclerosis
FTT. *See* Failure to thrive
Functional gastrointestinal disorders (FGIDs), 134, 151
Functional heart disease, 86, 99–100
Functional heart murmurs, 86, 87*t*
Fungal infections, superficial, 77, 77*f*, 77*t*
FUO. *See* Fever of unknown origin
Furosemide, 66, 251

G6PD deficiency. *See* Glucose-6-phosphate dehydrogenase deficiency
Gabapentin, 268*t*
Galactosemia, 321
Galeazzi sign, 280
Gammaglobulin administration, 226
Gastric lavage, 357
Gastroenteritis, 163–164
Gastroenterology, 134–148
  abdominal pain, 134–135, 141
  appendicitis, 135–136
  constipation, 141–142
  diarrhea, 63, 139–141, 140*t*, 144
  emesis, 136–137, 138*t*
  gastroesophageal reflux, 137–139
  gastrointestinal bleeding, 142–147, 143*t*, 145*f*, 146*t*
  liver disease, 147–148
Gastroesophageal reflux (GER), 137–139
Gastroschisis, 34
Gaucher disease, 322
GBS. *See* Guillain–Barré syndrome
GCS. *See* Glasgow Coma Scale
Generalized epilepsy, 262
Generalized seizures, 262*t*, 263, 265*t*
Generalized tonic–clonic (GTC) seizures, 262*t*, 263
Genetic disorders, 315–322, 315*t*
  chromosomal disorders, 317–320, 318*t*
  environmental factors of, 315, 316*t*
  genetic factors of, 315
  metabolic disorders, 268, 320–322
  molecular cytogenic disorders, 320
  single-gene disorders, 315–320, 316*t*–318*t*
Genital herpes simplex virus infection, 167–168
Genitalia, 20
Gentamicin, 30, 136, 162, 168, 177, 298
GER. *See* Gastroesophageal reflux
Gestational age, 18
Giannoti-Crosti syndrome, 74
Giardia, 151, 152
Giardia lamblia, 141, 164, 237
Giardiasis, 164
Glasgow Coma Scale (GCS), 346, 347*t*, 351, 353
Global developmental delay, 258
Glomerulonephritis, 240, 300–302, 310, 313
Glucocorticoids, 249, 251
Glucose-6-phosphate dehydrogenase (G6PD)
  assay, 182
  deficiency, 190
Glycogen storage disease (GSD), 321
Gonorrhea, 168–169, 286
Gower's sign, 279
Granulocytes, 193
  infusions, 199
Graves disease, 246
Gray matter disorders, 260
Great arteries, D-transposition of, 89–90, 90*f*
Griseofulvin, 77*t*
Gross motor, 256, 257*t*
  delay, 276, 278
Group A streptococcus (GAS; *Streptococcus pyogenes*), 83, 85, 173, 175
Growth chart, 57
Growth hormone, 319
GSD. *See* Glycogen storage disease
GTC seizures. *See* Generalized tonic–clonic seizures
Guillain–Barré syndrome (GBS), 270, 279
Gummas, 167
Gynecomastia, 41

H_1-histamine blockers, 228
H2RAs. *See* Histamine-2 receptor antagonists
Haemophilus influenzae, 176, 334
Haemophilus influenzae type b (Hib) vaccine, 12*f*, 159, 162, 331
Hagedorn (NPH) insulin, 242
Hallucinogens, 50*t*
Halo nevi, 80
Hand-foot-and-mouth disease, 74, 156
Hashimoto thyroiditis, 246
Hay fever, 228
Hb Barts, significance on newborn screening, 201, 203
Head computed tomography (CT), 364, 366
Head shapes, abnormal, 274
Head trauma, 345
Headache, 268–270
HEADSS assessment, 54, 56
Health supervision partnership, 1
Heart block, 101, 101*f*
Heart disease. *See* Cardiology
Heart murmurs, 86, 87*t*
Heart rates, 86, 87*t*, 350, 352
Hemangiomas, 82, 84
Hematology
  anemia, 146, 179–183, 180*t*–181*t*
  blood product transfusion, 199–200
  hemostasis disorders, 193–199
  macrocytic anemias with decreased red cell production, 191–192
  microcytic anemias with decreased red blood cell production, 183–186, 183*t*–184*t*
  normocytic anemias with decreased red cell production, 186
  normocytic anemias with increased red cell production, 186–191
  white blood cell disorders, 192–193
Hematuria, 300–302
Hemizygous, 317
Hemolysis, 203
Hemolytic anemia, 186–187
Hemolytic uremic syndrome (HUS), 164, 302
Hemophilia A, 196–197, 197*t*
Hemophilia B, 196–197, 197*t*
Hemophilus influenza B, 239
Hemoptysis, 126
Hemorrhagic strokes, 270

Hemostasis disorders, 193
Henoch-Schönlein purpura (HSP), 230*t*, 234–235, 238, 240, 301
nephritis, 313
Heparin, 196, 199, 270
Hepatitis, 165–166, 165*t*–166*t*, 166*f*
Hepatitis A virus vaccine, 12*f*, 165
Hepatitis B virus vaccine, 12*f*, 165
Hepatolenticular degeneration. *See* Wilson disease
Hepcidin, 186
Hereditary angioedema, 229
Hereditary nephritis. *See* Alport syndrome
Heroin, 50*t*
Herpangina, 156
Herpes, 41
Herpes simplex (HSV) encephalitis, 264, 268
Herpes simplex virus (HSV), 23*t*, 167–168
Herpes zoster, 74–75, 84
Heterozygous, 315
Hip
developmental dysplasia of, 280, 281*f*
pain, 290, 292
Hirschsprung disease, 142
Histamine-2 receptor antagonists (H2RAs), 135, 139, 144
HLA-B27, 240
HLHS. *See* Hypoplastic left heart syndrome
Hodgkin lymphoma, 206*f*–207*f*, 211–213, 212*t*
Holliday-Segar method, 63
Homicide, 10
Homocystinuria, 321
Homozygous, 315
Hordeolum, 330
HSP. *See* Henoch-Schönlein purpura
HSV. *See* Herpes simplex virus
HSV encephalitis. See Herpes simplex (HSV) encephalitis
Humalog insulin, 242
Human immunodeficiency virus (HIV), 24*t*, 169–170
enzyme-linked immunosorbent assay (ELISA) test, 174, 177
Human papillomavirus (HPV), 54, 56, 177
Humoral immunity disorders, 225*t*, 226
Hurler syndrome, 322
Hyaline membrane disease, 41. *See also* Respiratory distress syndrome
Hydralazine, 102*f*, 305
Hydroceles, 20, 297
Hydrocephalus, 273–274
Hydrocortisone, 65, 111, 249
Hydronephrosis, 295
Hydroxychloroquine, 233–234
Hydroxylase deficiency, 248–249
Hyperadrenocorticism, 249
Hyperbilirubinemia, 30
Hypercalcemia, 251
Hyperchloremic metabolic acidosis, 302–303, 303*f*
Hyperglycemia, 242
Hyperkalemia, 65–66, 66*f*, 70, 72, 254
calcium gluconate infusion in treating, 70, 72
cation exchange resin administration for managing, 70, 72–73
Hyperleukocytosis, 208–209
Hypernatremia, 65
Hyperoxia test, in cyanotic neonate, 89
Hyperphagia, 323, 325
Hyperpigmented lesions, 80, 80*f*
Hyperpnea, 67
Hypertension, 60, 304–305, 304*t*
diuretic use for, 310, 313
Hypertensive encephalopathy, 305
Hyperthyroidism, 246
Hypertonic dehydration, 64
Hypertonic saline infusion, for correcting electrolyte deficit, 69, 71
Hypertrophic obstructive cardiomyopathy, 100
Hypnotics, 340
Hypoadrenocorticism, 247–248
Hypocalcemia, 250–251, 253
Hypoglycemia, 40, 241–242
Hypokalemia, 66, 66*f*, 302
Hypomagnesemia, 67
Hyponatremia, 65. *See also* Syndrome of hyponatremia with inappropriate increased secretion of vasopressin
in infants, 69, 71
water restriction in, 71
Hypoparathyroidism, 250–251
Hypoplastic left heart syndrome (HLHS), 92–93, 93*f*
Hypospadias, 20, 296–297
Hypotension, 63, 347, 352
Hypothyroidism, 246, 252, 254
Hypotonic dehydration, 64
Hypovolemic shock, 64, 341, 343
Hypoxia, 132

IBD. *See* Inflammatory bowel disease
Ibuprofen, 74, 84, 195, 247, 270, 279, 355*t*, 357*t*, 365
ICS. *See* Inhaled corticosteroids
Idiopathic hypertrophy subaortic stenosis. *See* Hypertrophic obstructive cardiomyopathy
Idiopathic scoliosis, 287
Ifosfamide, 217
IgA nephropathy, 301
Imiquimod, 75
Immune thrombocytopenia, 194–195
Immunizations. *See* Vaccinations
Immunodeficiency syndromes, 224–227, 225*t*
Immunologic classification, of leukemias, 205–206
Immunology, 224–227, 225*t*
Imprinting disorders, 319–320
Inactivated poliovirus vaccine (IPV), 12*f*
Incomplete atrioventricular canal defect, 95–96
Indomethacin, 96, 304
Infancy
apnea of, 128*t*, 129
health supervision in, 2*t*–9*t*
Infant feeding, 57–60, 58*t*–60*t*
Infant mortality rate, 35
Infantile colic, 364, 366
Infantile glaucoma, 335
Infantile hemangiomas, 81, 82, 84
in lumbosacral region, 82, 84
Infantile seborrhea, 19, 41
Infants
daily fluid and electrolyte requirements, 69, 71
with DDH, 289, 291–292
hyponatremia in, 69, 71
physical examination of, 18–22
requiring vitamin D supplementation, 61, 62
vitamin D for, 38, 41
Infections, 189, 199
Infectious conjunctivitis, 329–330, 330*t*
Infectious disease, 154–172. *See also* Urinary tract infections
bacteremia and sepsis, 155–170, 157*t*, 158*f*–159*f*, 161*t*–163*t*, 165*t*–166*t*, 166*f*
of bone, 285
conjunctivitis, 329–330, 330*t*
of endocardium, 98–99
fever of unknown origin, 154–155
hordeolum and chalazion, 330
of joint, 286–287
of myocardium, 99
other sexually transmitted, 168
periorbital cellulitis, 331
pinworm, 164
skin manifestations of, 74–76, 75*f*
vaccinations, 162, 165, 331
viral, 74–76, 75*f*, 99, 139, 170–172, 170*t*, 271
Infectious mononucleosis, 157–158, 158*f*
Inflammatory bowel disease (IBD), 144–147, 146*t*
family history of, 151
Infliximab, 85, 235
Influenza vaccines, 12*f*. *See also* *Haemophilus influenzae* type b (Hib) vaccine
Infratentorial tumors, 213*t*, 214
Inhalants, 44*t*, 50*t*

Inhaled corticosteroids (ICS), 117*t*, 122, 123*t*–124*t*, 124
Injury, 351, 353
- emergency management of, 336–349, 337*t*, 338*f*, 339*t*, 340*f*, 341*t*–342*t*, 345*f*, 346*t*–347*t*, 348*f*
- fire, prevention of, 15, 17
- prevention of, 15, 17, 354–362

Innate immune system, 224
Inotropes, 99
INSS. *See* International Neuroblastoma Staging System
Insulin resistance, 60, 242–243
Insulin therapy, 66, 126, 242–243
Intellectual disability, 258
Intensive phototherapy, 33
Interferons, 154
Intermittent diarrhea, 149, 151
International Neuroblastoma Staging System (INSS), 215, 215*t*
Interrupted aortic arch, 93–94, 93*f*
Interstitial lung disease, 127–128
Intolerance, of feeding, 58
Intracranial injuries, from child abuse, 361
Intrauterine growth retardation (IUGR), 19, 40
Intravascular volume depletion in children, 350, 352
Intravenous antibiotics, 126
Intravenous immunoglobulin (IVIG), 80, 98–99, 226, 234–235, 270
Intrinsic renal failure, 305–306, 306*t*
Intussusception, 136
Ipecac, 138*t*, 354
Iphosphamide, 208*t*
Ipratropium, 125
Iron, 185, 307, 356*t*
Iron-deficiency anemia, 183–184, 201, 203
- cause, 201, 203

Iron overload, 200
Ischemic strokes, 270
Isoniazid, 57
Isoproterenol, 102*f*
Isotonic dehydration, 64
Isotretinoin, 78, 79*f*, 316*t*
IUGR. *See* Intrauterine growth retardation
IVIG. *See* Intravenous immunoglobulin

Janz syndrome. *See* Juvenile myoclonic epilepsy
Jaundice, 30–33
JDM. *See* Juvenile dermatomyositis
JIA. *See* Juvenile idiopathic arthritis
Joint infection, 286–287
Juvenile dermatomyositis (JDM), 230*t*, 233–234
Juvenile idiopathic arthritis (JIA), 230–232, 230*t*–231*t*
Juvenile myoclonic epilepsy, 278

Karyotype, 323, 325
Kawasaki disease, 98, 230*t*, 234–235, 235*t*, 238, 240
- complication of, 238, 240
- erythrocyte sedimentation rate (ESR) in, 238, 240

Kayexelate, 72–73
Kerions, 82, 85
Kernicterus, 31–32, 39, 42
Kernig sign, 163
Ketoconazole, 251
Kidney. *See* Nephrology
Klinefelter syndrome, 319
Klumpke paralysis, 21
Knee, radiograph of, 220, 222
Koebner phenomenon, 78, 83, 85
Kyphosis, 287

Labetalol, 102*f*, 305
Labyrinthine, viral infection of, 271
Lactase deficiency, 134
Lactated Ringers, 352
- infusion of, 69, 71

Lactobacillus, 141
Lactoferrin, 57
Lactulose, 142
Lamivudine. *See* 3TC
Lamotrigine, 264, 265*t*–268*t*, 279
Language delay, 13, 15, 16, 256
Large for gestational age (LGA), 19
Laryngomalacia, 114
Laryngotracheobronchitis, 158–159, 159*f*
Late-onset 21-OH deficiency, 253, 255
Late onset sepsis, 30
Laxatives, 68, 135
Lead poisoning, 11, 11*t*, 141, 183
Legg-Calvé-Perthes disease, 282, 283*f*
Lennox–Gastaut syndrome, 278
Leptomeningeal angiomatosis. *See* Sturge–weber syndrome
Leukemia, 205–211, 206*f*–207*f*, 209*t*–210*t*. *See also* Acute lymphoblastic leukemia (ALL)
- diagnosis of, 220, 222
- symptoms of, 220, 222

Leukocoria, 328–329
Leukocyte adhesion deficiency (LAD), 227
Leukocytes. *See* White blood cells disorders
Leukocytosis, 193
Leukodystrophies, 260
Leukotriene receptor antagonists (LTRAs), 122, 123*t*–124*t*, 124, 228
Leuprolide, 250
Levetiracetam, 264, 265*t*–268*t*
Levothyroxine, 245, 246
LGA. *See* Large for gestational age
Lidocaine, 80, 107*f*, 342*t*
Limp, 281–284, 282*f*–284*f*, 282*t*
Linear scleroderma, 230*t*, 234
Liquid nitrogen, 75
Lisdexamfetamine, 259
Lisinopril, 244
Lithium, 27*t*, 57, 67*t*, 316*t*
Liver disease, 147–148
Long QT syndrome, 104, 104*f*
Loperamide, 152
Lorazepam, 264, 267*t*, 278
Low-molecular-weight heparin, 270
Lower airway obstructive disease, 115–127, 116*t*–121*t*, 122*f*, 123*t*–124*t*, 125*t*, 126*f*
LSD, 50*t*
LTRAs. *See* Leukotriene receptor antagonists
Lumbar puncture (LP), 261
- for pseudotumor cerebri, 277, 279

Lung disease, restrictive, 127–128
Lupus nephritis, 233
Lyme disease, 171–172
Lymphoblastic leukemia, 205–211, 206*f*–207*f*, 209*t*–210*t*
Lymphoma
- Hodgkin, 206*f*–207*f*, 211–213, 212*t*
- non-Hodgkin, 206*f*–207*f*, 211

Lysosomal storage disorders, 322

Maalox, 80
Macrocephaly, 274
Macrocytic anemias, 180*t*, 191–192
Macrolide antibiotics, 136, 154
Magnesium, 66–67, 107*f*
Magnesium hydroxide, 142
Magnetic resonance imaging (MRI)
- of brain, 277, 279
- to evaluating spinal canal, 82, 84

Maintenance fluids, 63–68, 64*t*, 66*f*, 67*t*
Malabsorption, 58
Male genitalia, 20
Malignant hyperthyroidism, 246
Malrotation, 137
Marijuana, 26*t*, 50*t*, 51, 56
Mastoiditis, 156
McArdle disease, 321
MCD. *See* Minimal change disease
MDMA, 50*t*
Measles, mumps, and rubella (MMR) vaccine, 12*f*
Mebendazole, 164
Meckel diverticulum, 144
Meconium aspiration syndrome (MAS), 27, 41
- diagnosis of, 38, 41

Meconium ileus, 126
Meconium-stained amniotic fluid, 27
Medicines. *See also* Neonatal medicine
- adolescent, 43–52
- psychotropic, 49

Megaloblastic macrocytic anemias, 180*t*, 191–192
Melphalan, 209*t*
Membranoproliferative glomerulonephritis (MPGN), 299–300, 299*t*, 301
Membranous nephropathy (MN), 299–300, 299*t*
Meningitis, 162–163, 162*t*–163*t*, 261
Meningoceles, 273
Meningococcal conjugate vaccine (MCV), 11
Meningococcal conjugate vaccines, quadrivalent (MCV4), 12, 54, 56
Mental retardation, 258
Mercaptopurine, 146, 208*t*, 209
Metabolic acidosis, 67–68, 67*t*, 302–303, 303*f*
Metabolic alkalosis, 68
Metabolic disorders, 268, 320–322
Metabolic syndrome, 60
Metatarsus adductus, 22, 42, 281
Metformin, 243
Methacholine, 120
Methanol, 67*t*, 356*t*
Methicillin, 154
Methicillin-resistant *Staphylococcus aureus* (MRSA), 177, 292
Methimazole, 247
Methotrexate, 79, 85, 146, 191, 208*t*, 209, 211, 218, 232, 234
Methylphenidate, 245, 259
Methylprednisolone, 234
Metronidazole, 136, 141, 164, 168–169
Microangiopathic hemolytic anemias, 194
Microcephaly, 274
Microcytic anemia, 180*t*
Midazolam, 264
Migraine headache, 268–269
Milia, 19, 41
Milk-protein intolerance, 61, 62
Mineral oil, 142
Mineralocorticoids, 248–249
Minimal change disease (MCD), 298–299, 299*t*, 310, 313
Minocycline, 78, 79*f*
Mitral regurgitation, 97–98
Mixed amphetamine salts, 259
MMR vaccine. *See* Measles, mumps and rubella vaccine
MN. *See* Membranous nephropathy
Modified Checklist for Autism for Toddlers (M-CHAT), 13, 15, 16–17, 258
Molecular cytogenic disorders, 320
Moles. *See* Hyperpigmented lesions
Molestation. *See* Sexual abuse
Molluscum contagiosum, 75, 75*f*, 84
Mometasone, 124
Mongolian spots, 19
Monocytes, 193
Montelukast, 124
Moro reflex, 22
Morphea, 234
Morphine sulfate, 92
Morphologic classification, of leukemias, 205
Motor vehicle injuries, 10
MPGN. *See* Membranoproliferative glomerulonephritis
Multicystic dysplastic kidney (MDK), 295
Multiple sclerosis, 279
Mupirocin, 76, 77
Muscular dystrophy, 276, 279
Musculoskeletal disorders. *See* Orthopedics
Myasthenia gravis (MG), 271
Mycophenolate mofetil, 233
Mycoplasma genitalium, 169
Myeloid leukemia, 205–211, 206*f*–207*f*, 209*t*–210*t*
Myelomeningocele, 273
Myocarditis, 99
Myringitis, 155

N-acetylcysteine, 355*t*
Nafcillin, 286
Naloxone, 356*t*–357*t*, 363, 365
Narcotics, 75, 141
Narrow-complex tachycardias, 102, 104–106, 104*f*, 105*f*
Nasal polyps, 125
Nasolacrimal duct obstruction, 329
Nedocromil, 123*t*–124*t*
Neglect, 360–361, 360*f*
Neisseria gonorrhoeae (gonorrhea), 18, 168, 174, 176–177, 286, 334
    urine NAAT for, 53, 55
Neisseria meningitidis, 174
Neonatal acne, 19
Neonatal medicine
    congenital anomalies, 33–34
    delivery, 22–27
    discharge criteria, 34
    health-maintenance visits, 35
    infant mortality, 35
    infant, physical examination of, 18–22
    jaundice, 30–33
    neonatal sepsis, 29–30
    newborn, distress in, 27–29
Neonatal sepsis, 29–30, 111
Neonatology, upper airway obstruction, 114–115
Nephritic syndrome, 300
Nephrogenic diabetes insipidus (NDI), 303–304
Nephrology, 295–309
    acute kidney injury, 305–307, 306*t*
    chronic kidney disease, 307–308
    cryptorchidism, 297
    enuresis, 308
    glomerulonephritis, 300–302
    hemolytic uremic syndrome, 302
    hydroceles and varicoceles, 297
    hypertension, 60, 304–305, 304*t*
    hypospadias, 296–297
    nephrogenic diabetes insipidus, 303–304
    nephrotic syndrome, 298–300, 299*t*
    posterior urethral valves, 295–296
    renal dysplasia and cystic diseases, 294–295
    renal tubular acidosis, 302–303, 303*f*
    testicular torsion, 297
    ureteropelvic junction obstruction, 295
    urinary tract infections, 295, 297–298, 299*f*
    vesicoureteral reflux, 295, 296*f*
Nephrotic syndrome, 298–300, 299*t*, 310, 313
    complications of, 313
Neural tube defects, 273
Neuroblastoma, 206*f*–207*f*, 214–216, 215*t*, 221, 223, 279
Neurodegenerative disorders, 260–261
Neurodevelopment, 256–258, 257*t*
    disabilities, 258–259
Neurofibromatosis, 272, 272*t*
Neurogenic (spinal) shock, 343
Neurology, 256–275
    encephalopathy, 264, 268, 269*t*, 305
    head shapes, abnormal, 274
    headache, 268–270
    hydrocephalus, 273–274
    ischemic/hemorrhagic strokes, 270
    neural tube defects, 273
    neurodegenerative disorders, 260–261
    neurodevelopment, 256–259, 257*t*
    phakomatoses, 272–273, 272*t*
    seizure and epilepsy, 261–264, 262*t*, 265*t*–267*t*
    weakness, 270–272
Neuromuscular disease, 127
Neutropenia, 193, 226–227
Neutrophils, 193
Nevi, 80, 80*f*
Newborn
    distress in, 27, 28*t*
    early discharge criteria, 34*t*
NHL. *See* Non-Hodgkin lymphoma
Nicardipine, 305
Nicotine replacement therapy, 51
Nifedipine, 305
Nitazoxanide, 141
Nitrofurantoin, 295, 298
Nitrogen mustard, 209*t*
Nitroprusside, 102*f*, 111, 305
NNRTIs. *See* Nonnucleoside analogue reverse transcriptase inhibitors

Non-Hodgkin lymphoma (NHL), 206f–207f, 211, 223
Nonalcoholic fatty liver disease (NAFLD), 148
Nonalcoholic steatohepatitis (NASH), 148
Nonbullous impetigo, 76
Noncommunicating hydrocephalus, 273–274
Nonfatal injuries, cause of, 10
Nonmegaloblastic macrocytic anemias, 180t
Nonnucleoside analogue reverse transcriptase inhibitors (NNRTIs), 170
Nonphysiologic jaundice, 30
Nonrhabdomyosarcomas, 219
Nonsteroidal anti-inflammatory drugs (NSAIDs), 79, 143, 143t, 233, 234, 299t, 306t
Normal saline, infusion of, 69, 71
Normocytic anemia, 180t
Noroviruses, 164
Norwood operation, 113
Nosocomial respiratory syncytial virus infection, 41
NPH insulin. *See* Hagedorn insulin
NSAIDs. *See* Nonsteroidal anti-inflammatory drugs
Nucleic acid amplification test (NAAT), 44
Nucleoside analogue reverse transcriptase inhibitor drugs, 170
Nursemaid's elbow, 285
Nutrition, 57–60, 58t–60t
Nystatin cream, 77

Obesity, 59–60, 60t
Obstipation, 141
Obstruction
  airway, 114–127, 116t–121t, 122f, 123t–124t, 125t, 126f, 358–359, 359f, 359t
  nasolacrimal duct, 329
  ureteropelvic junction, 295
Obstructive shock, 343
Obstructive sleep apnea (OSA), 115
Occult bacteremia, 155
Office visit, for adolescent, 43–44, 44t
Ofloxacin, 330
OI. *See* Osteogenesis imperfecta
Oligoarticular Juvenile Idiopathic Arthritis (JIA), 231, 231t, 238, 240
  characteristics, 238, 240
  physical examination findings in, 238, 240
  tests, 238, 240
Omalizumab, 124, 124t
Omphalocele, 34
Oncology, 205–219, 206f–207f, 208t
  bone tumors, 206f–207f, 216–218
  central nervous system tumors, 206f–207f, 213–214, 213t–214t
  Hodgkin lymphoma, 206f–207f, 211–213, 212t
  leukemia, 205–211, 206f–207f, 209t–210t
  neuroblastoma, 206f–207f, 214–216, 215t
  non-Hodgkin lymphoma, 206f–207f, 211
  retinoblastoma, 206f–207f, 218, 328–329
  soft tissue sarcomas, 206f–207f, 218–219
  Wilms tumor, 206f–207f, 216, 217t
Ondansetron, 141, 152
Ophthalmia neonatorum, 329, 330t
Ophthalmology, 327–331
  amblyopia, 327
  hordeolum and chalazion, 330
  infectious conjunctivitis, 329–330, 330t
  leukocoria, 328–329
  nasolacrimal duct obstruction, 329
  ophthalmia neonatorum, 329, 330t
  periorbital cellulitis, 331
  strabismus, 327
  vision screening, 327, 328t
Opiates, 26t, 356t, 365
Opioids, 340
Oral acyclovir, 84
Oral contraceptives, 78, 79f, 169, 304t
Oral corticosteroid (prednisone), 130, 132
Oral griseofulvin, 82, 85
Oral metronidazole, 150, 152
Oral rehydration therapy (ORT), 64, 137
Orbital cellulitis, 331
Organophosphates, 356t
Ornithine transcarbamylase deficiency (OTC), 321–322
ORT. *See* Oral rehydration therapy; Orthodromic reentrant tachycardia
Orthodromic reentrant tachycardia (ORT), 102–104, 104f
Orthopedics, 280–288
  achondroplasia, 287
  common fractures in children, 284–285, 285f
  developmental dysplasia of hip, 280–281, 281f
  foot deformities, 280–281
  idiopathic scoliosis, 287
  limp, 281–284, 282f–284f, 282t
  Osgood–Schlatter disease, 287
  osteogenesis imperfecta, 287, 288t
  osteomyelitis, 285–286
  septic arthritis, 286–287
  subluxation of radial head, 285
Ortolani maneuver, 291–292
Ortolani provocative tests, 280, 281f
OSA. *See* Obstructive sleep apnea
Osgood–Schlatter disease, 287
Osmotic fragility testing, 187
Osteogenesis imperfecta (OI), 287, 288t
Osteogenic sarcoma, 217–218
Osteomyelitis, 285–286
Osteonecrosis, 290, 292
Osteopenia, 53, 55
Osteosarcoma, 217–218, 220, 222
  characteristic of, 220, 222
OTC. *See* Ornithine transcarbamylase deficiency
Otitis externa, 155
Otitis media, 155–156
Ova and parasites (O&P) testing, 150, 152
Overweight, 59
Oxacillin, 77, 286
Oxcarbazepine, 264, 265t, 268t
Oxycodone, 363, 365

Packed red blood cells (PRBCs) transfusion, 199
  complications of, by irradiation, 202, 204
Palivizumab, 160
Pamidronate, 251, 287
Papilledema, 269
Papular acrodermatitis of childhood. *See* Giannoti-Crosti syndrome
Paralysis, 270–272
Parents Evaluation of Developmental Status (PEDS), 11
Partial airway obstruction, 358, 359f
Partial seizures, 262, 262t, 265t
Parvovirus, 23t
Patau syndrome. *See* Trisomy 13
Patent ductus arteriosus (PDA), 96, 97f
Pathologic fractures, 284
Patient-centered medical home, 1
PCD. *See* Primary ciliary dyskinesia
PCOS. *See* Polycystic ovary syndrome
PCP. *See* Phencyclidine
PDA. *See* Patent ductus arteriosus
Pectus carinatum, 127
Pectus excavatum, 127
Pediatric abuse/neglect, 364, 366
Pediatrics
  anticipatory guidance, 1–10
  cardiopulmonary arrest for, 350, 352
  dental development and care, 13
  developmental milestones, 11–13
  effective communication skills in, 1
  family-centered partnerships, 1
  health supervision, in infancy and childhood, 1, 2t–9t
  language delay, 13
  parent–child interaction, observation of, 1
  screening, 10–11
  vaccinations, 11

Pelvic inflammatory disease (PID), 53, 56, 168, 174, 176
  organisms responsible for, 176–177
Penicillamine, 316t
Penicillin G, 167, 172
Penicillins, 79, 154, 157, 188, 190, 287, 331
Perennial allergens, 239
Perimembranous, 94
Periodic fever, apthous stomatitis, pharyngitis, adenitis syndrome (PFAPA), 235
Periodic fever syndromes (PFS), 235
Periorbital cellulitis, 331
Peripheral pulmonic stenosis (PPS), 37, 40
Peritoneal dialysis, 307
Persistent pulmonary hypertension of newborn (PPHN), 88
Pertussis, 160
Petit mal seizures. *See* Absence epilepsy
PFA. *See* Platelet Function Analyzer
PGE1. *See* Prostaglandin E1
pH management, 63–68
Phagocyte stimulating factors, 154
Phagocytic immunity disorders, 225t, 226–227
Phakomatoses, 272–273, 272t
Pharyngitis, streptococcal, 156–157, 157t
Phencyclidine (PCP), 50t
Phenobarbital, 191, 198, 264, 267t, 268t
Phenothiazine, 141
Phenylacetate, 322
Phenylbutazone, 192
Phenylketonuria (PKU), 321
Phenytoin, 27t, 147, 191, 198, 264, 268, 268t, 278, 316t
Phonetic disorders, 13
Physical abuse, 360
Physical dependence, 50
Physiologic anemia of infancy, 179
Physiologic jaundice, 30
Physostigmine, 355t, 365
Pickwickian syndrome, 115
PID. *See* Pelvic inflammatory disease
Pimecrolimus cream, 228
Pink eye. *See* Infectious conjunctivitis
Pinworm infection, 164
Piperacillin/tazobactam monotherapy, 136
Pityriasis rosea, 76, 84
PKU. *See* Phenylketonuria
Platelet Function Analyzer (PFA), 197
Platelet transfusions, 199
Platelets disorders, 193–196
Pneumococcal polysaccharide vaccine (PPSV), 11
Pneumococcal vaccines, 12f
Pneumocystis carinii. *See Pneumocystis jirovecii*
Pneumocystis jirovecii, 176
Pneumonia, 112, 151, 160–162, 161t
Pneumothorax, 126–127
Point tenderness, 284
Poisoning, 10, 16
  acute, 354–357, 355f–357f
  lead, 141, 183
Polyarticular JIA, 230t, 231t
Polycystic kidney disease, 294
Polycystic ovary syndrome (PCOS), 78
Polyethylene glycol, 135, 142
Polyhydramnios, 34
  cause of, 22
Polymyxin-bacitracin, 330
Polysomnography, 115
Pompe disease, 322
Pontine glioma, 279
Positional plagiocephaly, 274
Posterior urethral valves (PUV), 295–296
  diagnosis of, 311, 314
Postrenal failure, 306–307, 306t
Poststreptococcal glomerulonephritis (PSGN), 156, 157, 301
  test for, 310, 313
  therapy for, 310, 313
Postviral enteritis, 149, 152
Potassium, levels of, 65–68, 66f
Potter sequence, 294
Potter syndrome, 25, 42
PPHN. *See* Persistent pulmonary hypertension of newborn
PPIs. *See* Proton pump inhibitors
PPSV. *See* Pneumococcal polysaccharide vaccine
Prader-Willi syndrome, 319–320, 324, 326
Pralidoxime chloride, 356t
Precocious puberty, 249–250
Prednisone, 211, 213, 234
Premature adrenarche, 252, 254
Premature beats, 100
Prematurity, retinopathy of, 328
Prerenal failure, 306t
Prerenal injury, 305–307
Presumed viral exanthems, 76, 76f
Prevention
  of hepatitis, 166
  of hypertension, 305
  of injury, 354–362
Primary adrenal insufficiency, 252, 254. *See also* Addison disease
Primary assessment, for emergency management, 336–340, 338f, 339t, 340f
Primary cardiomyopathy, 112
Primary ciliary dyskinesia (PCD), 127, 130, 132
Primary enuresis, 308
Primary hemostasis, 193
Primary hypertension. *See* Essential hypertension
Primary nocturnal enuresis, 308
Primary systemic vasculitis, 230t, 234–235, 235t
Primary tension headache, 268
Primary varicella, 82, 84
Probiotics, 141
Procainamide, 105f–106f, 106, 341, 342t
Procarbazine, 213
Progesterone administration, 319
Prone sleeping position, 366
Propranolol, 81, 105f, 247
Propylthiouracil (PTU), 247
Prostaglandin E1 (PGE1), 89, 91–93, 97, 109, 110, 111, 113, 343
  side effect of treatment with, 109, 111
Protease inhibitors, 170
Proteinuria, 299–300
Proton pump inhibitors (PPIs), 135, 139, 145f
Pseudoephedrine, 228
Pseudomonas aeruginosa, 286
Pseudoseizures, 264
Pseudotumor cerebri, 270
  management of, 277, 279
  risk factor for, 277, 279
  tests, 277, 279
Psoriasis, 78–79, 82
  Group A streptococcus, triggering, 83, 85
  Koebner phenomenon and, 83, 85
  treatment options for, 83, 85
Psoriatic arthritis, 231t, 232
Psychological dependence, 50
Psychotropic medicines, 49
PTU. *See* Propylthiouracil
Pubertal delay, 250
Puberty, 43–44, 46f, 46t, 47f–48f, 249–250
Pulmonary embolism, 198–199
Pulmonary function testing, 114
Pulmonary hypertension, 27, 127
Pulmonic stenosis, critical, 97
Pulmonology, 114–129
  apnea of infancy, 128t, 129
  diagnostic techniques for pediatric pulmonology, 114
  lower airway obstructive disease, 115–127, 116t–121t, 122f, 123t–124t, 125t, 126f
  restrictive lung disease, 127–128
  upper airway obstructive disease, 114–115
Pulse oximetry, 89, 115, 124, 130
Pulseless ventricular tachycardia, 106, 107f
PUV. *See* Posterior urethral valves
Pyelonephritis, 176, 297–298, 299f
Pyloric stenosis, 137
Pyrantel pamoate, 164
Pyridostigmine, 271
Pyridoxine, 321

Quinidine, 190

Radial head, subluxation of, 285
Radiograph, 114
of airway obstruction, 358, 359*f*
aspiration syndrome, 128
of asthma, 122, 122*f*
of croup, 159*f*
of cystic fibrosis, 126, 126*f*
of Ebstein anomaly, 92*f*
of epiglottitis, 159*f*
of knee, 220, 222
of Legg-Calvé-Perthes disease, 284*f*
of slipped capital femoral epiphysis, 284, 284*f*
of transposition of great arteries, 90*f*
Radioiodine, 247, 316*t*
Rapidly progressive glomerulonephritis, 301
Rash. *See* Dermatology
RDS. *See* Respiratory distress syndrome
Rebound headaches, 268
Recombinant erythropoietin, 307
Recombinant human deoxyribonuclease, 126
Recombinant human granulocyte-colony stimulating factor (rhG-CSF), 227
Rectal bleeding, 143*t*
Red blood cell, anemias with decreased production, 183–186, 183*t*–184*t*
Red reflex, 328
Reiter syndrome, 168
Renal agenesis, 294
Renal dysplasia and cystic diseases, 294–295
Renal tubular acidosis (RTA), 302–303, 303*f*, 311, 314
Renal tumor. *See* Wilms tumor
Repetitive hand wringing, 261
Replacement fluid, 65
Reproductive health, 44, 46*f*, 46*t*, 47*f*–48*f*
Respiratory acidosis, 68
Respiratory alkalosis, 68
Respiratory distress syndrome (RDS), 29, 41
Respiratory syncytial virus (RSV), 159
Restrictive lung disease, 127–128
Retained fetal lung liquid syndrome, 29. *See also* Transient tachypnea of the newborn (TTN)
Reticulocyte count, normal range for, 203
Retinoblastoma, 206*f*–207*f*, 218, 328–329
Retinoic acid, 27*t*
Retinoids, 78, 79*f*
Retinopathy of prematurity (ROP), 328
Retractile testes, 20, 41
Rett syndrome, 261
Reye syndrome, 74, 264
Rh incompatibility, 31
Rhabdomyosarcomas, 218, 223
Rheumatic fever, 156–157, 157*t*
Rheumatic heart disease, 97–98
Rheumatoid factor, 240
Rheumatology, 229–235, 230*t*–231*t*, 233*t*, 235*t*
rhG-CSF. *See* Recombinant human granulocyte-colony stimulating factor
Rhinitis, allergic, 228
Rhinovirus, 132
Rhonchi, 20
Rickets, 57, 58*t*
Rickettsia rickettsia, 177
Rifampin, 174, 178
Rigid bronchoscopy, 359, 363, 366
Rituximab, 195
RMSF. *See* Rocky mountain spotted fever
Rocky Mountain spotted fever (RMSF), 171, 174, 177
Rocuronium, 340
ROP. *See* Retinopathy of prematurity
Roseola infectiosum, 170
Rotavirus (RV), 149, 151, 164
treatment for, 149, 151–152
vaccines, 12*f*
RSV. *See* Respiratory syncytial virus
RTA. *See* Renal tubular acidosis
Rubella, 24*t*, 84

Sacral dimples, 37, 40
Salbutamol, 122
Salicylate, 67*t*, 143, 340, 356*t*
Salicylic acid, 75
Salmon patch, 19
Salmonella, 151
Salter–Harris classification, 284, 285*f*
SAMPLE mnemonic, 340, 353
Sarcomas, 206*f*–207*f*, 216–217, 218–219
SBS. *See* Shaken baby syndrome
Scald burns, prevention of, 14, 16
Scarlet fever, 157, 173, 175
SCFE. *See* Slipped capital femoral epiphysis
Scheuermann disease, 287
SCID. *See* Severe combined immunodeficiency disease
Scoliosis, 287
Screening
for lead poisoning, 11, 11*t*
in pediatrics, 10
for tuberculosis (TB), 11
vision, 327, 328*t*
Seasonal influenza vaccine, 54, 56
Secondary adrenal insufficiency, 247, 252, 254
Secondary amenorrhea, 48
Secondary assessment, for emergency management, 342
Secondary cardiomyopathy, 112
Secondary enuresis, 308
Secondary hemostasis, 193
Secondary hypertension, 304–305, 304*t*
Sedatives, 271, 340, 356*t*
Seizures, 65, 214, 261–264, 262*t*, 265*t*–267*t*, 276, 278, 366
Selective IgA deficiency, 226
Selective serotonin reuptake inhibitors, 49
Selenium sulfide, 77, 77*t*
Sensorineural hearing loss, causes of, 16
Sepsis, 155–170, 157*t*, 158*f*–159*f*, 161*t*–163*t*, 165*t*–166*t*, 166*f*
Septal defects, 94–95, 94*f*
Septic arthritis (SA), 286–287
diagnosis of, 290, 292
Staphylococcus aureus in, 292
Septic shock, 343, 351, 353
Serial manipulations and casting, for congenital clubfoot, 289, 291
Serum osmolarity, 365
Severe combined immunodeficiency disease (SCID), 224
Sex chromosome abnormalities, 319–320
Sexual abuse, 360
Sexual development, 44, 46*f*, 46*t*, 47*f*–48*f*
Sexual Maturity Rating scale, 44
Sexually transmitted infections (STIs), 174
SGA. *See* Small for gestational age
Shagreen patches, 272
Shaken baby syndrome (SBS), 360
Shingles. *See* Herpes zoster
Shock, 64, 341–343, 341*t*
Short stature, 244–246
SIADH. *See* Syndrome of hyponatremia with inappropriate increased secretion of vasopressin
Sickle cell disease, 188–189, 188*t*, 202, 204
Sickle-β^+-thalassemia (Sβ^+), 202, 204
SIDS. *See* Sudden infant death syndrome
Silent carriers, 185
Silver nitrate, 329
Silver sulfadiazine, 359
Simple febrile seizures, 261
Simple partial seizures, 262, 262*t*
Single-gene disorders, 315–320, 316*t*–318*t*
Single palmar crease, 323, 325
Sinus bradycardia, 101, 101*f*
Sinus node dysfunction, 101, 101*f*
Sinus tachycardia, 104, 104*f*
Sinusitis, 156
Sjögren syndrome, 230*t*, 234
SJS. *See* Stevens–Johnson syndrome
Skin. *See* Dermatology
SLE. *See* Systemic lupus erythematosus
Sleep apnea. *See* Obstructive sleep apnea
Slipped capital femoral epiphysis (SCFE), 284, 284*f*, 290, 293
treatment for, 290, 293
Slipped capital femoral epiphysis, 284, 284*f*
SMA. *See* Spinal muscle atrophy
Small for gestational age (SGA), 18, 37, 40

Snuffles, 167
Social/emotional development, 256, 257*t*
Sodium, 65
Sodium bicarbonate, 66, 67, 92, 342*t*, 356*t*–357*t*
Sodium sulfacetamide, 330
Soft tissue sarcomas (STS), 206*f*–207*f*, 218–219
Sorbitol, 142
Sotalol, 106
Spasmus nutans, 263
Spastic cerebral palsy, 260, 260*t*
Speech delay, 256
Speech disorders, 13
Spherocytosis, 187–188
Spina bifida, 273
Spina bifida occulta, 273
Spinal muscle atrophy (SMA), 271, 279
Spironolactone, 78
Spitting up, 136
Spitz nevus, 80
Splenic sequestration, 189
Spontaneous bacterial peritonitis, 300
Spontaneous pneumothorax, 126–127
Squaric acid dibutylester, 75
Stanford-Binet test, 258
Staphylococcal scalded skin syndrome, 76–77
Staphylococcus aureus, 175, 286, 292
Staphylococcus epidermidis, 274
Status epilepticus, 264
Steroidogenesis, 248, 248*f*
Steroids, 44*t*, 68, 75–76, 79, 124, 127, 143, 157, 209, 228–229, 245, 247, 249, 284, 300–301, 330, 343
Stevens–Johnson syndrome (SJS), 79
Stool culture, 150, 152
Stork bite, 19
Strabismic amblyopia, 332, 334
Strabismus, 327
Strep throat. *See* Streptococcal pharyngitis
Streptococcal pharyngitis, 156–157, 157*t*
Streptococcus pneumoniae, 173, 175, 239, 334
Streptococcus pyogenes, 83, 85, 173, 175
Streptococcus viridans, 175
Streptomycin, 316*t*
Stress dosing, 249
Stress fractures, 284
Strokes, 189, 270
Structural heart disease, 86, 97–99
STS. *See* Soft tissue sarcomas
Sturge–Weber syndrome, 272–273
Stuttering. *See* True dysfluency
Styes. *See* Hordeolum; Chalazion
Subacute thyroiditis, 247
Subdural brain hemorrhage, 345*f*, 346*t*
Subluxation, of radial head, 285
Substance use and abuse, 50–51, 50*t*–51*t*
Succinylcholine, 340
Sudden infant death syndrome (SIDS), 10, 129, 139, 361, 364, 366
Suicide, 10, 51–52
  risk factors for, 54, 56
Sulfamethoxazole, 227
Sulfonamides, 79, 154, 192, 226
Sumatriptan, 270, 279
Superficial fungal infections, 77, 77*f*, 77*t*
Supportive therapy, for primary varicella, 82, 84
Supratentorial tumors, 213*t*, 214
Supraventricular tachycardia (SVT), 102–107, 105*f*, 109, 111, 341, 342*t*
  adenosine administration, 109, 112
  diagnosis of, 109, 112
  patients with unstable hemodynamics
    undergoing synchronized cardioversion, 110, 112
Surfactant deficiency, 29
SVT. *See* Supraventricular tachycardia
Sweat test, 130–131, 132
Sympathomimetics, 100*t*, 228–229
Synchronized cardioversion, in SVT, 110, 112
Syncope, 263
Syndrome of hyponatremia with inappropriate increased secretion of vasopressin (SIADH), 244
Synovitis, 230, 286
Syphilis, 25*t*, 166–167, 177
Systemic JIA, 231*t*, 232, 240
Systemic lupus erythematosus (SLE), 230*t*, 232–233, 233*t*, 313
Systemic sclerosis, 230*t*, 234
Systolic blood pressure, 350, 352

T-cell immunity disorders, 224–225
T1DM. *See* Type 1 diabetes mellitus
T2DM. *See* Type 2 diabetes mellitus
Tachyarrhythmias, 100, 102–107, 103*f*–107*f*
Tachycardia, 63
Tacrolimus, 228
Talipes equinovarus, 22, 281
Tanner staging system, 46*t*, 47*f*–48*f*. *See also* Sexual Maturity Rating scale
TAPVC. *See* Total anomalous pulmonary venous connection
Tazarotene, 78
Tdap (tetanus and diphtheria toxoids and acellular pertussis), 54, 56
TEC. *See* Transient erythroblastopenia of childhood
Technetium-99, 34
TEF. *See* Tracheoesophageal fistula
TEN. *See* Toxic epidermal necrolysis
Tension headache, 268
Tension pneumothorax, 353
Teratogenic substances, congenital exposure to, 25, 26*t*, 27*t*
Teratogens, 315
Terbutaline, 125
Tertiary assessment, for emergency management, 340–341
Testes, descent of, 297
Testicular torsion, 297
Testosterone-like drugs, 316*t*
Testosterone therapy, 319
Tet spells, 92
Tetracycline, 78, 79*f*, 154, 316*t*
Tetralogy of Fallot (TOF), 91–92, 91*f*
Tetrathiomolybdate, 147
Thalassemia, 184–185, 184*t*
Thalidomide, 316*t*
Theophylline, 123*t*–124*t*, 124, 138*t*, 356*t*
Thiazide, 68, 302, 304
Thin membrane disease. *See* Benign familial hematuria
Thioguanine, 208*t*
Thoracentesis, 173, 176
3TC (lamivudine), 170
Throat culture, 173, 175
Thrombocytopenia-absent radius (TAR) syndrome, 194
Thrombocytopenia, immune, 194–195
Thyroid dysfunction, 246–247
Thyroid nodule, 247
Tick bite, 171
Tick paralysis, 271
Tinea infections, 77, 77*f*, 77*t*
TNF inhibitors, 235
Tobacco, 26*t*, 44*t*, 51, 51*t*
Tobramycin, 126
TOF. *See* Tetralogy of Fallot
Topiramate, 264, 265*t*, 267*t*–268*t*
Torticollis, 21
Total anomalous pulmonary venous connection (TAPVC), 90
Tourette complex, 263
Toxic epidermal necrolysis (TEN), 79–80
Toxic synovitis, 286
Toxoplasmosis, 25*t*
Tracheoesophageal fistula (TEF), 33, 132
Tracheomalacia, 127
Transfusion-associated acute lung injury (TRALI), 199
Transfusion-associated circulatory overload (TACO), 204
Transfusion-associated graft-versus-host disease (TA-GVHD), 200, 202, 204
Transfusional hemochromatosis, 204
Transient erythroblastopenia of childhood (TEC), 186, 203
Transient hypogammaglobulinemia of infancy, 226
Transient neonatal pustular melanosis, 40
Transient synovitis, 290, 292

Transient tachypnea of the newborn (TTN), 28*t*, 29, 38, 41
Transposition of the great arteries (TGA), 111
Trauma. *See also* Head trauma
  from adolescent violence, 51–52
  limp from, 281
Traumatic injuries, 10
Tremor, 263
Treponema pallidum, 167, 177
Tretinoin, 78
Trichomonas vaginalis, 168–169, 177
Trichomoniasis, 169
Trichophyton tonsurans, 82, 84
Tricuspid atresia, 90–91
Tricyclic antidepressants, 100*t*, 244, 357*t*
Tricyclic psychotropic agents, 135
Trientine, 147
Trimethadione, 316*t*
Trimethoprim, 191, 227
Trimethoprim-polymyxin B, 330
Trimethoprim-sulfamethoxazole, 76, 164, 170, 227, 295, 298
Trisomy 13, 318–319, 318*t*
Trisomy 18, 318, 318*t*
Trisomy 21, 318
True dysfluency, 13, 256
Truncus arteriosus, 89, 324, 325–326
Tuberous sclerosis, 272
Tumor lysis syndrome, 208
Tumor necrosis factor receptor-associated periodic fever syndrome (TRAPS), 235
Tumors. *See* Oncology
Turner syndrome, 96, 245–246, 319
22q11.2 deletion syndrome, 89, 320, 326
Type 1 diabetes mellitus (T1DM), 241–242
Type 2 diabetes mellitus (T2DM), 242–243

Ulcerative colitis, 144–147, 146*t*
Umbilical hernias, 20
Unilateral thoracic exanthem, 76, 76*f*
Uniparental disomy, 319
Upper airway obstructive disease, 114–115
Upper endoscopy and colonoscopy, for Crohn's disease, 150, 153
Ureteropelvic junction obstruction (UPJO), 295
Urinary tract infections (UTIs), 295, 297–298, 299*f*
Urine drug screen, 363, 365
Urine nucleic acid amplification test (NAAT), for diagnosing *N. gonorrhoeae* and C. *trachomatis*, 53, 55
Urine tests, for cannabis intake, 54, 56
Urology. *See* Nephrology
Ursodeoxycholic acid, 148
Urticaria, 229, 239
UTIs. *See* Urinary tract infections

Vaccinations, 11, 162, 165, 331
Vaginal candidiasis, 169
Vaginosis, 169
Valacyclovir, 74
Valproate, 316*t*
Valproic acid, 27*t*, 147, 191, 264, 265*t*–266*t*, 268*t*, 273
Vancomycin, 141, 162, 163, 177, 306, 331
Variable expressivity, 316
Varicella, 74–75, 75*f*, 170*t*
  incubation period for, 82, 84
  treating with supportive therapy, 82, 84
  vaccine, 12*f*, 74
Varicella zoster virus, 24*t*
Varicella zoster–immune globulin, 84
Varicoceles, 297
Varus, 289, 291
Vascular access, 340, 340*f*
Vasculitis, primary systemic, 230*t*, 234–235
Vaso-occlusion, 188
Vasoactive agents, 145*f*
Vasoconstrictors, 92
Vasodilators, 99, 301, 305
Vasopressin, 308. *See also* Syndrome of hyponatremia with inappropriate increased secretion of vasopressin
  normal regulation of, 243
Vasopressors, 343
VATER syndrome, 320
Vecuronium, 340
Ventricular fibrillation (VF), 104, 104*f*, 106, 341, 342*t*
Ventricular septal defect (VSD), 94–95, 94*f*
Ventricular tachycardia (VT), 104, 104*f*, 106, 106*f*, 341, 342*t*, 348
Verrucae, 75–76, 75*f*
Versed, 340
Vesicoureteral reflux (VUR), 295, 296*f*
VF. *See* Ventricular fibrillation
Vigabatrin, 267*t*
Vincristine, 81, 141, 208*t*, 209, 211, 213, 216, 217, 217*t*
Violence, in adolescent population, 51–52
Viral gastroenteritis, 112
Viral infection, 74–76, 75*f*, 99, 139, 170–172, 170*t*, 271
Vision screening, 327, 328*t*
Visual-motor, 256, 257*t*
Vitamin B_{12} deficiency, 183, 191
Vitamin D, 38, 41
  deficiency, 250–251
  supplementation, 57, 307
Vitamin K deficiency, 198
Volvulus, 137
Vomiting. *See* Emesis
von Gierke disease, 321
von Willebrand disease, 197–198
VSD. *See* Ventricular septal defect
VT. *See* Ventricular tachycardia
Vulvovaginal infections, 168–169
VUR. *See* Vesicoureteral reflux

Warfarin, 198, 316*t*
Warts. *See* Verrucae
Water deprivation test, 253, 255
Water regulation, disorders of, 243–244
Weakness, 270–272
Wechsler scales, 258
Werdnig-Hoffmann disease. *See* Spinal muscle atrophy
White blood cells disorders, 192–193
White matter disorders, 260
Whole bowel irrigation, 354
Whooping cough. *See* Pertussis
Wide-complex tachycardias, 102–104, 106, 106*f*–107*f*
Wilms tumor, 206*f*–207*f*, 216, 217*t*, 221, 223
Wilson disease, 147
Wiskott-Aldrich syndrome, 194, 226
Wolff-Parkinson-White syndrome, 92, 102–104, 103*f*, 106

X-linked agammaglobulinemia, 226
X-linked disorders, 317, 317*t*

Zafirlukast, 124
Zidovudine (AZT), 169
Zileuton, 124*t*
Zonisamide, 265*t*, 268*t*